TOCOTRIENOLS
VITAMIN E BEYOND TOCOPHEROLS

Contents

Foreword

Fat-soluble vitamins have their root in the 1913 discovery by Elmer V. McCollum, Thomas B. Osborne and Lafayette B. Mendel, who isolated a growth-producing substance from egg yolks. The *substance* appeared quite different from the water-soluble vitamins already discovered. In 1916, McCollum went on to show that at least two factors were responsible for the normal growth of rats, factors he named fat-soluble A and water-soluble B. McCollum therefore is credited with initiating the custom of labeling vitamins by letters. Vitamin E was discovered in 1922 in green leafy vegetables by University of California researchers Herbert Evans and Katherine Bishop. In 1924, Sure named it vitamin E.

In 1926, the February 15th issue of *TIME* magazine reported that:

> From the University of California, Drs. Herbert M. Evans and K. S. Bishop last week announced through the California State Board of Health the influence of the mysterious Vitamin X which they now have renamed E. This vitamin stimulates reproduction in animals, prevents sterility. It is a complex organic compound, like the four other known vitamins, and occurs in lettuce, wheat germs, alfalfa and egg yolk. Because humans eat largely of these foods, the discovery has little bearing on their habits.

Although it was eight decades ago that we thought we were successful in demystifying the X-factor in vitamin E, it is my observation that a considerable fraction of today's nutritional community assume that vitamin E is synonymous with tocopherol. In fact, natural vitamin E includes eight chemically distinct molecules: α-, β-, γ- and δ-tocopherol; and α-, β-, γ- and δ-tocotrienol. However, until less than 5 years ago, the authoritative *Merck Manual* defined vitamin E as the following: "Vitamin E (tocopherol) is a generic term for compounds that have a 6-chromanol ring, an isoprenoid sidechain, and the biologic activity of α-tocopherol. The vitamin E group contains α-, β-, γ-, and δ-tocopherols, which vary in extent to which the chromanol ring is methylated." Note the omission of tocotrienols.

In the current literature, more than 95% of all studies on vitamin E are directed toward the specific study of α-tocopherol. The other forms of natural vitamin E remain poorly understood. The abundance of α-tocopherol in the human body and the comparable efficiency of all vitamin E molecules as antioxidants led biologists to neglect the non-tocopherol vitamin E molecules as topics for basic and clinical research. Recent developments warrant a serious reconsideration of this conventional wisdom. The tocotrienol subfamily of natural vitamin E possesses powerful neuroprotective, anti-cancer and cholesterol lowering properties that are often not exhibited by tocopherols. Current developments in vitamin E research clearly indicate that members of the vitamin E family are not redundant with respect to their biological functions. α-Tocotrienol, γ-tocopherol and δ-tocotrienol have emerged as vitamin E molecules with functions in health and disease that are clearly distinct from that of α-tocopherol. At nanomolar concentration, α-tocotrienol, not α-tocopherol, prevents neurodegeneration. On a concentration basis, this finding represents the most potent of all biological functions exhibited by any natural vitamin E molecule. In light of the emergent literature, the *Merck Manual* seems to have recognized the incompleteness of its definition cited above and currently has included tocotrienols to define vitamin E as: "Vitamin E is a group of compounds (including tocopherols and tocotrienols) that have similar biologic activities. The most biologically active is α-tocopherol, but β-, γ-, and δ-tocopherols, four tocotrienols and several stereoisomers may also have important biologic activity." Here, that α-tocopherol is most biologically active begs further consideration. For example, this does not seem to be true for the neuroprotective properties of vitamin E.

A rapidly expanding body of evidence supports that members of the vitamin E family are functionally unique. In recognition of this fact, title claims in manuscripts should be limited to the specific form of vitamin E studied. For example, evidence for toxicity of a specific form of tocopherol in excess may not be used to conclude that high-dosage "vitamin E" supplementation may increase all-cause mortality. Such conclusion incorrectly implies that tocotrienols are toxic as well under conditions where tocotrienols were not even considered. The current state of knowledge warrants strategic investment into the lesser known forms of natural vitamin E. I laud the efforts of the American Oil Chemists' Society for their investment in publishing this first-ever volume dedicated to the biology of the tocotrienol forms of natural vitamin E.

Professor Chandan K. Sen
Columbus, Ohio

Acknowledgments

The encouragement and research support of Mr. H. B. and Jocelyn Wallace through research grants from the Jocelyn Wallace Research Foundation to Ronald Ross Watson was vital to the book's conception and publication. The Wallace Research Foundation has been important in supporting research on nutrition and health promotion in the aged for decades, leading to this book. The work of editorial assistant Bethany L. Stevens in communicating with authors and working with the manuscripts and the publisher was critical to the successful completion of the book and is much appreciated. Her daily responses to queries and collection of manuscripts and documents were extremely helpful. Support for her work was graciously provided by the National Health Research Institute and AOCS. This was part of their efforts to educate scientists and the lay public on the health and economic benefits of nutrients in the diet as well as supplements. It came from inspiration and ideas from their Vitamin E symposium at the American Oil Chemists' Association meeting in 2006. Finally, Nguyen T. Nga of the Arizona Health Sciences library was instrumental in finding the authors and their addresses in the early stages of the book's preparation.

Editors

Ronald Ross Watson has edited 68 biomedical books including *The Encyclopedia of Vitamin E.* He has published more than 500 papers, and presently directs or has directed several National Institutes of Health (NIH)-funded biomedical grants relating to alcohol and disease, particularly immune function and cardiovascular effects. Professor Watson was director of a NIH-funded Alcohol Research Center for 5 years. The main goal of the center was to understand the role of ethanol-induced immunosuppression on immune function and disease resistance in animals. He is an internationally recognized alcohol researcher, nutritionist and immunologist. He also initiated and directed other NIH-associated work at the University of Arizona College of Medicine. Professor Watson attended the University of Idaho, but graduated from Brigham Young University in Provo, Utah, with a degree in chemistry in 1966. He completed his Ph.D. degree in 1971 in biochemistry from Michigan State University, and his postdoctoral schooling was completed at the Harvard School of Public Health in nutrition and microbiology, including a two-year postdoctoral research experience in immunology. Dr. Watson is a distinguished member of several national and international nutrition, immunology and cancer societies.

Victor R. Preedy is currently a professor in the Department of Nutrition and Dietetics, King's College London. He directs studies regarding nutrition and the biochemical aspects of food health and toxicity. He graduated in 1974 from the University of Aston with a combined honors degree in biology and physiology with pharmacology. He gained his Ph.D. in 1981 in the field of nutrition and metabolism, specializing in protein turnover. In 1992, Dr. Preedy received his membership in the Royal College of Pathologists, based on his published works, and in 1993, gained a D.Sc. degree for his outstanding contribution to protein metabolism. At the time, he was one of the university's youngest recipients of this distinguished award. Professor Preedy was elected as a Fellow to the Royal College of Pathologists in 2000. Since then, he has been elected as a Fellow to the Royal Society for the Promotion of Health (2004) and the Royal Institute of Public Health (2004). Professor Preedy specializes in the field of alcohol studies within the confines of a nutrition and food environment as a senior academic member of the Department of Nutrition and Dietetics. He has published more than 550 articles that include in excess of 150 peer-reviewed manuscripts based on original research and 75 reviews, as well as 12 books including *The Encyclopedia of Vitamin E.*

Contributors

Bruce Blumberg
Department of Developmental and Cell Biology
University of California
Irvine, California

Jiao Cao
The State Key Laboratory of Molecular Biology
Institute of Biochemistry and Cell Biology
Shanghai Institutes for Biological Sciences
Chinese Academy of Sciences
Shanghai, China

Dallas L. Clouatre
NOW Health Group
Bloomingdale, Illinois

Dipak K. Das
Cardiovascular Research Center
University of Connecticut School of Medicine
Farmington, Connecticut

Manika Das
Cardiovascular Research Center
University of Connecticut School of Medicine
Farmington, Connecticut

Samarjit Das
Cardiovascular Research Center
University of Connecticut School of Medicine
Farmington, Connecticut

Takahiro Eitsuka
Faculty of Applied Life Sciences
Niigata University of Pharmacy and Applied Life Sciences
Niigata, Japan
and
Food and Biodynamic Chemistry Laboratory
Graduate School of Agricultural Science
Tohoku University
Sendai, Japan

Charles E. Elson
Department of Nutritional Sciences
University of Wisconsin-Madison
Madison, Wisconsin

Sanchita P. Ghosh
The Henry M. Jackson Foundation for the Advancement of Military Medicine
Rockville, Maryland
and
Armed Forces Radiobiology Research Institute
Bethesda, Maryland

Liva Harinantenaina
Graduate School of Biomedical Sciences
Division of Medicinal Chemistry
Program for Pharmaceutical Sciences
Hiroshima University
Hiroshima, Japan

Martin Hauer-Jensen
University of Arkansas Medical Sciences
and
Central Arkansas Veteran's Healthcare System
Little Rock, Arkansas

Tiffany Hsu
Department of Developmental and Cell Biology
University of California
Irvine, California

Jahangir Iqbal
Department of Anatomy and Cell Biology
SUNY Downstate Medical Center
Brooklyn, New York

Qing Jiang
Interdepartmental Nutrition Program
Department of Foods and Nutrition
Purdue University
West Lafayette, Indiana

Kameran R. Johnson
Department of Developmental and Cell Biology
University of California
Irvine, California

Vijaya Juturu
Research and Development
Nutrition 21, Inc.
Purchase, New York

Savita Khanna
Laboratory of Molecular Medicine
Department of Surgery
Davis Heart and Lung Research Institute
The Ohio State University Medical Center
Columbus, Ohio

Amy Kosowski
NOW Health Group
Bloomingdale, Illinois

K. Sree Kumar
Uniformed Services University of the Health Sciences
Armed Forces Radiobiology Research Institute
Bethesda, Maryland

Neil E. Levin
Department of Nutrition
NOW Foods
Bloomingdale, Illinois

Mohammad Minhajuddin
Department of Pediatrics
University of Rochester Medical Center
Rochester, New York

Teruo Miyazawa
Food and Biodynamic Chemistry Laboratory
Graduate School of Agricultural Science
Tohoku University
Sendai, Japan

Yoshiyuki Mizushina
Laboratory of Food & Nutritional Sciences
Department of Nutritional Science
Kobe-Gakuin University
Kobe, Japan

Huanbiao Mo
Department of Nutrition and Food Sciences
Texas Woman's University
Denton, Texas

Anne M. Mueller
American River Nutrition, Inc.
Hadley, Massachusetts

Yuji Naito
Medical Proteomics and Inflammation and Immunology
Kyoto Prefectural University of Medicine
Kyoto, Japan

Kiyotaka Nakagawa
Food and Biodynamic Chemistry Laboratory
Graduate School of Agricultural Science
Tohoku University
Sendai, Japan

Bee-Hong Ng
R&D Division
Hovid Bhd
Ipoh, Perak, Malaysia

Etsuo Niki
Human Stress Signal Research Center
National Institute of Advanced Industrial Science and Technology
Osaka, Japan

Noriko Noguchi
Faculty of Life and Medical Sciences
Department of Medical Life Systems
Doshisha University
Kyoto, Japan

Paola Palozza
Institute of General Pathology
Catholic University
Rome, Italy

Wei Qi
Institute for Nutritional Sciences
Shanghai Institutes for Biological Sciences
Chinese Academy of Sciences
Shanghai, China

Sashwati Roy
Laboratory of Molecular Medicine
Department of Surgery
Davis Heart and Lung Research Institute
The Ohio State University Medical Center
Columbus, Ohio

Yoshiro Saito
Human Stress Signal Research Center
National Institute of Advanced Industrial Science & Technology
Osaka, Japan
and
Faculty of Life and Medical Sciences
Department of Medical Life Systems
Doshisha University
Kyoto, Japan

Alexander G. Schauss
Natural and Medicinal Products Research
AIBMR Life Sciences
Puyallup, Washington

Chandan K. Sen
Laboratory of Molecular Medicine
Department of Surgery
Davis Heart and Lung Research Institute
The Ohio State University Medical Center
Columbus, Ohio

Akira Shibata
Food and Biodynamic Chemistry Laboratory
Graduate School of Agricultural Science
Tohoku University
Sendai, Japan

Rossella Simone
Institute of General Pathology
Catholic University
Rome, Italy

Bao-Liang Song
The State Key Laboratory of Molecular Biology
Institute of Biochemistry and Cell Biology
Shanghai Institutes for Biological Sciences
Chinese Academy of Sciences
Shanghai, China

Phumon Sookwong
Food and Biodynamic Chemistry Laboratory
Graduate School of Agricultural Science
Tohoku University
Sendai, Japan

Elizabeth S. Stuart
Department of Microbiology
University of Massachusetts-Amherst
Amherst, Massachusetts

Paul W. Sylvester
College of Pharmacy
University of Louisiana at Monroe
Monroe, Louisana

Barrie Tan
American River Nutrition, Inc.
Hadley, Massachusetts

Nantiga Virgona
Project for Complementary Factors
National Institute of Health and Nutrition
Tokyo, Japan

Jia-Woei Wong
R&D Division
Hovid Bhd
Ipoh, Perak, Malaysia

Tomohiro Yano
Project for Complementary Factors
National Institute of Health and Nutrition
Tokyo, Japan

Hiromi Yoshida
Laboratory of Food & Nutritional Sciences
Department of Nutritional Science
Kobe-Gakuin University
Kobe, Japan

Yasukazu Yoshida
Human Stress Signal Research Center
National Institute of Advanced Industrial Science & Technology
Osaka, Japan

Toshikazu Yoshikawa
Medical Proteomics
and
Inflammation and Immunology
Kyoto Prefectural University of Medicine
Kyoto, Japan

Kah-Hay Yuen
School of Pharmaceutical Sciences
Universiti Sains Malaysia
Penang, Malaysia

Henryk Zielinski
Division of Food Science
Institute of Animal Reproduction and Food Research of Polish Academy of Sciences
Olsztyn, Poland

Part A

Introduction and Overview

1 Tocotrienols: A Review

Alexander G. Schauss

CONTENTS

1.1 INTRODUCTION

Vitamin E is a generic name for the family of eight major and four minor compounds that have been found to possess vitamin E activity. The major compounds are: d-α-tocopherol, d-β-tocopherol, d-γ-tocopherol, d-δ-tocopherol, and d-α-tocotrienol d-β-tocotrienol and d-γ-tocotrienol. Essentially, the family of vitamin E compounds primarily found in cell membranes and blood plasma is a major lipid-soluble chain-breaking antioxidant. A prime difference between tocopherol and tocotrienol is that the latter possesses three double bonds in its isoprenoid side chain: tocopherol has a saturated hydrocarbon phytyl tail, while tocotrienol has an unsaturated farnesyl isoprenoid tail. This 6-hydroxychroman moiety with a lipid-soluble side chain constitutes what is called vitamin E. Another difference is that tocopherols do not have tocotrienol's cholesterol-lowering properties and may actually interfere with its cholesterol-lowering activity (Qureshi et al., 1996; Tan, 2005). See Figure 1.1.

Tocotrienols down-regulate 3-hydroxy-3-methylglutaryl coenzyme A (HMG-CoA) reductase activity, which is the rate limiting activity in the mevalonate pathway that contributes to the synthesis of cholesterol (Brown and Goldstein, 1980; Parker et al., 1990; Pearce et al., 1992).

Palm oil, rice bran oil (and its fatty acid distillate), barley and, particularly, Annatto (*Bixa orellana*, family: Bixaceae), are the primary sources of tocotrienols. The latter contains nearly 100% tocotrienols, including desmethyl tocotrienols, and is virtually free of any tocopherols. Annatto extract, available for dietary supplements, contains two tocotrienol isomers: 10% γ-tocotrienol and 90% δ-tocotrienol. Palm oil contains a larger concentration of tocotrienols than all other natural sources except Annato.

To understand the delay in discovering the health-giving properties of tocotrienols, it is useful to know that until the late 1980s most of the experiments on vitamin E and carcinogenesis (i.e., antitumor and antiproliferation activity) and hyperlipidemias (inhibition of cholesterol biosynthesis) involved the use of tocopherols owing to the ready availability of tocopherols as the major source of vitamin E. Given the history behind vitamin E research, it is understandable how the tocotrienols failed to get the attention they deserved.

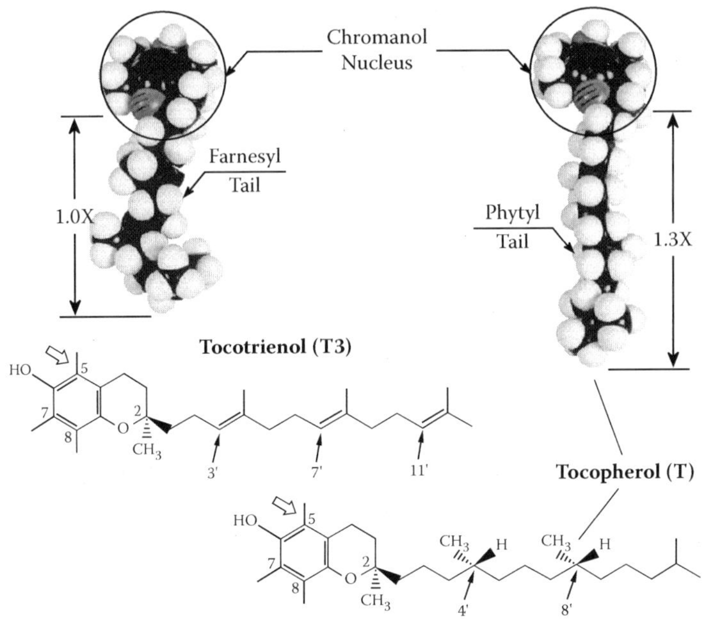

Methyl Group Position(s)	Tocotrienol*	Tocopherol*
5,7,8 - Trimethyl	alpha-T3 (58864-81-6)	alpha-T (59-02-9)
5,8 - Dimethyl	beta-T3 (490-23-3)	beta-T (16698-35-4)
7,8 - Dimethyl	gamma-T3 (14101-61-2)	gamma-T (54-28-4)
8 - Monomethyl	delta-T3 (25612-59-3)	delta-T (119-13-1)

*CAS number in parenthesis

FIGURE 1.1 Molecular and chemical structures of vitamin E.

Research interest in vitamin E began following the discovery of this vitamin by Herbert Evans after the appearance of an unrecognized substance necessary for reproduction that was published in a paper that appeared 1922 in *Science* (Evans and Bishop, 1922). Once identified, it was referred as containing tocopherols; the term comes from the Greek words *tokos*, which means "offspring" and *phero*, which means "to bear." Hence, tocopherol means "to bear children."

Fourteen years later, in 1936, Evans and colleagues reported on the isolation of an alcohol α-tocopherol found in wheat germ oil (Evans et al., 1936). The discovery was confirmed by Fernholz in 1937 (Fernholz, 1937, 1938). Recognition of vitamin E's antioxidant activity and existence in various foodstuffs was reported the same year by Emerson and Olcott (Emerson et al., 1937).

Beginning in the late 1930s, the brothers Wilfrid and Evan Shute, both Canadian physicians, began giving patients large doses of vitamin E, usually above 800 IU a day. The Shute brothers reported on numerous benefits of vitamin E at various medical conferences and in papers published in various medical journals. However, Harvard University's *Medical Letter* wrote a highly critical article in 1950 about the use of what was then perceived as an unnecessary and possibly "dangerous" megadose of vitamin E, going so far as to state that vitamin E had no therapeutic value for treating heart disease or any other disease or condition (Di Cyan, 1972). This opinion circulated widely and carried considerable weight within the medical establishment, discouraging scientists and physicians from further researching vitamin E. Ironically, in 1993, Harvard University's School of Medicine reported on the benefit of vitamin E based on two large prospective studies that found an association between increased consumption of vitamin E and a reduced risk of coronary heart disease in both men and women that appeared in the *New England Journal of Medicine* (Stampfer, et al., 1993; Rim et al., 1993). In the first study, the investigators found that during an 8-year follow-up period, women who had taken 100 IU or more per day of vitamin E for at least 2 years had a 46% lower risk of having a heart attack. In the second study involving men, they showed a 37% lower risk. Both papers concluded that it was nearly impossible to obtain a sufficient amount of vitamin E from the diet, hence supplementation might be recommended. No mention was made of the Shute brothers' work on some 30,000 patients for whom they had observed similar benefits in terms of reduction of heart disease or in the treatment of angina pectoris more than 40 years earlier (Shute, 1959).

In 1959, when Dr. Evan Shute reported on his observations of a wide range of benefits related to vitamin E, the average diet in North America provided about 20 mg (30 IU) a day of vitamin E. In the same year, the Recommended Daily Allowance (RDA) for vitamin E was set at 30 IU. In 1974, the RDA was lowered to 15 IU a day. The reasons for this change are discussed in a review of the evolution of RDA's for nutrients such as vitamin E written in 1986 (Horwitt, 1986).

Of even greater interest is that the author who summarized the evidence in support of a lower level of vitamin E in 1974 (Horwitt, 1974) was the same author of a paper that in 1991 urged that higher levels of vitamin E be consumed via supplementation than the RDA in vogue at the time (Horwitt, 1991). These changes in opinion that were among the forces that influenced perceptions about the benefits of vitamin E in previous years illustrate the paradigm shift that transpired between the 1960s and 1970s and recommendations some 20 years later.

It is worth noting that in reviewing the writings and works of the Shute brothers, including a text titled *Alpha Tocopherol in Cardiovascular Disease*, published in 1954, and *The Heart and Vitamin E*, in 1956, they never wavered in support of further research on vitamin E, despite constant criticism from mainstream medicine. In many ways the controversy they stirred for many years keeps vitamin E a subject of debate within medicine.

A timeline of the Shute brothers' discoveries and observations of a therapeutic benefit for vitamin E is as follows:

- 1936—angina
- 1940—fibroids, endometriosis and atherosclerosis
- 1945—hemorrhages of the skin and mucosal membranes and decreased requirement for insulin
- 1947—therapy for gangrene, Buerger's disease (an inflammation of blood vessels), retinitis and choroditis
- 1948—lupus erythematosus and shortness of breath
- 1950—varicose veins and severe burns to the skin

It would be interesting to see how many of these therapeutic associations to vitamin E are related more so to the tocotrienols than to the tocopherols.

The Shute brothers' bitterness at how their clinical research was ignored and attacked, despite the publication of 120 papers in the medical literature, comes across in a work they published in 1985 (Shute and Shute, 1985), in which they wrote:

> It was nearly impossible now for anyone who valued his future in Academe to espouse Vitamin E, prescribe it or advise its use. That would make a man a "quack" at once. This situation lasted for many years. In the United States, of course, the closure of the J.A.M.A. pages against us and tocopherol meant that it did not exist. It was either in the U.S. medical bible or it was nought. No amount of documentation could budge medical men from this stance. Literature in the positive was ignored and left unread. Individual doctors often said: "If it is as good as you say, we would all be using it." But nothing could induce them as persons of scientific background to make the simplest trial on a burn or coronary. (p. 146)

1.2 THE EMERGENCE OF RESEARCH ON TOCOTRIENOLS

Identification of tocopherol compounds beyond α-tocopherol started in 1947 with the isolation of δ-tocopherol in soybean oil (Stern et al., 1947).

The discovery of tocotrienols was first reported by Pennock and colleagues in 1964, followed soon thereafter by Whittle and colleagues describing the discovery and isolation of δ-tocotrienol 2 years later (Pennock et al., 1964; Whittle et al., 1966).

The biological significance of tocotrienols, however, was not clearly appreciated until the early 1980s, when its ability to lower lipids was first reported. During the following decade, evidence appeared suggesting an inhibitory role of tocotrienols against cancers. A review of the series of discoveries that led to its recognition as a potential therapeutic agent in the 1980s is described by Sylvester and Theriault (Sylvester and Theriault, 2003). During the 1990s, the differential biological properties of tocopherols and tocotrienols began to be more clearly delineated, especially for γ- and δ-tocopherol and γ- and δ-tocotrienol.

A number of health-related biological properties of tocotrienols have been identified, including its anticancer, anticholesterolemic, antihypertensive, antioxidant, immunomodulatory and neuro-protective properties, each of which would be worth reviewing.

1.2.1 Anticancer

Initial evidence of tocotrienol's anti-cancer properties was reported in 1989 in rodents. Sundram and colleagues studied the effect of tocotrienol-rich palm oil on mammary carcinogensis in female rats and demonstrated it could prevent chemically induced mammary tumorigenesis (Sundram et al., 1989). In the same year, intraperitoneally injected tocotrienol was shown to prevent proliferative activity and growth of transplanted tumors (Komiyama et al., 1989). Beginning in 1991, it was reported that tocotrienol had chemopreventive properties in both mammary tumor and hepatic tumor models, confirmed as a chemopreventive in 1993 (Guthrie et al., 1993, 1994). The following year, palm tocotrienols were found to reduce the severity of hepatocarcinogenesis following treatment of rats with 2-acetylaminofluorene (AAF) and diethylnitrosamine (DEN) (Gould et al., 1991; Ngah et al., 1991; Rahmat et al., 1993). Tocotrienol attenuated the impact of both carcinogens in rats.

In 1994, it was reported that palm-oil-derived tocotrienols were found to suppress activation of the Epstein-Barr virus's early antigen expression in PMA-activated EBV-genome-carrying human lymphoblastoid Raji cells (Goh et al., 1994). Alpha- and γ-tocopherols and dimers of γ-tocotrienol or γ-tocopherol lacked this activity.

In 1995, tocotrienol, but not tocopherol, was found to suppress the growth of human breast cancer cell line *in vitro* (Nesaretnam et al., 1995). This discovery was followed by the work of Elson and Qureshi, who reported that isoprenoid-mediated suppression of mevalonate synthesis depleted tumor tissues of two intermediate products: farnesyl pyrophosphate and geranylgeranyl pyrophosphate. Both contribute post-translationally into growth control-associated proteins (Elson and Qureshi, 1995).

Further evidence of tocotrienols' anticancer properties appeared between 1997 and 1999. Tocotrienols were shown to inhibit the proliferation of human estrogen receptor-negative MDA-MB-435 and human MCF-7 breast cancer cells *in vitro*, either alone or in combination with tamoxifen (Guthrie et al., 1997) and to suppress the growth of murine B16 melanomas both *in vitro* and *in vivo* in mice (He et al., 1997). In 1998, further support for its inhibitory properties against breast cancer was reported based on a study that showed tocotrienols inhibit the growth of human breast cancer cells *in vitro* irrespective of estrogen receptor status (Nesaretnam et al., 1998). The mechanism behind this effect was partially resolved when it was reported in 1999 that isoprenoids can initiate apoptosis and cell-cycle arrest *in vitro* in human and murine tumor cells (Mo and Elson, 1999), as supported by additional evidence the same year that tocotrienols are effective apoptotic inducers in human breast cancer cell lines (Yu et al., 1999).

1.2.2 Anticholesterol

Tocotrienols are farnesylated benzopyrans that exhibit hypocholesterolemic activity *in vitro* and *in vivo*. The chiral (natural) and racemic (synthetic) tocotrienols exhibit nearly identical inhibition of cholesterogenesis and HMG-CoA reductase suppression properties *in vitro* and *in vivo*. However, it is the delta and gamma isomers found in tocotrienols that are effective at reducing elevated cholesterol due to the position of methyl groups at the head of the molecule. (Tocotrienols with lesser levels of methyl groups are called desmethyl tocotrienols.)

Early evidence of tocotrienols' inhibiting cholesterogenesis was first observed in chickens and reported by Qureshi and colleagues (Qureshi et al., 1986). Speculation, later supported by others, was that the three double bonds in the isoprenoid chain were necessary for the inhibition of cholesterogenesis. Within several years of this finding, a study in pigs confirmed its hypocholesterolemic properties. The first study reported in 1991 in pigs with inherited hyperlipidemias found that tocotrienols added to the feed reduced the concentration of plasma cholesterol, apolipoprotein B, thromboxane B_2 and platelet factor 4 (Qureshi et al., 1991).

Initial evidence of its benefit as an anticholesterolemic in humans appeared in the same year. Qureshi and colleagues studied tocotrienols derived from palm oil in humans and reported in 1991 lowered serum cholesterol in those diagnosed with hypercholesterolemia. The same year, Tan and colleagues also found tocotrienols lowered serum total cholesterol and low-density lipoprotein (LDL) cholesterol (Tan et al., 1991).

Between 1992 and 1994, Pearce and Parker and colleagues reported that tocotrienols regulate cholesterol production in mammalian cells by posttranscriptional suppression of HMG-CoA reductase via a process that was distinctively different from other known mechanisms of inhibition involving cholesterol biosynthesis in mammalian cells *in vitro* (Pearce et al., 1992; Parker et al., 1993). These studies found that synthetic and natural tocotrienols had nearly identical biosynthesis inhibition and HMG-CoA reductase suppression. They also demonstrated that two tocotrienol analogues, 2-methyltocotrienol and 8-bromotocotrienol, had the same degree of reduction in low-density-lipoprotein (LDL) cholesterol as natural tocotrienols (Pearce et al., 1992).

In 1993, the ability of tocotrienols to act as a anti-cholesterolemic agent was found to be partially due to its ability to spare plasma tocopherol as demonstration in the rat (Watkins et al., 1993). Further understanding of this property came about through the work of two groups who reported their findings in 1994 and 1995. Pearce and colleagues reported that in studying HepG2 they determined that the farnesyl side chain and the methyl/hydroxy substitution pattern of gamma-tocotrienol was responsible for HMG CoA reductase suppression (Pearce et al., 1994).

Human studies of tocotrienols' hypocholesterolemic benefit first appeared in 1994 and 1995 with the work of Qureshi and colleagues and Teoh and colleagues, who demonstrated lowered serum plasma cholesterol levels in rabbits fed an atherogenic diet and in hypocholesterolemic subjects, respectively (Qureshi et al., 1995; Teoh et al., 1995). Teoh's team studied the effects of tocotrienols on serum cholesterol, lipid peroxides, and aorta atheroma in rabbits fed an atherogenic diet for 12 weeks. They found that tocotrienols were significantly more effective in preventing an increase in serum low-density lipoprotein (LDL) and total cholesterol. A significant increase of serum lipid peroxides was also suppressed. Both tocopherols and tocotrienols significantly protected against atheroma in rabbit aorta, but tocotrienol was more effective. However, in 1999, a study conducted in males at risk for cardiovascular disease found no benefit following tocotrienol supplementation on lipid markers (Mensink et al., 1999). Nevertheless, in the same year, two studies encouraged further examination of its benefit in humans with hyperlipidemias. Among these studies was that of Theriault and colleagues, which found γ-tocotrienol effected Apolipoprotein B synthesis, degradation, and secretion in HepG2 cells, possibly as a result of decreased ApoB translocation into the endoplasmic reticulum lumen (Theriault et al., 1999). Through the work of Qureshi and colleagues in chickens, reported in 2000, it was discovered that the number and position of the methyl substitutes in tocotrienols can affect not only the hypocholesterolemic properties of the chroman moiety better than α-tocopherol, but also explain their influence on tocotrienols' anticancer, antitumor, and antioxidant properties (Qureshi et al., 2000).

As mentioned earlier, another difference between tocopherols and tocotrienols is that tocopherols do not have tocotrienols' cholesterol-lowering properties and may actually interfere with its cholesterol-lowering activity (Qureshi et al., 1996). This difference, unknown until the mid-1990s, may explain why attempts to demonstrate α-tocopherol's benefits to cardiovascular health have been equivocal (Tan et al., 1991; Mensink et al., 1999; Qureshi et al., 2002; Mustad et al., 2002; Yu et al., 2006). In 2006, it was reported that only the δ- and γ-tocotrienol moieties stimulate degradation of HMG-CoA reductase (Song et al., 2006).

1.2.3 Antioxidant

In 1991 it was reported by Serbinova and colleagues that tocotrienols were better antioxidants than α-tocopherol *in vitro* (Serbinova et al., 1991). The authors concluded that α-tocotrienols possess around 50 times higher antioxidant activity against iron-induced lipid peroxidation and 6.5 times greater protection of cytochrome P-450 against oxidative damage than α-tocopherol. The following year, Kagan and colleagues discovered why using human LDL-cholesterol *in vitro* facilitated antioxidant recycling of vitamin E (Kagan et al., 1992). Further elucidation of this finding was reported a year later by Suarna and colleagues (Suarna et al., 1993). Studying humans, they found that dietary tocotrienols were incorporated into lipoproteins and reacted with peroxyl radicals as efficiently as corresponding tocopherol isomers.

That same year, Suzuki and colleagues reported that tocotrienols are not only located closer to the cell membrane surface but more so than tocopherol (Sukuzi et al., 1993). This *in vitro* observation was confirmed the same year in plasma in rats fed an atherogenic diet to determine whether α-tocopherol and γ-tocotrienol would reduce the concentration of plasma cholesterol, triglycerides, and fatty acid peroxides (Watkins et al., 1993). The consumption of these vitamin E moieties resulted in significant decreases in plasma cholesterol, low-density lipoprotein (LDL) cholesterol, very-low-density lipoprotein (VLDL) cholesterol and triglycerides. Similar results were reported in 1993 in humans in a study conducted by the Heart Research Group in Australia. In this study, dietary supplementation with palm oil-derived tocotrienol resulted in a dose-dependent increase in α- and γ-tocotrienol in both plasma and circulating lipoproteins (Suarna et al., 1993). The study also found these tocotrienols were more efficient free radical scavengers within circulating lipoproteins than tocopherols.

In 1995, evidence of a neuroprotective effect from the antioxidant activity of tocotrienols was reported by Kamat and Devasagayam. Using palm oil tocotrienols, they found tocotrienols to be potent inhibitors of protein oxidation and lipid peroxidation in rat brain mitochondria (Kamat and Devasagayam, 1995). In the same year, Tomeo and colleagues reported on a study they performed in which tocotrienols were administered to patients with carotid stenosis and hyperlipidemia, and observed an inhibitory effect on the progression of carotid atherosclerosis, which they concluded was due to its antioxidant properties (Tomeo et al., 1995).

Additional associations between tocotrienol and its antioxidant activity emerged in 1999, following a study by Newaz and Nawal in spontaneously hypertensive rats. They observed a reduction in blood pressure and lipid peroxidation, and an increase in total antioxidant status in serum, suggesting a possible role for tocotrienols in the treatment of hypertension (Newaz and Nawal, 1999). Their findings supported earlier work in rats by Koba and colleagues in which they found that tocotrienols were superior to α-tocopherol in suppressing the age-related increase in systolic blood pressure in spontaneously hypertensive rats (Koba et al., 1992).

Which vitamin E moieties are responsible for tocotrienols' antioxidant effects was determined in 2000 by Qureshi and colleagues, when they showed that the methyl substitutes in tocotrienols affected their antioxidant activity in chickens, rather than the tocopherols (Qureshi et al., 2000). This finding was supported by the work of Adachi and Ishii the same year, showing α-tocopherol acetate did not demonstrate an antiaging antioxidant effect in *C. elegans* (Adachi and Ishii, 2000).

1.2.4 Other Biological Properties

Ikeda and colleagues demonstrated that there was preferential absorption of α-tocotrienol by γ- and δ-tocotrienols and α-tocopherol in lymphatic transport in rats (Ikeda et al., 1996).

In a study by Hosomi and colleagues on the affinity for α-tocopherol transfer protein (α-TTP) as a determinant of the biologica activities of vitamin E analogs, they reported that α-TTP binds α-tocotrienol with 11% efficiency compared with α-tocopherol (Hosomi et al., 1997).

Gu and colleagues studied the dietary effect of tocotrienols in rats on the immune function of spleen and mesenteric lymph node lymphocytes. They found that tocotrienol feeding affected the proliferation and function of these lymphocytes, suggesting the possibility that tocotrienols had an immunomodulatory effect (Gu et al., 1999).

An examination of tocotrienols' effect on epithelial cells has found that both normal and preneoplastic and neoplastic mammary epithelial cells preferentially absorbed them compared with tocopherols in mice (McIntyre et al., 2000a, 2000b).

Sen and colleagues conducted a study in mice and found evidence of a neuroprotective effect of tocotrienols (Sen et al., 2000). Glutamate toxicity is mediated by ROS, a major contributor to cell death in the nervous system. The study by Sen's group found that tocotrienols protect against glutamate-induced neuronal death in mice by suppressing inducible pp60 c-Src kinase activation. Further work by the same investigators found that tocotrienol, but not tocopherol, completely protected neurons by an antioxidant-independent mechanism involving the two major targets of tocotrienol in the neuron, not only c-Src kinase, but also 12-lipoxygenase (Sen, Khanna and Roy, 2004). More significantly, the work of O'Byrne and colleagues determined earlier that the neuroprotective properties could occur at nanomolar concentrations following tocotrienol supplementation in humans (O'Byrne, 2000). Although initially there was doubt up to the late 1990s that, if tocotrienol could pass through the blood–brain barrier, experimental evidence emerged in 2002 that dietary intake of palm-oil-derived tocotrienol does reach the brain and finds its way into the cerebrospinal fluid, even at a dose as low as 5 mg/kg of body weight when taken over an extended period of time (Roy et al., 2002). This suggests that tocotrienol may provide neuroprotection by its antioxidant action as a major lipid-soluble, chain-breaking antioxidant in the body at 100 nM (1/10th of the concentration achieved in the plasma of all vitamin E compounds) (Sen, Khanna and Roy, 2004).

1.3 SUMMARY

A considerable body of studies have demonstrated that tocotrienol moieties possess antioxidant, anticholesterolemic, antiatherosclerotic, anticancer, antitumor, antihypertensive, immunomodulatory and neuroprotective properties. For example, when tocotrienols become incorporated into circulating human lipoproteins, they react with peroxyl radicals as effectively as tocopherol isomers. When all of its attributes are taken together, it is becoming clear that tocotrienols' benefits are significantly greater than α-tocopherol, which for decades received far more attention by the research community than the tocotrienols. The shift in attention from tocopherols to tocotrienols is partially due to the latter's having superior distribution in the fatty bilayers of the cell membrane as a lipid-soluble chain-breaking antioxidant. Alpha-tocotrienol's higher antioxidant property is partially due to its higher recycling efficiency from chromanoxyl radicals.

What has been lacking is sufficient understanding of the mechanisms by which tocotrienol works, other than the known suppression of HMG-CoA reductase responsible for mediating cholesterol synthesis. Hence, by publication of this work on tocotrienol, we are given not only a wealth of information on what is known about tocotrienols and its range of biological properties, but also recently discovered mechanisms of action. All of this knowledge brought together by leading investigators in vitamin E will hopefully increase needed recognition of the importance of tocotrienols in the prevention and maintenance of human health.

Tocotrienols are found throughout the plant kingdom. Unfortunately, data is still limited as to the concentration of tocotrienol moieties in foods sufficient to guide the discerning consumer on which foods provide the richest sources of tocotrienols (Eitenmiller and Lee, 2004), rather than just "vitamin E." This comes at a time when much has been learned about the molecular and chemical structure of vitamin E and the different attributes and properties of the tocopherols and tocotrienols. Once such compositional information breaking down the tocopherols and tocotrienols (based on their methyl group position) found in food becomes available, humans can select foods richest in those foodstuffs capable of providing the highest intakes of the desired vitamin E moiety of interest. This is especially important as tocotrienols are found in a wide range of foods, including fruits, vegetables and grains, nuts, seeds, meats, eggs and a variety of edible oils and fats. As recognition of the importance of tocotrienols grows, it will be interesting to see the net effect on the incidence and prevalence of certain diseases as the percentage of vitamin E as γ-tocopherol from corn- and soy-derived products decreases and tocotrienol-rich foods increase.

REFERENCES

Adachi H. and Ishii N. 2000;, Effects of tocotrienols on lifespan and protein carbonylation in *caenorhabditis elegans. J Gerontol*: Series A, *Biol Sci Med Sci*, 55: B280–B285.

Brown MS and Goldstein JL. 1980; Multivalent feedback control of HMG CoA reductase, a control mechanism coordinating isoprenoid synthesis and cell growth. *J Lipid Res*, 21: 505–517.

Di Cyan, E. 1972. *Vitamin E and Aging.* Pyramid Books: New York.

Eitenmiller R and Lee J. 2004. *Vitamin E: Food Chemistry, Composition and Analysis,* Marcel Dekker: New York, pp. 425–505.

Elson CE and Qureshi AA. 1995. Coupling the cholesterol- and tumor-suppressive actions of palm oil to the impact of its minor constituents on 3-hydroxy-3-methylglutaryl coenzyme A reductase activity. *Prostag Leukotr Essent Fatty Acids,* 52: 205–207.

Emerson OH et al. 1937. The chemistry of vitamin E: tocopherols from various sources. *J Bio Chem*, 122: 99–107.

Evans HM and Bishop KS. 1922. On the existence of a hitherto unrecognized dietary factor essential for reproduction. *Science*, 56: 650–651.

Evans HM et al. 1936. The isolation from wheat germ oil of an alcohol alpha-tocopherol, having the properties of vitamin E. *J Biochem,* 113: 319–332.

Fernholz E. 1937. The thermal decomposition of alpha-tocopherol. *J Am Chem Soc*, 59: 1154–1155.

Fernholz E. 1938. On the constitution of alpha-tocopherol. *J Am Chem Soc*, 60: 700–705

Goh SH et al. 1994. Inhibition of tumor promotion by various palm-oil tocotrienols. *Int J Cancer*, 57: 529–531.

Gould MN, et al. 1991. A comparison of tocopherol and tocotrienol for the chemoprevention of chemically induced rat mammary tumors. *Am J Clin Nutr*, 53; 1068S–1070S.

Gu JY et al. 1999. Dietary effect of tocopherols and tocotrienols on the immune function of spleen and mesenteric lymph node lymphocytes in Brown Norway rats. *Biosci Biotechnol Biochem,* 63: 1697–1702.

Guthrie N et al. 1993. Inhibition of breast cancer cell growth by tocotrienols. *FASEB J,* 7: A70.

Guthrie N et al. 1997. Inhibition of proliferation of estrogen receptor-negative MDA-MB-435 and -positive MCF-7 human breast cancer cells by palm oil tocotrienols and tamoxifen, alone and in combination. *J Nutr,* 127: 544S–548S.

Guthrie N et al. 1994. Inhibition of proliferation of human breast cancer cells by individual tocotrienols from palm oil. *Proc Ann Meet Assoc Cancer Res,* 35: A3749.

He L et al. 1997. Isoprenoids suppress the growth of murine B16 melanomas in vitro and in vivo. *J Nutr*, 127: 668–674.

Horwitt MK 1974. Status of human requirements for vitamin E. *Am J Clinl Nutr*, 27: 1182–93.

Horwitt MK. 1986. Interpretations of requirements of thiamin, riboflavin, niacin-tryptophan, and vitamin E plus comments on balance studies and vitamin B-6. *Am J Clin Nutr*, 44: 973–85.

Horwitt MK 1991. Data supporting supplementation of humans with vitamin E. *J Nutr*, Vol. 121, pp. 424–29.

Hosomi A et al. 1997. Affinity for alpha-tocopherol transfer protein as a determinant of the biological activities of vitamin E analogs. *FEBS Lett*, 409: 105–108.

Ikeda I et al. 1996. Lymphatic transport of alpha-, gamma- and delta-tocotrienols and alpha-tocopherol in rats. *Int J Vit Nutr Res*, 66: 217–221.

Kagan VE et al. 1992. Recycling of vitamin E in human low density lipoproteins. *J Lipid Res*, 33: 385–397.

Kamat JP and Devasagayam TP. 1995. Tocotrienols from palm oil as potent inhibitors of lipid peroxidation and protein oxidation in rat brain mitochondia. *Neurosci Lett*, 195: 179–182.

Khor HT and Chieng DY. 1996. Effect of dietary supplementation of tocotrienols and tocopherols on serum lipids in the hamster. *Nutr Res*, 16: 1391–1401.

Koba K et al. 1992. Effects of alpha-tocopherol and tocotrienols on blood pressure and linoleic acid metabolism in the spontaneously hypertensive rat (SHR). *Biosci Biotechnol Biochem*, 56: 1420–1423.

Komiyama K et al. 1989. Studies on the biological activity of tocotrienols. *Chem Pharmaceut Bull*, 37: 1369–1371.

McIntyre BS et al. 2000a. Antiproliferative and apoptic effects of tocopherols and tocotrienols on normal mouse mammary epithelial cells. *Lipids*, 35. 171–180.

McIntyre BS et al. 2000b. Antiproliferative and apoptic effects of tocopherols and tocotrienols on preneoplastic and neoplastic mouse mammary epithelial cells. *Proc Soc Exp Biol Med*, 224: 292–301.

Mensink RP et al. 1999. A vitamin E concentrate rich in tocotrienols had no effect on serum lipids, lipoproteins, or platelet function in men with mildly elevated serum lipid concentrations. *Am J Clin Nutr*, 69: 213–219.

Mo H and Elson CE. 1999. Apoptosis and cell–cycle arrest in human and murine tumor cells are initiated by isoprenoids. *J Nutr*, 129: 804–813.

Mustad VA et al. 2002. Supplementation with 3 compositionally different tocotrienol supplements does not improve cardiovascular disease risk factors in men and women with hypercholesterolemia. *Am J Clin Nutr*, 76: 1237–1243.

Nesaretnam K et al. 1995. Effect of tocotrienols on the growth of a human breast cancer cell line in culture. *Lipids*, 30: 1139–1143.

Nesaretnam K et al. 1998. Tocotrienols inhibit the growth of human breast cancer cells irrespective of estrogen receptor status. *Lipids*, 33: 461–469.

Newaz MA and Nawal NN. 1999. Effect of gamma-tocotrienol on blood pressure, lipid peroxidation and total antioxidant status in spontaneously hypertensive rats. *Clin Exp Hypertens*, 21: 1297–1313.

Ngah WZ et al. 1991. Effect of tocotrienols on hepatocarcinogenesis induced by 2–acetylaminofluorene in rats. *Am J Clin Nutr*, 53. 1076S–1081S.

O'Byrne D et al. 2000. Studies of LDL oxidation following alpha-, gamma-, or delta-tocotrienyl acetate supplementation of hypercholesterolemic humans. *Free Radic Biol Med*, 29: 834–845.

Olcott HS and Emerson OH. 1937. Antioxidants and autoxidation of fats: The antioxidant properties of tocopherols. *J Am Chem Society*, 59: 1008–1009.

Parker RA et al. 1990. Tocotrienols descrease cholesterol synthesis in HEPG2 cells by a novel post–transcriptional suppression of HMGCoA reductase. *FASEB J*, 4: A1744.

Parker RA et al. 1993. Tocotrienols regulate cholesterol production in mammalian cells by post–transcriptional suppression of 3-hydroxy-3-methylglutaryl-coenzyme A reductase. *J Biol Chem*, 268: 11230 11238.

Pearce BC et al. 1992. Hypcholesterolemic activity of synthetic and natural tocotrienols. *J Med Chem*, 36: 1420–1423.

Pearce BC, Parker RA, Deason ME et al. 1992. Hypocholesterolemic activity of synthetic and natural tocotrienols. *J Med Chem*, 35: 3595–3606.

Pearce BC et al. 1994. Inhibitors of cholesterol biosynthesis. 2. Hypocholesterolemic and antioxidant activities of benzopyran and tetrahydronaphthalene analogues of the tocotrienols. *J Med Chem*, 37: 526–541.

Pennock JF et al. 1964. Reassessment of tocopherol chemistry. *BBRC*, 17: 542–548.

Qureshi AA et al. 1986. The structure of an inhibitor of cholesterol biosynthesis isolated from barley. *J Biol Chem*, 261: 10544–10550.

Qureshi AA et al. 1991. Dietary tocotrienols reduce concentrations of plasma cholesterol, apoliopoprotein B, thromboxane B2, and platelet factor 4 in pigs with inherited hyperlipidemias. *Am J Clin Nutr*, 53: 1042S–1046S.

Qureshi AA et al. 1995. Response of hypercholesterolemic subjects to administration of tocotrienols. *Lipids*, 30: 1171–1177.

Qureshi AA et al. 1996. Dietary alpha-tocopherol attenuates the impact of gamma–tocotrineol on hepatic 3-hydroxy-3-methylglutaryl coenzyme A reductase activity in chickens. *J Nutr*, 126: 389–394.

Qureshi AA et al. 2000. Isolation and identification of novel tocotrienols from rice bran with hypocholesterolemic, antioxidant, and antitumor properties. *J Agric Food Chem,* 48: 3130–3140.

Qureshi AA et al. 2002. Dose-dependent suppression of serum cholesterol by tocotrienol-rich fraction (TRF25) of rice bran in hypercholesterolemic humans. *Atherosclerosis,* 161: 199–207.

Rahmat A et al. 1993. Long-term administration of tocotrienols and tumor-marker enzyme activities during hepatocarcinogenesis in rats. *Nutrition,* 9: 229–232.

Rim EB et al. 1993. Vitamin E consumption and the risk of coronary disease in men. *New Engl J Med,* 328: 1450–1456.

Roy S et al. 2002. Simultaneous detection of tocopherols and tocotrienols in biological samples using HPLC–coulometric electrode array. *Meth Enzymol,* 352: 326–332.

Sen CK et al. 2000. Molecular basis of vitamin E action: tocotrienol potently inhibits glutamate-induced pp60(c-Src) kinase activation and death of HT4 neuronal cells. *J Biol Chem,* 275: 13049–13055.

Sen CK, Khanna S and Roy S. 2004. Tocotrienol: The natural vitamin E to defend the nervous system. *Ann NY Acad Sci,* 1031: 127–142.

Serbinova E et al. 1991. Free radical recycling and intramembrane mobility in the antioxidant properties of alpha-tocopherol and alpha-tocotrienol. *Free Rad Biol Med,* 10: 263–275.

Shute E and Shute CM. 1985. *The Vitamin E Story.* Welch Publ: Burlington, ON.

Shute E. 1959. The current status of alpha tocopherol in cardiovascular disease. In: *Vitamin E: Your Key to a Health Heart.* Bailey H (Ed.) *ARC Books*: New York.

Song BL et al. 2006. Insig-dependent ubiquitination and degradation of 3-hydroxy-3-methylglutaryl coenzyme a reductase stimulated by delta- and gamma-tocotrienols. *J Biol Chem,* 281: 25,054–25,061.

Stampfer MJ et al. 1993. Vitamin E consumption and the risk of coronary disease in women. *New Engl J Med,* 328: 1449–1449.

Stern MG et al. 1947. Delta-tocopherol I: Isolation from soybean oil and properties. *J Am Chem Soc,* 69: 869–874.

Suarna C et al. 1993. Comparative antioxidant activity of tocotrienols and other natural lipid-soluble antioxidants in a homogeneous system, and in rat and human lipoproteins. *Biochim Biophys Acta,* 1166: 163–170.

Sukuzi YJ et al. 1993. Structural and dynamic membrane propetrties of alpha-tocopherol and alpha- tocotrienol: Implication to the molecular mechanism of their antioxidant potency. *Biophys Acta,* 1166: 163–170.

Sundram et al. 1989. Effect of dietary palm oils on mammary carcinogenesis in female rats induced by 7,12–dimethylbenz(a)anthracene. *Cancer Res,* 49: 1447–1451.

Sylester P and Theriault A. 2003. Role of tocotrienols in the prevention of cardiovascular disease and breast cancer. *Curr Topics Nutr Res,* 1(2): 121–136.

Tan B. 2005. Appropriate spectrum vitamin E and new perspectives on desmethyl tocopherols and tocotrienols. *J Am Nutraceut Assoc,* 8: 35–42.

Tan DT et al. 1991. Effect of a palm-oil–vitamin E concentrate on the serum and lipoprotein lipids in humans. *Am J Clin Nutr,* 53: 1027S 1030S.

Teoh MK et al. 1995. Protection by tocotrienols against hypercholesterolemia and atheroma. *Med J Malaysia,* 50: 117.

Theriault A et al. 1999. Effects of gamma-tocotrienol on ApoB synthesis, degradation, and secretion in HepG2 cells. *Arterioscler Thromb Vasc Biol,* 19: 704–712.

Tomeo AC et al. 1995. Antioxidant effects of tocotrienols in patients with hyperlipidemia and carotid stenosis. *Lipids,* 30: 1179–1183.

Watkins E et al. 1993. Gamma-tocotrienol as a hypocholesterolemic and antioxidant agent in rats fed atherogenic diets. *Lipids,* 28: 1113–1118.

Whittle KJ et al. 1966. The isolation and properties of delta–tocotrienol from Hevea latex. *Biochem J,* 100: 138–145.

Yu SG et al. 2006. Dose response impact of various tocotrienols on serum lipid parameters in 5-week-old female chickens. *Lipids,* 41: 453–461.

Yu W et al. 1999. Induction of apoptosis in human breast cancer cells by tocopherols and tocotrienols. *Nutr Cancer,* 33: 26–32.

2 Tocotrienols in Vitamin E: Hype or Science?

Neil E. Levin and Dallas L. Clouatre

CONTENTS

2.1 INTRODUCTION

News media coverage of vitamin E can affect perceptions of this essential oil-soluble nutrient; not just by the public, but also within the scientific community. Critical analysis combined with the ability to repeat experiments ultimately will triumph in leading to an enhanced scientific understanding, but "media myths" often are self-referential and scarcely dented by subsequent study results. And, even if science is self-correcting in the long run ... that, of course, is the rub—in the long run. In the short term, hope, hype and experimental science all compete to define a topic, with accuracy often suffering. Science is not practiced in isolation from society. This fact is abundantly clear in the controversy currently raging over vitamin E. Unconscious biases and the multiplication of variables challenge the designers of review articles such as meta-analyses, the conclusions of which frequently and irrationally get touted as overturning all previous scientific studies, especially if an unexpected conclusion emerges.

The case for vitamin E as protective against heart disease, cancer and a number of other conditions not long ago was thought to have been open and shut, with further clinical trials expected merely to dot the i's and cross the t's. Vitamin E, it was believed, is a winner. Many physicians used it themselves, though relatively fewer actually recommended it to their patients. More recently still, after years of hope and hype, the pendulum swung in the other direction so far that a journal editorial could ask rhetorically, "Is there any hope for vitamin E?" as the authors surveyed vitamin E's rise and fall as a potential cancer and cardiovascular cure-all.[1] As with most pendular swings, the truth is somewhere in the middle.

Disputes frequently turn on fine distinctions. In this instance, which vitamin E is it that is supposed to have succeeded or failed? There is the common d–α tocopherol, extracted from vegetable oils. But there are, after all, a total of eight different naturally occurring forms within the vitamin E family and an additional seven largely physiologically inactive forms created in the synthesis of dl–α-tocopherol. One half of the entire vitamin E family, the tocotrienols, furthermore, has been the subject of less than 1% of the studies and papers published on the topic.[2]

These distinctions immediately suggest several questions that need to be addressed. First, what led to the extraordinary hype and then disappointment associated with vitamin E studies in the past? Second, was/is the disappointment warranted or is the disillusionment as unwarranted as was the initial hope and hype? Third, will the bad-press fate of the tocopherol side of the vitamin E family befall the tocotrienol side?

2.2 ALPHA-TOCOPHEROL AND THE VITAMIN E FAMILY

2.2.1 Tocopherols and Tocotrienols

Vitamin E is the collective name for a family of fat-soluble compounds and generically includes all entities that exhibit the biological activity of d–α-tocopherol. Aside from d–α-tocopherol, there exist also β-, γ and δ tocopherol. These forms (isomers) are variations of the same chemical constituents with slightly different structures. Closely related members of the family include α, β-, γ, and δ tocotrienol. Natural vitamin E is a mixture of tocopherols and tocotrienols (α-, β-, γ-, δ-tocopherol, and α-, β-, γ-, δ-tocotrienol). The naturally occurring forms are predominantly in the stereoisomeric d-forms; with the synthesized dl-form actually a mixture of eight isomers, only one of which is d–α-tocopherol. Most research has focused on α-tocopherol, but the other isomers are now gaining attention, especially γ-tocopherol and the tocotrienols. Common to all the isomers is a chromanic nucleus (6-chromanol) with an aliphatic side chain (C16). The side chain is saturated for tocopherols (with three chiral centers in the RRR stereoisomeric configuration) and unsaturated for tocotrienols (only one chiral center with three double bonds at 3', 7', and 11' positions).[3] Tocotrienols have an isoprenoid instead of a phytyl side chain. It may be the case that the double bonds in the isoprenoid side chain allow tocotrienols to move more freely and more efficiently within cell membranes than do tocopherols, especially in tissues with saturated fatty layers, such as the brain and liver.[4] This hints at a superior ability of tocotrienols to perform certain functions in the body.

The number of methyl groups and the pattern of methylation of the chromanol ring primarily distinguish the tocopherols and tocotrienols. Alpha-tocopherol and α-tocotrienol each have three methyl groups, β- and γ-tocopherols and tocotrienols have two methyl groups, whereas δ-tocopherol and tocotrienol have one methyl group. Independent of dietary sources of vitamin E, only α-tocopherol is actively maintained in human plasma due to the fact that the hepatic α-tocopherol transfer protein (α-TTP) selectively recognizes α-tocopherol and mediates its secretion into the circulation.[5] Yet γ-tocopherol may constitute a higher percentage of common diets.

2.2.2 Great Expectations

Even more than is true of vitamin C, within the research community vitamin E has been viewed as "the" antioxidant for preventing damage to biological systems. Theories linking oxidative damage to aging and to various disease states date back only to the 1940s. Johan Bjorksten, a research chemist working for a branch of Eastman Kodak, first observed a similarity between the aging of film materials and the aging of human tissues in 1941. He surmised that the common point is the damage to both by free radicals and that in living organisms this damage results in the cross-linking of protein molecules, including the RNA and DNA strands that reproduce all the proteins in the body. Denham Harman of the University of Nebraska put such observations to experimental tests starting in the 1950s, and thus began the popularization of free radical and antioxidant theories of health.

To be sure, the earliest promotion of vitamin E for cardiovascular functioning, starting in the 1940s, did not draw upon the antioxidant theory.[6] However, in the 1950s, researchers discovered that a vitamin E deficiency in humans leads to oxidative damage to lipids.[7] This was followed by the end of the next decade with arguments that vitamin E is a biological antioxidant.[8] Indeed, some observers declared, "[i]n human blood plasma and erythrocyte ghost membranes vitamin E is the major, and possibly the only, chain-breaking antioxidant."[9] By 1989, α-tocopherol was declared to possess near optimal activity as a chain-breaking antioxidant.[10] Alpha-tocopherol, usually in its synthetic form, was viewed as being most active as an antioxidant and therefore assumed to be most protective against oxidative damage in biological systems.

With what seemed the clear backing of *in vitro* and animal work, open clinical trials were conducted that yielded encouraging results. Evidence suggested that men taking at least 100 IU vitamin E per day for at least 2 years exhibited a significantly reduced risk of coronary disease.[11] This level is higher than found in the typical American diet. Similar results were found with women, with vitamin E intake proving to be protective, but only after approximately 2 years.[12] Likewise, the US Nurses' Health Study and the US Health Professionals' Follow-up Study, which found 34% and 39% reductions, respectively, in the risk of having a cardiac event for those taking vitamin E supplements in doses of 100 IUs or greater for at least 2 years, were in line with the accepted dictum that benefits usually take at least 2 years to manifest in cardiovascular treatments.[13] Even protection against the progression of coronary artery atherosclerosis was directly observed.[14]

Through the end of the 1990s, it appeared that the great expectations for vitamin E would be realized. Cancer studies seemed similarly promising. The α-Tocopherol, β-Carotene Cancer Prevention (ATBC) Study demonstrated a 32% reduction in prostate cancer incidence in smokers in response to daily supplementation with α tocopherol at 50 mg per day (74.5 IU) synthetic α-tocopheryl acetate.[15] Significant prevention also was found in the case of colorectal cancer.[16]

However, before the decade ended, there already were hints of things to come. The Iowa Women's Health Study found that only vitamin E from food, not from supplements, was associated with fewer cardiac events.[17] Similar results emerged from a study lasting 7 years involving 34,486 post-menopausal women. That study showed that the amount of vitamin E supplied in the diet, predominantly γ-tocopherol, but not supplemental α tocopherol, was inversely correlated to deaths from cardiovascular disease (CVD).[18]

2.2.2.1 Vitamin E's Fall from Grace

An easy set of assumptions allowed for α-tocopherol, either in its synthetic or its purified naturally derived forms, to be taken as the active vitamin E, though the NIH notes that the synthetic form is only about half as effective as the natural form. As a result of the fact that α-tocopherol transfer protein (α-TTP) selectively recognizes α-tocopherol and mediates its secretion into the circulation, and thus ensures that it is the predominant form found in serum and tissues, and for other reasons, α tocopherol was accepted as the most active form of vitamin E and as the most significant in protecting against oxidative stress. The unique vitamin action of α-tocopherol, combined with its prevalence in the human body and the similar efficiency of tocopherols as chain-breaking antioxidants, led biologists to almost completely discount the "minor" vitamin E molecules as topics for basic and clinical research.[19]

Indeed, α-tocopherol fit so nicely into the pure oxidative stress theory of illness that the hopes of theory were practically taken as evidence for this compound. Hence, there always was an aura of excessive expectation in many quarters, including scientific ones. The fact that supplementation with α-tocopherol might block and deplete other members of the E family, such as γ-tocopherol, was ignored, just as was the possibility that the activities of these other E family members might not be tied directly to their chemical antioxidant aspects, but rather reflect anti-inflammatory, antineoplastic and natriuretic functions.[20]

If one were to choose a date, the refutation of excessive hopes hit first in 2005 via somewhat questionable meta-analyses and then rapidly was picked up by the media at large.[21] Publication of negative long-running clinical studies followed. Two decades of experimental and epidemiological data had given support to the notion that vitamin E supplementation might prevent cancer and cardiovascular events; yet well-controlled clinical trials had not borne out these expectations. The Heart Outcomes Prevention Evaluation (HOPE) trial and its follow-up lasted a total of 7 years and included a daily dose of natural-source vitamin E (400 IU) or matching placebo. Results were negative.[22] The researchers' conclusion? "In patients with vascular disease or diabetes mellitus, long-term vitamin E supplementation does not prevent cancer or major cardiovascular events and may increase the risk for heart failure."

These two articles are fairly representative of the recent attack on vitamin E and refutations flowed quickly. Regarding the 2005 Miller et al. meta-analysis, consider:

- Trials were excluded in which there were fewer than 12 deaths.
- The trials tested high dosages in adults with chronic diseases and should not be applied to healthy adults.
- Some trials included multivitamin combinations.
- The findings do not clearly establish that the lowest dosage of supplements is associated with increased risk of mortality, nor any reliable dose-dependent risk.
- A major review in response found that clinical trial evidence shows vitamin E supplements appear safe for most adults in amounts ≤1600 IU/day, even when considering the original data reviewed by the Miller meta-analysis.[23]

Similarly, the HOPE authors[22] relegate findings of a lower risk of cancer in the E group to chance, yet arbitrarily treat a similarly slight increase in cardiovascular risk as important. Complicating the analysis is the fact that the group getting vitamin E included somewhat greater numbers of current smokers, more diabetics and more patients taking β–blockers, but fewer taking lipid-lowering medications, which were also ignored in reaching sensational conclusions. In other words, the groups may not have met standard criteria for randomization of these confounding variables.

The battle over vitamin E's safety and efficacy now has been joined, with new meta-analyses again casting doubt on efficacy and safety.[24] With the inclusion of more recent results, clinical trials supplementing antioxidant vitamins continue to yield conflicting results.[25] Even seemingly positive trials have come out with mixed results. For instance, on the one hand, in spite of the fact that the authors play down the benefit with regard to cardiovascular deaths, there was a significant 24% reduction in CVD mortality over a period of more than 10 years in the recently reported Women's Health Study in subjects taking 600 IU α-tocopherol ("natural source," but not further defined) every other day versus placebo.[26] On the other hand, cardiovascular events were *not* significantly reduced and neither was the overall rate of death.

It may not be possible to fairly sort out whether vitamin E does or does not inhibit cancer and heart disease based upon current data because of the biases currently built into the available data. Almost all large trials have been conducted with either synthetic α-tocopherol or "natural source" α-tocopherol, which still leaves out the other seven members of the chemical family that exist in foods. Matters actually are worse than this. Current supplement practices actively detract from the possible benefits from other members of the vitamin E family. Supplementation with α-tocopherol clearly depresses γ-tocopherol levels, whereas γ-tocopherol has little effect on α-tocopherol.[27,28,29,30] Lest one think that the negative impact of α-tocopherol is limited to other tocopherols, research shows that α-tocopherol attenuates the impact of γ-tocotrienol as well.[31]

2.2.3 Redemption by Tocotrienol?

The ratio of α-tocopherol to γ-tocopherol is higher in subjects with cardiovascular disease than in those without.[32,33] These findings support the contention that a true dietary spectrum of vitamin E and family members other than α-tocopherol likely are heart-protective despite the conflicting clinical results with α tocopherol. But what about the lesser-known side of the family, the tocotrienols?

In one trial, tocotrienols, but not α-tocopherol, significantly extended the average life span of nematodes as much as 19% and reduced protein carbonylation.[34] An interesting finding, to be sure, but not one that can be compared easily with other data.

Tocotrienols, primarily γ- and δ-tocotrienols, have been shown to be able to reduce both total cholesterol and the low-density lipoprotein cholesterol fractions. Most trials have found that tocotrienols can significantly lower blood cholesterol levels even in subjects who already have adopted low-fat diets. In a study published in the journal *Lipids* in 1997, supplementing with 200–220 mg/day of tocotrienols reduced cholesterol levels an additional 10–13% in 4 weeks in men who followed a special cholesterol-lowering diet and previously had reduced their cholesterol levels by 5–7% by means of the diet alone. This indicates that the combined use of diet and tocotrienol supplementation was able to reduce cholesterol levels by 15–20% in men with elevated readings within less than 8 weeks.[35] A more recent study showed that a dose of 100 mg/day of tocotrienol-rich fraction (TRF25) of stabilized and heated rice bran produces maximum decreases of 20, 25, 14 ($P<0.05$) and 12%, respectively, in serum total cholesterol, LDL-cholesterol, apolipoprotein B and triglycerides compared with the baseline values, "suggesting that a dose of 100 mg/day TRF25 plus AHA Step-1 diet may be the optimal dose for controlling the risk of coronary heart disease in hypercholesterolemic human subjects."[36]

Clinical work is just as impressive. In an 18-month trial, 50 patients with carotid stenosis were randomly assigned to receive either 160 mg daily of palm tocotrienols (γ- and α-forms) with 64 mg of α-tocopherol or palm oil only as a placebo. After 6 months, the dosage in the treatment group was increased to 240 mg mixed tocotrienols with 96 mg of α-tocopherol. At the end of the study, ultrasound scans of the carotid artery showed that none of the patients in the control group had improved during the trial and 10 showed a worsening of their condition, whereas, in the tocotrienol group, atherosclerosis was reduced and blood flow to the brain improved in 7 of 25 patients. Only two patients in this group showed worsened conditions. No adverse side effects were reported in either group.[37]

Tocotrienols are effective in lowering serum total and LDL-cholesterol levels by inhibiting the hepatic enzymic activity of 3-hydroxy-3-methylglutaryl-coenzyme A (HMG-CoA) reductase through the post-transcriptional mechanism. Alpha-tocopherol, however, has an opposite effect on this enzyme's activity. Because tocotrienols are also converted to tocopherols *in vivo*, some researchers argue that it is necessary to not exceed a certain dose, as this would be counter-productive.[38]

A growing body of work shows that γ-tocotrienol reduces oxidative neurodegeneration, glutamate-induced cell death, homocysteine-induced damage, tumor angiogenesis, hyperlipidemia and atherosclerosis.[39,40,41] The tocotrienols more generally exert anti-aging effects; acting on immunoregulation, cellular homeostasis, adhesion molecules and tumor growth.[42,43] Extremely interesting is the potential benefit of γ-tocotrienol in hypertension. Whereas one of the complaints raised against high-dosage α-tocopherol supplementation is a possible temporary elevation in blood pressure, γ-tocotrienol appears to exert the opposite effect and undergoes metabolism to a hormone form that releases excess fluid from the body.[44,45]

Yet to be undertaken with tocotrienols are the large-scale and long-term clinical trials seen with α-tocopherol. Nevertheless, more is known about the comparative effects of the different members of the E family than in the past, with some promising results. Tocotrienols exhibit some distinct advantages over α-tocopherol, not the least of which is stability of tissue levels with long-term usage, but also rapid return more or less to baseline after cessation of supplementation, something not true of α-tocopherol.[46]

2.3 CONCLUSION

In spite of the controversies over vitamin E supplementation, some of which are dependent on questionable meta-analyses of previously published dissimilar data that come to conclusions that differ from those of the original researchers, the underdeveloped field of tocotrienol research is still very promising.

While criticism of the techniques and results of meta-analyses are far less well known as these controversial reviews, some critiques are quite authoritative.[23] One publication has even catalogued the many errors found in both the science and the media coverage of the science, particularly where unexpected or controversial conclusions are reached that create long-lasting myths that never seem to acknowledge the relatively lower value of meta-analyses to more rigorous scientific reports. That review also noted the tendency to treat nutrients as drugs, using a model of administering a single nutrient and looking for a drug-like effect. This ignores the fact that nutrients, especially antioxidants, are both synergistic and co-dependent, and biologically work far better as a family than as individual chemicals. [47] This lack of understanding—or respect—for the very nature of nutrients complicates any analysis of clinical studies in this field.

Additionally, confusion over all of the possible natural and synthetic forms of vitamin E isomers may lead some to conclude that the same potential cautions, however overblown or tentative, should apply to both α-tocopherol and all the other natural tocopherols and tocotrienols. In fact, a recent review noted that desmethyl forms of tocotrienols and tocopherols, namely the γ- and δ-forms, were significantly different from the predominant α and relatively scarce β-forms. The paper concluded that an appropriate spectrum of these eight natural isomers, with the desmethyl forms dominating, should provide the benefits long associated with vitamin E found in foods without the risks associated with α tocopherol dominance caused by supplementation with a single isomer (or synthetic dl-α-tocopherol's combination of eight isomers). [48]

In short, the several stereoisomers of natural vitamin E administered in proper balance as tocopherols and tocotrienols may provide better cardiovascular and lipid benefits than α-tocopherol-only supplements by better mimicking nature and improving the range of biological activities performed by these substances. Also, combining vitamin E complexes with other supporting antioxidants is more nutritive than the single-entity drug model that often seems to fail vitamins, especially antioxidants.

It is unfortunate that sensational reports seem to be continually cited as references by reporters, regulators and researchers while more rigorous corrections are ignored and uncited. Flawed science accepted as a new paradigm somehow has a charmed life, at least for a while. With conflicting studies changing perceptions of the vitamin that was yesterday's media darling and news reports prematurely jumping in to declare its era at an end, it's no wonder so many people are so confused about vitamin E in particular, and nutrition science in general.

Finally, the hierarchy of clinical trial methodology ranked by robustness, where test tube studies rank lower than animal or human models, where diet surveys rank lower than blood work, and where primary trials rank higher than meta-analyses that inevitably introduce additional variables, should always be considered before a new report erroneously erases and causes a collective amnesia as to past scientific successes. Even if the media don't understand these truths, impartial scientists should. For science to live up to its definition of being self-correcting, it must be impartial and aware of potential flaws that can be corrected over time.

REFERENCES

1. Brown BG, Crowley J. 2005. Is there any hope for vitamin E? *JAMA*. Mar 16;293(11):1387–90.
2. Sen CK, Khanna S, Roy S. 2006. Tocotrienols: Vitamin E beyond tocopherols. *Life Sci. Mar* 27;78(18):2088–98.
3. Munteanu A., Zingg JM, Azzi A. 2004. Anti-atherosclerotic effects of vitamin E—myth or reality? *J Cell Mol Med*. Jan-Mar; 8(1), 59–76.
4. Suzuki YJ, Tsuchiya M, Wassall SR, Choo YM, Govil G, Kagan VE, Packer L. 1993. Structural and dynamic membrane properties of alpha-tocopherol and alpha -tocotrienol: Implication to the molecular mechanism of their antioxidant potency. *Biochemistry* Oct 12;32(40):10692–9.
5. Kaempf-Rotzoll DE, Traber MG, Arai H. 2003. Vitamin E and transfer proteins. *Curr Opin Lipidol*. Jun;14(3):249–54.
6. Vogelsang A., Shute E. V. 1946. Effect of vitamin E in coronary heart disease. *Nature* (Lond.), 157, 772.
7. Horwitt MK, Harvey CC, Duncan GD, Wilson WC. 1956. Effects of limited tocopherol intake in man with relationships to erythrocyte hemolysis and lipid oxidations. *Am J Clin Nutr*. Jul-Aug;4(4):408–19.

8. Green J, Bunyan J. 1969. Vitamin E and the biological antioxidant theory. *Nutr Abstr Rev*;39 (2):321–45.
9. Burton GW, Cheeseman KH, Doba T, Ingold KU, Slater TF. 1983. Vitamin E as an antioxidant in vitro and in vivo. *Ciba Found Symp.*;101:4–18.
10. Burton GW, Ingold KU. 1989. Vitamin E as an in vitro and in vivo antioxidant. *Ann N Y Acad Sci.*;570:7–22.
11. Rimm EB, Stampfer MJ, Ascherio A, Giovannucci E, Colditz GA, Willett WC. 1993. Vitamin E consumption and the risk of coronary heart disease in men. *N Engl J Med.* May 20;328(20):1450–6.
12. Stampfer MJ, Hennekens CH, Manson JE, Colditz GA, Rosner B, Willett WC. 1993. Vitamin E consumption and the risk of coronary disease in women. *N Engl J Med.* May 20;328(20):1444–9.
13. Emmert DH, Kirchner JT. 1999. The role of vitamin E in the prevention of heart disease. *Arch Fam Med.* Nov-Dec;8(6):537–42.
14. Hodis HN, Mack WJ, LaBree L, Cashin-Hemphill L, Sevanian A, Johnson R, Azen SP. 1995. Serial coronary angiographic evidence that antioxidant vitamin intake reduces progression of coronary artery atherosclerosis. *JAMA.* Jun 21;273(23):1849–54.
15. Heinonen OP, Albanes D, Virtamo J, Taylor PR, Huttunen JK, Hartman AM, Haapakoski J, Malila N, Rautalahti M, Ripatti S, Maenpaa H, Teerenhovi L, Koss L, Virolainen M, Edwards BK. 1998. Prostate cancer and supplementation with α-tocopherol and β-carotene: incidence and mortality in a controlled trial. *J Natl Cancer Inst.* Mar 18;90(6):440–6.
16. Albanes D, Malila N, Taylor PR, Huttunen JK, Virtamo J, Edwards BK, Rautalahti M, Hartman AM, Barrett MJ, Pietinen P, Hartman TJ, Sipponen P, Lewin K, Teerenhovi L, Hietanen P, Tangrea JA, Virtanen M, Heinonen OP. 2000. Effects of supplemental alpha-tocopherol and beta-carotene on colorectal cancer: Results from a controlled trial (Finland) *Cancer Causes Control.* Mar;11(3):197–205.
17. Emmert DH, Kirchner JT. 1999. The role of vitamin E in the prevention of heart disease. *Arch Fam Med.* Nov-Dec;8(6):537–42.
18. Kushi LH, Folsom AR, Prineas RJ, Mink PJ, Wu Y, Bostick RM. 1996. Dietary antioxidant vitamins and death from coronary heart disease in postmenopausal women. *N Engl J Med*;334:1156–1162.
19. Hensley K, Benaksas EJ, Bolli R, Comp P, Grammas P, Hamdheydari L, Mou S, Pye QN, Stoddard MF, Wallis G, Williamson KS, West M, Wechter WJ, Floyd RA. 2004a. New perspectives on vitamin E: Gamma-tocopherol and carboxyelthylhydroxychroman metabolites in biology and medicine. *Free Radic Biol Med.* Jan 1;36(1):1–15.
20. Hensley K, Benaksas EJ, Bolli R, Comp P, Grammas P, Hamdheydari L, Mou S, Pye QN, Stoddard MF, Wallis G, Williamson KS, West M, Wechter WJ, Floyd RA. 2004b. New perspectives on vitamin E: γ-tocopherol and carboxyethylhydroxychroman metabolites in biology and medicine. *Free Radic Biol Med.* Jan 1;36(1):1–15.
21. Miller ER 3rd, Pastor-Barriuso R, Dalal D, Riemersma RA, Appel LJ, Guallar E. 2005. Meta-analysis: High-dosage vitamin E supplementation may increase all-cause mortality. *Ann Intern Med.* Jan 4;142(1):37–46.
22. Lonn E, Bosch J, Yusuf S, Sheridan P, Pogue J, Arnold JM, Ross C, Arnold A, Sleight P, Probstfield J, Dagenais GR. 2005. HOPE and HOPE-TOO Trial Investigators. Effects of long-term vitamin E supplementation on cardiovascular events and cancer: a randomized controlled trial. *JAMA.* Mar 16;293(11):1338–47.
23. Hathcock JN, Azzi A, Blumberg J, Bray T, Dickinson A, Frei B, Jialal I, Johnston CS, Kelly FJ, Kraemer K, Packer L, Parthasarathy S, Sies H, Traber MG. 2005. Vitamins E and C are safe across a broad range of intakes. *Am J Clin Nutr.* Apr;81(4):736–45.
24. Bjelakovic G, Nikolova D, Gluud LL, Simonetti RG, Gluud C. 2007. Mortality in randomized trials of antioxidant supplements for primary and secondary prevention: Systematic review and meta-analysis. *JAMA.* Feb 28;297(8):842–57.
25. Riccioni G, Bucciarelli T, Mancini B, Di Ilio C, Capra V, D'Orazio N. 2007. The role of the antioxidant vitamin supplementation in the prevention of cardiovascular diseases. *Expert Opin Investig Drugs.* Jan 16(1), 25–32.
26. Lee IM, Cook NR, Gaziano JM, Gordon D, Ridker PM, Manson JE, Hennekens CH, Buring JE. 2005. Vitamin E in the primary prevention of cardiovascular disease and cancer: The Women's Health Study: A randomized controlled trial. *JAMA.* Jul 6;294(1):56–65.
27. Sundl I, Resch U, Bergmann AR, Roob JM, Winklhofer-Roob BM. 2004. The decrease in γ-tocopherol in plasma and lipoprotein fractions levels off within two days of vitamin E supplementation. *Ann N Y Acad Sci.* Dec;1031:378–80.

28. Handelman GJ, Machlin LJ, Fitch K, Weiter JJ, Dratz EA. 1985. Oral alpha-tocopherol supplements decrease plasma gamma-tocopherol levels in humans. *J Nutr.* Jun;115(6):807–13.
29. Baker H, Handelman GJ, Short S, Machlin LJ, Bhagavan HN, Dratz EA, Frank O. 1986. Comparison of plasma alpha and gamma tocopherol levels following chronic oral administration of either all-rac-alpha-tocopheryl acetate or RRR-alpha-tocopheryl acetate in normal adult male subjects. *Am J Clin Nutr.* Mar;43(3):382–7.
30. Galli F, Lee R, Atkinson J, Floridi A, Kelly FJ. 2003. Gamma-tocopherol biokinetics and transformation in humans. *Free Radic Res.* Nov;37(11):1225–33.
31. Qureshi AA, Pearce BC, Nor RM, Gapor A, Peterson DM, Elson CE. 1996. Dietary alpha-tocopherol attenuates the impact of gamma-tocotrienol on hepatic 3-hydroxy-3-methylglutaryl coenzyme A reductase activity in chickens. *J Nutr.* Feb;126(2):389–94.
32. Ruiz Rejon F, Martin-Pena G, Granado F, Ruiz-Galiana J, Blanco I, Olmedilla B. 2002. Plasma status of retinol, alpha- and gamma-tocopherols, and main carotenoids to first myocardial infarction: Case control and follow-up study. *Nutrition.* Jan;18(1):26–31.
33. Nojiri S, Daida H, Mokuno H, Iwama Y, Mae K, Ushio F, Ueki T. 2001. Association of serum antioxidant capacity with coronary artery disease in middle-aged men. *Jpn Heart J.* Nov;42(6):677–90.
34. Adachi H, Ishii N. 2000. Effects of tocotrienols on life span and protein carbonylation in Caenorhabditis elegans. *J Gerontol A Biol Sci Med Sci.* Jun;55(6):B280–5.
35. Qureshi AA, Bradlow BA, Brace L, Manganello J, Peterson DM, Pearce BC, Wright JJ, Gapor A, Elson CE. 1995. Response of hypercholesterolemic subjects to administration of tocotrienols. *Lipids.* Dec;30(12):1171–7.
36. Qureshi AA, Sami SA, Salser WA, Khan FA. 2002. Dose-dependent suppression of serum cholesterol by tocotrienol-rich fraction (TRF25) of rice bran in hypercholesterolemic humans. *Atherosclerosis.* Mar;161(1):199–207.
37. Tomeo AC, Geller M, Watkins TR, Gapor A, Bierenbaum ML. 1995. Antioxidant effects of tocotrienols in patients with hyperlipidemia and carotid stenosis. *Lipids.* Dec;30(12):1179–83.
38. Qureshi AA, Sami SA, Salser WA, Khan FA. 2002. Dose-dependent suppression of serum cholesterol by tocotrienol-rich fraction (TRF25) of rice bran in hypercholesterolemic humans. *Atherosclerosis.* Mar;161(1):199–207.
39. Das S, Nesaretnam K, Das DK. 2007. Tocotrienols in cardioprotection. *Vitam Horm.*;75:285–99.
40. Khanna S, Roy S, Ryu H, Bahadduri P, Swaan PW, Ratan RR, Sen CK. 2003. Molecular basis of vitamin E action: Tocotrienol modulates 12-lipoxygenase, a key mediator of glutamate-induced neurodegeneration. *J Biol Chem.* Oct 31;278(44):43508–15.
41. Miyazawa T, Tsuzuki T, Nakagawa K, Igarashi M. 2004 Antiangiogenic potency of vitamin E. *Ann N Y Acad Sci.* Dec;1031:401–4.
42. Nesaretnam K, Ambra R, Selvaduray KR, Radhakrishnan A, Canali R, Virgili F. 2004. Tocotrienol-rich fraction from palm oil and gene expression in human breast cancer cells. *Ann N Y Acad Sci.* Dec;1031:143–57.
43. Schaffer S, Muller WE, Eckert GP. 2005. Tocotrienols: Constitutional effects in aging and disease. *J Nutr.* Feb;135(2):151–4.
44. Hattori A, Fukushima T, Imai K. 2000. Occurrence and determination of a natriuretic hormone, 2,7,8-trimethyl-2-(beta-carboxyethyl)-6-hydroxy chroman, in rat plasma, urine, and bile. *Anal Biochem.* Jun 1;281(2):209–15.
45. Newaz MA, Nawal NN. 1999. Effect of gamma-tocotrienol on blood pressure, lipid peroxidation and total antioxidant status in spontaneously hypertensive rats (SHR). *Clin Exp Hypertens.* Nov;21(8):1297–313.
46. Patel V, Khanna S, Roy S, Ezziddin O, Sen CK. 2006. Natural vitamin E alpha-tocotrienol: Retention in vital organs in response to long-term oral supplementation and withdrawal. *Free Radic Res.* Jul;40(7):763–71.
47. Levin N. 2005. Land of confusion: How poor science and misleading media coverage create public confusion about how dietary supplements affect health. *J App Nutr,* 55(1):8–15.
48. Tan B. 2005. Appropriate spectrum vitamin E and new perspectives on desmethyl tocopherols and tocotrienols. *J Am Nutraceut Assn.* 8(1):35–4.

Part B

Sources

3 Tocotrienols: Distribution and Sources Cereals—Role in Human Health

Henryk Zielinski

CONTENTS

3.1 INTRODUCTION

Vitamin E is the main lipid-soluble antioxidant in the human body. Vitamin E is not a single compound but refers to at least four tocopherols (T) and four tocotrienols (T3) (Figure 3.1). They cannot be synthesized by the human body, and therefore must be obtained from the diet.

All of them consist of a chromanol ring and a hydrophobic side chain, which is a phytyl in tocopherols and an isoprenyl with three double bonds in tocotrienols. Tocopherols and tocotrienols (referred to as tocols) are further separated into individual compounds assigned by the Greek letter prefixes (α, β, γ, δ) depending on the number and position of methyl substitution on the chromanol ring.

When the vitamin E activity in a food product is evaluated, a sum of the different structures, or vitamers, is calculated, taking into account their relative biological activities. For this reason, all eight vitamers are usually quantified together. Tocopherols and tocotrienols are well recognized for their effective inhibition of lipid oxidation in foods and biological systems and each homologue shows, to a different extent, vitamin E activity. *In vivo* study has clearly shown that vitamin E prevents lipid peroxidation in humans. Lipid peroxidation is generally viewed as a damaging process that contributes to many chronic diseases as well as to aging. When evaluating the scientific literature it is critical to know what form of vitamin E is being used in a study.

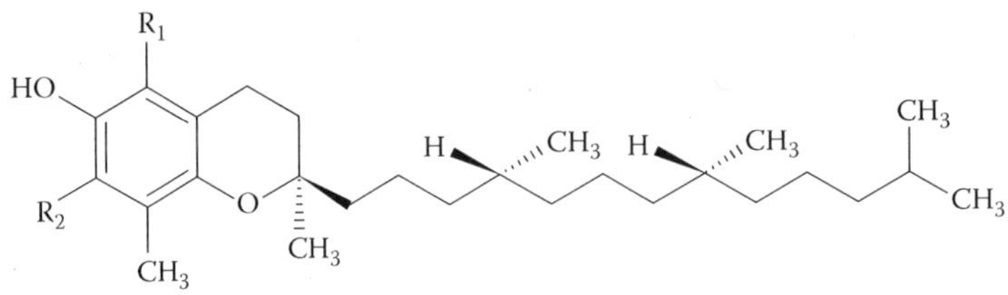

	R_1	R_2
α-analog	$-CH_3$	$-CH_3$
β-analog	$-CH_3$	–H
γ-analog	–H	$-CH_3$
δ-analog	–H	–H

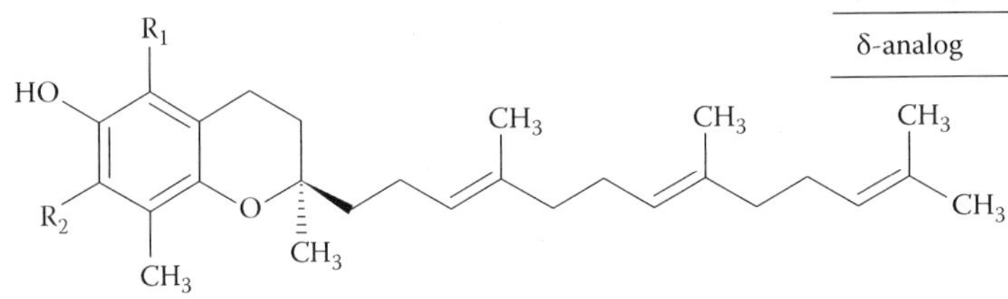

FIGURE 3.1 Detailed chemical structures of tocopherols (top) and tocotrienols (bottom). The canonical structures are shown.

Dietary vitamin E is primarily γ-T, whereas the vitamin E in supplements is predominantly α-T (natural or synthetic). Synthetic vitamin E is the most common form found in supplements and the most common form used in research. The abundance of α-T in the human body and the comparable efficiency of all vitamin E molecules as antioxidants, led biologists to neglect the non-tocopherol vitamin E molecules as topics for basic and clinical research. Recent developments warrant a serious reconsideration of this conventional wisdom (Schaffer et al., 2005). Most studies compare the activities of tocotrienols with those of tocopherols ("classical vitamin E"). However, some biological effects are unique only for tocotrienols. Although the absorption mechanisms are essentially the same for all vitamin E analogs, tocotrienols are degraded to a greater extent than tocopherols (Birringer et al., 2002). As reflected in their structural similarity, tocopherols and tocotrienols are well recognized for their antioxidative effect (Kamal-Eldin and Appelqvist, 1996).

Despite the fact that the latest North American guidelines consider α-T to be the only biologically active form of vitamin E and discount other vitamers, the biological importance of tocotrienols have gained attention (Anon, 2000). Unfortunately, up till now, only just over 1% from of the 24,000 papers on vitamin E listed in PubMed relate to tocotrienols (Sen et al., 2006).

3.2 NATURAL SOURCES OF TOCOTRIENOLS

A little is known about the distribution of tocotrienols in the plant kingdom. In nearly all green plant tissues α-T is the major vitamin E form, although the presence of low levels of tocotrienols has been reported in needles of *Picea* sp. (spruce) (Franzen et al., 1991). In non-green plant parts, especially seeds and fruits, γ-T is preferentially found instead of α-T.

Limited available data suggest a somewhat unusual and restricted distribution of tocotrienols. They are found in the seeds of monocotyledonous and dicotyledonous plants, including *Gevuina avellana* Mol. (Chilean hazelnut), *Bixa orellana* L. (Annato), *Carum carvi* L. (caraway), *Orobanche sp.* L., some Vietnamese plants, *Calophyllum sp.* L., *Juglans regia* L. and *Vitis vinifera* L. (Horvath et al., 2006). Previously, the bioconversion of tocotrienols to tocopherols in plants via methylation and reducing reactions has been suggested, based on the notion that tocotrienols may be intermediates in the biosynthesis of α-tocopherol (Pennock, 1983). The research showed that δ-T3 is a precursor of β-T3 but not of the other tocotrienols. Among tocopherols, γ-T is a precursor of α-T (Dörmann, 2003).

Recently, genes were identified that encode the key enzymes of the tocochromanol biosynthesis pathway. These include homogentisate phytyl transferases (Collakova and DellaPenna, 2001; Venkatesh et al., 2006), cyclase (Porfirova et al., 2002), and methyl transferases (Shintani et al., 2002; Cheng et al., 2003). Homogentisate geranyl transferaze (HGGT) has been identified as a key enzyme pathway of tocotrienol biosynthesis. The gene encoding HGGT was found in three monocotyledonous plants (*Oryza* sp., *Hordeum* sp. and *Triticum* sp.).

Tocotrienols are found in abundance in plant foods such as rice bran or palm oil. Edible oils originating from plants are rich sources of tocotrienols. Crude palm oil extracted from the fruits of oil palm (*Elaeis guineensis*) particularly contains a high amount of tocotrienols (up to 800 mg kg^{-1}), mainly consisting of γ-T3 and α-T3. It also contains the most potent form of all commercially available tocotrienol: δ-T3 (Theriault et al., 1999).

Such cereal grains as oat, barley, rye, wheat, corn and rice are the major sources of tocopherols and tocotrienols in human nutrition. They have a potentially beneficial distribution of the vitamers within the kernels characterized by the higher content of tocotrienols than tocopherols. Therefore, cereal-based products contribute significantly to the dietary intake of tocotrienols (Andlauer & Furst, 1999; Slavin, 2000; Qureshi et al., 2000; Goffman and Bohme, 2001; Panfili et al., 2003a).

1.3 ANALYSIS OF TOCOTRIENOLS AND TOCOPHEROLS IN CEREALS

The structural complexity and the wide variation in biological activity of the different vitamin E vitamers necessitate reliable analytical techniques for the isolation, separation, differentiation and quantification of individual components in mixtures derived from various cereal matrices. High-performance liquid chromatography (HPLC) provides a convenient method for quantification and characterization purposes of vitamin E. Several HPLC methods are available, and attempts to independently analyze tocopherols and tocotrienols have been performed on both normal and reversed phase columns (Abidi, 2000). Although reversed phase columns are generally known to have the advantages of better stability and longer durability than normal phase columns, the latter are more efficient in separating beta and gamma isomers of tocopherols and tocotrienols. Moreover, they provide the possibility of operating with organic solvents, allowing a high solubility of lipids.

Considering the qualitative and quantitative variability of tocopherols and tocotrienols in cereal grains, the use of normal phase columns is required for the analysis of all vitamin E homoloques. A fluorescence detector is preferred over an ultraviolet one in tocopherol and tocotrienol analyses because of its specificity and sensitivity (Abidi, 2000). As lipophilic substances, tocols are intimately associated with lipid components of the sample matrix. Therefore, the various sample preparation procedures serve to liberate tocols from the sample matrix and extract them into a solvent that is compatible with the chromatographic system.

The sample preparation methods for tocotrienols and tocopherols analysis fall into two categories: nonsaponification (solvent extraction) and saponification methods (alkaline hydrolysis). In cereals, tocopherols and tocotrienols are extracted by either a direct solvent method or by saponification followed by extraction. Extraction with organic solvents disrupts the structures to which the vitamers are attached and solubilizes them. *n*-Hexane is the commonly used solvent, but more polar solvent mixtures are also used, e.g., ethyl acetate in *n*-hexane or acetone (Ueda and Igarashi, 1987; Eitenmiller and Landen, 1999; Ruperez et al., 2001). Saponification, involving the heating of the sample in a strong alkaline environment, reduces the amount of organic extractables in a sample. This is accomplished by hydrolysis of lipid esters to more hydrophilic fatty acids and alcohols, which, in a solvent system extraction, will remain in the aqueous phase. This decreases the load of material that will be extracted with tocols into the organic phase and injected into the analytical column. Tocopherols and tocotrienols are relatively unstable in alkaline conditions, and care must be taken to avoid their destruc-

TABLE 3.1
Recommended Analytical Procedure for the Determination of Tocopherols and Tocotrienols

Procedure step	Description
Preparing the sample for saponification	0.5 g sample, 0.1 g ascorbic acid, 5 mL ethanol, 2 mL water flushing with nitrogen
Saponification	0.5 mL KOH solution, 100°C, 25 min.
Extraction and purification of non-saponificable lipids	2.5 mL ethanol, 2.5 mL water 3 × 10 mL n-hexane:ethyl acetate (8:2) washing the extract 3 times with water and evaporating to dryness
Preparing the samples for HPLC analysis	2 mL ethanol and 2 mL n-hexane Evaporating to dryness Dissolving the resideue in 5 mL n-hexane
Normal phase HPLC analysis with fluorescence detector	Inertsil silica column 5 μm, 250 × 4.6 mm with silica guard column, temperature of the column oven 30°C, isocratic elution, mobile phase containing 3% of 1, 4-dioxane and 97% of n-hexane, flow rate 2 mL/min, detection at excitation λ = 292 nm and emission λ = 325 nm.

tion. They are protected by addition of antioxidants to the sample, flushing the saponification vessel with nitrogen and working under subdued light (Eitenmiller and Landen, 1999). Panfili et al. (2003a) determined tocotrienols and tocopherols in cereals using the normal phase HPLC. Hot saponification followed by solvent extraction provided significantly higher tocols recovery. When compared with the saponification method, solvent extraction without saponification provided tocol recoveries varying from 68% for β-T to 100% for γ-T3 and δ-T. In methanol extraction, these recoveries ranged from 57% for α-T3 and γ-T3 to 93% for α-T. These findings, in accord with those of previous works (Wang et al., 1998; Fratianni et al., 2002), show that, to quantify total tocols from cereals, a saponification procedure, which transforms the tocol esters into their corresponding alcohols, is needed. Recently, a recommended analytical procedure for extraction and determination of tocotrienols and tocopherols was established by Ryynänen et al. (2004) (Table 3.1).

The use of supercritical fluid extraction has also been proposed as an alternative method for the determination of vitamers of vitamin E from cereal and cereal-based products (Fratianni et al., 2002; Panfili et al., 2003b). Others means of separation include gas chromatography and most recently, capillary electrochromatography (Abidi et al., 2002). Electrochemical detection is also applied as a sensitive detector for tocotrienols and tocopherols after HPLC separation (Yamauchi et al., 2002), while mass spectroscopy (MS) in combination with HPLC assists in identification of tocols (Strohschein et al., 1999).

In summary, the lack of a standardized method for the extraction and analysis of tocols has led to a wide variation in quantities and qualities of the various tocols reported. In particular, apart from reversed phase chromatographic analysis, which is not able to resolve beta and gamma isomers of tocopherols and tocotrienols, also some normal phase methods are not able to separate the couple γ-T/β-T3, and this could lead to a misinterpretation in the identification of the different isomers (Abidi, 2000).

3.4 TOCOTRIENOLS: DISTRIBUTION AND SOURCE CEREALS

The principal cereal crops grown in the world are wheat, barley, oats, rye, rice and corn. In a generalized model for all cereal grains, the kernel comprises an embryo. Around the embryo is the endosperm, most of which is referred to as the starchy endosperm. The starchy endosperm is surrounded by the aleurone layer, which mainly comprises protein and lipids. Enclosing the endosperm

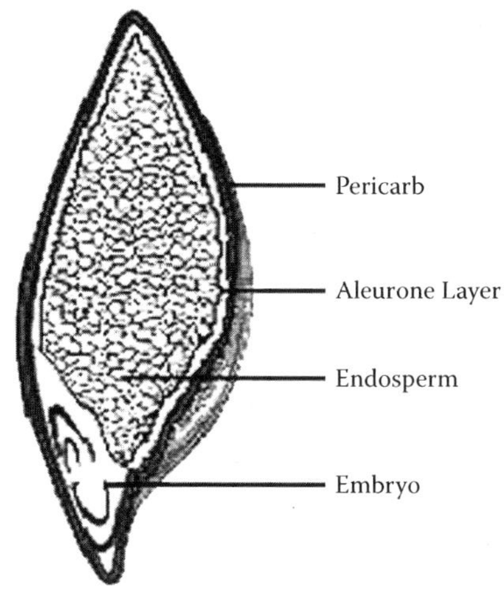

FIGURE 3.2 A generalized model of the kernel for all cereal grains.

and embryo is the protective seed coat, referred to as pericarb (Figure 3.2). In the case of barley, oat and rice grains, the kernels are surrounded by protective hulls. The hull-less barley genotypes and naked oats do not contain this fraction. The removal of the rice hull results in brown rice.

The function of tocotrienols and tocopherols in cereal is certainly related to the distribution of these compounds in the kernel. In corn, barley, oat, rye and wheat, tocopherols are mainly present in the germ fraction, whereas the tocotrienols are present in the pericarb and endosperm fraction (Peterson and Qureshi, 1993; Zielinski et al., 2001a). Due to the lipophilic properties of tocols, it is likely that tocotrienols are part of the lipid fraction of starch granules (Kaukovirta-Norja et al., 1997).

Cereal grains are the second most important source of tocotrienols and tocopherols in our diet, following the group of vegetable oils with exception of palm and coconut oils. In contrast to the majority of vegetable oils, cereals are a unique source because they contain more tocotrienols than tocopherols. The percentage contribution of tocotrienols and tocopherols to the tocols content in the whole grain of the main cereals is illustrated in Figure 3.3.

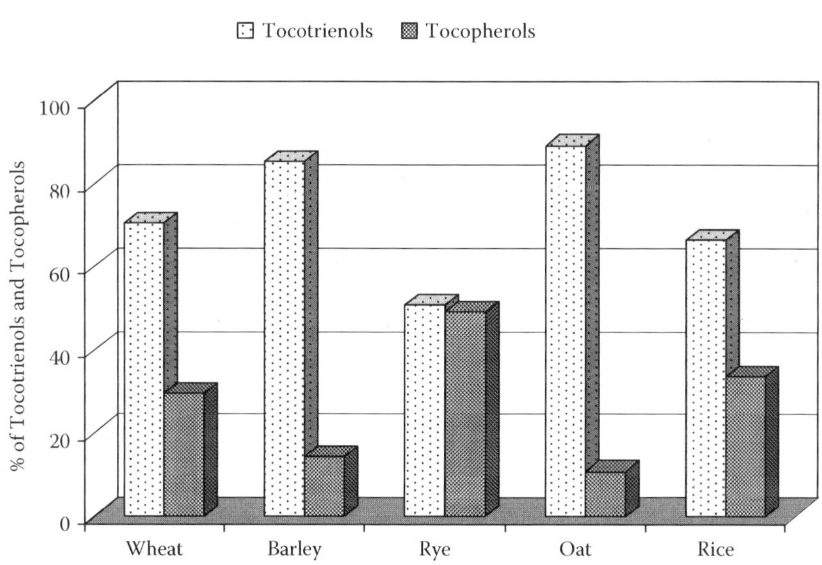

FIGURE 3.3 Contribution of tocopherols and tocotrienols to the tocol content in the whole grain of the main cereals (adapted from Chen and Bergman, 2005 and Zielinski et al., 2001a).

The content of total tocols, percentage contribution of tocopherols (T) and tocotrienols (T3), and percentage contribution of α- β-, γ- and δ-tocotrienol to total tocotrienols content in the main cereals grains is shown in Table 3.2.

3.4.1 Distribution and Fraction of Tocotrienols in Barley Grain

Historically, barley and oats were important human foodstuffs in addition to their role as animal feed, and, in the case of barley, as a raw material for brewing. By 1900, human consumption of barley and oats was restricted to the agricultural laboring classes of continental Europe and some Asian countries where wheat production was impossible.

Barley (*Hordeum vulgare* L.) is one of the best sources of tocotrienols and tocopherols. The total tocols concentration reportedly ranges from 30.5 to 80.6 mg kg^{-1} (Työppönen and Hakkaranen, 1985). The whole, cleaned barley sample had the composition of tocols similar to that reported for 30 genotypes from USDA Western Regional Spring Barley Nursery (Peterson and Qureshi, 1993). Alpha-tocotrienol was the predominant isomer (20.40 mg kg^{-1}), with substantial quantities of α-tocopherol (5.94 mg kg^{-1}), β-tocotrienol (5.02 mg kg^{-1}), γ-tocotrienol (4.36 mg kg^{-1}) and δ-tocotrienol (0.79 mg kg^{-1}) (Peterson, 1994). The total tocotrienols content in barley measured 83% of tocols concentration. Similar results were reported by Holasova et al., (1995) for 13 European barley genotypes, in which tocotrienol fraction was about 75% of all tocols. The barley fractions, namely hull, endosperm and germ, contained different level of tocotrienols. The richest fraction was endosperm (95% of tocols), then hull (63% of tocols) and germ (about 10% of tocols (Table 3.3).

The milling process of barley into flour with different extraction rates causes a decrease in tocotrienol concentration, depending on the type of flour obtained, with the lowest concentration in white flour. For this reason, it can be proposed to increase tocols amount in barley flour by mechanical means (milling, sieving, air-classifying) with the aim of employing it as an ingredient in food (Wang et al., 1993) or extracting the pure compound using techniques such as supercritical carbon dioxide extraction for high-grade specialty products for cosmetic and health use (Colombo et al., 1998). The development of high tocol barley cultivars would favor the application of such techniques by food industries, but the lack of knowledge of genotype potential, in terms of tocol productivity, has limited the possible application of this cereal as a primary tocol source. This is particularly true for hull-less barley, which has been largely investigated for its soluble-fiber [(1→3, 1→4)-β-D-glucan)] content and which seems to be the most promising type of barley for the food industry (Bhatty, 1999; Cavallero et al., 2002).

The pearling flour fraction (20% of the kernel weight) contained the highest concentrations of α-tocotrienol (61% of total tocols), indicating this barley byproduct as the richest source of tocotrienols. The barley byproducts consist of the abraded material, containing hull, aleurone, and subaleurone tissues (bran). The high content of all tocols found in this fraction reflect their concentration in the outer layer of the kernel. Each of the tocotrienols was at least twice as concentrated in the byproduct as in whole barley; they formed about 75% of total tocols (Peterson, 1994). The oil and total vitamin E levels in barley are lower than those in most other grains, but the concentration of tocotrienols in barley grain is higher, with a favorable distribution of the most biologically active homologues. Other technological processes such as malting and germination of barley have no influence on tocotrienol concentration when compared with barley grain. In contrast, the spent barley grain contained at least threefold higher levels of tocotrienol than did the barley or malt (Peterson, 1994).

In summary, barley byproduct and brewers' spent grains are rich sources of tocotrienols (above 91% and 83% of tocols). This attribute could make them valuable additions to food products, particularly for persons attempting to reduce serum cholesterol levels through diet modification.

TABLE 3.2

Content of Total Tocols, Percentage Tocopherols and Tocotrienols and Percentage of α- β-, γ- and δ-Tocotrienol in Total Tocotrienols Content in the Main Cereal Grains

Family	Common name	Total tocols (mg kg^{-1})	% of T	% of T3	Percentage of total tocotrienols (%) α-T3	β-T3	γ-T3	δ-T3	References
Poaceae (Hordeum vulgare L.)	Barley	58.5	20.4	79.6	71.3	15.3	11.5	1.9	Peterson and Qureshi, 1993
		70.9	26.6	73.4	83.4	–	14.8	1.9	Wang et al., 1993
		40.5	16.5	83.5	73.6	14.4	10.6	1.4	Peterson, 1994
		67.5	25.1	74.9	74.3	11.3	14.4	–	Holasova et al., 1995
		27.0	14.2	85.8	73.8	5.7	20.5	–	Zieliński et al., 2001a
		76.1	20.8	79.2	66.8	14.4	17.3	1.5	Panfili et al., 2003a
		54.4	22.0	78.0	72.5	9.4	16.3	1.8	Cavallero et al., 2004
		19.2	29.7	70.3	79.2	17.8	–	3.0	Choi et al., 2007
Poaceae (Avena sativa L.)	Oat	25.9	38.4	61.6	93.2	5.4	1.3	–	Peterson and Qureshi, 1993
		29.2	34.0	65.9	90.1	9.9	–	–	Holasova et al., 1995
		15.1	10.8	89.2	19.9	80.1	–	–	Zieliński et al., 2001a
		80.1	22.8	77.2	91.3	8.7	–	–	Panfili et al., 2003a
		15.8	54.4	45.6	58.3	–	29.2	12.5	Horvath et al., 2006
Poaceae (Triticum sp.)	Wheat	46.9	35.0	65.0	13.4	86.6	–	–	Holasova et al., 1995
		27.4	17.3	82.7	4.6	95.4	–	–	Zieliński et al., 2001a
		45.0	45.3	54.7	20.3	79.7	–	–	Horvath et al., 2006
Poaceae (Secale cereale)	Rye	37.6	36.3	63.7	63.2	36.1			Holasova et al., 1995
		27.9	49.3	50.7	42.0	58.0			Zieliński et al., 2001a
Poaceae (Zea mays L.)	Corn	66.9	74.6	25.4	31.2	–	66.5	2.3	Panfili et al., 2003a
Poaceae (Oryza sativa L.)	Rice	269.3	28.4	72.4	53.9	–	46.1	–	Bergman and Xu, 2003
		302.01	33.5	66.5	25.9	–	71.4	2.7	Chen et al., 2005
	White rice	7.4	10.8	89.2	12.1	–	87.9	–	Choi et al., 2007
	Brown rice	26.4	20.5	79.5	26.7	–	73.3	–	Choi et al., 2007
	Black rice	93.7	57.1	42.9	34.3	–	65.7	–	Choi et al., 2007
Poaceae (Amaranthus ssp.)	Amaranths	17.6	29.1	70.9	1.0	73.7	24.4	0.9	Lehmann et al., 1994
Poaceae (Amaranthus ssp.)	Sorghum	17.9	83.3	16.7	70.0	-	26.7	3.3	Choi et al., 2007

TABLE 3.3
Total Tocols, Percentage of Tocopherols and Tocotrienols, and Percentage of α-, β-, γ- and δ-Tocotrienol in Total Tocotrienols Content in Barley

Fraction	Total tocols (mg kg^{-1} d.m.)	Contribution of tocopherols (%)	Contribution of tocotrienols (%)	Percentage of total tocotrienols			
				α-T3	β-T3	γ-T3	δ-T3
Hull	28.9	37.0	63.0	75.0	12.9	11.5	0.5
Germ	206.5	90.3	9.7	0	100	0	0
Endosperm	33.3	3.6	96.4	73.0	14.0	11.6	1.4

Source: After Peterson, 1994.

3.4.2 Distribution and Fraction of Tocotrienols in Oat Grain

Oat-based foods have long been recognized for their health benefits, and it is now generally accepted knowledge that oats make a significant contribution to human health. There are several species of oats, but only two of them are of significant commercial importance. Seventy-five percent of world oat production is of the *avena sativa* species, while most of the remaining production is of the *avena byzantina* species. The *avena nuda* species may gain importance in the future because of its hull-less characteristics. The oat seeds are covered with a thick hull (except *avena nuda*, which is enclosed in a papery sheath). Traditionally, only the whole oat groat was used for human food, but recently grain fraction, such as the bran and even the hull, have entered the human food supply.

Total tocol concentration in oat ranges from about 20 to 30 mg kg^{-1}, with α-tocotrienol as the predominant homoloque (Peterson and Quershi, 1993; Lasztity, 1998). Similar contents were reported by Holasova et al. (1995) for seven European oat genotypes, in which the tocotrienol fraction made up about 66% of all tocols. The oat endosperm was the location for almost all tocotrienols, mainly for α-T3 and β-T3, whereas the germ was poor in tocotrienols, but almost all tocopherols were located in this fraction, mainly α-T and γ-T. The oat hulls were almost devoid of tocopherols, whereas a small quantity of tocotrienols were present (Peterson, 1995) (Table 3.4).

This was in contrast with barley, where hulls had considerable quantities of all eight homologues (18.2 mg kg^{-1}). The differential distribution of tocotrienols and tocopherols between germ and endosperm was confirmed by other authors (Zielinski et al., 2001a).

3.4.3 Distribution and Fractions of Tocotrienols in Wheat

Wheat varieties differ with respect to optimal growing conditions, color of the kernel, hardness and composition. The varieties planted in the late summer or fall intended to mature the following summer are called winter wheats. These include red and white as well as hard and soft varieties. Wheat varieties planted in spring for harvesting in late summer are known as spring varieties and these include durum as well as hard red and hard and soft wheat varieties.

Total tocol concentration in wheat genotypes ranges from about 35 to 46 mg kg^{-1}, whereas tocotrienol fraction contributes about 65–71% of all tocols. Beta-tocotrienol is the predominant homoloque (56–67% of all tocols) whereas α-tocotrienol contributes about 3–10% of total tocols (Holasova et al., 1995; Holasova 1997; Zielinski et al., 2001a). In wheat kernel fractions, α-tocotrienol was mostly in bran, whereas β-tocotrienol was equally distributed between the bran and the endosperm (Morrison et al., 1982).

Wheat bran, composed mainly of the outer layers of the seed coat, pericarb and aleurone layer, and containing very little starchy endosperm, is prepared by roller milling. In this process, bran and germ are removed, yielding starchy endosperm. Wheat bran contains about twofold higher level of tocols than noted in wheat kernel, and tocotrienols form more than 70% of total tocols. The ratio

TABLE 3.4
Total Tocols Content, Percentage Contribution of Tocopherols and Tocotrienols and Percentage of α-, β-, γ- and δ-Tocotrienol in Tocotrienols Content in Oat Fractions

Fraction	Total tocols ($mg\ kg^{-1}$ d.m.)	Contribution of tocopherols (%)	Contribution of tocotrienols (%)	Percentage of total tocotrienols			
				α-T3	β-T3	γ-T3	δ-T3
Hull	2.7	31.5	68.5	74.9	0	17.5	7.6
Germ	131.2	97.6	2.4	0	45.8	48.4	5.8
Endosperm	41.9	10.0	90.0	92.4	6.3	0.7	0.6

Source: After Peterson, 1995.

of tocotrienols to tocopherols content (T3/T) is therefore the highest in bran fraction (2.85) and the lowest in germ fraction (0.06) whereas in the kernel it ranged from 1.8–2.4 (Holasova 1997; Zielinski et al., 2001a).

The sequence of milling, sifting and aspiration processes produces a number of flours with defined ash content. With lowering ash content between whole meal flour and white flours the tocotrienols content is decreased. White wheat flour type 450 is the poorest source of tocols (17.4 mg kg^{-1}) as well as tocotrienols (12.4 mg kg^{-1}) (Holasova, 1997).

3.4.4 Distribution and Fraction of Tocotrienols in Rye

Total tocol concentration in rye genotypes ranges from about 17 to 39 mg kg^{-1}, whereas tocotrienol fraction contributes about 52–71% of all tocols. Alpha- and β-tocotrienol are the predominant homoloques and contribute about 21–40% and 19–20% of total tocols, respectively (Table 3.5) (Holasova et al., 1995; Holasova 1997; Zielinski et al., 2001a; Zielinski et al., 2007).

In rye kernel fractions α-tocotrienol was mostly in the bran, whereas β-tocotrienol was equally distributed between the bran and the endosperm (Holasova, 1997). Rye bran contains about threefold higher level of tocols than are noted in rye kernel, and tocotrienols form about 86% of total tocols. The ratio of tocotrienols to tocopherols content (T3/T) is therefore the highest in the bran fraction and lowest in the germ fraction (Holasova, 1997; Zielinski et al., 2001a; Zielinski et al., 2007).

In the process of rye grain milling, the bran and germ are removed, yielding starchy endosperm. The proportion of the original rye that is ultimately converted to flour is referred to as the extraction rate. The extraction rate has an impact on the quality of different types of flour obtained. Whole meal rye flour (extraction rate of 100%) is the most popular for bread baking, however, rye flour

TABLE 3.5
Total Tocols Content, Percentage of Tocopherols and Tocotrienols and Percentage of α-, β-, γ- and δ-Tocotrienol to Total Tocotrienols Content in Three Rye Varieties

Fraction	Total tocols ($mg\ kg^{-1}$ d.m.)	Contribution of tocopherols (%)	Contribution of tocotrienols (%)	Percentage of total tocotrienols			
				α-T3	β-T3	γ-T3	δ-T3
Whole grain	20.8	44.6	55.4	57.1	42.9	-	-
Endosperm with embryo	18.8	41.2	58.8	54.3	45.7	-	-
Pericarb	25.8	10.6	89.4	62.7	37.3	-	-

Source: After Zielinski et al., 2007.

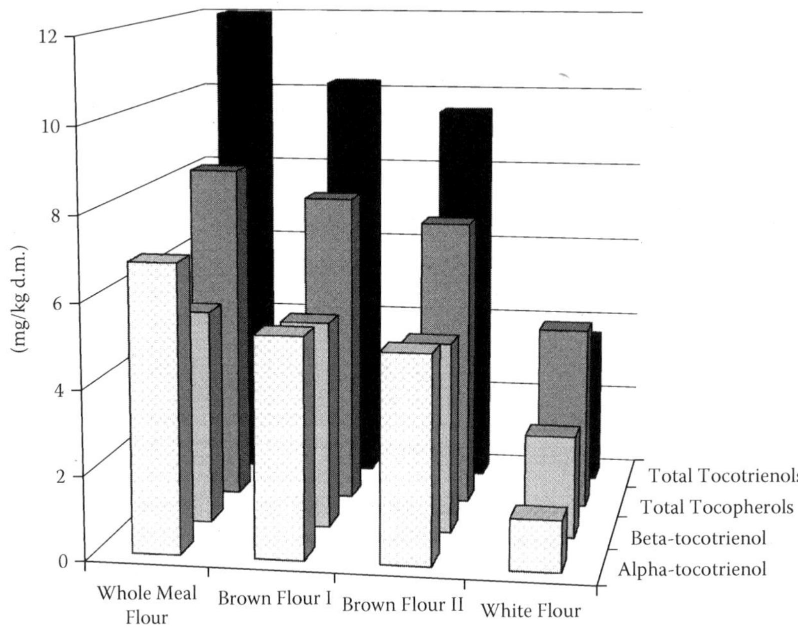

FIGURE 3.4 Content of total tocotrienols, total tocopherols and α-T3 and β-T3 in different types of rye flours. Whole meal, brown flour I, brown flour II and white flour mean rye flours with extraction rate of 100, 95, 90 and 70%, respectively. Elaborated from Michalska et al., 2007a.

with an extraction rate of about 80% is widely used as well. The milling process causes a decrease of both tocotrienols and tocotrienols, as shown on Figure 3.4.

The ratio of tocotrienols to tocopherols (T3/T) was the highest in rye flours, with an extraction rate of 90–100%, whereas light flour was the poorest source of tocopherols and tocotrienols. The provided data support the current trend to increase the number of rye products from wholemeal or brown flours.

3.4.5 Distribution and Fraction of Tocotrienols in Corn

Corn is primarily used as an animal feed crop, but it is also used in human nutrition, especially in developing countries. A number of food ingredients are obtained from corn. Among them are corn grits, corn meal and corn flour. The latest is an ingredient of ready-to-eat breakfast cereals as well as a component in numerous dry mixes such as those for pancakes, muffins or doughnuts. The total tocopherols content of 30 mg kg^{-1} was found in 44 varieties of sweet and dent (field) corn lines with a range of 7–86 mg kg^{-1}. The α-, γ-, and δ-tocopherols were identified in all varieties and averaged 8, 20, and 1 mg kg^{-1}, respectively (Kurilich and Juvik, 1999). Grams et al. (1970) reported that tocols are mainly distributed in the germ (up to 90%) with the pericarb and endosperm accounting for about 5% each. Nearly all (96%) of the α- and γ-tocopherols were found in the germ, while tocotrienols were predominantly found in the endosperm. Higher content of tocopherols and tocotrienols can be found in corn oils, which have around 880 mg kg^{-1} tocopherols. Gamma-tocopherol accounted for 57% of the tocols, followed by α-tocopherol (28%), γ-tocotrienol (6%), α-tocotrienol (5%), δ-tocotrienol (3%) and β-tocotrienol (1%). The total tocotrienols contribution of 15% to tocols content indicate that both corn and corn oil are rather poor sources of tocotrienols.

3.4.6 Distribution and Fraction of Tocotrienols in Rice

Rice, an important staple food for over half of the world's population, is grown and harvested in more than 100 countries. Total tocol concentration in seven rice cultivars grown in four states of the southern U.S has ranged from 241 to 309 mg kg^{-1}. The content of tocotrienols has been shown to be almost three times higher than tocopherols. Alpha-tocotrienols and γ-T3 are the predominant homologues and contribute about 39% and 33% of total tocols, respectively (Bergman and Xu, 2003). Averaged across all samples, the content of α-T3 > γ-T3 > α-T > γ-T. The milling of rice includes the removal of the hull to produce brown rice, and following this, the removal of bran by polishing of kernels leaving white rice, composed mainly of starchy endosperm. This process removes significant amounts of tocols and simultaneously produces rice bran, the fraction rich in tocotrienols.

Brown rice was reported to contain different levels of tocols as well as tocotrienols. Choi et al. (2007) reported about 26 mg kg^{-1} of tocols (wet weight basis), in which both α-T3 and γ-T3 formed approximately 80%. Aquilar-Garcia et al. (2007) noted a twofold higher level of tocols, also with 80% contribution of tocotrienols. In contrast, white rice (7.4 mg kg^{-1} of tocols) was reported as a poor source of tocotrienols (89% contribution of tocotrienols) (Choi et al., 2007). This indicates that rice bran milling byproducts are a really rich source of tocotrienols. The bran is composed of pericarb, seed coat, nucellus, aleurone layers and germ. Tocols content in rice bran originated from the U.S. long grain rice variety; a conventional U.S. medium grain variety ranged from 285 to 290 mg kg^{-1} and tocotrienols formed about 63–67% of tocols. Tocotrienols contained mainly β-T3 and γ-T3 (70–73 % of total T3) followed by α-T3 (24–27% of total T3), and small quantity of δ-T3 (about 5% of T3) (Chen and Bergman, 2005). Milling duration and thickness of the kernel have an impact on tocotrienol levels in rice bran. Longer milling duration generally resulted in lower levels of tocotrienols, tocopherols and oryzanols, because bran collected by longer milling durations contains more endosperm and less of the tocol-rich aleurone layer and the germ. The thicker kernel tends to contain higher levels of tocotrienols than thinner kernels (Rohrer and Siebenmorgen, 2004). The rice bran from the short milling duration (10 s) of two long-grain rice cultivars contained 242 mg kg^{-1} of tocols with tocotrienols and tocopherol contribution of 73.5 and 26.5%, respectively (Rohrer and Siebenmorgen, 2004). The rice bran oil contains very high levels of tocols (about 608 mg kg^{-1}), in which 56% is tocopherols and 44% is tocotrienols (Weicheng et al., 1996).

3.5 GENOTYPE AND ENVIRONMENT EFFECTS ON TOCOTRIENOLS

The tocotrienols content in cereal grains might be influenced by genetics, location and weather conditions during growing and harvesting seasons, the state of maturity and handling after harvest (Piironen et al., 1986). Peterson and Qureshi (1993) studied the grains of 12 oat and 30 barley genotypes originating from three locations for tocotrienols and tocopherols content. The researchers found that significant genotype differences existed for most tocols in both species. Location differences were significant for oats but not for barley. Only a small percentage of the variance was associated with the interaction of genotype and location. Alpha-tocotrienol and α-T were the predominant tocol isomers in both species, β-T3 and γ-T3 were also present in significant amounts in barley (Table 3.1). Cavallero et al. (2004) investigated the presence of tocol homologues in hulled and hull-less barley as influenced also by genotype and location. Both factors significantly influenced the amount of tocols in barley kernel, with genotype having the greater effect for most homologues; however, no genotype versus location interaction was observed for total tocotrienols or total tocopherols. Bergman and Xu (2003) quantified the effects of genetics versus environment on the tocotrienols and tocopherols of seven rice cultivars grown in four states in the southern U.S. during a 2-year period. They found that total E vitamers content ranged from 179 to 389 mg kg^{-1}, and tocotrienols were 72.5% of the total E vitamers content. The growing environment had a greater effect on tocotrienols and tocopherols levels than did genotype.

3.6 EFFECT OF PROCESSING ON TOCOTRIENOLS CONTENT IN CEREAL-BASED PRODUCTS

Nutritional factors are widely considered to be critical for human health, however, the health-promoting capacity of cereal-based products strictly depends on their processing history. Processing is

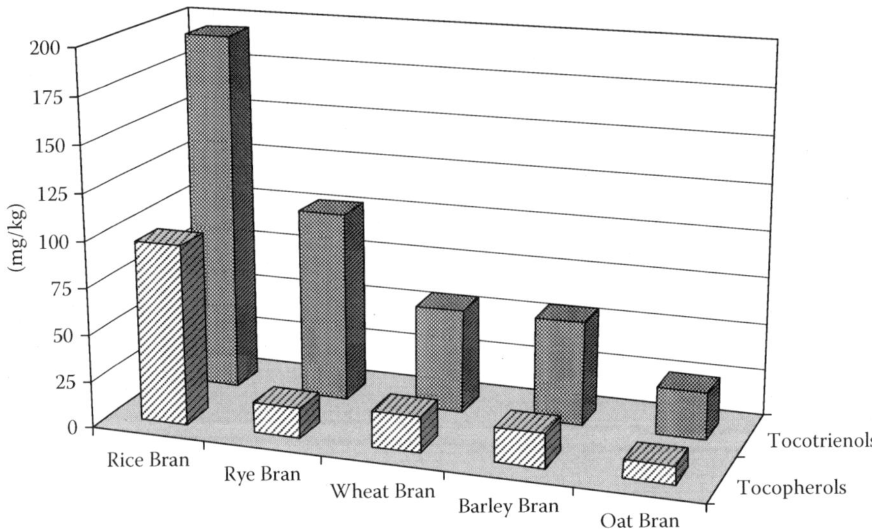

FIGURE 3.5 Content of total tocotrienols and tocopherols in bran obtained from rice (adapted from Chen and Bergman, 2005), rye, wheat (adapted from Holasova, 1997), barley (adapted from Peterson, 1994) and oats (adapted from Peterson, 1995).

expected to affect content and bioavailability of tocols. Milling and baking are the most common techniques used in grain processing for human food.

3.6.1 Effect of Milling and Storage on Tocotrienols Level in Cereal Brans

In the process of milling, bran and germ are removed, yielding starchy endosperm. The sequence of milling, sifting and aspiration processes used result in final flours of varying composition with defined ash content. The principal nutritional benefit of processing is to increase the bioavailability of the nutrients present in the grain. Essentially, this is brought about by making the cereal grain a better substrate for digestive enzymes. This is achieved at either a physical or chemical level. In the milling process, the grains may be fractionated into different types of flour. With decreasing extraction rates in milling, more and more of the outer grain layers are removed. Because tocotrienols are mainly present in the pericarb and endosperm fraction, the bran fractions can be considered a rich source of tocotrienols. According to the available literature, the content of tocotrienols and tocopherols in bran obtained from the main cereals is shown on Figure 3.5.

The storage of rice bran affect the tocotrienols levels. The order of losses of E vitamers in raw rice bran after 35 days was α-T (57.5%) > α-T3 (56.8%) > γ-T3 (39.6%) > γ-T (34.9%) > δ-T3 (34.0%) > β-T (33.4%) > δ-T (32.9%). This established that α-T and α-T3 were less stable than the other E vitamers during storage. After 1 year storage, 73% of the total vitamin E content of rice bran was lost as follows: γ-T3 (77.9%) > α-T (74.7%) > α-T3 (72.4%) > δ-T3 (69.0%) > γ-T (60.1%) > β-T (58.6%) > δ-T (57.0%). These losses were higher than in other cereal grains and brans during storage (Shin et al., 1997).

3.6.2 Effect of Thermal Treatment: Extrusion and Baking

Cereal-based foods intended for human consumption must undergo some form of thermal processing. It can be simply boiling the grain or its meal in water or it may cover complex systems involving breadmaking procedures followed by mechanical processing and subsequent traditional baking or extrusion cooking. In general, during conventional baking of flour products (generally, temperatures close to 200°C or higher for several minutes), more intense processing conditions are applied than with the extrusion process.

TABLE 3.6
Mean Content of Total Tocols, Percentage Contribution of Tocopherols and Tocotrienols and Percentage Contribution of α-, β-, γ- and δ-Tocotrienol to Total Tocotrienols in Raw and Extruded Whole Grains

Material	Total tocols ($mg\ kg^{-1}$ d.m.)	Contribution of tocopherols (%)	Contribution of tocotrienols (%)	Percentage of total tocotrienols			
				α-T3	β-T3	γ-T3	δ-T3
Wheat	27.8	30.4	69.7	14.6	85.4	–	–
After extrusion 120°C	8.6	20.7	79.4	3.4	96.6	–	–
160°C	6.2	15.9	84.1	0.4	99.6	–	–
200°C	9.3	22.7	77.3	7.2	92.8	–	–
Barley	18.7	16.8	83.2	68.1	14.6	17.3	–
After extrusion 120°C	3.5	6.5	93.5	52.9	23.3	23.8	–
160°C	3.8	9.2	90.8	47.3	26.5	26.2	–
200°C	3.1	8.7	91.3	39.2	30.4	30.4	–
Rye	27.7	47.3	52.7	59.4	40.6	–	–
After extrusion 120°C	6.1	25.3	74.7	45.2	54.8	–	–
160°C	8.9	39.8	60.2	50.7	49.3	–	–
200°C	8.7	31.3	68.7	55.6	44.4	–	–
Oat	11.5	22.4	77.6	15.4	84.6	–	–
After extrusion 120°C	7.3	21.6	78.4	27.3	73.0	–	–
200°C	1.0	39.4	60.6	1.7	98.3	–	–

Source: After Zielinski et al., 2001b.

Extrusion cooking is a relatively recent form of food processing. Most extruders act as heat exchangers, and also shape and form food products. Mixing, dehydration, pasteurization and sterilization are other unit operations that typically occur during extrusion. Extrusion can produce safe, lightweight, shelf-stable foods that can be stored for use during famines and natural disasters. Little is known about tocotrienol retention during extrusion of cereal grain because most work carried out was related to retention of tocopherols. We noted a significant decrease in tocopherols and tocotrienols after extrusion cooking of whole meal flour of wheat, rye, dehulled oat and dehulled barley (Zielinski et al., 2001b). Extrusion caused approximately three times as large a decrease in wheat, rye and oat tocotrienols, and even higher in dehulled barley (five times). Simultaneously, tocopherols were also decreased in a wider range, from three times (wheat and oat) up to barley (10 times). The least resistant for extrusion cooking were α-T and α-T3. The remaining tocols were more stable; however, the degree of their degradation was up to 50% (Table 3.6).

One positive fact found was that the ratio of tocotrienols to tocopherols was increased after extrusion cooking, indicating that tocotrienols remain the main retained isomers of vitamin E. This shows that tocotrienols are more resistant to hydrothermal conditions than are tocopherols.

Michalska et al. (2007b) studied the effect of baking on the tocols content in rye bread manufactured from rye flours with different extraction rates (Table 3.7).

The tocotrienols content noted in rye bread ranged from 3.38 $mg\ kg^{-1}$ d.m. to 0.38 $mg\ kg^{-1}$ d.m., whereas content of tocopherols, depending on the flour extraction rate taken for the breadmaking, ranged from 3.42 $mg\ kg^{-1}$ d.m. to 1.19 $mg\ kg^{-1}$ d.m. The main rye bread fraction of tocotrienols was formed by α-T3 and β-T3. The highest level of tocotrienols and tocopherols was in bread with flour extraction rate of 100%. This level was comparable with the data obtained for commercial wheat bakery products in which content of tocotrienols and tocopherols was 3.25 $mg\ kg^{-1}$ d.m. and 3.02 $mg\ kg^{-1}$ d.m., respectively.

TABLE 3.7
Mean Content of Total Tocols and Percentages of Tocopherols, Tocotrienols and Ratio of α- β, γ- and δ-Tocotrienol to Total Tocotrienols in Rye and Wheat Bakery Products

Bread/flour extraction rate	Total tocols (mg kg^{-1} d.m.)	Contribution of tocopherols (%)	Contribution of tocotrienols (%)	Percentage of total tocotrienols α-T3	β-T3	γ-T3	δ-T3
Rye bread/100%	6.8	50.3	49.7	54.7	45.3	–	–
Rye bread/95%	2.1	48.9	51.2	38.7	61.3	–	–
Rye bread/90%	2.1	57.8	42.2	40.2	59.8	–	–
Rye bread/70%	1.7	76.9	23.0	36.8	63.2	–	–
Wheat roll/65%	6.3	48.2	51.8	16.3	70.0	–	–

Source: After Michalska et al., 2007b.

Data showed that the content of tocotrienols and tocopherols in bakery products strongly depends on both refining and thermal processes. The losses of tocotrienols and tocopherols may also occur due to the sourdough fermentation of rye dough when in contact with air (Katina et al., 2005). That is why the food industry is obliged to add vitamin E to bakery products, because bakeries prefer rather light flours for breadmaking. Instead of vitamin E, researchers incorporated brewers' spent grains into bread and cookies at levels that produced products of acceptable quality (Pentice at al., 1978). The incorporation of rice bran into food products for humans could also be utilized provided that the bran is stabilized immediately after milling to prevent the formation of free fatty acids caused by cell wall lipases.

This stabilization of rice bran can be reached by heating with an extruder oven, or by microwave, freezing or treatment with chemicals. The most common stabilization is with an extruder. After heat treatment at 100°C for 30 min., rice bran obtained from three varieties still showed significant amounts of tocotrienols. Their content ranged from 155 to 163 mg kg^{-1} and contributed 72–79% of tocols. Gamma tocotrienol formed more than 80% of tocotrienols. The heat treatment due to inactivate endogenous lipases caused a decrease in tocotrienol levels by aproximately 20% (Aquilar-Garcia et al., 2007) when compared with untreated rice bran (Chen and Bergman, 2005; Rohrer and Siebenmorgen, 2004). The order of stability of the E vitamers in extruded rice bran for 110–140°C extrusion temperatures was γ-T3 < α-T < α-T3 < γ-T < δ-T3 < β-T < δ-T (Shin et al., 1997).

3.7 HEALTH EFFECT OF TOCOTRIENOLS IN HUMANS

Cereal grains contribute significant quantities of energy, protein, selected micronutrients and non-nutrients to a human diet. Therefore, cereal and cereal-based foods represent the bulk of all foods consumed (Edge et al., 2005). Nutritionists worldwide recommend an increased intake of whole-grain products and dietary fiber (Adams and Engstrom, 2000; Lang and Jebb, 2003). In 43 out of 45 epidemiological studies, whole grains in particular have been shown to reduce the risk of cancer (Slavin et al., 2000). It is hypothesized that the biological activities of natural antioxidants and other phytochemicals in the whole grains, in addition to digestion-resistant polysaccharides, contribute to risk reduction (Temple, 2000). Now that consumers are increasingly interested in health and their knowledge of the relationship between diet and well-being has been raised, cereal-based products are likely to gain interest and popularity (Andlauer and Furst, 1999).

The role of tocotrienols and tocopherols in diet is essential because of the multiprotective effect of these bioactive compounds. Tocotrienols have a variety of novel beneficial functions (Hood, 1998; Theriault et al., 1999; Schaffer et al., 2005). They possess excellent antioxidant activity *in vitro* and are able to suppress reactive oxygen species (ROS) production more efficiently than tocopherols (Mutalib et al., 2003). Biological activities of tocols are generally believed to be due to their antioxidant action by inhibiting lipid peroxidation in biological membranes. However, tocotrienols are a member of a wider bioactive compounds family that includes phenolic acids, flavonoids, aventramides, lignans, tocopherols, carotenoids, melatonin, inositol phosphates, glutathione and thioaminoacids, as well as macro- and microelements and selenomethionine for humans (Edge et al., 2005). Although antioxidants and their function in cereal grains and grain products are known, their potential contribution to health through diet has essentially been ignored (Miller et al., 2000; Zielinski, 2002; Zielinski et al., 2007).

Alpha-tocopherol has been labeled the most efficient antioxidant for breaking free radical-driven chain reaction. Recent results indicate that α-T3 is at least three times more efficient as a scavenger of peroxyl radicals than α-T (Packer, 1995). Tocotrienols destroy nitrite, a component whose presence in the food chain is associated with some types of stomach cancer (Andlauer and Furst, 1999). In addition, tocotrienols show promising non-antioxidant activity in various *in vitro* and *in vivo* models. Most notable are the interactions of tocotrienols with the mevalonate pathway leading to the lowering of serum cholesterol levels (Qureshi et al., 2002), the prevention of cell adhesion to endothelial cells (Chao et al., 2002) and the suppression of tumor cell growth and glutamate-induced neurotoxicity (Khanna et al., 2003). Tocotrienols were shown to inhibit the growth of human breast cancer cells in culture (Nesarettnam et al., 1998) irrespective of estrogen receptor status (Guthrie et al., 1997). They also inhibit atherosclerotic lesions (Qureshi et al., 2001a). Tocotrienols have also been suggested to have neuroprotective effects independent of their antioxidant activity (Packer et al., 2001).

Tocotrienols have been the focus of growing research interest as unique nutritional compounds for their hypocholesterolemic action by inhibiting cholesterol biosynthesis (Qureshi et al., 1997; Hood, 1998; Theriault et al., 1999). This action was reported in chickens, swine and human subjects (Qureshi et al., 1986; Qureshi et al., 1991a–c). Tocotrienols may act as the inhibitors of the HMG-CoA reductase, a rate-limiting enzyme involved with cholesterol synthesis (Packer et al., 1993). The number and localization of the methyl groups of their chroman rings influence their biological activities, δ-T3 being the most potent cholesterol synthesis inhibitor, followed by γ-T3 and α-T3 (Qureshi and Qureshi, 1993). The oat-soluble fiber from oat bran and oatmeal, when added to the daily diet, tends also to lower serum low-density lipoprotein cholesterol and total blood cholesterol, particularly in individuals with initially greater levels of serum cholesterol (Davidson et al., 1991; Shinnick et al., 1991; Wood, 1994). The various mechanisms have been postulated for the effects of oat bran and other soluble-fiber sources on blood cholesterol concentrations. There are two potential sources of blood and tissue cholesterol: *de novo* synthesis and dietary absorption; both sources are subject to possible regulatory mechanisms. Regulation of the removal of cholesterol can occur only through major pathway conversion to bile acids followed by excretion in feces.

Tocotrienols-rich fractions from rice bran reportedly lower plasma total and LDL cholesterols levels in humans (Qureshi et al., 1997; Qureshi et al., 2001a). Moreover, other studies demonstrated that whole-fat rice bran at the same dietary level of oat bran is equal or even better for the prevention of diet-induced hypercholesterolemia and the development of early aortic atherosclerosis in hamsters (Qureshi et al., 2001b; Wilson et al., 2002).

The fate of supplemental tocotrienols and the relationships among intestinal absorption, blood levels and tissue distribution is still not fully understood. Even with relatively high doses of tocotrienols in animals or humans, sustained plasma levels of tocotrienols have not been observed (Hayes et al., 1993). In contrast, Weber et al. (1991) showed that dietary intervention with ingredients from brewer's spent grain increased the concentration of blood tocotrienol and lowered cholesterol in hypercholesterolemic human subjects.

There is growing evidence that the greatest advantage of a tocopherol- and tocotrienol-rich diet is achieved when various E vitamers are administered concurrently. Alpha-tocopherol supplementation alone has little effect on mammary tumors, and evidently other vitamers such as α-, γ- and δ-tocotrienols reduce the risk of breast cancer (Schwenke, 2002). The ratios of the individual tocotrienols and tocopherols play an important role in determining the hypocholesterolemic, antioxidant and antitumor properties of palm oil and rice bran (Qureshi et al., 2000; Qureshi et al., 2002). For example, α-T and α-T3 had opposite effects on the cholesterol metabolism of chicks, a higher ratio of tocotrienols to tocopherols being optimal (Qureshi et al., 1989). Therefore, the higher ratio of tocotrienols to tocopherols in the diet seems to be important in the metabolic regulation of cholesterol (Qureshi et al., 1989).

U.S. Pharmacopoeia and Food and Drug Administration (FDA) have not assigned vitamin activity to tocotrienols for their use in commercial products but commercial preparations of palm oil tocotrienols have been available for some time, and microencapsulated tocotrienols from rice bran are also now being marketed (Pszczola, 2001).

REFERENCES

Abidi, S.L. 2000. Chromatographic analysis of tocol-derived lipid antioxidants. *J. Chromatogr.* A, 881, 197–216.

Abidi, S.L., Thiam, S., Warner, I.M. 2002. Elution behavior of unsaponifitable lipids with various capillary electrochromatographic stationary phases. *J. Chromatogr.* A, 949, 195–207.

Adams, J.F., Engstrom, A. 2000. Dietary intake of whole grain vs. recommendations. *Cereal Foods World,* 45, 75–78.

Andlauer, W., Furst P. 1999. Does cereal reduce the risk of cancer? *Cereal Foods World,* 44, 76–78.

Anon. 2000. Subcommittee on Upper Reference Levels of Nutrients and Interpretation and Uses of Dietary Reference Intakes, and the standing Committee on the Scientific Evaluation of Dietary Reference Intakes. Food and Nutrition Board, Vitamin E. In *Dietary Reference Intakes for Vitamin C, Vitamin E, Selenium, and Carotenoids. Panel on Dietary Antioxidants and Related compounds,* Institute of Medicine, National Academy Press, Washington, DC, pp. 186–283.

Aquilar-Garcia, C. Gavino, G., Baragano-Mosqueda, M., Hevia, P., Gavino, V.C. 2007. Correlation of tocopherol, tocotrienol, γ-oryzanol and total polyphenol content in rice bran with different antioxidant capacity assays. *Food Chem.,* 102, 1228–1232.

Bergman, C.J., Xu, Z. 2003. Genotype and environment effects on tocopherols, tocotrienols, and γ-oryzanol contents of southern U.S. rice. *Cereal Chem.*, 80, 446–449.

Bhatty, R.S. 1999. The potential of hull-less barley. *Cereal Chem.*, 76, 589–599.

Birringer, M., Pfuger, P., Kluth, D., Landes, N., Brigelius-Flohe, R. 2002. Identities and differences in the metabolism of tocotrienols and tocopherols in HepG2 cells. *J. Nutr.*, 132, 3113–3118.

Cavallero, A., Empilli, S., Brighenti, F., Stanca, A.M. 2002. High (1→3, 1→4)–β–glucan barley fractions in bread making and their effects on human glycemic response. *Cereal Chem.*, 36, 59–66.

Cavallero, A., Gianinetti, A., Finocchiaro, F., Delogu, G., Stanca, A.M. 2004. Tocols in hull-less and hulled barley genotypes grown in contrasting enviroments. *J. Cereal Sci.,* 39, 175–180.

Chao, J.T., Gapor, A., Theriault, A. 2002. Inhibitory effect of delta-tocotrienol, a HMG CoA reductase inhibitor, on monocyte–endothelial cell adhesion. *J. Nutr. Sci. Vitamol.*, 48, 332–337.

Chen, M.-H., Bergman, C.J. 2005. A rapid procedure for analyzing rice bran tocopherol, tocotrienol and γ-oryzanol contents. *J. Food Compos. Anal.,* 18, 139–151.

Cheng, Z., Sattler, S., Maeda, H., Sakuragi, Y., Bryant, D.A., DellaPenna, D. 2003. Highly divergent methyltransferases catalyze a conserved reaction in tocopherol and plastoquinone synthesis in cyanobacteria and photosynthetic eukaryotes. *Plant Cell*, 15, 2343–2356.

Choi, Y., Jeong, H.-S., Lee, J. 2007. Antioxidant activity of methanolic extractys from some grains consumed in Korea. *Food Chem.*, 103, 130–138.

Collakova, E., DellaPenna, D., 2001. Isolation and functional analysis of homogentisate phytyltransferase from *Synechocystis* sp. PCC 6803 and Arabidopsis. *Plant Physiol.*, 127, 1113–1124.

Colombo, M.L., Corsini, A., Mossa, A., Sala, L., Stanca, M. 1998. Supercritical carbon dioxide extraction, fluorimetric and electrochemical HPLC detection of vitamin E from *Hordeum vulgare* L. *Phytochem. Analysis*, 9, 192–195.

Davidson, M.H., Dugan, L.D., Burns, J.H., Bova, J., Story, K., Drennan, K.S. 1991. The hypocholesterolemic effects of β–glucan in oatmeal and oat bran. *J. Am. Med. Assoc.,* 265, 1833–1839.

Dörmann, P. 2003. Corn with enhanced antioxidant potential. *Nat. Biotech.,* 21, 1015–1016.

Edge, M.S., Jones, J.M., Marquart, L. 2005. A new life for whole grains. *J. Am. Diet. Assoc.,* 15 (12), 1856–1860.

Eitenmiller, R.R., Landen, W.O. Jr. 1999. Vitamin E: Tocopherols and tocotrienols. In *Vitamin Analysis for the Health and Food Science.* Eitenmiller, R.R., Landen, W.O., Eds., CRC Press, Boca Raton, FL, 109–148.

Franzen, J., Bausch, J., Glatzle, D., Wagner, E. 1991. Distribution of vitamin E in spruce seedlings and mature tree organs, and within the genus. *Phytochemistry,* 30, 147–151.

Fratianni, A., Caboni, M.F., Irano, M., Panfili, G. 2002. A critical comparison between traditional methods and supercritical carbon dioxide extraction for the determination of tocochromanols in cereals. *Eur. Food Res. Technol.,* 215, 353–358.

Goffman, F.D., Bohme T. 2001. Relationship between fatty acid profile and vitamin E content in maize hybrids (*Zea mays* L.). *J. Agric. Food Chem.,* 49, 4990–4994.

Grams, G., Blessin, C., Inglett, G. 1970. Distribution of tocopherols within the corn kernel. *J. Amer. Oil Chem. Soc.,* 47, 337–339.

Guthrie, N., Gapor, A., Chambers, A.F., Carroll, K.K. 1997. Inhibition of proliferation of estrogen receptor-negative MDA-MB-435 and -positive MCF-7 human breast cancer cells by palm oil tocotrienols and tamoxifen, alone and in combination. *J. Nutr.,* 127, 544s–548s.

Hayes, K.C., Pronczuk, A., Laing, J.S. 1993. Differences in the plasma transport and tissue concentration of tocopherols and tocotrienols: Observation in humans and hamsters. *Proc. Soc. Exp. Biol. Med.,* 202, 353–360.

Holasova, M. 1997. Distribution of tocopherols and tocotrienols in the main products of wheat and rye milling. *Potrav. Vedy,* 15, 343–350.

Holasowa, M., Velisek, J., Davidek, J. 1995. Tocopherol and tocotrienol contents in cereal grains. *Czech J. Food Sci.,* 13, 409–417.

Hood, R.L. 1998. Tocotrienols in metabolism. In *Phytochemicals—A New Paradigm.* Bidlack W.R., Omaye S.T., Meskin M.S., Jahner D. (Eds.), Technomic, Lancaster, PA, 33–51.

Horvath, G., Wessjohann, L., Bigirimana, J., Jansen, M., Guisez, Y., Caubergs, R., Horemans, N., 2006. Differential distribution of tocopherols and tocotrienols in photosynthetic and non-photosynthetic tissues. *Phytochemistry,* 67, 1185–1195.

Kamal-Eldin, A., Appelqvist, L.A. 1996. The chemistry and antioxidant properties of tocopherols and tocotrienols. *Lipids,* 31, 671–701.

Katina, K., Arendt, E., Liukkonen, K.-H., Autio, K., Flander, L., Poutanen, K. 2005. Potential of sourdough for healthier cereal products. *Trends Food Sci. Technol.* 16, 104–112.

Kaukovirta-Norja, A., Reinikainen, P., Olkku, J., Laakso, S. 1997. Starch lipids of barley and malt. *Cereal Chem.,* 74, 733–738.

Khanna, S., Roy, S., Ryu, H., Bahadduri, P., Swaan, P.W., Ratan, R.R., Sen, C.K. 2003. Molecular basis of vitamin E action: tocotrienol modulates 12–lipoxygenase, a key mediator of glutamate-induced neurodegeneration. *J. Biol. Chem.,* 278, 43508–43515.

Kurilich, A., Juvik, J. 1999. Quantification of carotenoid and tocopherols antioxidants in *Zea mays. J. Agric. Food Chem.,* 47, 337–339.

Lang, R., Jebb, S.A. 2003. Who consumes whole grains, and how much? *Proc. Nutr. Soc.,* 62, 123 127.

Lasztity, R. 1998. Oat grain—a wonderful reservoir of natural nutrients and biologically active substances. *Food Rev. Int.,* 14, 99–119.

Lehmann, J.W., Putnam, D.H., Qureshi, A.A. 1994. Vitamin E in grain amaranths (*Amaranthus* spp.). *Lipids,* 29, 177–181.

Michalska, A., Ceglińska, A., Zieliński, H. 2007a. Bioactive compounds in rye flours with different extraction rates. *Eur. Food Res. Technol.,* DOI 10.1007//s00217-006-0452-4.

Michalska, A., Ceglińska, A., Amarowicz, R., Piskuła, M.K., Szawara-Nowak, D., Zieliński, H. 2007b. The antioxidant contents and antioxidative properties of traditional rye breads. *J. Agric. Food Chem., 55,* 734–740.

Miller, H.E., Rigelhof, F., Marguart, L., Prakash, A., Kanter, M. 2000. Antioxidant content of whole grain breakfast cereals, fruits and vegetables. *J. Am. Coll. Nutr.,* 19, 312–319.

Morrison, R., Coventry, A.M., Barnes, P.J. 1982. The distribution of acyl lipids and tocopherols in flour millstreams. *J. Sci. Food Agric.,* 33, 925–933.

Mutalib, M.S.A., Khazaai, H., Wahle, K.W.J. 2003. Palm–tocotrienol rich fraction (TRF) is more effective inhibitor of LDL oxidation and endothelial cell lipid peroxidation than alpha–tocopherol in vitro. *Food Res. Int.,* 36, 405–413.

Nesaretnam, K., Stephen, R., Dils, R., Dabre, P. 1998. Tocotrienols inhibit the growth of human breast cancer cells irrespective of estrogen receptor status. *Lipids,* 33, 461–469.

Packer, L. 1995. Nutrition and biochemistry of the lipophylic antioxidants, vitamin E and carotenoids. In *Nutrition, Lipids, Health, and Disease*, Ong A.S.H., Niki E., Packer L., Eds., American Oil Chemists' Society: Champaign, IL, 8–35.

Packer, L., Weber, S.U., Rimbach, G. 2001. Molecular aspects of alpha-tocotrienol antioxidant action and cell signaling. *J. Nutr.,* 131, 369–373.

Packer, R.A., Pearce, R.W., Clark, D.A., Gordon, J., Wright, J.K. 1993. Tocotrienols regulate cholesterol production in mammalian cells by post-transcriptional suppression of 3-hydroxy-3-methylglutaryl coenzymeA reductase. *J. Biol. Chem.,* 268, 11230–11238.

Panfili, G., Fratianni, A., Irano, M. 2003a. Normal phase high-performance liquid chromatography method for the determination of tocopherols and tocotrienols in cereals. *J. Agric. Food Chem.*, 51, 3940–944.

Panfili, G., Cinquanta, L., Fratianni, A., Cubadda, R. 2003b. Extraction of wheat germ oil by supercritical CO2, oil and defatted cake characterization. *J. Am. Oil Chem. Soc.* 80, 157–161.

Pennock, J.F. 1983. The biosynthesis of chloroplastic terpenoid quinines and chromanols. *Biochem. Soc. Trans.*, 11, 504–510.

Pentice, N., Kissell, L.T., Lindsay, R.C., Yamazaki, W.T. 1978. High-fiber cookies containing brewer's spent grain. *Cereal Chem.*, 55, 712–721.

Peterson, D.M. 1994. Barley tocols: Effects of milling, malting and mashing. *Cereal Chem.,* 71, 42–44.

Peterson, D.M. 1995. Oat tocols: Concentration and stability in oat products and distribution within the kernel. *Cereal Chem.,* 72 *(1),* 21–24.

Peterson, D.M., Qureshi, A.A. 1993. Genotype and environment effects on tocols of barley and oats. *Cereal Chem.,* 70, 157–162.

Piironen, V., Syvaoja, E.I., Varo, P., Salminek, K., Koivistoinen, P. 1986. Tocopherols and tocotrienols in cereal products from Finland. *Cereal Chem.,* 63, 78–81.

Porfirova, S., Bergmuller, E., Tropf, S., Lempke, R., Dormann, P. 2002. Isolation of an Arabidopsis mutant lacking vitamin E and identification of a cyclase essential for all tocopherol biosynthesis. *Proc. Natl. Acad. Sci.,* 99, 12495–12500.

Pszczola, D.E. 2001. Diverse strategies help promote ingredient products. *Food Technol.*, 55, 77–99.

Qureshi, A.A., Bradlow, B.A., Salser, W.A., Brace, L.D. 1997. Novel tocotrienols of rice bran modulate cardiovascular disease risk parameters of hypercholesterolemic humans. *J. Nutr. Biochem.*, 8, 290–298.

Qureshi, A.A., Burger, W.C., Peterson, D.M., Elson, C.E. 1986. The structure of an inhibitor of cholesterol biosynthesis isolated from barley. *J. Biol. Chem.,* 261, 10544–10550.

Qureshi, A.A., Chaudhary, V., Weber, F.E., Chicoye, E., Qureshi, N. 1991a. Effects of brewer's grain and other cereals on lipid metabolism in chickens. *Nutr. Res.*, 11, 159–162.

Qureshi, A.A., Qureshi, N., Wright, J.J.K., Shen, Z., Kramer, G., Gapor, A., Chong, Y.H., Dewitt, G., Ong, A.S.H., Peterson, D.M., Bradlow, B.A. 1991b. Lowering serum cholesterol in hypercholesterolemic humans by tocotrienols (palmvitee). *Am. J. Clin. Nutr.,* 53, 1021–1026.

Qureshi, A.A., Qureshi, N., Hasler-Rapacz, J.O., Weber, F.E., Chaudhary, V., Crewshaw, T.D., Gapor A., Ong, A.S.H., Chong, Y.H., Peterson D., Rapacz J. 1991c. Dietary tocotrienols reduce concentrations of plasma cholesterol, apolipoprotein B., tromboxane B2, and platelet factor 4 in pigs with inherited hyperlipidemias. *Am. J. Clin. Nutr.,* 53, 1042–1046.

Qureshi, A.A., Salser, W.A., Parmar, R., Emeson, E.E. 2001a. Novel tocotrienols of rice bran inhibit atherosclerotic lesions in C57BL/6 ApoE-deficient mice. *J. Nutr., 131,* 2606–2618.

Qureshi A.A.,Sami S.A., Salser W.A., Khan F.A. 2001b. Synergistic effect of tocotrienols–rich fraction of rice bran and lovastatin on lipid parameters in hypercholesterolemic humans. *J. Nutr. Biochem.,* 12, 318–329.

Qureshi, A.A., Mo, H., Packer, L., Peterson, D.M. 2000. Isolation and identification of novel tocotrienols from rice bran with hypocholesterolemic, antioxidant, and antitumor properties. *J. Agric. Food Chem.,* 48, 3130–3140.

Qureshi, A.A., Peterson, D.M., Elson, C.E., Mangels, A.R., Din, Z.Z. 1989. Stimulation of avian cholesterol metabolism by α-tocopherol. *Nutr. Rep. Inter.,* 40, 993–1001.

Qureshi, A.A., Sami, S.A., Salser, W.A., Khan, F.A. 2002. Dose-dependent suppression of serum cholesterol by tocotrienol–rich fraction (TRF25) of rice bran in hypercholesterolemic humans. *Artherosclerosis,* 161, 199–207.

Qureshi, N., Qureshi, A.A. 1993. Tocotrienols, novel hypocholesterolemic agents with antioxidant properties. In *Vitamin E in Health and Disease*, Packer L., Fuchs J., Eds., Dekker: New York, 247–268.

Rohrer, C.A., Siebenmorgen, T.J. 2004. Nutraceutical concentrations within the bran of various rice kernel thickness fractions. *Biosyst. Eng.,* 88(4), 453–460.

Ruperez, F.J., Martin, D., Herrera, E., Barbas, C. 2001. Chromatographic analysis of α–tocopherol and related compounds in various matrices. *J. Chromatogr. A.*, 935, 45–69.

Ryynänen, M., Lampi, A.-M., Salo-Vaananen, P., Ollilainen, V., Piironen, V. 2004. A small-scale sample preparation method with HPLC analysis for determination of tocopherols and tocotrienols in cereals. *J. Food Compos. Anal.,* 17, 749–765.

Schaffer, S., Müller, W.E., Eckert, G.P. 2005. Tocotrienols: Constitutional effects in aging and disease. *J. Nutr.*, 135, 151–154.

Schwenke, D.C. 2002. Does the lack of tocopherols and tocotrienols put women at increased risk of breast cancer? *J. Nutr. Biochem.*, 13, 2–20.

Sen, C.K., Khanna, S., Roy, S. 2006. Tocotrienols: Vitamin E beyond tocopherols. *Life Sci.*, 78, 2088–2098.

Shin, T.-S., Godber, J.S., Martin, D.E., Wells, J.H. 1997. Hydrolitic stability and changes in E vitamers and oryzanol of extruded rice bran during storage. *J. Food Sci.*, 62 (4), 704–709.

Shinnick, F.L., Mathews, R., Ink, S. 1991. Serum cholesterol reduction by oats and other fiber sources. *Cereal Foods World*, 36, 815–821.

Shintani, D.K., Cheng, Z., DellaPenna, D. , 2002. The role of 2-methyl-6-phytylbenzoquinone methyltransfrase in determining tocopherol composition in *Synechocystis* sp. PCC 6803. *FEBS Lett.* 511, 1–5.

Slavin, J.L. 2000. Mechanisms for the impact of whole grain foods on cancer risk. *J. Am. Coll. Nutr.,* 19, 300–307.

Slavin, J., Marquart, L., Jacobs, D. Jr. 2000. Consumption of whole-grain foods and decreased risk of cancer: Proposed mechanisms. *Cereal Foods World, 45*, 54–58.

Strohschein, S., Rentel, C., Lacker, T., Bayer, E., Albert, K. 1999. Separation and identification of tocotrienol isomers by HPLC-MS and HPLC-NMR coupling. *Anal. Chem.,* 71, 1780–1785.

Temple, N.J. 2000. Antioxidants and disease: More questions than answers. *Nutr. Res.,* 20, 449–459.

Theriault, A., Chao, J.T., Wang, Q., Gapor, A., Adeli, K. 1999. Tocotrienols: A review of its therapeutic potential. *Clin. Biochem.,* 32, 309–319.

Työppönen, J.T., Hakkaranen, R.V.J. 1985. Thermal stability of vitamin E in barley. *Acta Agric. Scand.,* 35, 136–142.

Ueda, T., Igarashi, O. 1987. New solvent system for extraction of tocopherols from biological specimens for HPLC determination and the evaluation of 2,2,5,7,8-pentamethyl-6-chromanol as an internal standard. *J. Micronutr. Anal.,* 3, 185–198.

Venkatesh, T.V., Karunanandaa, B., Free, D.L., Rottnek, J.M., Baszis, S.R., Valentin, H.E. 2006. Identification and characterization of an Arabidopsis homogentisate phytyltransferase paralog. *Planta*, 12, 1–11.

Wang, C., Ning, J., Krishnan, P.G., Matthees, D.P. 1998. Effects of steeping conditions during wet-milling on the retentions of tocopherols and tocotrienols in corn. *J. Am. Oil Chem. Soc.* 75, 609–613.

Wang, L., Xue, Q., Newman, R.K., Newman, C.W. 1993. Enrichment of tocopherols, tocotrienols and oil in barley fractions by milling and pearling. *Cereal Chem.,* 70 *(5)*, 499–501.

Weber, F.E., Chaudhary, V.K., Qureshi, A.A. 1991. Suppression of cholesterol biosynthesis in hypercholesterolemic subjects by tocotrienol of barley ingredients made from brewers grain. *Cereal Foods World,* 36, 680–684.

Weicheng, H., Wells, J., Shin, T.-S., Godber, J.S. 1996. Comparison of isopropanol and hexane for extraction of vitamin E and oryzanols from stabilized rice bran. *J. Amer. Oil Chem. Soc.,* 73, 1653–1656.

Wilson, T., Idreis, H.M., Taylor, C. M., Nicolosi, R.J. 2002. Whole fat rice bran reduces the development of early aorthic atherosclerosis in hypercholesterolemic hamsters compared with wheat bran. *Nutr. Res.,* 22, 1319–1332.

Wood, P.J. 1994. Evaluation of oat bran as a soluble fibre source. Characterization of oat β–glucan and its effect on glycaemic response. *Carbohydr. Polym.,* 25, 331–336.

Yamauchi, R., Noro, H., Shimoyamada, M., Kato, K., 2002. Analysis of vitamin E and its oxidation products by HPLC with electrochemical detection. *Lipids,* 37, 515–522.

Zieliński, H. 2002. Low molecular weight antioxidants in the cereal grains. *Pol. J. Food Nutr. Sci.,* 11/52, 3–9.

Zieliński, H., Ceglińska, A., Michalska, A. 2007. Antioxidants content and properties as quality indices of rye cultivars. *Food Chem.,* 104, 980–988.

Zieliński, H., Ciska, E., Kozłowska, H. 2001a. The cereal grains: Focus on vitamin E. *Czech J. Food Sci.*, 19, 182–188.

Zielinski, H., Kozlowska, H., Lewczuk, B. 2001b. Bioactive compounds in the cereal grains before and after hydrothermal processing. *Inn. Food Sci. Emerg. Technol.*, 2/3, 159–169.

4 Tocotrienols in Plants: Sources and Importance

Liva Harinantenaina

CONTENTS

4.1 INTRODUCTION

The recent results of the investigations of vitamin E appear to substantiate the pharmacological and clinical studies of its tocotrienol (T3) analogs. To offer contributions on the sources of T3s in plants and their importance, this chapter focuses on the distribution of T3s in the plant kingdom based on literature surveys and phytochemical investigations of some plants I have studied. The occurrence of T3s in the plant classes Pteridophyta, Gymnospermae and Angiospermae is discussed. Apart from the well known plants containing T3s, among all grains, wheat germ, olives, barley, beans, nuts, rice bran oil and palm oils, several have been found to biosynthesize T3s. References were collected to define the role, importance and origin of T3s in plants. The importance of T3s in common human diseases is also discussed.

4.2 DEFINITION

4.2.1 Vitamin E: Tocotrienols

T3s, together with tocopherols, compose the vitamin E family. Natural T3s display the four different forms or isomers, α-, β-, γ- and δ- tocotrienols. Although both tocopherols and T3s are present and play very important roles in the plant kingdom, most of the literature to date has focused mainly on tocopherols.

4.2.2 Structures of Tocotrienols, the Vitamin E Analogs

T3s, the primary forms of Vitamin E, are amphiphilic lipids consisting of a polar chromanol head and a lipophylic isoprenoid side chain (Figure 4.1). All of the four forms of T3s can occur in plants and their structures differ from each other with regard to the numbers and positions of methyl groups on the aromatic chromanol head group (A, Figure 4.1). T3s differ from tocopherols in terms of the double bonds in the side chain, which are geranylgeranyl and phytyl, respectively.

4.3 BIOSYNTHESIS TOCOTRIENOLS

The biosynthesis of tocopherols and T3s *in planta* is localized in the plastids of seeds and the chloroplasts of leaves. Unlike tocopherols, the biosynthesis of T3s in the plant kingdom has not been well characterized. However, based on the similarity of the tocotrienol side chain and geranylgeranyl diphosphate (GGDP), they are believed to be derived from the condensation of a compound derived from tyrosine called homogentisic acid (HGA) and GGDP (Figure 4.2) (Soll et al., 1980; Schultz et al., 1985; Collakova and DellaPenna, 2001). GGDP are synthesized via the nonmevalonate pathway of plastid isoprenoid synthesis (Dormann, 2003). The reaction can be thus suggested to be catalyzed by HGA geranylgaranyl transferase (HGGT) enzyme.

In 2003, Cahoon and co-workers identified and isolated the cDNAs for divergent forms of HGA phytyl transferase (HPT) from tocotrienol-accumulating seeds (Cahoon et al., 2003). The full-length cDNA for a 408-amino acids polypeptide with 45–50% identity of the reported *A. thaliana*, soybean, corn and rice HPTs was obtained. The design of the isolation was based on the similarity of the HPT and HGGT substrates, which implies the similarities between the HPT and HGGT enzymes amino acid sequences. Since HPTs from several monocot and dicot as well as *Synechocytis sp* cyanobacterium have been determined (Collakova and DellaPenna, 2001; Savidge et al., 2002), the alignment of amino acid sequences of HPT-related enzymes revealed at least three short domains of partially conserved residues. These domains were used in amplifying HPT-related cDNA sequences from tocotrienols accumulating tissues. Expression of these cDNAs is shown to confer tocotrienol biosynthetic ability to transgenic plant tissue in a manner consistent with that of HGGT. Moreover, large increases in amounts of tocol products (vitamin E) could be observed in leaves and seeds of transgenic plants.

Northern blot analyses also showed that mRNA for the corresponding gene is abundant in seed-enriched tocotrienols. The full length of cDNA for HPT-related sequences from developing tocotrienols enriched rice and wheat seeds have been also determined. The findings provided a method for producing tocotrienols in transgenic plants and demonstrated the first evidence for the synthesis of tocotrienols through the HGGT-catalyzed pathway. The authors had concluded that although the polypeptides from barley, wheat and rice seeds are related to HPTs, they correspond to a structurally distinct enzyme class and might have shared common ancestors (Figure 4.3). Interestingly, normal *A. thaliana* leaves do not accumulate T3s, but using the isolated HGGTs in transgenic *A. thaliana* leaves, (10- to 15-fold) tocotrienols could be manufactured. Also, using this method, massive T3s production in corn seed (6-fold) was detected. Noteworthy, this experience demonstrated an increase mainly of γ-tocotrienols (Cahoon et al., 2003). Rippert and his group (Rippert et al. 2004) demonstrated that the synthesis of *p*-hydroxyphenylpyruvate (HPP) is a limiting step for the accumulation of Vitamin E in plants. The efficiency in bolstering the biosynthesis of T3s in the leaves was observed during genetic engineering of the metabolic pathways in plants, by increasing the flux of HPP and homogentisate due to the expression of the yeast prephenate dehydrogenase gene in *nicotianna tobaccum* (tobacco) that already overexpresses the *Arabidopsis* HPP dioxygenase coding gene.

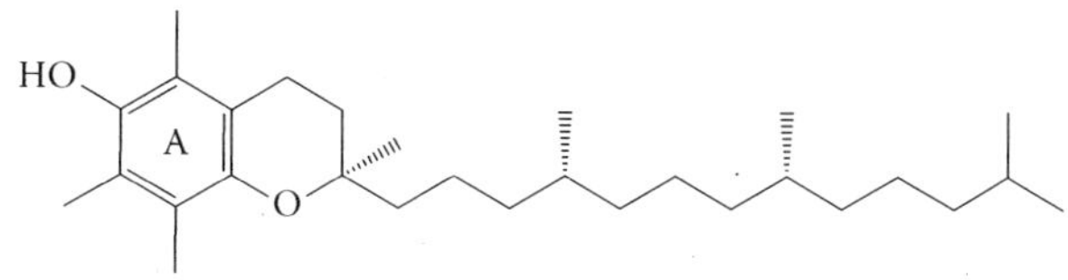

α-Tocopherol (1)

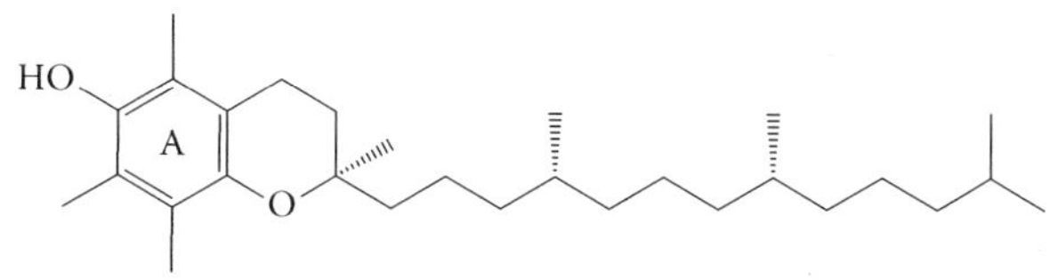

β-Tocopherol (2)

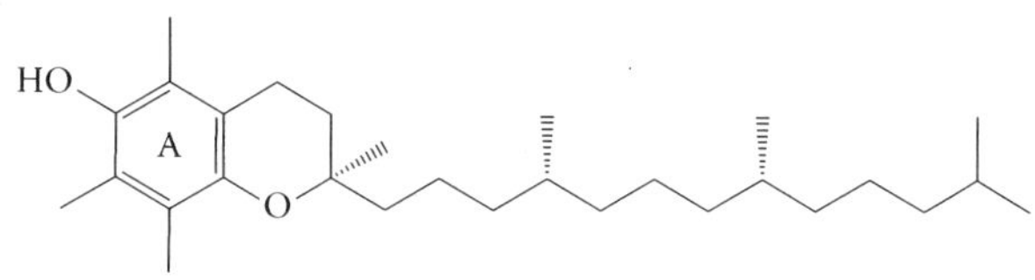

γ-Tocopherol (3)

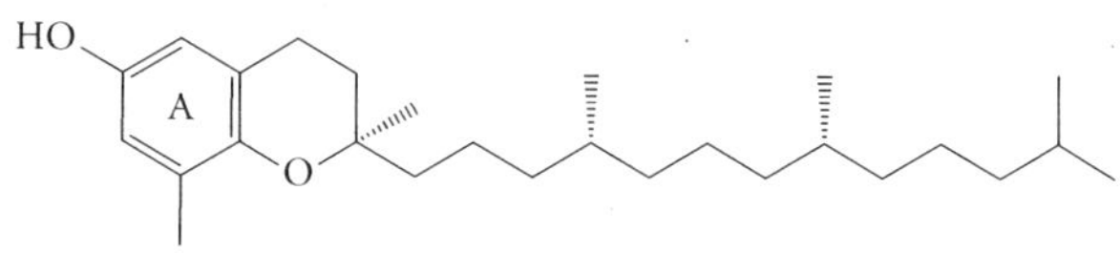

δ-Tocopherol (4)

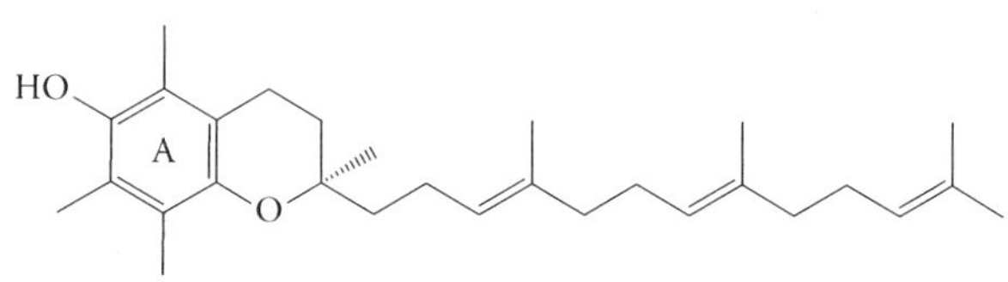

α-Tocotrienol (5)

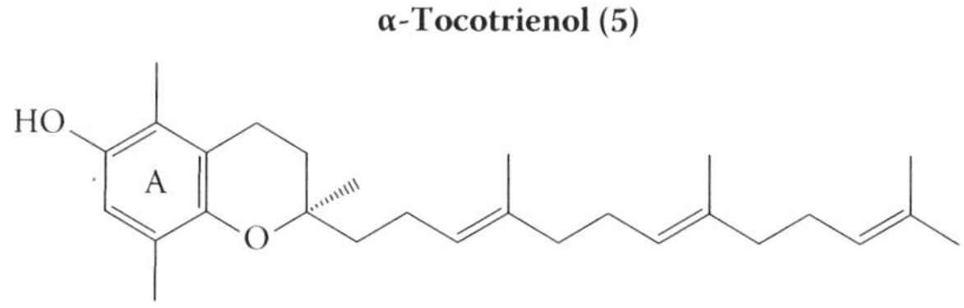

β-Tocotrienol (6)

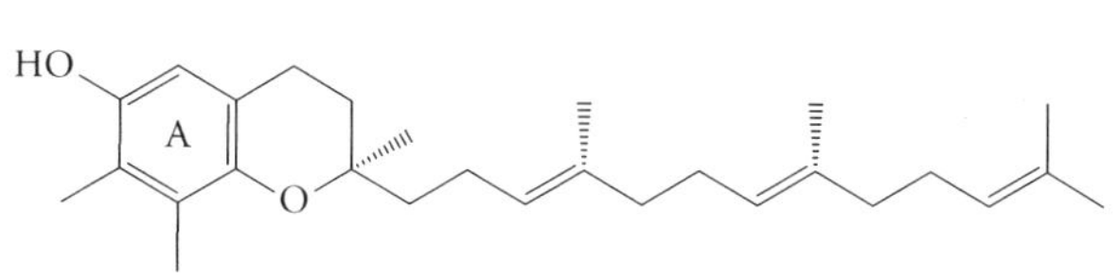

γ-Tocotrienol (7)

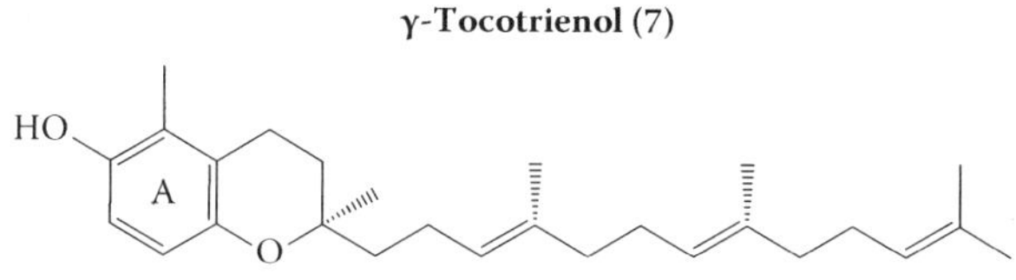

δ-Tocotrienol (8)

FIGURE 4.1 Structures of tocopherols and tocotrienols.

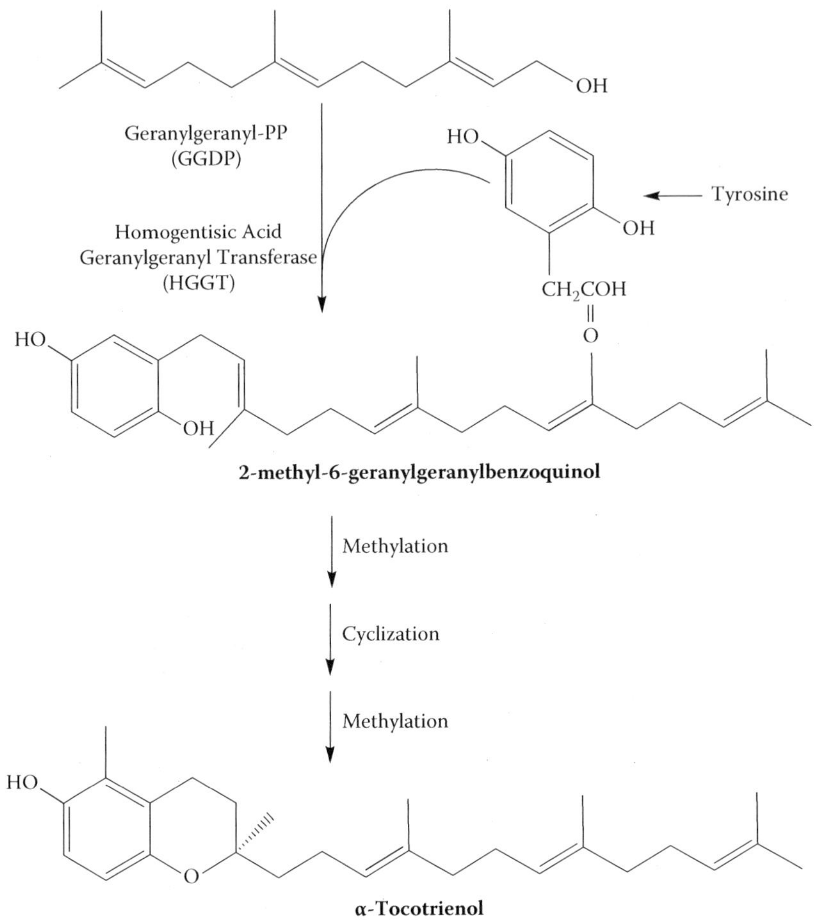

FIGURE 4.2 Biosynthesis of tocotrienols.

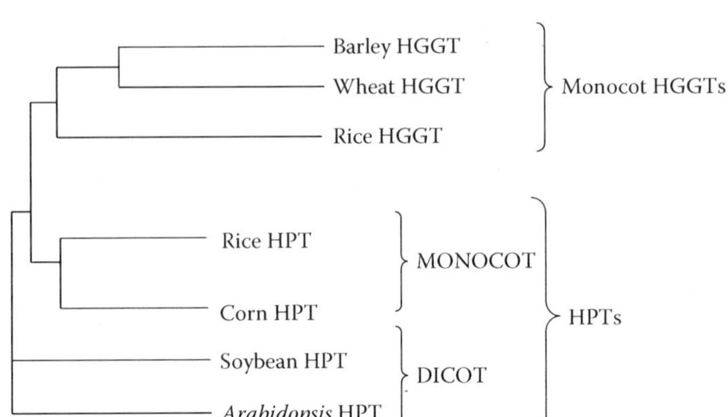

FIGURE 4.3 Classification resulting from phylogenetic analysis of HPT and HGGT amino acid sequences.

4.4 ROLE OF TOCOTRIENOLS IN PLANTS

Unlike tocopherols, there is very little literature describing the role of T3s in plants. Based on the structural similarities, the role of T3s is often assumed to be comparable with that of tocopherols. *In planta* T3s together with tocopherols appear to play a role in the physiological phenomena of plant growth, development and senescence, and to interact with the signal cascades that convey abiotic and biotic stress signals (Horvath et al., 2006a).

Havaux and his group have demonstrated the protection properties of tocopherols against photoinhibition and photooxidative stress in *Arabidopsis thaliana* (Havaux et al., 2005). Although all members of vitamin E have antioxidant properties, each analog has a different level of activity. T3s are a more potent antioxidant than other forms of vitamin E (Chandan et al. 2006). The factors that determine the high antioxidant activity of T3s' compared with α-tocopherols have been suggested (Serbinova et al., 1991) to be due to:

- Uniformity of the distribution in membrane bilayer
- The stronger disordering of membrane lipids
- Their more effective collision with radicals
- The greater recycling activity of chromanoxyl radical
- The correlation of the recycling activity with inhibition of lipid peroxidation

More likely, these proprieties enhance the interaction of chromanols with plant lipid radicals. Tocotrienols incorporated into plant cellular membranes inhibit peroxidations of lipids during seed dormancy, germination and early seedling development, and scavenge the chain propagating peroxyl radical. Compared with α-tocopherol, the activity of T3s in liposomes is 1.5-fold higher (Packer et al. 2001). Since protection of cytochrome P-450 against oxidative damage of α-tocotrienol has been observed in rat liver microsomal membranes (Serbinova et al., 1991), similar or at least related phenomena could possibly occur *in planta*.

Horvath and co-workers reported the differential distribution of tocopherols and tocotrienols in photosynthetic tissues (Horvath et al., 2006b). They found the transience accumulation of low levels of T3s in the young coleoptiles of plant species whose seeds contained T3s. Also, from their data, photosynthetically active tissues have been shown to contain only transient tocotrienol. As mentioned earlier, the majority of these tissues do not biosynthesize T3s, since no HGGT was found in the wild plant. Therefore, the low levels of T3s found in young coleoptiles can be elucidated to be transported mainly from the seeds or from T3s biosynthesizing tissues. T3s biosynthesis has been detected in these seeds during T3s accumulation and in an endosperm fraction isolated at 75 days after flowering (Horvath et al., 2006a). Undoubtedly, the protection of such tissues against sunlight is one of the roles of T3s in plants. In the study of the accumulation of T3 and tocopherol during development of caryopses from barley (*Hordeum vulgare* L.), Falk and scientists in the University of Kiel, Germany, reported that tocochromanols and lipids accumulated in parallel until 80% of the final dry weight of the barley kernels was reached. Later on, the tocochromanol content did not change while the lipid content decreased. Generally, only about 13% of the tocochromanols were found in the germ fraction, whereas the pericarp fraction contained about 50% and the endosperm fraction about 37% of the tocochromanols. About 85% of the tocochromanols were T3s in both cultivars. This finding proved the important role of T3s in seed protection (Falk et al. 2004).

4.5 DISTRIBUTION OF TOCOTRIENOLS IN THE PLANT KINGDOM

Tocopherols are present in all higher plants. T3s in contrast seem to be the constituents of a limited number of plant species. They are highly abundant in mature seeds of monocots, fruits of dicots, and latex of *Hevea brasiliensis* (Willd. ex A. Juss. Müll. Arg) (d'Auzac et al., 1989).

Table 4.1 exhibits plants reported to biosynthesize T3s. Apart from the studies on the occurrence of tocochromanols in *Pinus* species (Franzen et al., 1991; Bagci and Karaagacli, 2004), the presence of T3s in Pderidophyta and other gymnospermae families has not yet been reported. Even though liverworts contain tocopherols, no literature describes their T3 content. Among the liverworts investigated, *Radula* species are a rich source of chromanols with prenyl side chain (Asakawa, 1995; Harinantenaina et al., 2006a). However, these species contain only tocopherols but not T3s. All eight Turkish pine species: *Pinus nigra* subsp. *pallasiana*, *P. nigra* subsp. *pallasiana* var. *pyramidata*, *P. halepensis*, *P. sylvestris*, *P. pinea*, *P. brutia*, *P. radiate*, *P. pinaster* (Bagci and Karaagacli, 2004) were shown to contain T3s although no fixed values were observed (Table 4.1).

Very few plant species are able to produce both tocopherols and T3s. *Vitis venenifera* L. cv. Albert Lavallée (Royal) is one of the examples. In the study of the accumulation of tocopherols and T3s during seed development of this plant, Horvath and his co-workers proved that T3s are located only in the endosperm of the seeds. T3s are accumulated in a sigmoid fashion during the maturation period of the seed development (Horvath et al., 2006a). Our recent investigations revealed the presence of δ-tocotrienol in the bark of three species of Madagascan medicinal plant from the genus *Cinnamosma* (Canellaceae): *Cinnamosma fragrans*, *Cinnamosma macrocarpa* and *Cinnamosma madagascariensis*. Among the three species, *C. macrocarpa* contains the highest amount of δ-tocotrienol (0.16%). Only about half of this amount was found in *C. fragrans* (ca 0.07), while the amount decreased 10-fold in *C. madagascariensis* (0.016%) (Harinantenaina and Takaoka, 2006, 2007a, and 2007b).

Recently, Amiguet and his group isolated δ-T3 from the bark of a newly discovered Canellaceae tree, *Pleodendron costaricense*, with a yield of 0.006% (Amiguet et al., 2006). The leaves of these plants have not yet been shown to contain δ-tocotrienol. Apart from the bioactive sesquiterpene dialdehydes of the Canellaceae species (Figure 4.4), the presence of δ-tocotrienol in a non-negligible amount in the bark is one of the reasons they are used in local traditional medicine (Harinantenaina et al., 2006, 2007a, and 2007b; Amiguet et al., 2006). The content of cytotoxic pungent drimane sesquiterpene dialdehydes (eg. 9, 10) in the bark is higher than that detected in the leaves. The high amount of δ-T3 in the bark can be thus elucidated to be used as detoxification of the pungent compounds in the host cells. Further investigation is, however, needed to prove this hypothesis. Gutifereae (Clusiaceae) family members contain plant species producing T3s and/or tocotrienol-like compounds. These plants are: *Callophyllum calaba* L., *Callophyllum inophyllum* L., *Garcinia virgata*, *Garcinia kola*, *Kielmeyera lathrophyton*, *K. reticulata*, *Tovomitopsis psycotriifolia*, *Clausia grandifolia* and *Clausia obdeltifolia* (Teixeira et al. 2006, Merza et al., 2004, crane et al., 2005).

4.6 ISOLATION AND STRUCTURAL DETERMINATION OF TOCOTRIENOLS

Although various literatures describe the method for the detection of T3s, few publications discuss their isolation. Soxhlet extraction using hexane by grinding the leaf and seed material in liquid nitrogen gave the highest extraction efficiency, while isolated chloroplasts showed the highest efficiency in liquid extraction with hexane and methanol (Horvath et al. 2006b). The use of high performance liquid chromatography (HPLC) equipped with normal phase column (Alltech Particil Pac, or silica gel packed system such as Agilent LiChroSpher Si 60) and UV detector is one of the best methods used to isolate T3s. Also, flash silica gel column chromatography (CC) using hexane/acetone, hexane/ethyl acetate, heptane/isopropanol gradient can afford T3s. Preparative thin layer chromatography (PTLC) with silica gel plate (Si gel 60 F_{254}, solvent system: hexane ethyl acetate: 4:1, Rf: 0.47) or with ODS (RP-18 F_{254} S, solvent system 100% aqueous methanol) is the easiest way to isolate T3s. An example of an isolation of a T3s: δ-tocotrienol from the Madagascan medicinal plant, *Cinnamosma fragrans*, a member of the Canellaceae family, is described in the following paragraphs.

TABLE 4.1
Plant Species Reported To Contain Significant Amount of Tocotrienols

	Common name	Organ	Tocotrienols (μg/g tissue or organ) α	β	γ	δ
		Gymnospermae				
Pinopsida						
Pinaceae		bark	nd	nd	nd	700
Pinus nigra subsp. *pallasiana*[1]		bark	nd	nd	nd	160
Pinus nigra subsp. *pallasiana* var. *pyramidata*[1]		bark	nd	nd	nd	1600
Pinus helepensis[1]		bark	nd	nd	nd	60
Pinus sylvastris[1]						
Pinus pinea[1]						
Pinus brutia[1]		seed	+	+	+	+
Pinus radiata[1]						
Pinus pinaster[1]		seed	+	+	+	+
		Magnoliidae				
Canellaceae						
Cinnamosma fragrans[2]		bark	nd	nd	nd	700
Cinnamosma madagascariensis[3]		bark	nd	nd	nd	160
Cinnamosma macrocarpa[4]		bark	nd	nd	nd	1600
Pleodendron costaricense[5]		bark	nd	nd	nd	60
		Eudicots				
Amaranthaceae						
Amaranthus hypochondriacus[6]	Amaranth	seed	+	+	+	+
Apiaceae						
Carum carvi L.[7]	Caraway	seed	+	+	+	+
Coriandrum sativum L.	Coriander	seed	6.0	bld	bld	tr.
Foeniculum vulgare L.[7]	Fennel	seed	+	+	+	+
Bixaceae						
Bixa orellana L.	Lipstick tree	seed	18.7	1.84	534.7	977.9
Clusiaceae						
Callophyllum calaba L.[8]		kernel	2.0	bld	130	103
Callophyllum inophyllum L.		kernel	2.0	bld	64.0	236.0
Garcinia virgata[9]		stem bark				
Garcinia kola[10]			+	+	+	+
Kielmeyera lathrophyton[10]			+	+	+	+
Kielmeyera reticulata[10]			+	+	+	+
Mammea seamensis[11]		seed				34
Euphorbiaceae						
Hevea brasiliesis Mull. Arg.	Rubber tree	latex	522.4	bld	196.7	1869.6

Continued

TABLE 4.1 (Continued)
Plant Species Reported To Contain Significant Amount of Tocotrienols

	Common name	Organ	Tocotrienols (μg/g tissue or organ)			
			α	β	γ	δ
Ericaceae						
Vaccinium macrocarpon Aiton[6]	Cranberry	seed	+	+	+	+
Hippocastanaceae						
Aesculus hippocastanum Hort.[12]	Horse Chestnuts	seed	97	nd	626	336
Juglandaceae						
Juglans regia L.[13]	Walnut	seed	bld	bld	bld	+
Lamiaceae						
Rosmarinus officinalis	Rosemary	seed	560.5	300.3	109.4	tr.
Proteaceae						
Gevuina avellana Mol.[14]	Chilean hazelnut	seed	0.4	Bld.	0.6	bld
Ranunculaceae						
Delphinium ajacis L.[12]	Larkspur	seed	566	153	Tr.	nd.
Sapindaceae						
Litchi chinensis Sonn.	Litchi	seed	bld	bld	3.37	488
Solanaceae						
Nicotiana tabacum L.[15]	Tobacco	seed	tr.	tr.	30	tr.
Vitaceae						
Vitis vinifera L.	Grape	seed, y.sl	5.0	bld	25.0	bld
	Monocotyledons					
Arecaceae						
Elaeis guineensis Jacq.[16]	Palm tree	fruit	4–193	0–234	0–526	0–123
Cocos nucifera	Coconut	seed	104.0	26.0	36.2	204
Poaceae						
Avena sativa L.[17]	Oat	seed, y.sl	4.2	tr.	2.1	0.9
Hordeum vulgare L.[17]	Barley	seed, y.sl	0.59	tr.	tr.	tr.
Oryza sativa L.[17]	Rice	seed, y.sl	0.4–3.33	0.02	1.7–5.14	0–0.35
Secale cereale L.[17]	Rye	seed, y.sl	1.97	0.38	0.57	bld
Triticum sp.	Wheat	seed, y.sl	5.0	19.6	bld	bld
Zea mays L.[18]	Maize	seed, y.sl	0–239	0–450	0–20	0–709

Note: y.sl–Young seedling, nd–Not detected, bld–Below detection limit, tr.–Traces–+: Reported or positively described to contain. (Horvath et al., 2006)

[1] Bagci, E. and Karaagacli, Y., 2004, [2]Harinantenaina, L. and Takaoka, S. 2006, [3]Harinantenaina et al., 2007b, [4]Harinantenaina et al., 2007a, [5]Amiguet et al., 2006. [6]Well known to contain vitamin E, [7]Aitzetmuller, K., 1997, [8]Crane, S. et al., 2005, [9]Merza, J. et al., 2004, [10]Teixeira, J.S.R., 2006, [11]Laphookhieo et al. 2006, [12]Matthaus, B. et al., 2003, [13]Amaral, J.S. et al. 2005, [14]Bertholi, C. et al., 1998, [15]Falk, J. et al., 2004, [16]Value in mg/kg oil. Firestone, D., 1999, [17]Horvath, G. et al., 2006, [18]Franzen, J. and Haass, M., 1991

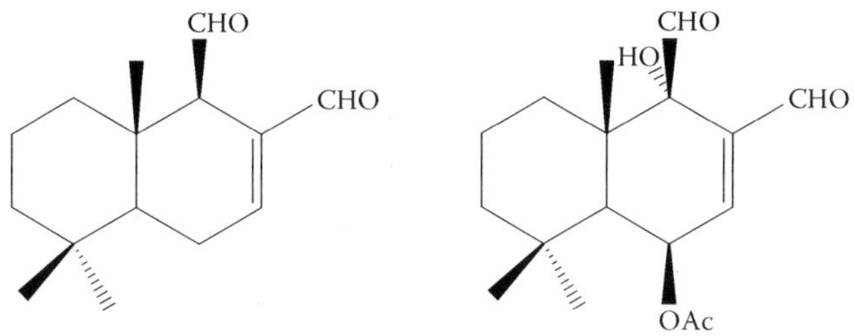

Polygodial (9) **Cinnamodial (10)**

FIGURE 4.4 Example of bioactive and cytotoxic pungent drimane sesuiterpene dialdehydes present in canellaceae family.

4.6.1 Isolation of δ-Tocotrienol in *Cinnamosma fragrans*

Cinnamosma fragrans was collected in Lakato (near Moramanga, a three hour drive from Antananarivo to the east, Madagascar) and identified by comparison with the authentic sample in the herbarium of PBZT (Parc Botanique et Zoologique de Tsimbazaza, Antananarivo, Madagascar).

4.6.1.1 Extraction and Isolation

Powdered *C. fragrans* (160 g) was extracted with MeOH (2 L) at room temperature for one week. The extract was filtered and concentrated *in vacuo* to yield brown residue. Precipitation of D-mannitol present in the extract was carried out by dissolving the residue in methanol. Evaporation of the remaining extract followed by suspension in water and partition with ethyl acetate gave 20 g of a residue (Figure 4.4). The latter was divided into seven fractions by column chromatography on silica gel (solvent system: hexane/ethyl acetate gradient, from 3:7 to 100% EtOAc). ODS column chromatography of the fraction 5 (solvent system: MeOH-H_2O, 9:1) afforded 10 fractions. Fraction 5-2 was applied in Sephadex CC (CH_2Cl_2_MeOH, 1:1) to give three fractions. δ-tocotrienol (103.5 mg) was obtained from preparative TLC in ODS (RP-18 F_{254} S, elution solvent: methanol) of the fraction 5-2-2.

4.6.1.2 Structural Determination

The structural determination of T3 was first described in detail by Goh and co-workers (Goh et al., 1990). Also, in this chapter, the structural elucidation of δ-tocotrienol isolated in our laboratory is taken as an example. The high resolution FAB (HRFAB) mass that displayed a quasi-molecular ion peak at 419.286 (requires, 419.20260) was in agreement with the molecular formula: $C_{27}H_{40}O_2$ of δ-tocotrienol. The nuclear magnetic resonance (NMR), one of the spectroscopic techniques used for determination of the structure of organic synthetic and organic natural product compounds, was utilized to elucidate the structure. The aromatic methyls (δ 2.1–2.25 ppm), the methyl of the chromanol ring at ca δ 1.25 ppm, the four double bond attached methyls signals at δ 1.6–1.7 ppm, the methylenic proton resonances (δ 5–5.4 ppm), and the aromatic proton signals (δ 6.2–7 ppm) are typical resonances usually observed in ^{1}H-NMR of T3s (Figure 4.6). The ^{13}C-NMR spectrum (Figure 4.7) exhibited signals for six aromatic carbons, two of which (δ 147.6 and 145.9 ppm: C-6, C-8a) bear oxygen atoms, five quaternary methyls and eight methylene including the two belonging to the chromanol ring (Table 4.2). The assignments of all carbons were based on the interpretation of the two dimensional NMR techniques: correlation heteronuclear single quantum coherence (HSQC) and heteronuclear multiple bond connectivity (HMBC) and correlation spectroscopy (COSY) (Figure 4.8).

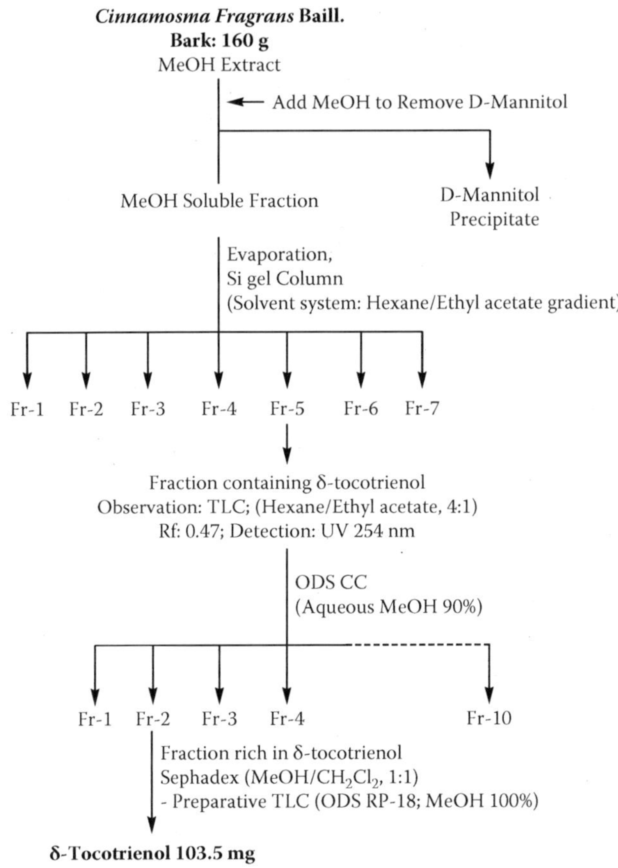

FIGURE 4.5 Isolation procedure of δ-tocotrienol.

4.7 IMPORTANCE AND USES

Research centered on large doses of oral tocotrienols *in vivo* or *in vitro* demonstrated that T3s have stronger activities than tocopherols (Packer et al. 2001). Apart from the well known vitamin proprieties of T3s, they have other biological activities.

4.7.1 Tocotrienols and Cosmetics

Human skin can be damaged by free radicals while exposed to ultraviolet (UV) in sunlight (photoaging) and to environmental chemicals. The biological activity of vitamin E has generally been associated with its antioxidant proprieties. Even though natural and synthetic forms of vitamin E have antioxidant significance, studies proved that natural forms are more potent and have a higher retention rate than their synthetic counterparts (Stone et al., 2003). Several reports describe the antioxidant activity of T3s when applied topically to skin (Packer et al., 2001). However, studies showed that the application of topical vitamin E may be detrimental to and even worsen the cosmetic appearance of a scar. Moreover, researchers concluded that vitamin E directly applied on skin does not appear to prevent scars (Baumann et al., 1999).

4.7.2 Tocotrienols and Aging

Vitamin E is important for normal function of the immune cells. Meydani and scientists from Jean Mayer USDA Human Nutrition Research Center on Aging at Tufts University, Boston, Massachu-

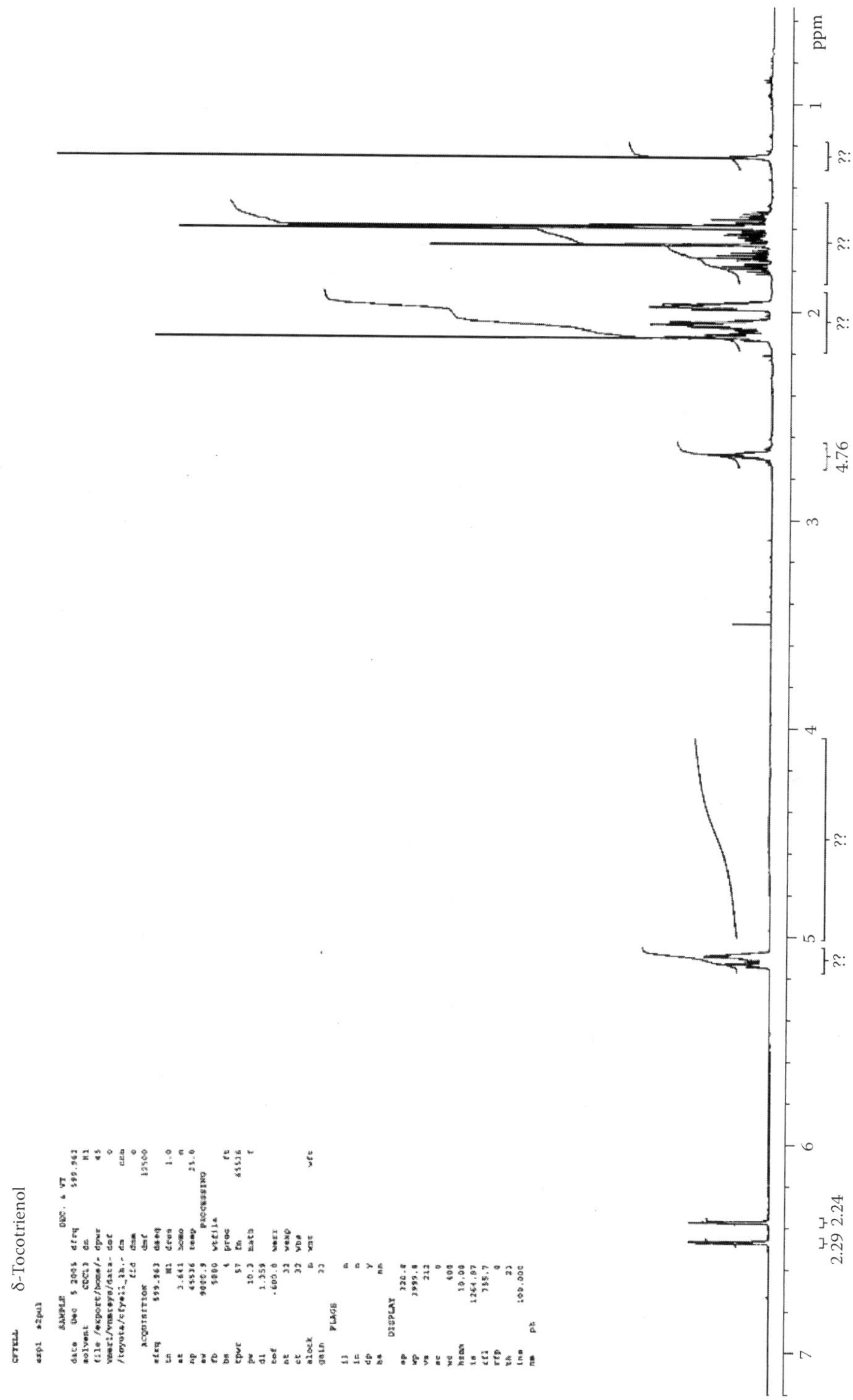

FIGURE 4.6 ^{1}H-NMR spectrum of δ-tocotrienol (in $CDCl_3$).

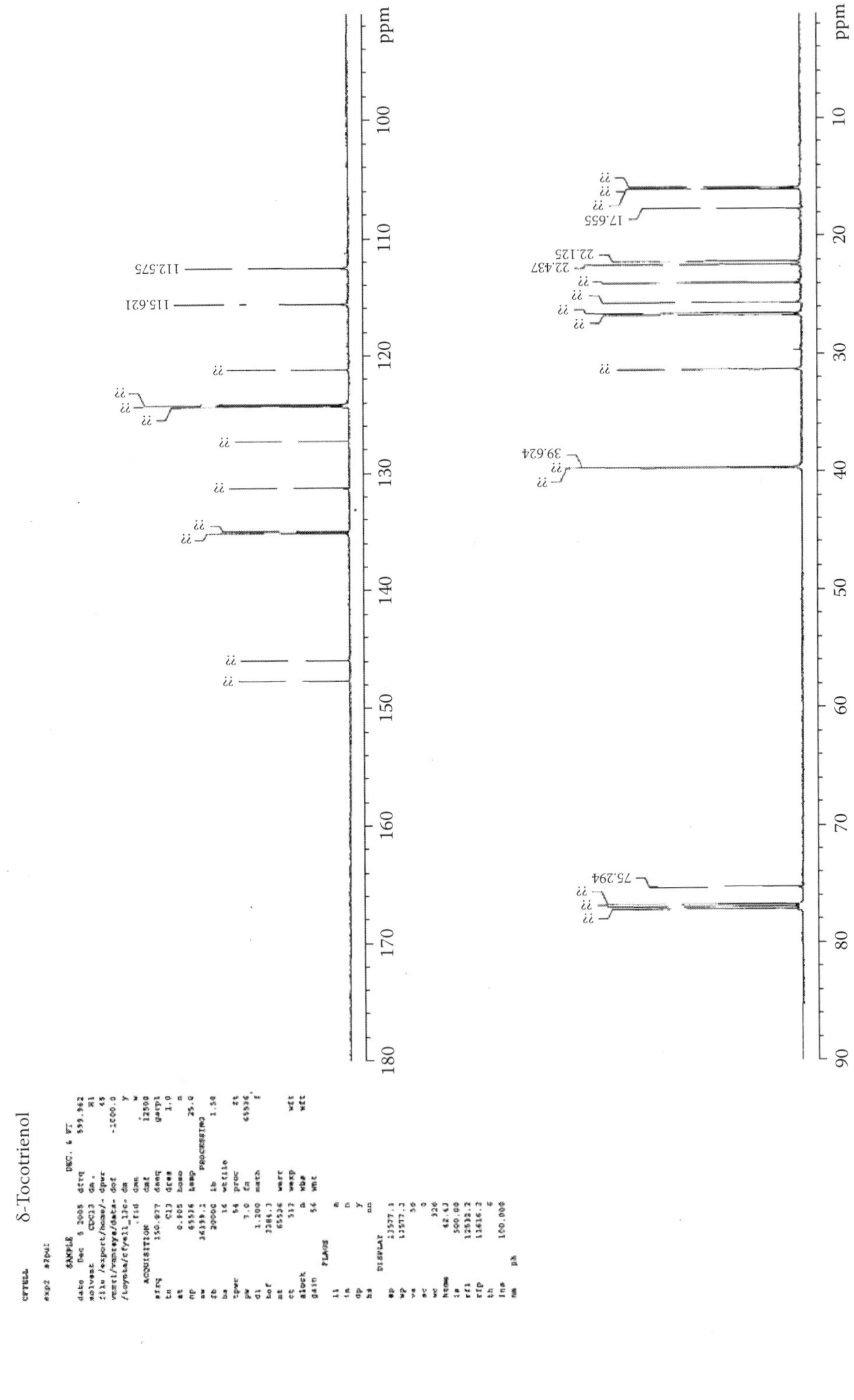

FIGURE 4.7 ^{13}C-NMR spectrum of δ-tocotrienol (in $CDCl_3$).

TABLE4. 2
^{1}H- and ^{13}C-NMR Spectral Data for δ-Tocotrienol (8, in $CDCl_3$)*

	8	
Position	H	C
2		75.3
3a	1.72 (dt, 13.4, 6.5)	31.3
3b	1.79 (dt, 13.4, 6.5)	
4	2.69 (m)	22.4
4a		121.2
5	6.37 (brd, 2)	112.5
6		147.6
7	6.47 (brd, 2)	115.6
8		127.3
8a		145.9
1'	1.98 (m)	39.6
2'	2.09 (m)	26.7
2'a	1.24 (s)	24.0
3'	5.11 (m)	124.3
4'		131.2
4'a	1.68 (s)	25.6
5'	1.98 (m)	39.6
6'	2.09 (m)	26.5
7'		124.4
8'a		134.9
8b	2.13 (s)	16.0
9'ab	1.98 (m)	39.6
10'ab	2.12 (m)	22.1
11'	5.11 (m)	124.2
12'		134.9
12'a	1.60 (s)	15.8
12'b	1.60 (s)	15.9

* Assignment based on HSQC, COSY and HMBC.

setts clearly demonstrated the molecular mechanisms, clinical implications, and immune response of vitamin E in the aged. Vitamin E supplementation above currently recommended levels has been shown to improve immune functions in the aged including delayed-type hypersensitivity skin response and antibody production in response to vaccination. The activity was mediated through increased production of interleukin (IL)-2, leading to enhanced proliferation of T cells, and through reduced production of prostaglandin E_2, a T-cell suppressive factor, as a result of a decreased peroxynitrite formation (Meydani et al., 2005).

4.7.3 Tocotrienols and Cholesterols

3-Hydroxy-3-methylglutaryl Coenzyme A (HMG-CoA) reductase (HMGR, EC 1.1.1.34) is the first rate-limiting enzyme in the isoprenoids and cholesterol synthesis. T3s side chain is thought to

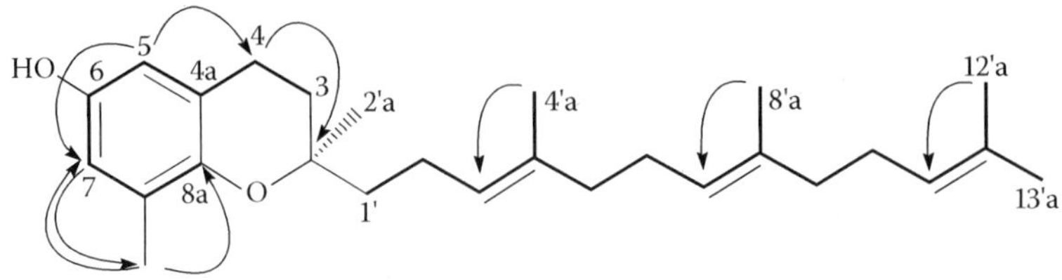

FIGURE 4.8 Important COSY (bold line) and HMBC (arrow: proton to carbon) correlations observed in compound 8.

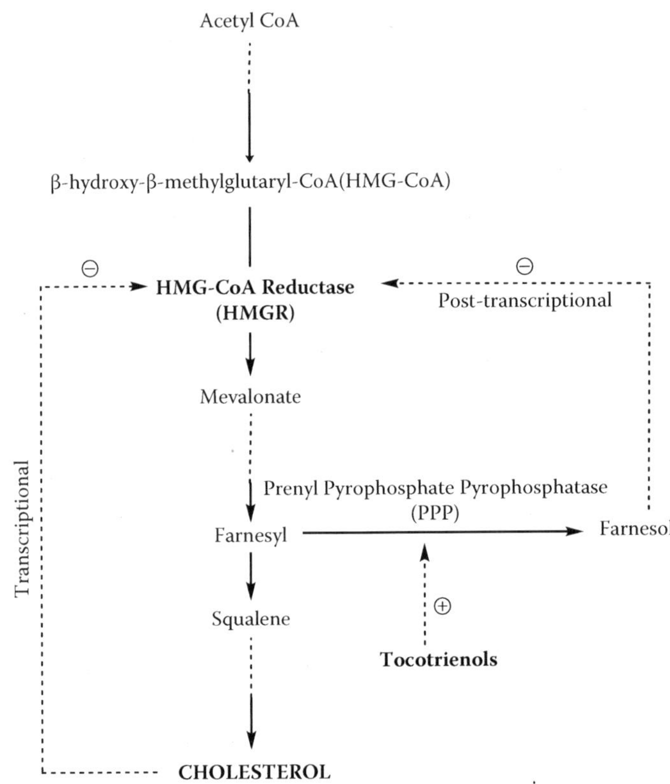

FIGURE 4.9 Mechanism of the cholesterol suppressive action of T3s.

induce prenyl pyrophosphate pyrophosphatase (PPP) to catalyze the dephosphorylation of farnesyl with a concomitant increase in cellular farnesol (Figure 4.9) (Theriault et al. 1999). The latter in turn down-regulates HMGR activity by a post-transcriptional process involving protein degradation. Noteworthy, the mechanism is different from that of cholesterol, which exerts a feedback transcriptional effect of HMGR activity.

There are several published reports on the hypocholesterolemic activity of T3s, only some of which are cited in this chapter. In 1986 Qureshi and co-workers demonstrated the cholesterol inhibitory proprieties of α-tocotrienol and its acetate derivative (Qureshi, 1986). Sixteen years later the same author reported that the suppression of serum cholesterol by the tocotrienol-rich fraction of rice bran in hypercholesterolemic human was dose-dependent, while hypercholesterolaemia was proved to be suppressed in rats (Qureshi, 2002). Furthermore, later investigations (Pearce et al., 1994) showed that T3s inhibit cholesterol-biosynthesis by involving posttranscriptional suppression of HMGR by imitating the action of putative non-sterol feedback inhibitors. The farnesyl side chain and the methyl/hydroxyl substitution are the important parts of the hypolipidemic action posttranscriptional suppression of (HMGR). The data suggest that the combination of γ-tocotrienol and α-tocopherol, as present in palm oil distillates, deserves further evaluation as a potential hypolipemic agent in hyperlipemic humans with atherogenic risk (Watkins et al. 1993).

4.7.4 Tocotrienols and Diseases

The health benefits of tocopherols have been studied extensively. However, recent findings have shown that T3s, the "vitamin E of the millennium" are responsible for the majority of the activity of vitamin E.

4.7.4.1 Tocotrienols, Diabetes and Obesity

Diabetes mellitus, the diseases that result from a deficiency or a failure of the normal action of insulin, which is dependent on the proper metabolism of the sugar in the diet, are common chronic diseases and a major contributor to the development of cardiovascular diseases. In the last decades, the number of cases of non-insulin-dependent diabetes mellitus has increased dramatically due to changes in lifestyle. Development of type 2 diabetes can be reduced by the intake of antioxidants in the diet. A T3s-rich diet decreased advanced glycosylation end-products in non diabetic rats and improved glycemic control in streptozotocin-induced diabetic rats (Wan Nazaimon and Khalid, 2002). Studies showed that risk of type 2 diabetes can be prevented by the intake of α, β, γ, δ-tocopherol, and β-tocotrienol. No data about the type 2 diabetes prevention proprieties of δ-tocotrienol are shown in the literature. Our study showed that δ-tocotrienol did not inhibit the activity of α-glucosidase enzyme (Harinantenaina et al., 2007a).

4.7.4.2 Tocotrienols and Cancer

The antioxidant proprieties of T3 are the main evidence for its anticancer activity. The superiority of T3s' chemopreventive activity compared with that of tocopherols in a rat mammary tumor model was reported (Gould et al., 1991). T3s showed proprieties of prevention of transplanted tumors chemically induced by mammary tumorigenesis, of mammal tumor and of hepatic tumor model (Komiyama et al., 1989, Sundram et al, 1989, Gould et al., 1989, Ngah et al., 1991, Rahmat et al., 1993). T3s suppress activation of early antigen expression of Epstein-barr virus in PMA-activated lymphoblastoid Raji cells growth of a human breast cancer cell line in culture (Goh et al. 1994, Nesaretnam et al, 1995). Iqbal and his group proved the suppression of 7,12-dimethylbenz[alpha]anthracene-induced carcinogenesis and diethylnitrosamine and 2-acetylaminofluorene-induced hepatocarcinogenesis in rats by tocotrienols-rich fraction isolated from rice bran oil (Iqbal et al., 2003 and 2004). Also, *in vitro* and *in vivo* studies demonstrated that the isoprenoid side chain suppressed the growth of murine B16 melanomas, and initiated apoptosis and cell-cycle arrest in human and murine tumor cells (He et al., 1997, Mo and Elson, 1999).

Naturally occurring T3s and RRR, δ-tocopherols have been proven to be effective apoptotic inducers for human breast cancer cells and in dRLh-84 hepatoma cells (Yu et al., 1999, Sakai et al. 2004). In mammary cancer cells, T3s-induced apoptosis is mediated through activation of the caspase-8 signaling pathway and is independent of caspase-9 activation (Shah et al., 2003). Studies showed that tocotrienol-rich palm oil prevented chemically induced mammary tumorigenesis in rats (Sundram et al. 1989). T3s inhibit the growth of ZR-75-1 breast cancer cells irrespective of estrogen receptor status (Nesaretnam et al. 1998 and 2000). T3s rich fraction of palm oil activated p53 modulated Bax/Bcl2 ratio and induced apoptosis independent of cell cycle association in colorectal cancer RKO cells (Agarwal et al., 2004). T3s also affect cell homeostasis which can be independent of their antioxidant activity (Nesaretnam et al., 2004). Investigation of the antiproliferative effect of T3s in PC3 and LNCaP prostate cancer cells suggests that the transformation of vitamin E to CEHC is mostly a detoxification mechanism, useful to maintain the malignant properties of prostate cancer cells (Conte et al., 2004).

4.7.4.3 Neuroprotective Effect of Tocotrienols

Studies with mice demonstrated that in contrast with tocopherols, α-tocotrienol protects against glutamate-induced neuronal death by suppressing inducible pp60 c-src kinase activation and inducible 12-lipoxygenase activation at nanomolar concentration (Sen et al., 2000, Khanna et al., 2003). Moreover, in the same paper, Sen and his group proved that α-tocotrienol provided the most potent neuroprotection among all vitamin E analogs and that the effects are independent of the antioxidant property. Osakada et al. demonstrated that among vitamin E, T3s, more precisely, α-tocotrienol, provided the most neuroprotection on cultured striatal neuron in rats (Osakada et al., 2004).

REFERENCES

Agarwal, M.K., Agarwal, M.L., Athar, M., Gupta, S. 2004. Tocotrienol-rich fraction of palm oil activates p53, modulates Bax/Bcl2 ratio and induces apoptosis independent of cell cycle association. *Cell Cycle*, 3, 205–211.

Aitzemuller, K. 1997. Antioxidative effects of Carum seeds. *J. Am. Oil. Chem. Soc.* 74. 185.

Amaral, J.S., Alves, M.R., Saebra, R.M., Oliviera, B.P. 2005. Vitamin E composition of walnuts (*Juglans regia* L.): A 3-year comparative study of different cultivars. *J. Agric. Food Chem.* 53, 5467–5472.

Amiguet, V.T., Petit, P., Ta, C.A., Nunez, R., Sanchez-Vindas, P., Alvarez, L.P., Smith, M.L., Arnason, J.T., Durst, T. 2006. Phytochemistry and antifungal properties of the newly discovered tree *Pleodendron costaricense*. *J. Nat. Prod.*, 69, 1005–1009.

Asakawa, Y. 1995. In W. Herz, G.W. Kirby, R.E, Moore, W. Steglich and Ch. Tamm, *Progress in the chemistry of organic natural product*, 65, 1–562.

d'Auzac, J., Jakob, J.L., Chrestin, H. Physiology of rubber tree latex. CRC press, Inc., Boca Raton, Florida, 1989.

Bagci, E., Karaagacli, Y. 2004. Fatty acid and tocochromanol patterns of Turkish pines. *Acta biologica cracoviensia Series Botanica*, 46, 95–100.

Baumann, L.S., Spencer, J. 1999. The effect of topical vitamin E on the cosmetic appearance of scars. *Derm. Surg.*, 25, 311–315.

Bertoli, C., Fay, L.B., Stancanelli, M., Gumy, D. Lambelet, P. 1998. Characterization of Chilean hazelnut (Genvuina avellana Mol.) seed oil. *J. Am. Oil Chem. Soc.*, 75, 1037–1040.

Cahoon, E.B., Hall, S.E, Ripp, K.G., Ganzke T.S., Hitz, W.D., Coughlan, S.J. 2003. Metabolic redesign of vitamin E biosynthesis in plants for tocotrienol production and increased antioxidant content. *Nature Biotechnol.*, 21, 1082–1087.

Chandan K.S., Khanna, S., Roy, S. 2006. Tocotrienols: Vitamin E beyond tocopherols. *Life Sci*, 78, 2088–2098.

Collakova, E., DellaPenna, D. 2001. Isolation and functional analysis of homogentisate phytyltransferase from *Synechocytis sp.* PCC 6803 and *Arabidopsis*. *Plant Physiol.* 127, 1113–1124.

Conte, C., Floridi, A., Aisa, C. et al. 2004. Gamma-tocotrienol metabolism and antiproliferative effect in prostate cancer cells. *Ann. New York Ac. Sc.* 1031: 391–394.

Crane, S., Aurore, G., Joseph, H., Mouloungui, Z., Bourgeois, P. 2005. Composition of fatty acids, triacylglycerols and unsaponifiable matter in *Calophyllum calaba* L. oil from Guadeloupe. *Phytochemistry*, 66, 1825–1831.

Dormann, P. 2003. Corn with enhanced antioxidant potential. *Nature Biotechol.*, 21, 1015–1016.

Falk, J., Krahnstover, A., Van der Kooij, T.A.W., Schlensog, M., Krupinska, K. 2004. Tocopherol and tocotrienol accumulation during development of caryopses from barley (*Hordeum vulgare* L.). *Phytochemistry*, 65, 2977–2985.

Franzen, J., Bausch, J., Glatzle, D., Wagner, E. 1991. Distribution of vitamin E in spruce seedlings and mature tree organs, and within the genus. *Phytochemistry*, 30, 147–151.

Franzen, J., Haass, M. 1991. Vitamin E content during development of some seedlings. *Phytochemistry*, 30, 2911–2913.

Goh, S.H., Hew, N.F, Ong, A.S.H., Choo, Y.M., Brumby, S. 1990. Tocotrienols from palm oil: Electron spin resonance spectra of tocotrienoxyl radicals. *J. Am. Oil Chem. Soc.*, 67, 250–254.

Goh, S.H., Hew, N.F, Norhanom, A.W. Yadav, M. 1994. Inhibition of tumor promotion by various palm-oil tocotrienols. *Inter. J. Cancer*, 57, 529–531.

Gould, M.N., Haag, J.D., Kennan, W.S., Tanner, M.A, Elson, C.E. 1991. A comparison of tocopherol and tocotrienol for the chemoprevention of chemically induced rat mammary tumors. *Am. J. Clin. Nutr.* 53 (4 Suppl.), 1068S–1070S.

Harinantenaina, L., Takahara, Y., Nishizawa, T., Kohchi, C., Soma, G.-I., Asakawa, Y. 2006. Chemical constituents of Malagasy liverworts, Part V: Prenyl bibenzyls and clerodane diterpenoids with nitric oxide inhibitory activity from *Radula appressa* and *Thysananthus spathulistipus*. *Chem. Pharm. Bull.* 54, 1046–1049.

Harinantenaina, L., Takaoka, S. 2006. Cinnafragrins A-C, dimeric and trimeric drimane sesquiterpenoids from *Cinnamosma fragrans*, and structure revision of capsicodendrin. *J. Nat. Prod.*, 69, 1193–1197.

Harinantenaina, L., Asakawa Y., De Clercq, E. 2007a. Cinnamacrins A-C, Cinnafragrin D and cytostatic metabolites with α-glucosidase inhibitory activity from *Cinnamosma macrocarpa*. *J. Nat. Prod.*, 70, 277–282.

Harinantenaina, L., Otsuka, H., Matsunami, K., Asakawa Y. 2007b. *Cinamosma madagascariensis* secondary metabolites and their α-glucosidase and aldose- reductase inhibitory activity. In preparation.

Havaux, M., Eymery, F., Porfirova, S., Rey, P., Dormann, P. 2005. Vitamin E protects against photoinhibition and photooxidative stress in *Arabidopsis thaliana*. *Plant Cell*, 17, 3451–3469.

He, L., Mo, H., Hadisusilo, S., Qureshi, A.A., Elson, C.E. 1997. Isoprenoids suppress the growth of murine B16 melanomas *in vitro* and *in vivo*. *J. Nutr.* 127, 668–674.

Horvath, G., Wessjohann, L., Bigirimana, J., Monica, H., Jansen, M., Guisez, Y., Caubergs, R., Horemans, N. 2006a. Accumulation of tocopherols and tocotrienols during seed development of grape (*Vitis vinifera* L. cv. Albert Lavallee). *Plant Physiol. Biochem.*, 44, 724–731.

Horvath, G., Wessjohann, L., Bigirimana, J., Jansen, M., Guisez, Y., Caubergs, R., Horemans, N. 2006b. Differential distribution of tocopherols and tocotrienols in photosynthetic and non-photosynthetic tissues. *Phytochemistry*, 67, 1185–1195.

Iqbal, J., Minhajuddin, M., Beg, Z.H. 2003. Suppression of 7,12-dimethylbenz[alpha] anthracene-induced carcinogenesis and hypercholesterolemia in rats by tocotrienol-rich fraction isolated from rice bran oil. *Eur. J. Canc. Prev.*, *12*, 515–520.

Iqbal, J., Minhajuddin, M., Beg, Z.H. 2004. Suppression of diethylnitrosamine and 2-acetylaminofluorene-induced hepatocarcinogenesis in rats by tocotrienol-rich fraction isolated from rice bran oil. *Eur. J. Canc. Prev.*, 13, 447–453

Khanna, S., Roy, S., Ryu, H., Bahadduri, P., Swan, P.W., Ratan, R.R., Sen, C.K. 2003. Molecular basis of vitamin E action: Tocotrienol modulates 12-lipoxygenase, a key mediator of glutamate-induced neurodegeneration. *J. Biol. Chem.*, 278, 43508–43515.

Komiyama, K., Iizuka, K., Yamaoka, M., Watanabe, H., Tsuchiya, N., Umezawa, I. 1989. Studies on the biological activity of tocotrienols. *Chem. Pharm. Bull.*, 37, 1369–1371.

Laphookhieo, S., Maneerat, W., Kiattansakul, R. 2006. Phenolic compounds from *Mammea siamensis* seeds. *Can. J. Chem.*, 84, 1546–1549.

Matthaus, B., Vosmann, K., Quoc Pham, L., Aitzemuller, K. 2003. Fatty acid and tocopherol composition of Vietnamese oilseeds. *J. Am. Oil Chem. Soc.*, 80, 1013–1020.

Merza, J., Aumond, M.C., Rondeau, D., Dumontet, V., Le Ray, A M., Seraphin D., Richomme, P. 2004. Prenylated xanthines and tocotrienols from *Garcinia virgata*. *Phytochemistry*, 65, 2915–2920.

Meydani, N.S., Han, S.N., Wu, Dayong. 2005. Vitamin E and immune response in the aged. *Imm. Rev.*, 205, 269–284.

Mo, H., Elson, C.E. 1999. Apoptosis and cell-cycle arrest in human and murine tumor cells are initiated by isoprenoids. *J. Nutr.*, 129, 804–813.

Nesaretnam, K., Guthrie, N., Chambers, A.F., Carroll, K.K. 1995. Effect of tocotrienols on the growth of a human breast cancer cell line in culture. *Lipids*, 30, 1139–1143.

Nesaretnam, K., Stephen, R., Dils, R., Darbre, P.D. 1998. Tocotrienols inhibit the growth of human breast cancer cells irrespective of estrogen receptor status. *Lipids*, 33, 461–569.

Nesaretnam, K., Dorasamy, S., Darbre, P.D. 2000. Tocotrienols inhibit the growth of ZR-75-1 breast cancer cells. *Int. J. Food Sci. and Nutr.*, 51(Suppl), S95–S103.

Nesaretnam, K., Ambra, R., Selvaduray, K.R., Radhakrishnan, A., Reimann, K., Razak, G., Virgili, F. 2004. Tocotrienol-rich fraction from palm oil affects gene expression in tumors resulting from MCF-7 cell inoculation in athymic mice. *Lipids*, 39, 459–467.

Ngah, W.Z., Jarien, Z., San, M.M., Marzuki, A., Top, G.M., Shamaan, N.A., Kadir, K.A. 1991. Effect of tocotrienols on hepatocarcinogenesis induced by 2-acetylaminofluorene in rats. *Am. J.Clin. Nutr.*, 53 (4 suppl.), 1076S–1081S.

Osakada, F., Hashino, A., Kume, T., Katsuki, H., Kaneko, S., Akaike, A. 2004. Alpha- tocotrienol provides the most potent neuroprotection among vitamin E analogs on cultures striatal neurons. *Neuropharmacology*, 47, 904–915.

Packer, L., Weber, S.U., Rimbach, G. 2001. Molecular aspects of α-Tocotrienol antioxidant action and cell signalling, *J. Nutr.*, 131, 369S–373S.

Pearce, B.C., Parker, R.A., Deason, M.E., Dischino, D.D., Gillespie, E., Qureshi, A.A, Volk, K., Wright, J.J. 1994. Inhibitors of cholesterol biosynthesis. 2. hypocholesterolemic and antioxidant activities of benzopyran and tetrahydronaphtalene analogues of the tocotrienols. *J. Med. Chem.* 37, 526–541.

Qureshi, A.A, Burger, W.C., Peterson, D.M., Elson, C.F. 1986. The structure of an inhibitor of cholesterol biosynthesis isolated from barley. *J. Biol. Chem.* 261, 10544–10550.

Qureshi, A.A, Sami, S.A., Salser, W.A, Khan, F.A. 2002. Dose dependent suppression of serum cholesterol by tocotrienol-rich fraction (TRF25) of rice bran in hypercholesterolemic humans. *Atherosclerosis.* 161, 199–207.

Rahmat, A., Ngah, W.Z., Shamaan, N.A., Gapor, A., Kadir, K.A. 1993. Long-term administration of tocotrienols and tumor marker enzyme activities during hepatocarcinogenesis in rats. *Nutrition*, 9, 229–232.

Rippert, P., Scimemi, C., Dubald, M., Matringe, M. 2004. Engineering plant shikimate pathway for production of tocotrienol and improving herbicide resistance. *Plant Physiology*, 134, 92–100.

Sakai, M., Okabe, M., Yamasaki, M., Tachibana, H., Yamada, K. 2004. Induction of apoptosis by tocotrienol in rat hepatoma dRLh-84 cells. *Anticancer Res.* 24(3a), 1683–1688.

Schultz, G., Soll, J., Fiedler, E., Schultze-Siebert, D. 1985. Synthesis of prenylquinones in chloroplasts. *Physiol. Plant.* 64, 123–129.

Serbinova, E., Kagan, V., Han, D., Packer, L. 1991. Free radical recycling and intramembrane mobility in the antioxidant properties of alpha-tocopherol and alpha-tocotrienol. *Free Rad. Biol. Med.,* 10, 263–275.

Shah, S., Gapor, A., Sylvester, P.W. 2003. Role of caspase-8 activation in mediating vitamin E-induced apoptosis in murine mammary cancer cells. *Nutr. Cancer*, 45, 236–246.

Soll, J., Kemmerling, M., Shultz, G. 1980. Tocopherols and plastoquinones synthesis in spinach chloroplasts subfractions. *Arch. Biochem. Biophys.* 204, 544–550.

Stone, W.L., LeClair, I., Ponder, T., Baggs, G., Reis, B.B. 2003. Infants discriminate between natural and synthetic vitamin E. *Am. J. Clin. Nutr.* 77, 899–906.

Sundram, K., Khor, H.T., Ong, A.S., Pathmanathan, R. 1989. Effect of dietary palm oil on mammary carcinogenesis in female rats induced by 7,12-dimethylbenz(a)anthracene. *Cancer Res.*, 49, 1447–1451.

Teixeira, J.S.R., Moreira, L.M., Guedes, M.L.S., Cruz, F.G. 2006. A new biphenyl from *Clusia melchiorii* and a new tocotrienol from *C. obdeltifolis. J. Braz. Chem. Soc.*, 17, 812–815.

Theriault, A., Chao, J-T., Wang, Q., Gapor, A., Adeli, K. 1999. Tocotrienol: A review of its therapeutic potential. *Clin. Biochem.*, 32, 309–319.

Wan Nazaimoon, W.M., Khalid, B.A. 2002. Tocotrienols-rich diet decreases advanced glycosylation endproducts in non-diabetic rats and improves glycemic control in streptozotocin-induced diabetic rats. *Malaysian J. Path.* 24, 77–82.

Watkins, T., Lenz, P., Gapor, A., Struck, M., Tomeo A., Bierenbaum M. 1993. γ-tocotrienol as a hypocholesterolemic and antioxidant agent in rats fed atherogenic diets. *Lipids*, 28, 1113–1118.

Yu, W., Simmons-Menchaca, M., Gapor, A., Sanders, B.G., Kline, K. 1999. Induction of apoptosis in human breast cancer cells by tocopherols and tocotrienols. *Nutr. Cancer,* 33, 26–32.

5 Vitamin E: Natural vs. Synthetic

Amy Kosowski and Dallas L. Clouatre

CONTENTS

5.1 INTRODUCTION

Discovered in 1922, Vitamin E was once thought to be a single molecule, namely alpha-tocopherol (α-TOH). Recent research, however, has shown that Vitamin E is actually a family of molecules, consisting of the tocopherols and the tocotrienols, all of which are important for defending the body against free radical attack, or oxidative stress. New evidence demonstrates that, although α-tocopherol is the most potent antioxidant of the tocopherol sub-family, the other members of the vitamin E family have their own unique functions, conferring equally important health benefits.

Aside from the issues stemming from the complex interplay of the eight natural vitamin E isomers, the use of synthetic forms of vitamin E in clinical studies by the scientific community, as well as by the general public, adds yet other complications. Because synthetic vitamin E supplements do not have the same biological activity as the natural vitamin E isomers, it is difficult to interpret these results alongside those from studies on dietary vitamin E, as well as those from studies using natural vitamin E supplements. Unfortunately, epidemiological studies, dietary intervention studies and other clinical studies tend to all be classified under the same umbrella of generic "vitamin E." Obviously, this practice has led to contradictory study results and a gross misunderstanding of the effects and functions of vitamin E in the body.

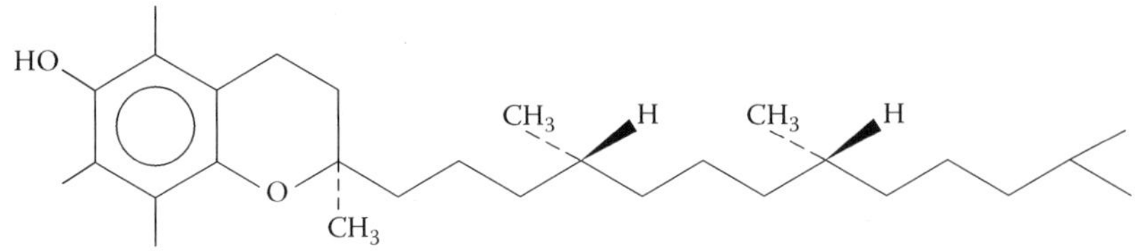

FIGURE 5.1 d-alpha-tocopherol.

This discrepancy has only recently been recognized in the literature. Attempts are currently being made to study these different forms and their specific effects. The use of synthetic forms of vitamin E is also being reconsidered. In addition, researchers are finally shifting away from their bias in favor of α-tocopherol and are recognizing the other tocopherols and the tocotrienols for their anti-inflammatory, cardioprotective and anti-cancer activities.

This chapter explores the different actions of the vitamin E isoforms, both natural and synthetic, as well as their utility in the prevention and mitigation of disease.

5.2 BACKGROUND

5.2.1 Basics of History and Structure

Since its discovery in 1922, vitamin E has had a mixed reception by the scientific community. Sometimes referred to disparagingly as the "sex vitamin" because of its role in the reproductive function of certain animals, such as rats—but not humans—this vitamin continues to elude definitive descriptions of its mechanisms of action in important areas of physiology.[1] Classic in this regard is the still raging controversy over vitamin E's place in the treatment of cardiovascular disease (CVD), for which it first was promoted as a therapy in the 1940s.[2] Despite a relative lack of clarity regarding its biochemical roles, the Food and Nutrition Board of the National Research Council established vitamin E as an essential vitamin in 1968. The consensus is that vitamin E is a major chain-breaking antioxidant that provides defense against lipid oxidation and protects cell membranes from free radical attack.

Vitamin E is the collective name for a family of fat-soluble compounds and generically includes all entities that exhibit the biological activity of d-alpha-tocopherol. Aside from d-alpha-tocopherol, there exist also beta-, gamma- and delta-tocopherol. Closely related members of the family include alpha-, beta-, gamma- and delta-tocotrienol. Natural vitamin E is a mixture of tocopherols and tocotrienols (α-, β-, γ-, δ-tocopherol, and α-, β-, γ-, δ-tocotrienol). Most research has focused on alpha-tocopherol, but the other isomers are gaining attention, especially gamma-tocopherol and the tocotrienols. Common to all the isomers is a chromanic nucleus (6-chromanol) with an aliphatic side chain (C16). The side chain is saturated for tocopherols (with three chiral centers in the RRR stereoisomeric configuration) and unsaturated for tocotrienols (only one chiral center with three double bonds at 3', 7', and 11' positions).[3]

5.3 FORMS OF VITAMIN E

Vitamin E chemistry, unlike the vitamin's role in physiology, is well worked out. The number of methyl groups and the pattern of methylation of the chromanol ring primarily distinguish the tocopherols and tocotrienols. Alpha-tocopherol and tocotrienol have three methyl groups, beta- and gamma-tocopherol and tocotrienol have two methyl groups, whereas delta-tocopherol and tocotrienol have one methyl group. Independent of dietary sources of vitamin E, only alpha-tocopherol is actively maintained in human plasma due to the fact that the hepatic alpha-tocopherol transfer protein (alpha-TTP) selectively recognizes alpha-tocopherol and mediates its secretion into the circulation.[4] This fact often is interpreted to mean that alpha-tocopherol is the most important member of the family in human physiology. However, especially in light of how well vitamin E is conserved by the body, it might mean simply that there is a minimum level of alpha-tocopherol absolutely required by physiology without indicating an order of importance beyond this minimum.

Unlike other vitamins, synthetic forms of vitamin E are not biochemically equivalent to natural forms because their molecular structures are not identical. Synthesized alpha-tocopherol (*all-rac*-alpha-tocopherol, [2, 5, 7, 8-tetramethyl-2RS-(4'RS, 8'RS, 12 trimethyltridecyl)-6-chromanol]) is not identical to the naturally occurring form, *RRR*-alpha-tocopherol [2, 5, 7, 8-tetramethyl-2R-(4'R, 8'R, 12 trimethyltridecyl)-6-chromanol]). Of the eight stereoisomers present in *all-rac*-alpha-tocopherol (*RRR-, RRS-, RSR-, RSS-, SRR-, SSR-, SRS-, SSS*), only one is found in nature and accounts for 12.5% of the total. The other seven isomers have different molecular structures possessing biological activities ranging from 21–90%.

High-dose supplementation with alpha-tocopherol alone depletes plasma and tissue gamma-tocopherol, whereas supplementation with gamma-tocopherol increases levels of both forms of E.[5] This finding is important because natural vitamin E demonstrates a higher bioavailability than do the synthetic forms. Studies in both animals and humans show a strong preference by the body for natural forms over synthetic and that natural forms are retained significantly longer. Animals preferentially incorporate *RRR*- over *all-rac*-alpha-tocopherol into milk, plasma and tissues.[6–8] It should be noted, however that the preference for natural vitamin E has been shown to be even stronger in humans than in animals.[9–12]

Two plentiful naturally occurring sources of d-alpha-tocopherol (*RRR*-alpha-tocopherol) are wheat germ oil and sunflower seed oil. However, much of the d-alpha-tocopherol found in supplements is derived from unrefined soy oil. Soy oil contains mainly gamma-tocopherol, hence a synthetic process is necessary to convert this into alpha-tocopherol, which is to say that alpha-tocopherol derived from soy oil is a semi-synthetic product properly termed "natural-source" alpha-tocopherol rather than "natural" alpha-tocopherol.

5.3.1 d-alpha-Tocopheryl Acetate and dl-alpha-Tocopheryl Acetate

Also known as *RRR*-alpha-tocopheryl acetate and 2R, 4', 8'R-d-alpha-tocopheryl acetate, this is the acetate ester of natural-source d-alpha-tocopherol obtained by the vacuum steam distillation and acetylation of edible vegetable oil products.

An all-synthetic form of alpha-tocopherol is dl-alpha-tocopheryl acetate, which is produced by reacting racemic isophytol with trimethylhydroquinone to form dl-alpha-tocopherol and then acetylating the product to yield dl-alpha-tocopheryl acetate. Eight stereoisomers are formed in the synthesis in equal amounts; only one of these is *RRR-alpha*-tocopherol. It and one other isomer are retained in the body by action of the alpha-tocopherol transfer protein (alpha-TTP).

5.3.2 d-alpha-Tocopherol Succinate and dl-alpha-Tocopherol Succinate

This is the succinate ester of natural-source d-alpha-tocopherol. It is insoluble in water, but is water-dispersible. It is the "dry" vitamin E sold in stores. Ingested d-alpha-tocopheryl succinate largely is hydrolyzed to d-alpha-tocopherol before absorption in the small intestine. dl-alpha-tocopheryl succinate is an all-synthetic form.

5.3.3 Mixed Tocopherols

Mixed tocopherols are mixtures of the natural tocopherol homologues: d-alpha-tocopherol, d-beta-tocopherol, d-gamma-tocopherol and d-delta-tocopherol present in their unesterified forms. Two types of mixed tocopherol products are available: high-alpha-mixed-tocopherols and low-alpha-mixed-tocopherols. The former contain mainly d-alpha-tocopherol with much smaller amounts of beta-, gamma- and delta-tocopherols. The latter contain gamma-tocopherol as the major tocopherol homologue.

5.4 VITAMIN E AGAINST OXIDATIVE STRESS IN DEGENERATIVE DISEASES?

The connection between antioxidants and health constitutes one of the most successful conjectures in modern science. Theories linking oxidative damage to aging and to various disease states date back only to the 1940s. Johan Bjorksten, a research chemist working for a branch of Eastman Kodak, first observed a similarity between the aging of film materials and the aging of human tissues in 1941. He surmised that the common point is the damage to both by free radicals and that in living organisms this damage results in the cross-linking of protein molecules, including the RNA and DNA strands, which reproduce all the proteins in the body. In the 1950s Denham Harman of the University of Nebraska put theory into practice by experimenting with the addition of antioxidants and other free radical deactivators to the diets of laboratory mice.

Research on vitamin E has tended to focus on its antioxidant actions in part because tocopherol in some ways is not a typical vitamin. For instance, it does not function as a cofactor. Moreover, cases of frank deficiency are rare. Deficiency is found in genetic abnormalities in which the alpha-tocopherol transfer protein is absent or defective. Likewise, deficiency is found in fat malabsorption syndromes, protein-calorie malnutrition, premature infants and hemodialysis patients. In adults, the manifestation of the usual hallmark of vitamin E deficiency, peripheral neuropathy, takes years to appear. Unlike what is normally expected of a vitamin, vitamin E is not associated with a disease with rapidly developing or unique symptoms.

Antioxidant roles for vitamin E are numerous. It is the major chain-breaking antioxidant in bodily tissues and the first line of defense against lipid peroxidation, it protects cell membranes at early stages of free radical attack, it is a free radical scavenger and interacts with other antioxidant nutrients within an antioxidant network, it inhibits the conversion of nitrites to nitrosamines.[13–16] These mechanisms and others suggest that vitamin E should be protective against diseases linked to oxidative stress.

Work undertaken over the last two to three decades initially appeared to support a role for vitamin E in reducing oxidative stress in a number of conditions, thereby indicating a mechanism for preventing or mitigating degenerative diseases. For instance, researchers had hoped that the discovery that vitamin E is the primary antioxidant found in circulating lipoproteins could be married to the hypothesis that antioxidants protect against atherosclerosis by limiting the oxidation of low-density lipoproteins in the arterial wall and thus prevent the pathological accumulation of plaque. Other oxidation-related mechanisms were proposed for the inhibition of carcinogenesis. However, unequivocal benefits at this late date have yet to be demonstrated. Extensive trials lasting even 6 years and more have yet to demonstrate that supplementation with vitamin E significantly reduces overall cardiovascular events or cancer. After so many failures, as one editorial title put it, "Is There Any Hope for Vitamin E?".[17]

5.5 VITAMIN E ON TRIAL

5.5.1 The Wrong E?

Findings from long-term studies that "in patients with vascular disease or diabetes mellitus, long-term vitamin E supplementation does not prevent cancer or major cardiovascular events and may increase the risk for heart failure," would seem to throw cold water not just on the antioxidant hypothesis of disease prevention, but upon vitamin E, as well.[18] Negative results of the breadth now being reported suggest that the whole paradigm is wrong, that the method of implementation remains inadequate to match the conditions under consideration or, perhaps, that protection (by vitamin E) depends on intake levels and other factors tailored to specific populations for specific circumstances.

One version of the third option is that the wrong vitamin E has been used in most clinical trials to date. A theme common to recent research findings is that members of the vitamin E family other than alpha-tocopherol are more protective against a wide range of physiologic deteriorations than is the substance classically treated as representing the entire family. Two hypotheses present themselves as explanations as to why natural vitamin E plausibly might be expected to be more effective than the synthetic vitamin. The first is that synthetic E, as is not true of other synthesized vitamins, for the most part consists of compounds not found in nature, hence fails to fulfill vitamin E's many possible roles in the body. The second hypothesis is that one or more of the seven members of the vitamin E family that are present in nature, but not in synthetic vitamin E, possess special qualities of their own not fully replicated by alpha-tocopherol, whether from natural or synthetic sources. These two explanations, quite obviously, are not mutually exclusive.

5.5.2 Complex Clinical and Epidemiological Findings

The hypothesis that vitamin E supplementation might significantly reduce the incidence and severity of various disease conditions associated with aging was not born of pure theory. Instead, substantial epidemiological trials strongly supported the likelihood of benefits, for instance, in the area of cardiovascular health.[19,20] These strong observational results were matched by bodies of *in vitro* and experimental evidence that appeared to support the basic premise that reductions in oxidative and free radical damage should lead, likewise, to reduced physiological decrements in a variety of conditions. The great surprise was that long-term clinical trials failed to support the antioxidant hypothesis. This was true not just in the case of vitamin E, but also with vitamin C, beta-carotene and a number of other antioxidants.

In each of the following conditions, different members of the vitamin E family, which is to say, "natural" vitamin E, usually have shown success even though alpha-tocopherol, almost always in the synthetic form, has yielded unremarkable results or even negative findings. From the perspective of the clinician and the experimental researcher, the first step in evaluating the relationship between natural and synthetic vitamin E is to determine that sufficient evidence exists to support a distinction in outcomes. Only if clinical and experiment results indicate substantial differences in outcomes does it become worthwhile to attempt to distinguish more fully the mechanisms involved.

5.5.2.1 Cardiovascular Disease

Cardiovascular disease (CVD) is the major degenerative disease in much of the world. The hypothesis that links vitamin E to the prevention of CVD postulates that the oxidation of unsaturated lipids in the low-density lipoprotein (LDL) particle initiates a complex sequence of events that leads to the development of atherosclerotic plaque (Pryor, 2000).[21] Evidence is strong for antioxidant benefits against CVD based on dietary intakes (Gaziano, 2004).[22] However, clinical trials supplementing antioxidant vitamins have yielded conflicting results (Riccioni, 2007).[23]

The report card is not entirely one of failure. Despite the fact that the authors play down the benefit with regard to cardiovascular deaths, there was a significant 24% reduction in CVD mortality over a period of over 10 years in the recently reported Women's Health Study in subjects taking 600 IU alpha-tocopherol (supposedly "natural source," but not further defined) every other day vs. placebo (Leeet al., 2005).[24] Still, cardiovascular events were *not* reduced and neither was the overall rate of death.

These findings should be compared with those from the U.S. Nurses' Health Study and the U.S. Health Professionals' Follow-up Study, which found 34% and 39% reductions, respectively, in the risk of having a cardiac event for those taking vitamin E supplements. Benefits were found in the case of those who took daily supplements of vitamin E in doses of 100 IUs or greater for at least 2 years, which is in line with the accepted dictum that benefits usually take at least 2 years to manifest in cardiovascular treatments. In contrast, the Iowa Women's Health Study found only vitamin E from food, not from supplements, was associated with fewer cardiac events.[25] Similar results emerged from a study lasting 7 years involving 34,486 post-menopausal women. That study showed that the amount of vitamin E supplied in the diet, predominantly gamma-tocopherol but, again, not supplemental alpha-tocopherol, was inversely correlated to deaths from CVD.[26]

One often observed problem with prospective studies of this type is that the benefits observed likely reflect healthier overall habits of self-selected individuals with, in this case, supplement intake as a marker rather than a cause. Another confounding factor is the specter that vitamin E (again, alpha-tocopherol) supplementation might reduce mortality rates only in those not already suffering from severe cardiovascular disease, yet produce negative results in those gravely ill.[27] Such an outcome already was suggested in the mid-1990s by the Cambridge Heart Antioxidant Study (CHAOS), which randomly assigned patients with proven coronary atherosclerosis to a treatment group receiving either 400 to 800 IU of vitamin E (natural alpha-tocopherol) daily or to a control group. There was a 47% reduction in total myocardial infarction, both fatal and nonfatal, in those who took either 400 IU or 800 IU of vitamin E daily, yet there actually was a trend toward greater mortality in those taking vitamin E.[28]

The case against the benefits for vitamin E supplementation is hardly conclusive, however, inasmuch as the form of the vitamin preponderantly used in the trials has been synthetic alpha-tocopherol and, in the few trials in which it was "natural," only the alpha-tocopherol form was used. No clinical trials to date have compared a mixed-tocopherol supplement with alpha-tocopherol alone. Nevertheless, several mechanisms are available to explain conflicting findings based upon total dietary vitamin E intake and supplementation with alpha-tocopherol alone. For instance, as CVD has a significant inflammatory aspect, the fact that excessive intakes of alpha-tocopherol are pro-oxidant and perhaps pro-inflammatory, whereas gamma-tocopherol is anti-inflammatory, provides an accessible explanation for the observed results.

Most observational studies based on the vitamin E content of the diet, which of necessity report on the full spectrum of natural vitamin E, support a heart-protective association. The amount of gamma-tocopherol found in plasma per se has not been shown to be protective.[29] This may be misleading because soybean oil, a major source of gamma-tocopherol in the diet, is also the primary starting point for the production of hydrogenated fats, and hence trans-fats, which are known factors in cardiovascular disease.[30] A different story emerges if the ratio of vitamin E fractions is considered. The ratio of alpha-tocopherol to gamma-tocopherol is higher in subjects with cardiovascular disease than in those without.[31,32] These findings support the contention that a true dietary spectrum of vitamin E and family members other than alpha-tocopherol are likely to be heart-protective despite the null clinical results with alpha-tocopherol.

5.5.2.2 Cancer

Similar to CVD, current general opinion is that overall scientific evidence does not support claims for protection against cancers through elevated intakes of vitamin E.[33] Not just supplement trials, but also direct physiologic measures have disappointed. Studies of plasma levels of tocopherols and several cancers, such as breast cancer, often have failed to yield significance.[34]

Nevertheless, there have been notable exceptions to the standard position. The Alpha-Tocopherol, Beta-Carotene Cancer Prevention (ATBC) Study demonstrated a 32% reduction in prostate cancer incidence in smokers in response to daily supplementation with alpha-tocopherol as 50 mg per day synthetic alpha-tocopheryl acetate.[35] Significant prevention also was found in the case of colorectal cancer.[36] A recent analysis by the same group found that higher serum levels of both alpha- and gamma-tocopherol were positively associated with protection from prostate cancer and that supplemental alpha-tocopherol increased this protection.[37] In this long-running Finnish study, vitamin E has not been reported to be protective against lung, pancreatic or urinary tract cancers.

In one large nested case control study of prostate cancer, statistically significant protective associations for high levels of alpha-tocopherol were observed only when gamma-tocopherol concentrations were high.[38] The meaning of this is not self-evident. In plasma, alpha-tocopherol will always be the major fraction due to the actions of the alpha-tocopherol transfer protein. Likewise, there is potential transformation from gamma- into alpha-tocopherol, which obviously would be a distorting factor in blood level tests.[39] Moreover, there is a problem in using North American and European data side by side as a result of different E fractions predominating in the diets. The U.S. diet is higher in gamma-tocopherol and the European diet is higher in natural alpha-tocopherol due to differences in oil sources.[40] As noted already, it is also necessary to factor in the greater use of hydrogenated oils, and hence greater trans-fat content, of the American diet concomitant with its greater gamma-tocopherol intake. Trans-fats are not univocally active as risk factors in all cancers. Even the particular chain lengths of trans-fatty acid may prove to be of varying importance in the development of different cancers.

With these various caveats in mind, it is quite possible that there is an outsized and positive role for natural vitamin E in protecting against a number of cancers. A *prima facie* case can be made for maintaining that at least one component in natural vitamin E, gamma-tocopherol, may be useful for the protection against prostate and aerodigestive tract cancers (cancers of the combined organs and tissues of the respiratory tract and the upper part of the digestive tract). Two studies of serum levels of gamma-tocopherol found these to be significantly inversely related to prostate cancer and a third found a trend in the same direction. Significant protection, likewise, was found in the case of aerodigestive tract cancers.[41] One early study found that women who consumed the most vitamin E from food sources, suggesting predominantly gamma-tocopherol, had a 60% reduction in the risk of breast cancer compared with women with the lowest consumption. Curiously, when total vitamin E intake was considered, thus including supplements presumably supplying alpha-tocopherol (indeed, most likely from synthetic sources), the risk of breast cancer was reduced by only 30%.[42] In any event, other epidemiological studies show that an increased dietary intake of vitamin E, mainly in the form of gamma-tocopherol, appears to be protective against breast, cervical and colon cancers.[43–47]

Because data on the role of vitamin E in cancer are drawn from such disparate study types, disparate dietary backgrounds and disparate types of E itself, it is worthwhile to look briefly at why results might vary so broadly. Protection against cancers is obviously very complex. For instance, protective nutrients may act directly by reducing the viability of tumor cells or indirectly by improving immune function. In an animal model, immune response was maximized by an intake of vitamin E greater than 50 mg/kg, whereas normal weight and growth required only 7.5 mg/kg (Bendichet al., 1986).[48]

The response of cell receptors that control cancer viability to different forms of vitamin E is similarly wide ranging. Tocopherols and other antioxidants may inhibit colon cancer by decreasing the formation of mutagens arising from the free radical oxidation of fecal lipids as well as by "non-antioxidant" mechanisms. In another animal model in which oxidative stress was increased by iron overload, rats fed gamma-tocopherol-supplemented diets had lower levels of fecal lipid hydroperoxides than rats fed the alpha-tocopherol-supplemented diets. Significantly, gamma-tocopherol was far better at upregulating peroxisome proliferator-activated receptor-gamma (PPAR-gamma) in this model, indicating better protection against colon cancer. In tests of apoptosis, treatment with RRR-gamma-tocopherol resulted in significant cell death for all colon cancer cell lines tested, whereas RRR-alpha-tocopherol did not.[49,50]

There is variation in the response of different cancer cell lines to different vitamin E preparations. In *in vitro* tests against estrogen-responsive MCF7 and estrogen-nonresponsive MDA-MB-435 human breast cancer cell lines in culture, naturally occurring tocotrienols and RRR-delta-tocopherol were effective apoptotic inducers whereas the other tocopherols (alpha-, beta-, and gamma-) and the acetate derivative of RRR-alpha-tocopherol (RRR-alpha-tocopheryl acetate) were ineffective.[51] Similarly, vitamin E succinate (RRR-alpha-tocopheryl succinate), but not RRR-alpha-tocopherol, can induce breast cancer cells, but not normal cells, to undergo apoptosis.[52] Curiously, in prostate cancer cell lines, it is gamma-tocopherol that most actively induces apoptosis, along with delta-tocopherol, tocotrienols and vitamin E succinate; RRR-alpha-tocopherol is inactive.[53–55] The predominant failure of even the natural form of alpha-tocopherol to yield benefits in these experiments, whereas various other natural isoforms were active, has implications for clinical trials conducted with conditions such as heart disease.

5.5.2.3 Alzheimer's Disease

Alzheimer's disease studies present a microcosm of the difficulties in determining the impact of vitamin E in preventing a condition plausibly held to be attributable to oxidative stress. Dutch researchers in 2002 published their finding that a high dietary intake of vitamin C and vitamin E may lower the risk of Alzheimer's disease.[56] Other researchers, likewise, found a reduced risk of Alzheimer's disease in subjects who supplemented with a combination of vitamins C and E.[57] Looking again at the Dutch study population, the argument for oxidative stress as an agent was strengthened by data that plasma levels of inflammatory proteins are increased before the clinical onset of dementia, Alzheimer's disease and vascular dementia.[58] Despite such positive data regarding dietary intakes of antioxidants and plausible mechanisms, reviewers of the body of available data typically conclude that there is not enough evidence from large well-designed studies to promote the use of vitamin E in Parkinson's disease, cataract, and Alzheimer's disease.[59]

Positive reports of benefits of vitamin E and other antioxidants for the prevention of the development of Alzheimer's disease usually, although not universally, are linked to dietary intakes, which is to say, natural vitamin E and the family of vitamin E compounds. In contrast, supplementation with synthetic alpha-tocopherol usually has not been associated with benefits.[60,61] These results suggest that the form of vitamin E, synthetic and limited to alpha-tocopherol vs. natural, consisting of a full complement of isoforms, is crucial. Researchers who have examined this hypothesis, in fact, have come to just this conclusion: tocopherol forms other than alpha-tocopherol alone may be important in the association of vitamin E intake and protection against developing Alzheimer's disease.[62]

5.5.2.4 Parkinson's Disease

Vitamin E's possible beneficial role in reducing the risk or altering the course of Parkinson's disease is strikingly similar to that observed in Alzheimer's disease. On the one hand, three large clinical studies of tocopherol (2 observational, 1 prospective randomized) reviewed in a recent paper failed to exhibit any benefit.[63] On the other hand, high dietary intakes of vitamin E (natural vitamin E) appear to reduce the risk of Parkinson's disease.[64,65] Of course, it cannot be ruled out definitively in this or in most other instance of protection by dietary vitamin E that a major source of the benefits observed could have been affected by other constituents in the diet for which vitamin E served as a marker.[66]

5.5.2.5 Arthritis

Osteoarthritis involves significant oxidative stress, albeit there is no agreement as to the role of such stress in either the etiology or the treatment of this condition. Higher oxygen-free-radical production, as evidenced by increased malonyldialdehyde and decreased glutathione, ascorbic acid, vitamin E and catalase activity, suggests a role for oxidative stress in osteoarthritis.[67] There is evidence that a high intake of antioxidants, especially vitamin C, may reduce the risk of cartilage loss and disease progression, yet the level of intake of antioxidant nutrients may not influence the rate of incidence.[68] Dietary assessment of patients with rheumatoid and osteoarthritis supports the contention that a marginal inadequacy of a number of nutrients, including vitamin E, may help to perpetuate these disease conditions.[69] However, randomized clinical trials testing the efficacy of vitamin E as a treatment for osteoarthritis and inflammatory arthritis have yielded contradictory results. According to one recent review, two shorter-term studies comparing supplementation with placebo were positive, whereas two longer-term studies were negative and two other trials suggested equivalence between vitamin E and diclofenac in the treatment of osteoarthritis.[70] Alpha-tocopherol is the form of vitamin E used in the trials reviewed. Presently, there is inadequate data available to support arguments either for or against natural vitamin E in this area.

5.5.2.6 Diabetes

Oxidative stress has been suggested to play a role in the development of diabetes, hypertension and vascular dysfunction. Moreover, oxidative stress not only is associated with the complications of diabetes, but also is linked to insulin resistance. *In vitro* models show that an increase in reactive oxygen species and free radicals can lead to the activation of multiple serine kinase cascades or to the inhibition of protein tyrosine phosphatases. These are normal signaling components of the cells that can become dysregulated by chronic or excessive exposure to reactive compounds. Dysregulation is a common feature in diabetes type 2.

Vitamin E has demonstrated benefits in areas such as insulin sensitivity and glucose disposal in many, but not all studies. One common distinguishing feature between trials indicating no benefit with vitamin E supplementation and those showing benefit is dosage level. An intake of alpha-tocopherol at the rate of 200 IU/day for 27 weeks, for instance, was not found to benefit insulin or other tested parameters.[71] Contrarily, trials supplementing vitamin E at the rate of 800 mg or more per day routinely demonstrate improvements in metabolic control in type 2 diabetics.[72,73]

Epidemiologically, vitamin E intake is significantly associated with a reduced risk of type 2 diabetes, with intakes of alpha-, gamma- and delta-tocopherol and beta-tocotrienol all inversely related to a risk of type 2 diabetes.[74] Considerable evidence exists to support roles for vitamin E family members other than alpha-tocopherol in protecting against diabetes and its complications. A mechanism for protection of insulin-secreting cells against functional inhibition by nitric oxide has been demonstrated for gamma-tocopherol.[75] Both human and animal data, similarly, support roles for the tocotrienols in reducing insulin resistance and improving glycemic control.[76,77] Mixed tocopherol supplementation in one trial proved superior to pure alpha-tocopherol for reducing stimulated neutrophil leukotriene B(4) production. However, it is important to note that dosage level is important. This trial used 500 mg/day, which appears to approach a lower limit for benefits. In addition, in patients with well-controlled diabetes, the study suggested that benefits in the area of reduced inflammation may be small.[78]

Studies have indicated that supplementing pure alpha-tocopherol may exert a negative effect on vitamin E metabolism as a whole and therefore, a diet rich in natural vitamin E may be more beneficial. For example, supplementing only with alpha-tocopherol in a clinical setting decreased red blood cell gamma-tocopherol, whereas supplementing with mixed tocopherols increased both serum alpha tocopherol and serum and cellular gamma-tocopherol.[79] Furthermore, in a cellular model, the inflammatory molecule nitric oxide inhibits insulin secretion and only gamma-tocopherol, but not alpha-tocopherol, was able to partially prevent this damage.[80]

5.5.2.7 Cataracts

Interest in preventing lens nuclear opacification has led to a number of trials examining the effects of antioxidant supplementation. The pattern of results is a familiar one. Studies utilizing vitamin E used alpha-tocopherol and often reported insignificant results. Even at an intake of 500 I.U. daily for 4 years, a prospective, randomized, double-masked, placebo-controlled clinical trial determined that the vitamin did not reduce the incidence of or progression of nuclear, cortical or posterior subcapsular cataracts.[81] Similarly, in another blinded trial, a high-dose formulation of vitamin C (500 mg/day), vitamin E (alpha-tocopherol, 400 I.U./day), and beta-carotene (15 mg/day) in a relatively well-nourished older adult population had no apparent effect on the 7-year risk of development or progression of age-related lens opacities or visual acuity loss.[82]

Such negative findings are at variance with positive findings from similarly large trials that tracked results with individuals who freely chose to supplement with antioxidant vitamins. In one such observational study of regular users of multivitamin supplements, the risk of nuclear opacification was reduced by one third and in regular users of vitamin E supplements and persons with higher plasma levels of vitamin E, the risk was reduced by approximately half.[83] Positive findings are fairly typical of long-term observational studies on vitamin E supplementation and cataract.[84]

Inasmuch as no studies have been performed with natural vitamin E or with other vitamin E components, no strong conclusions can be drawn as to the value of natural vs. synthetic E with regard to cataracts. Still, the positive observational studies suggest that other dietary factors self-selected in the vitamin supplement-using populations are at work and of major significance.

5.5.3 Antioxidant, Pro-Oxidant or Cell Signal?

Several contrasts present themselves between natural and synthetic vitamin E in the clinical trials. Two, in particular, are of interest. First, it would appear that natural vitamin E and certain single homologues of the family, particularly gamma-tocopherol, offer benefits not found with synthetic vitamin E. Second, synthetic vitamin E in many studies exhibited benefits in trials lasting approximately 2 years, but not in longer trials. Perhaps these two contrasts are linked?

An excess of alpha-tocopherol long has been known to reduce gamma-tocopherol and delta-tocopherol in serum and tissues.[85,86] It is primarily gamma-tocopherol, not alpha-tocopherol, which protects the membranes of cells, including brain cells, from peroxynitrite damage.[87] Studies of peroxynitrite, a powerful mutagenic oxidant and nitrating species, have confirmed that tocopherol balance is essential.[88] Tests in which nitrite-based oxidative stress in brain tissue is examined have shown that protection of brain nerve mitochondria can be significantly enhanced by gamma-tocopherol but not by alpha-tocopherol.[89–92] Despite alpha-tocopherol's actions, generally regarded as antioxidant, gamma-tocopherol is required to effectively remove peroxynitrite-derived metabolites because the peroxynitrite-trapping structure of the vitamin is blocked in alpha-tocopherol. Hence the conclusion of one set of researchers was that "because large doses of dietary alpha-tocopherol displace gamma-tocopherol in plasma and other tissues, the current wisdom of vitamin E supplementation with primarily alpha-tocopherol should be reconsidered."[93]

This interaction of alpha- and gamma-tocopherol at the cell membrane goes far to explain why several large multiyear studies using synthetic vitamin E or even only natural-source alpha-tocopherol found no benefit to heart patients although shorter studies had been positive. So does the fact that excessive alpha-tocopherol, far from being protective, can act as a pro-oxidant.[94]

Potentially more unfortunate still is the possibility that long-term alpha-tocopherol excess may result in damage to the mitochondrial respiratory chain. The antioxidant activity of alpha-tocopherol in lipid membranes can lead to the irreversible formation of alpha-tocopheryl quinone (TQ) in those same membranes. TQ has been shown to be able to interfere with the electron transfer function of ubiquinone to cytochrome c and a reduction in the rate respiratory activities in the mitochondria.[95,96]

One other matter needs to be brought up in closing—the over-determined nature of vitamin E analysis limited to models based on redox potential and radical scavenging. Vitamin E acts by inhibiting smooth muscle cell proliferation, platelet aggregation, monocyte adhesion, the uptake of oxidized LDL, cytokine production and so forth—all effects that are *not* the result of the antioxidant activity of the tocopherols, but rather of targeted molecular actions by this family of compounds. Likewise, the tocopherols influence the activity of several key enzymes that affect pathways involving COX-2, 5-lipooxygenase, nitric oxide synthase, superoxide dismutase, etc.[97–100]

5.6 CONCLUSION

It is clear that vitamin E, as a family of related molecules, has a number of functions in the body that are not limited to antioxidant activity. Furthermore, a number of recent studies have shown significant differences between natural-source and synthetic vitamin E. They have also shown that natural-source vitamin E is more efficiently retained by the body than its synthetic counterpart. The human body therefore has a preference for natural-source vitamin E over synthetic vitamin E. In addition, the different vitamin E isomers can affect the levels of other isomers, as well as the levels and efficiency of other antioxidants in the body.

What is not entirely clear, however, is whether specific combinations of isomers will maximize vitamin E activity. Because the activities of all of these isoforms have not been determined, and because these isomers are studied in isolation, the data regarding their health benefits have been contradictory, incomplete and perhaps even misleading. Moreover, results of epidemiological studies suggest that dietary forms, and therefore isomer ratios found in nature, may be the most beneficial. Research focused on naturally occurring forms and ratios of vitamin E isomers may provide important insight into not only their functions, but also their interactions and possible synergy.

REFERENCES

1. Brigelius-Flohe R, Kelly FJ, Salonen JT, Neuzil J, Zingg JM, Azzi A. 2002. The European perspective on vitamin E: Current knowledge and future research. *Am J Clin Nutr.* Oct;76(4):703–16.
2. Vogelsang A, Shute EV. Effect of vitamin E in coronary heart disease. *Nature* (Lond.) 1946, 157, 772.
3. Munteanu A, Zingg JM, Azzi A. 2004. Anti-atherosclerotic effects of vitamin E—myth or reality? *J Cell Mol Med.* Jan–Mar, 8(1), 59–76.
4. Kaempf-Rotzoll DE, Traber MG, Arai H. 2003. Vitamin E and transfer proteins. *Curr Opin Lipidol.* Jun;14(3):249–54.
5. Jiang Q, Christen S, Shigenaga MK, Ames BN. 2001. Gamma-tocopherol, the major form of vitamin E in the US diet, deserves more attention. *Am J Clin Nutr;* 74:714–22.
6. Meglia GE, Jensen SK, Lauridsen C, Persson Waller K. 2006. Alpha-tocopherol concentration and stereoisomer composition in plasma and milk from dairy cows fed natural or synthetic vitamin E around calving. *J Dairy Res.* May;73(2):227–34.
7. Jensen SK, Norgaard JV, Lauridsen C. 2006. Bioavailability of alpha-tocopherol stereoisomers in rats depends on dietary doses of all-rac- or RRR-alpha-tocopheryl acetate. *Br J Nutr.* Mar;95(3):477–87.
8. Lauridsen C, Engel H, Jensen SK, Craig AM, Traber MG. 2002. Lactating sows and suckling piglets preferentially incorporate RRR- over all-rac-alpha-tocopherol into milk, plasma and tissues. *J Nutr.* Jun;132(6):1258–64.
9. Clifford AJ, de Moura FF, Ho CC, Chuang JC, Follett J, Fadel JG, Novotny JA. 2006. A feasibility study quantifying in vivo human alpha-tocopherol metabolism. *Am J Clin Nutr.* Dec;84(6):1430–41.
10. Stone WL, LeClair I, Ponder T, Baggs G, Reis BB. 2003. Infants discriminate between natural and synthetic vitamin E. *Am J Clin Nutr.* Apr;77(4):899–906.
11. Burton GW, Traber MG, Acuff RV, Walters DN, Kayden H, Hughes L, Ingold KU. 1998. Human plasma and tissue alpha-tocopherol concentrations in response to supplementation with deuterated natural and synthetic vitamin E. *Am J Clin Nutr.* Apr;67(4):669–84.
12. Kiyose C, Muramatsu R, Kameyama Y, Ueda T, Igarashi O. 1997. Biodiscrimination of alpha-tocopherol stereoisomers in humans after oral administration. *Am J Clin Nutr.* Mar;65(3):785–9.
13. Janisch KM, Milde J, Schempp H, Elstner EF. 2005. Vitamin C, vitamin E and flavonoids. *Dev Ophthalmol.* 38, 59–69.
14. Niki E, Noguchi N. 2004. Dynamics of antioxidant action of vitamin E. *Acc Chem Res.* Jan, 37(1), 45–51.
15. Herrera E, Barbas C. 2001. Vitamin E: Action, metabolism and perspectives. *J Physiol Biochem.* Mar, 57(2), 43–56.
16. Gotoh N, Noguchi N, Tsuchiya J, Morita K, Sakai H, Shimasaki H, Niki E. 1996. Inhibition of oxidation of low density lipoprotein by vitamin E and related compounds. *Free Radic Res.* Feb, 24(2), 123–34.
17. Brown BG, Crowley J. 2005. Is there any hope for vitamin E? *JAMA.* Mar 16;293(11):1387–90.
18. Lonn E, Bosch J, Yusuf S, Sheridan P, Pogue J, Arnold JM, Ross C, Arnold A, Sleight P, Probstfield J, Dagenais GR. 2005. HOPE and HOPE–TOO Trial Investigators. Effects of long-term vitamin E supplementation on cardiovascular events and cancer: A randomized controlled trial. *JAMA.* Mar 16;293(11):1338–47.

19. Stampfer MJ, Hennekens CH, Manson JE, Colditz GA, Rosner B, Willett WC. 1993. Vitamin E consumption and the risk of coronary disease in women. *N Engl J Med.* 328:1444–1449.
20. Rimm EB, Stampfer MJ, Ascherio A, Giovannucci E, Colditz GA, Willett WC. 1993. Vitamin E consumption and the risk of coronary heart disease in men. *N Engl J. Med.* 328:1450–1456.
21. Pryor WA. 2000. Vitamin E and heart disease: basic science to clinical intervention trials. *Free Radic Biol Med.* Jan 1, 28(1), 141–64.
22. Gaziano JM. 2004. Vitamin E and cardiovascular disease: Observational studies. *Ann N Y Acad Sci.* Dec, 1031, 280–91.
23. Riccioni G, Bucciarelli T, Mancini B, Di Ilio C, Capra V, D'Orazio N. 2007. The role of the antioxidant vitamin supplementation in the prevention of cardiovascular diseases. *Expert Opin Investig Drugs.* Jan, 16(1), 25–32.
24. Lee IM, Cook NR, Gaziano JM, Gordon D, Ridker PM, Manson JE, Hennekens CH, Buring JE. 2005. Vitamin E in the primary prevention of cardiovascular disease and cancer: The Women's Health Study: a randomized controlled trial. *JAMA.* Jul 6;294(1):56–65.
25. Emmert DH, Kirchner JT. 1999. The role of vitamin E in the prevention of heart disease. *Arch Fam Med.* Nov–Dec;8(6):537–42.
26. Kushi LH, Folsom AR, Prineas RJ, Mink PJ, Wu Y, Bostick RM. 1996. Dietary antioxidant vitamins and death from coronary heart disease in postmenopausal women. *N Engl J Med.* 334:1156–1162.
27. Hayden KM, Welsh–Bohmer KA, Wengreen HJ, Zandi PP, Lyketsos CG, Breitner JC2007. Cache County Investigators. Risk of mortality with vitamin E supplements: The Cache County study. *Am J Med.* Feb;120(2):180–4.
28. Emmert DH, Kirchner JT. 1999. The role of vitamin E in the prevention of heart disease. *Arch Fam Med.* Nov–Dec;8(6):537–42.
29. Evans RW, Shaten BJ, Day BW, Kuller LH. 1998. Prospective association between lipid soluble antioxidants and coronary heart disease in men. The Multiple Risk Factor Intervention Trial. *Am J Epidemiol.* Jan 15;147(2):180–6.
30. Steinhart H, Rickert R, Winkler K. 2003. Trans fatty acids (TFA): Analysis, occurrence, intake and clinical relevance. *Eur J Med Res.* Aug 20;8(8):358–62.
31. Ruiz Rejon F, Martin–Pena G, Granado F, Ruiz–Galiana J, Blanco I, Olmedilla B. 2002. Plasma status of retinol, alpha- and gamma-tocopherols, and main carotenoids to first myocardial infarction: Case control and follow-up study. *Nutrition.* Jan;18(1):26–31.
32. Nojiri S, Daida H, Mokuno H, Iwama Y, Mae K, Ushio F, Ueki T. 2001. Association of serum antioxidant capacity with coronary artery disease in middle-aged men. *Jpn Heart J.* Nov;42(6):677–90.
33. Brown BG, Crowley J. 2005. Is there any hope for vitamin E? *JAMA.* Mar 16;293(11):1387–90.
34. Tamimi RM, Hankinson SE, Campos H, Spiegelman D, Zhang S, Colditz GA, Willett WC, Hunter DJ. 2005. Plasma carotenoids, retinol, and tocopherols and risk of breast cancer. *Am J Epidemiol.* Jan 15;161(2):153–60.
35. Heinonen OP, Albanes D, Virtamo J, Taylor PR, Huttunen JK, Hartman AM, Haapakoski J, Malila N, Rautalahti M, Ripatti S, Maenpaa H, Teerenhovi L, Koss L, Virolainen M, Edwards BK. 1998. Prostate cancer and supplementation with alpha-tocopherol and beta-carotene: incidence and mortality in a controlled trial. *J Natl Cancer Inst.* Mar 18;90(6):440–6.
36. Albanes D, Malila N, Taylor PR, Huttunen JK, Virtamo J, Edwards BK, Rautalahti M, Hartman AM, Barrett MJ, Pietinen P, Hartman TJ, Sipponen P, Lewin K, Teerenhovi L, Hietanen P, Tangrea JA, Virtanen M, Heinonen OP. 2000. Effects of supplemental alpha-tocopherol and beta-carotene on colorectal cancer: Results from a controlled trial (Finland) *Cancer Causes Control.* Mar;11(3):197–205.
37. Weinstein SJ, Wright ME, Pietinen P, King I, Tan C, Taylor PR, Virtamo J, Albanes D. 2005. Serum alpha-tocopherol and gamma-tocopherol in relation to prostate cancer risk in a prospective study. *J Natl Cancer Inst.* Mar 2;97(5):396–9.
38. Helzlsouer KJ, Huang HY, Alberg AJ, Hoffman S, Burke A, Norkus EP, Morris JS, Comstock GW. Association between alpha-tocopherol, gamma-tocopherol, selenium, and subsequent prostate cancer. 2000. *J Natl Cancer Inst.* Dec 20;92(24):2018–23.
39. Wagner KH, Kamal-Eldin A, Elmadfa I. Gamma-tocopherol—an underestimated vitamin? *Ann Nutr Metab.* 2004;48(3):169–88.
40. Wagner KH, Kamal-Eldin A, Elmadfa I. 2004. Gamma-tocopherol—an underestimated vitamin? *Ann Nutr Metab.* 48(3):169–88.
41. Dietrich M, Traber MG, Jacques PF, Cross CE, Hu Y, Block G. 2006. Does gamma-tocopherol play a role in the primary prevention of heart disease and cancer? A review. *J Am Coll Nutr.* Aug;25(4):292–9.

42. London SJ, Stein EA, Henderson IC, Stampfer MJ, Wood WC, Remine S, Dmochowski JR, Robert NJ, Willett WC. 1992. Carotenoids, retinol, and vitamin E and risk of proliferative benign breast disease and breast cancer. *Cancer Causes Control*. Nov;3(6):503–12.
43. Kushi LH, Fee RM, Sellers TA, Zheng W, Folsom AR. 1996. Intake of vitamins A, C, and E and postmenopausal breast cancer. The Iowa Women's Health Study. *Am J Epidemiol*. Jul 15;144(2):165–74.
44. Zhang S, Hunter DJ, Forman MR, Rosner BA, Speizer FE, Colditz GA, Manson JE, Hankinson SE, Willett WC. 1999. Dietary carotenoids and vitamins A, C, and E and risk of breast cancer. *J Natl Cancer Inst*. Mar 17;91(6):547–56.
45. Giuliano AR, Papenfuss M, Nour M, Canfield LM, Schneider A, Hatch K. 1997. Antioxidant nutrients: associations with persistent human papillomavirus infection. *Cancer Epidemiol Biomarkers Prev*. Nov;6(11):917–23.
46. Goodman MT, Kiviat N, McDuffie K, Hankin JH, Hernandez B, Wilkens LR, Franke A, Kuypers J, Kolonel LN, Nakamura J, Ing G, Branch B, Bertram CC, Kamemoto L, Sharma S, Killeen J. 1998. The association of plasma micronutrients with the risk of cervical dysplasia in Hawaii. *Cancer Epidemiol Biomarkers Prev*. Jun;7(6):537–44.
47. Stone WL, Papas AM. 1997. Tocopherols and the etiology of colon cancer. *J Natl Cancer Inst*. Jul 16;89(14):1006–14.
48. Bendich A, Gabriel E, Machlin LJ. 1986. Dietary vitamin E requirement for optimum immune responses in the rat. *J Nutr*. 116, 675–681.
49. Campbell SE, Stone WL, Lee S, Whaley S, Yang H, Qui M, Goforth P, Sherman D, McHaffie D, Krishnan K. 2006. Comparative effects of RRR-alpha- and RRR-gamma-tocopherol on proliferation and apoptosis in human colon cancer cell lines. *BMC Cancer*. Jan 17, 6, 13.
50. Stone WL, Krishnan K, Campbell SE, Qui M, Whaley SG, Yang H. 2004. Tocopherols and the treatment of colon cancer. *Ann N Y Acad Sci*. Dec, 1031, 223–33.
51. Yu W, Simmons–Menchaca M, Gapor A, Sanders BG, Kline K. 1999. Induction of apoptosis in human breast cancer cells by tocopherols and tocotrienols. *Nutr Cancer*. 33(1):26–32.
52. Kline K, Yu W, Sanders B.G. 2004. Vitamin E and breast cancer. *J Nutr*. Dec, 134(12 Suppl), 3458S–3462S.
53. Crispen PL, Uzzo RG, Golovine K, Makhov P, Pollack A, Horwitz EM, Greenberg RE, Kolenko VM. 2007. Vitamin E succinate inhibits NF-kappaB and prevents the development of a metastatic phenotype in prostate cancer cells: implications for chemoprevention. *Prostate*. May 1, 67(6), 582–90.
54. Jiang Q, Wong J, Fyrst H, Saba JD, Ames BN. 2004. Gamma-tocopherol or combinations of vitamin E forms induce cell death in human prostate cancer cells by interrupting sphingolipid synthesis. *Proc Natl Acad Sci USA*. Dec 21, 101(51), 17825–30.
55. Srivastava JK, Gupta S. 2006. Tocotrienol-rich fraction of palm oil induces cell cycle arrest and apoptosis selectively in human prostate cancer cells. *Biochem Biophys Res Commun*. Jul 28, 346(2), 447–53.
56. Engelhart MJ, Geerlings MI, Ruitenberg A, van Swieten JC, Hofman A, Witteman JC, Breteler MM. 2002. Dietary intake of antioxidants and risk of Alzheimer disease. *JAMA*. Jun 26, 287(24), 3223–9.
57. Zandi PP., Anthony JC., Khachaturian AS., Stone SV, Gustafson D, Tschanz JT, Norton MC, Welsh–Bohmer KA, Breitner JC. 2004. Cache County Study Group. Reduced risk of Alzheimer disease in users of antioxidant vitamin supplements: The Cache County Study. *Arch Neurol*. Jan, 61(1), 82–8.
58. Engelhart MJ, Geerlings MI, Meijer J, Kiliaan A, Ruitenberg A, van Swieten JC, Stijnen T, Hofman A, Witteman JC, Breteler MM. 2004. Inflammatory proteins in plasma and the risk of dementia: the rotterdam study. *Arch Neurol*. May, 61(5), 668–72.
59. Pham DQ, Plakogiannis R. 2005. Vitamin E supplementation in Alzheimer's disease, Parkinson's disease, tardive dyskinesia, and cataract: Part 2. *Ann Pharmacother*. Dec, 39(12), 2065–72.
60. Boothby LA, Doering PL. 2005. Vitamin C and vitamin E for Alzheimer's disease. *Ann Pharmacother*. Dec, 39(12), 2073–80.
61. Fillenbaum GG., Kuchibhatla MN., Hanlon JT., Artz MB, Pieper CF, Schmader KE, Dysken MW, Gray SL. 2005. Dementia and Alzheimer's disease in community-dwelling elders taking vitamin C and/or vitamin E. *Ann Pharmacother*. Dec, 39(12), 2009–14.
62. Morris MC, Evans DA, Tangney CC, Bienias JL, Wilson RS, Aggarwal NT, Scherr PA. 2005. Relation of the tocopherol forms to incident Alzheimer disease and to cognitive change. *Am J Clin Nutr*. Feb, 81(2), 508–14.
63. Weber CA, Ernst ME. 2006. Antioxidants, supplements, and Parkinson's disease. *Ann Pharmacother*. May, 40(5), 935–8.

64. Etminan M, Gill SS, Samii A. 2005. Intake of vitamin E, vitamin C, and carotenoids and the risk of Parkinson's disease: A meta-analysis. *Lancet Neurol.* Jun, 4(6), 362–5.
65. de Rijk MC, Breteler MM, den Breeijen JH, Launer LJ, Grobbee DE., van der Meche FG, Hofman A. 1997. Dietary antioxidants and Parkinson disease. The Rotterdam Study. *Arch Neurol.* Jun, 54(6), 762–5.
66. Zhang SM, Hernan MA, Chen H, Spiegelman D, Willett WC, Ascherio A. 2002. Intakes of vitamins E and C, carotenoids, vitamin supplements, and PD risk. *Neurology.* Oct 22, 59(8), 1161–9.
67. Surapaneni KM, Venkataramana G. 2007. Status of lipid peroxidation, glutathione, ascorbic acid, vitamin E and antioxidant enzymes in patients with osteoarthritis. *Indian J Med Sci.* Jan;61(1):9–14.
68. McAlindon TE, Jacques P, Zhang Y, Hannan MT, Aliabadi P, Weissman B, Rush D, Levy D, Felson DT. 1996. Do antioxidant micronutrients protect against the development and progression of knee osteoarthritis? *Arthritis Rheum.* Apr;39(4):648–56.
69. Kowsari B, Finnie SK, Carter RL, Love J, Katz P, Longley S, Panush RS. 1983. Assessment of the diet of patients with rheumatoid arthritis and osteoarthritis. *J Am Diet Assoc.* Jun;82(6):657–9.
70. Canter PH, Wider B, Ernst E. 2007. The antioxidant vitamins A, C, E and selenium in the treatment of arthritis: A systematic review of randomized clinical trials. *Rheumatology* (Oxford). May 23; [Epub ahead of print].
71. Boshtam M, Rafiei M, Golshadi ID, Ani M, Shirani Z, Rostamshirazi M. 2005. Long term effects of oral vitamin E supplement in type II diabetic patients. *Int J Vitam Nutr Res.* Sep;75(5):341–6.
72. Gokkusu C, Palanduz S, Ademoglu E, Tamer S. 2001. Oxidant and antioxidant systems in niddm patients: Influence of vitamin E supplementation. *Endocr Res.* Aug;27(3):377–86.
73. Paolisso G, D'Amore A, Galzerano D, Balbi V, Giugliano D, Varricchio M, D'Onofrio F. 1993. Daily vitamin E supplements improve metabolic control but not insulin secretion in elderly type II diabetic patients. *Diabetes Care.* Nov;16(11):1433–7.
74. Montonen J, Knekt P, Jarvinen R, Reunanen A. 2004. Dietary antioxidant intake and risk of type 2 diabetes. *Diabetes Care.* Feb;27(2):362–6.
75. Sjöholm A, Berggren PO, Cooney RV. 2000. Gamma-tocopherol partially protects insulin-secreting cells against functional inhibition by nitric oxide. *Biochem Biophys Res Commun.* Oct 22;277(2):334–40.
76. Baliarsingh S, Beg ZH, Ahmad J. 2005. The therapeutic impacts of tocotrienols in type 2 diabetic patients with hyperlipidemia. *Atherosclerosis.* Oct;182(2):367–74.
77. Wan Nazaimoon WM, Khalid BA. 2002. Tocotrienols-rich diet decreases advanced glycosylation end-products in non-diabetic rats and improves glycemic control in streptozotocin-induced diabetic rats. *Malays J Pathol.* Dec;24(2):77–82.
78. Wu JH, Ward NC, Indrawan AP, Almeida CA, Hodgson JM, Proudfoot JM, Puddey IB, Croft KD. 2007. Effects of alpha-tocopherol and mixed tocopherol supplementation on markers of oxidative stress and inflammation in type 2 diabetes. *Clin Chem.* Mar;53(3):511–9.
79. Clarke MW, Ward NC, Wu JH, Hodgson JM, Puddey IB, Croft KD. 2006. Supplementation with mixed tocopherols increases serum and blood cell gamma-tocopherol but does not alter biomarkers of platelet activation in subjects with type 2 diabetes. *Am J Clin Nutr.* Jan;83(1):95–102.
80. Sjöholm A, Berggren PO, Cooney RV. 2000. Gamma-tocopherol partially protects insulin-secreting cells against functional inhibition by nitric oxide. *Biochem Biophys Res Commun.* 277:334–340.
81. McNeil JJ, Robman L, Tikellis G, Sinclair MI, McCarty CA, Taylor HR. 2004. Vitamin E supplementation and cataract: Randomized controlled trial. *Ophthalmology.* Jan;111(1):75–84.
82. Age-Related Eye Disease Study Research Group. 2001. A randomized, placebo-controlled, clinical trial of high-dose supplementation with vitamins C and E and beta carotene for age-related cataract and vision loss: AREDS report no. 9. *Arch Ophthalmol.* Oct;119(10):1439–52.
83. Leske MC, Chylack LT Jr, He Q, Wu SY, Schoenfeld E, Friend J, Wolfe J. 1998. Antioxidant vitamins and nuclear opacities: The longitudinal study of cataract. *Ophthalmology.* May;105(5):831–6.
84. Jacques PF, Taylor A, Moeller S, Hankinson SE, Rogers G, Tung W, Ludovico J, Willett WC, Chylack LT Jr. 2005. Long-term nutrient intake and 5–year change in nuclear lens opacities. *Arch Ophthalmol.* Apr;123(4):517–26.
85. Huang HY, Appel LJ. 2003. Supplementation of diets with alpha-tocopherol reduces serum concentrations of gamma- and delta-tocopherol in humans. *J Nutr.* Oct;133(10):3137–40.
86. Handelman GJ, Machlin LJ, Fitch K, Weiter JJ, Dratz EA. 1985. Oral alpha-tocopherol supplements decrease plasma gamma-tocopherol levels in humans. *J Nutr.* Jun;115(6):807–13.
87. Jiang Q, Ames BN. 2003. Gamma-tocopherol, but not alpha-tocopherol, decreases proinflammatory eicosanoids and inflammation damage in rats. *FASEB J.* May;17(8):816–22.

88. Christen S, Woodall AA, Shigenaga MK, Southwell-Keely PT, Duncan MW, Ames BN. Gamma-tocopherol traps mutagenic electrophiles such as NO(X) and complements alpha-tocopherol: Physiological implications. *Proc Natl Acad Sci USA*. 1997. Apr 1;94(7):3217–22.
89. Jiang Q, Ames BN. 2003. Gamma-tocopherol, but not alpha-tocopherol, decreases proinflammatory eicosanoids and inflammation damage in rats. *FASEB J.* May;17(8):816–22.
90. Jiang Q, Lykkesfeldt J, Shigenaga MK, Shigeno ET, Christen S, Ames BN. 2002. Gamma-tocopherol supplementation inhibits protein nitration and ascorbate oxidation in rats with inflammation. *Free Radic Biol Med.* Dec 1;33(11):1534–42.
91. Williamson KS, Gabbita SP, Mou S, West M, Pye QN, Markesbery WR, Cooney RV, Grammas P, Reimann-Philipp U, Floyd RA, Hensley K. 2002. The nitration product 5-nitro-gamma-tocopherol is increased in the Alzheimer brain. *Nitric Oxide.* Mar;6(2):221–7.
92. Jiang Q, Christen S, Shigenaga MK, Ames BN. 2001. Gamma-tocopherol, the major form of vitamin E in the US diet, deserves more attention. *Am J Clin Nutr.* Dec;74(6):714–22.
93. Jiang Q, Christen S, Shigenaga MK, Ames BN. 2001. Gamma-tocopherol, the major form of vitamin E in the US diet, deserves more attention. *Am J Clin Nutr.* Dec;74(6):714–22.
94. Thomas SR, Neuzil J, Stocker R. 1996. Cosupplementation with coenzyme Q prevents the prooxidant effect of alpha-tocopherol and increases the resistance of LDL to transition metal–dependent oxidation initiation. *Arterioscler Thromb Vasc Biol.* May;16(5):687–96.
95. Gregor W, Staniek K, Nohl H, Gille L. 2006. Distribution of tocopheryl quinone in mitochondrial membranes and interference with ubiquinone-mediated electron transfer. *Biochem Pharmacol.* May 28;71(11):1589–601.
96. Gille L, Gregor W, Staniek K, Nohl H. 2004. Redox-interaction of alpha-tocopheryl quinone with isolated mitochondrial cytochrome bc1 complex. *Biochem Pharmacol.* Jul 15;68(2):373–81.
97. Zingg JM, Azzi A. 2004. Non-antioxidant activities of vitamin E. Curr Med Chem.. May;11(9):1113–33.
98. Azzi A, Gysin R, Kempna P, Munteanu A, Negis Y, Villacorta L, Visarius T, Zingg JM. 2004. Vitamin E mediates cell signaling and regulation of gene expression. *Ann N Y Acad Sci.* Dec;1031:86–95.
99. Rimbach G, Minihane AM, Majewicz J, Fischer A, Pallauf J, Virgli F, Weinberg PD. 2002. Regulation of cell signaling by vitamin E. *Proc Nutr Soc.* Nov;61(4):415–25.
100. Packer L, Weber SU, Rimbach G. 2001. Molecular aspects of alpha-tocotrienol antioxidant action and cell signalling. *J Nutr.* Feb;131(2):369S–73S.

Part C

Chemistry of Tocotrienols

6 Angiogenesis Inhibition

Kiyotaka Nakagawa, Akira Shibata,
*Phumon Sookwong and Teruo Miyazawa**

CONTENTS

6.1 INTRODUCTION

Vitamin E occurs naturally in eight different forms: α-, β-, γ- and δ-isomers of both tocopherol (Toc) and tocotrienol (T3). Tocopherol has a phytyl side chain attached to a chroman ring, whereas the tail of T3 is an unsaturated isoprenoid chain. Tocopherol is abundantly present in common vegetable oils and nuts, whereas T3, a minor plant constituent, is particularly abundant in rice bran (Sookwong et al., 2007), palm and wheat germ (Sundram et al., 2002). Some recent investigations have shown that T3 has better antioxidative (Serbinova et al., 1991; Suzuki et al., 1993), antihypercholesterolemic (Parker et al., 1993), anticancer (McIntyre et al., 2000) and neuroprotective (Sen et al., 2000; Khanna et al., 2003) activities than Toc. These findings suggest that T3 may serve as a food component with better health benefits.

Recently, we found the inhibitory effect of T3 on angiogenesis by measuring proliferation, migration and tube formation of endothelial cells (Inokuchi et al., 2003; Miyazawa et al., 2004a; Miyazawa et al., 2004b; Nakagawa et al., 2004; Mizushina et al., 2006). Because angiogenesis is of fundamental importance in pathological states (e.g., diabetic retinopathy, rheumatic arthritis and tumor growth) (Kim et al., 1993), T3 is expected to have potential use as functional food for prevention of angiogenic disorders. In this chapter, we discuss the anti-angiogenic effect of T3 and its mechanism, which were evaluated by *in vitro* cell studies and *in vivo* egg and animal models.

6.2 *IN VITRO* STUDY OF ANGIOGENESIS INHIBITION BY T3

The angiogenic process is involved with endothelial cell proliferation, migration and tube formation (Folkman and Klagsbrun, 1987). Tocotrienols at a low micromolar range (2–35 μM) inhibited proliferation and tube formation of bovine aortic endothelial cells (BAEC) (Figure 6.1) (Inokuchi et al., 2003). The inhibitory potency of T3 isomers was as follows; δ- > β- > γ- > α-T3. It is reported that plasma T3 concentration in an acetate supplemented-hypercholesterolemic human was around 1.0 μM (O'Byrne et al., 2000). Therefore, the concentration range of T3 (2–35 μM) that we used in

* Corresponding author: Teruo Miyazawa

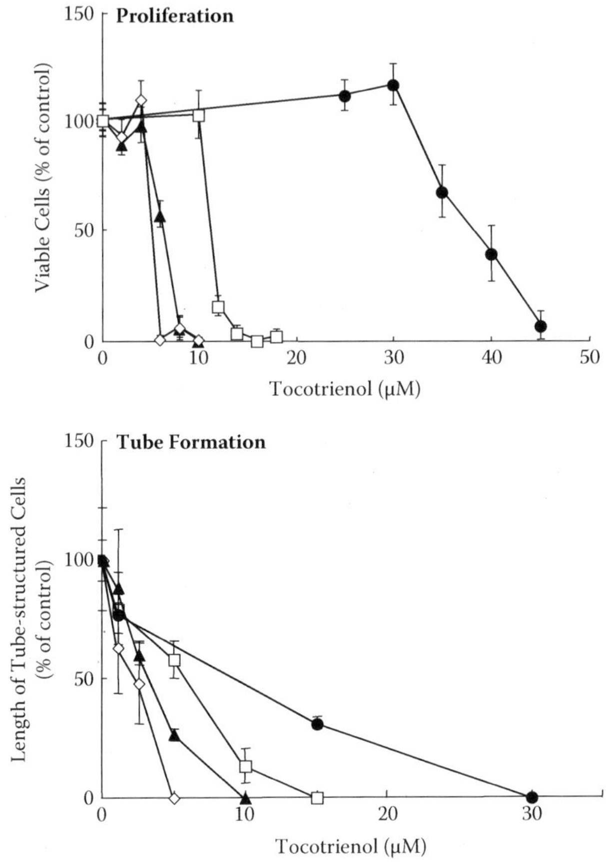

FIGURE 6.1 Effects of increasing concentrations of T3 on the proliferation and tube formation of BAEC. In the assay of BAEC proliferation, cells were incubated in medium containing α– (●), β– (▲), γ– (□) or δ–T3 (◇) at concentrations from 0 (control) to 45 μM for 24 h. The viable cells were then assessed by WST–1. In the assay of BAEC tube formation, cells were cultured between collagen gel layers in the absence (control) or presence of α– (●), β– (▲), γ– (□) or δ–tocotrienol (◇) at various concentrations. After 72 h, the length of tube-structured cells was determined. Values are means ± S.D.

our *in vitro* experiments (Inokuchi et al., 2003) was comparable to the concentration of T3 detected in the plasma of hypercholesterolemic humans.

In contrast to T3, Toc did not show any effect on BAEC proliferation and tube formation. These results suggested that T3 may be a better bioactive compound than Toc in terms of anti-angiogenesis. Structurally, T3 and Toc can be distinguished by considering their side chains and it has been reported that the unsaturated side chain of T3 allows it to pass through cell membranes more efficiently and at a faster rate than the saturated phytyl side-chain of Toc (Traber and Packer, 1995). For this reason, it can be possibly thought that the greater anti-angiogenic effect of T3 may be due, in part, to their effective incorporation into BAEC.

6.3 ANTI-ANGIOGENIC MECHANISM OF T3

The inhibitory mechanisms of T3 on angiogenesis have not been fully clarified. One of our recent studies (Miyazawa et al., 2004b) showed that the anti-angiogenic effect of T3 acted via its inhibition of the growth factor (e.g., vascular endothelial growth factor (VEGF) and fibroblast growth factor [FGF])-stimulated cell proliferation, migration and tube formation of human umbilical vein endothe-

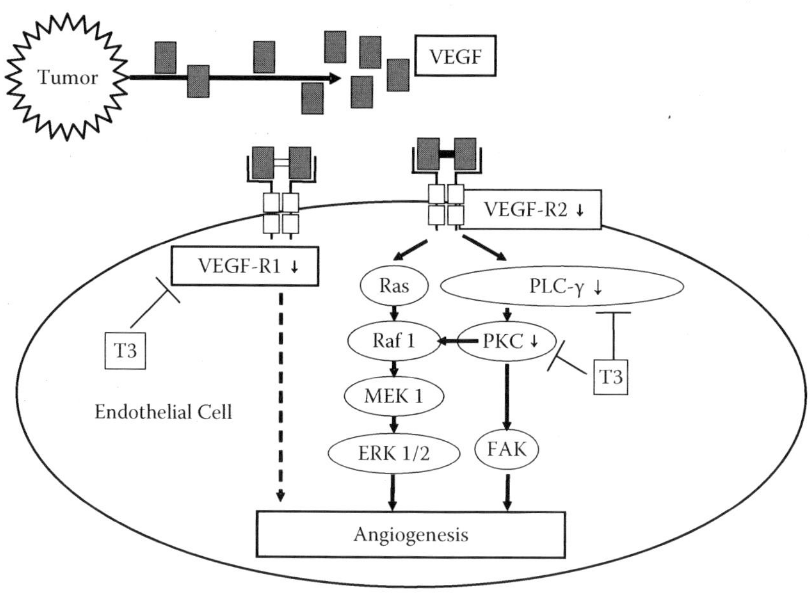

FIGURE 6.2 A postulated anti-angiogenic mechanism of T3. Based on DNA chip analysis, T3 down-regulates the expression of VEGF receptor (VEGFR) in endothelial cells, blocks intracellular VEGF signaling (PLC-γ and PKC) and causes inhibition of angiogenesis.

lial cells (HUVEC). DNA chip analysis revealed that T3 specifically down-regulated the expression of VEGF receptor (VEGFR) (Figure 6.2) (Nakagawa et al., 2004). Since it is well known that VEGF regulates angiogenesis by binding to VEGFR (Kim et al., 1993; Folkman and Klagsbrun, 1987), T3 could block the intracellular signaling of VEGF via the down-regulation of VEGFR, which results in the inhibition of angiogenesis. On the other hand, some studies report that 3-hydroxy-3-methylglutarate (HMG)-CoA reductase inhibitors (i.e., statins) interfered with angiogenic processes both *in vitro* and *in vivo* (Vincent et al., 2001; Park et al., 2002). It would be possible for the anti-angiogenic effect of T3 because T3 is known to have an inhibitory effect of HMG-CoA reductase (Parker et al., 1993). We also assumed another possibility about the anti-angiogenic effect of T3 by discussing its antioxidant property. That is because T3 was reported to be a better antioxidant than Toc (Serbinova et al., 1991; Suzuki et al., 1993) and Tang and Meydani (2001) demonstrated that Toc prevented the oxidative stress-induced tube formation of human microvascular endothelial cells. On the basis of these reports (Serbinova et al., 1991; Suzuki et al., 1993; Tang and Meydani, 2001), it is implied that inhibition of angiogenesis by T3 might be related to its antioxidant activity. However, the inhibitory mechanism of T3 is still suggestive, so further detailed studies are needed to fully clarify the mechanism.

6.4 *IN VIVO* STUDY OF ANGIOGENESIS INHIBITION BY T3

One of the problems faced by angiogenesis researchers has been the difficulty of finding suitable methods for assessing the effects of angiogenic regulators (Carolyn et al., 2004). The chick chorioallantoic membrane (CAM) assay is probably the most widely used *in vivo* assay for studying angiogenesis (Ribatti et al., 1996). The dorsal air sac (DAS) model is designed to be used in an examination of the *in vivo* effects of substances against the angiogenic response triggered by cancer cells (Yonekura et al., 1999). The advantages of DAS assay are a technically simple and natural environment in which to study blood vessels. We chose these reliable methods and used them in the evaluation of the anti-angiogenic effect of T3 in our *in vivo* study (Miyazawa et al., 2004b).

In the CAM assay, a pellet containing T3 was placed on the CAM. After the incubation, angiogenic response was evaluated by measuring the avascular zone in the CAM. As the result, T3

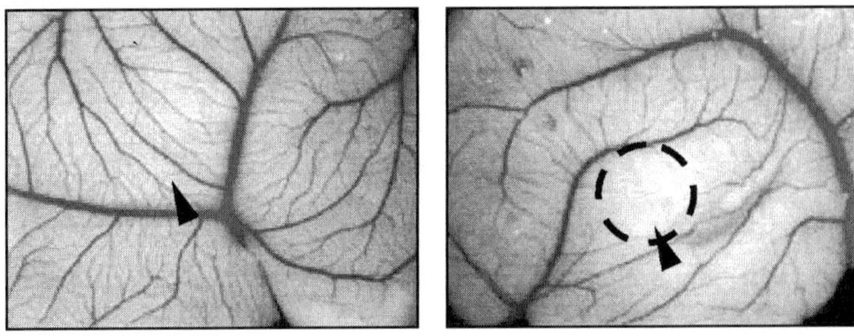

FIGURE 6.3 Photographs of the CAM vascular network following treatment with vehicle (ethylene-vinyl acetate copolymer, control) or with δ-T3 (500 μg/egg). δ-T3-free vehicle did not show any anti-angiogenic effect, _while δ-T3 treatment on CAM resulted in the suppression of embryonic angiogenesis, causing a significant avascular zone.

(125–1000 μg/egg) exhibited a dose-dependent inhibition in angiogenesis (Figure 6.3) (Miyazawa et al., 2004b). In contrast, Toc did not show the effect at the same dosage. In the DAS assay, DLD-1 human colon carcinoma cells were injected into a chamber ring. This chamber was implanted into a dorsal air sac produced in a mouse (ICR). A T3-rich oil (Tocomin 50; Carotech, Malaysia) was orally administrated to the mouse once a day at a T3 dose of 1.2–4.4 mg/day for 5 days. After that, the implanted chamber was removed and angiogenic response was assessed by counting newly formed capillary vessels. It was found that oral administration of T3 (4.4 mg/day) suppressed the tumor cell-induced angiogenesis (Miyazawa et al., 2004b). In the DAS model, Toc showed very weak inhibition effect.

The results indicate that T3 has potential as a therapeutic dietary supplement for preventing angiogenic disorders. In one of our animal studies, it was found that T3 orally administrated to rats was distributed into the blood stream and various tissues (Kawakami et al., 2007). This data would be advantageous for application of T3 preventive medical purposes. The possibility for using T3 for its anti-angiogenic property is now being investigated in clinical studies (see section 6.6).

6.5 SUMMARY

In this chapter, we discussed the anti-angiogenic effect of T3 and its mechanism from the fundamental data of *in vitro* cell studies and *in vivo* CAM and DAS models. We found that among the vitamin E group, T3 performed a potent anti-angiogenic function *in vitro* and *in vivo*. Our data showed that the anti-angiogenic effect of T3 was attributable in part to regulation of intracellular VEGF signaling in endothelial cells, but the inhibitory mechanism of T3 is still controversial and further detailed studies are required.

6.6 PROSPECTIVE

Anti-angiogenic therapy was established as a novel strategy for treatment of cancers, diabetic retinopathy and rheumatic arthritis. Currently, a considerable number of works are being undertaken to screen potential anti-angiogenic compounds. The dietary constituents, including curcumin (Thaloor et al., 1998), flavonoids (Cao and Cao, 1999), N-acetylcysteine (Cai et al., 1999), vitamin D (Mantell et al., 2000) and conjugated fatty acids (Masso-Welch et al., 2002, Tsuzuki et al., 2007) have been shown to inhibit angiogenesis *in vitro* and/or *in vivo*. As shown in the present study, T3 represents as a member of a new class of dietary-derived anti-angiogenic compounds. Angiogenic inhibitors derived from natural products have an advantage in that they are non-toxic at physiological doses, can be given orally and can be easily obtained or manufactured. As one of our goals is to prepare a large amount of high-quality T3 for its anti-angiogenic benefits, we are studying many related fields such as farming T3-rich rice paddies and the technology for a large-scale preparation of rice bran T3 (Sookwong et al., 2007). The rice bran T3 will be used not only as the material for human trials and animal studies but also as the functional food.

ACKNOWLEDGMENTS

This study was supported in part by a Grant-in-Aid from the Bio-oriented Technology Research Advancement Center of the National Agricultural and Biological Research Organization, Japan.

REFERENCES

Cai, T., Fassina, G., Morini, M., Aluigi, M.G., Masiello, L., Fontanini, G., D'Agostini, F., De Flora, S., Noonan, D.M., Albini, A. 1999. N-acetylcysteine inhibits endothelial cell invasion and angiogenesis. *Lab. Invest.* 79, 1151–1159.

Cao, Y., Cao, R. 1999. Angiogenesis inhibited by drinking tea. *Nature* 398, 381.

Carolyn, A.S., Stephen, M.S., Simon, T., Russell, H., Nicola, J.B., Claire, E.L. 2004. Current methods for assaying angiogenesis *in vitro* and *in vivo*. *Int. J. Exp. Path.*, 85, 233–248.

Folkman, J., Klagsbrun, M. 1987. Angiogenic factors. *Science*, 235, 442–447.

Inokuchi, H., Hirokane, H., Tsuzuki, T., Nakagawa, K., Igarashi, M., Miyazawa, T. 2003. Anti-angiogenic activity of tocotrienol. *Biosci. Biotechnol. Biochem.*, 67, 1623–1627.

Kawakami, Y., Tsuzuki, T., Nakagawa, K., Miyazawa, T. 2007. Distribution of tocotrienols in rats fed a rice bran tocotrienol concentrate. *Biosci. Biotechnol. Biochem.*, 71, 464–471.

Khanna, S., Roy, S., Ryu, H., Bahadduri, P., Swaan, P.W., Ratan, R.R., Sen., C.K. 2003. Molecular basis of vitamin E action. Tocotrienol modulates 12-lipoxygenase, a key mediator of glutamate-induced neurodegeneration. *J. Biol. Chem.*, 278, 43508–43515.

Kim, K.J., Li, B., Winer, J., Armanini, M., Gillett, N., Phillips, H.S., Ferrara, N. 1993. Inhibition of vascular endothelial growth factor–induced angiogenesis suppresses tumor growth *in vivo*. *Nature*, 362, 841–844.

Mantell, D.J., Owens, P.E., Bundred, N.J., Mawer, E.B., Canfield, A.E. 2000. 1α,25-Dihydroxyvitamin D3 inhibits angiogenesis *in vitro* and *in vivo*. *Circ. Res.*, 87, 214–220.

Masso-Welch, P.A., Zangani, D., Ip, C., Vaughan, M.M., Shoemaker, S., Ramirez, R.A., Ip, M.M. 2002. Inhibition of angiogenesis by the cancer chemopreventive agent conjugated linoleic acid. *Cancer Res.*, 62, 4383–4389.

McIntyre, B.S., Briski, K.P., Gapor, A., Sylvester, P.W. 2000. Antiproliferative and apoptotic effects of tocopherols and tocotrienols on preneoplastic and neoplastic mouse mammary epithelial cells. *Proc. Soc. Exp. Biol. Med.*, 224, 292–301.

Miyazawa, T., Inokuchi, H., Hirokane, H., Tsuzuki, T., Nakagawa, K., Igarashi, M. 2004a. Anti-angiogenic potential of tocotrienol *in vitro*. *Biochemistry* (Mosc), 69, 67–69.

Miyazawa, T., Tsuzuki, T., Nakagawa, K., Igarashi, M. 2004b. Antiangiogenic potency of vitamin E. *Ann. N.Y. Acad. Sci.*, 1031, 401–404.

Mizushina, Y., Nakagawa, K., Shibata, A., Awata, Y., Kuriyama, I., Shimazaki, N., Koiwai, O., Uchiyama, Y., Sakaguchi, K., Miyazawa, T., Yoshida, H. 2006. Inhibitory effect of tocotrienol on eukaryotic DNA polymerase lambda and angiogenesis. *Biochem. Biophys. Res. Commun.*, 339, 949–955.

Nakagawa, K., Eitsuka, T., Inokuchi, H., Miyazawa, T. 2004. DNA chip analysis of comprehensive food function: Inhibition of angiogenesis and telomerase activity with unsaturated vitamin E, tocotrienol. *Biofactors*, 21, 5–10.

O'Byrne, D., Grundy, S., Packer, L., Devaraj, S., Baldenius, K., Hoppe P.P., Kraemer, K., Jialal, I., Traber, M.G. 2000. Studies of LDL oxidation following α–, γ–, or δ–tocotrienyl acetate supplementation of hypercholesterolemic humans. *Free Radic. Biol. Med.*, 29, 834–845.

Park, H.J., Kong, D., Iruela-Arispe, L., Begley, U., Tang, D., Galper, J.B. 2002. 3-Hydroxy-3-methylglutaryl coenzyme A reductase inhibitors interfere with angiogenesis by inhibiting the geranylgeranylation of RhoA. *Circ. Res.*, 91, 143–150.

Parker, R.A., Pearce, B.C., Clark, R.W., Gordon, D.A., Wright, J.J. 1993. Tocotrienols regulate cholesterol production in mammalian cells by post-transcriptional suppression of 3-hydroxy-3-methylglutaryl-coenzyme A reductase. *J. Biol. Chem.*, 268, 11230–11238.

Ribatti, D., Vacca, A., Roncali, L., Dammacco, F. 1996. The chick embryo chorioallantoic membrane as a model for *in vivo* research on angiogenesis. *Int. J. Dev. Biol.*, 40, 1189–1197.

Sen, C.K., Khanna, S., Roy, S., Packer, L. 2000. Molecular basis of vitamin E action. Tocotrienol potently inhibits glutamate-induced pp60c-src kinase activation and death of ht4 neuronal cells. *J. Biol. Chem.*, 275, 13049–13055.

Serbinova, E., Kagan, V., Han, D., Packer, L. 1991. Free radical recycling and intramembrane mobility in the antioxidant properties of α-tocopherol and α-tocotrienol. *Free Radic. Biol. Med.*, 10, 263–275.

Sookwong, P., Nakagawa, K., Murata, K., Kojima, Y., Miyazawa, T. 2007. Quantitation of tocotrienol and tocopherol in various rice brans. *J. Agric. Food Chem.*, 55, 461–466.

Sundram, K., Thiagarajan, T., Gapor, A., Basiron, Y. 2002. Palm tocotrienols: New antioxidants for the new millennium. *Inform*, 13, 634–640.

Suzuki, Y.J., Tsuchiya, M., Wassall, S.R., Choo, Y.M., Govil, G., Kagan, V.E., Packer, L. 1993. Structural and dynamic membrane properties of α-tocopherol and α-tocotrienol: Implication to the molecular mechanism of their antioxidant potency. *Biochemistry*, 32, 10692–10699.

Tang, F.Y., Meydani, M. 2001. Green tea catechins and vitamin E inhibit angiogenesis of human microvascular endothelial cells through suppression of IL–8 production. Nutr. *Cancer*, 41, 119–125.

Thaloor, D., Singh, A.K., Sidhu, G.S., Prasad, P.V., Kleinman, H.K., Maheshwari, R.K. 1998. Inhibition of angiogenic differentiation of human umbilical vein endothelial cells by curcumin. *Cell Growth Differ.*, 9, 305–312.

Traber, M.G., Packer, L. 1995. Vitamin E: Beyond antioxidant function. *Am. J. Clin. Nutr.*, 62, 1501S–1509S.

Tsuzuki, T., Shibata, A., Kawakami, Y., Nakagawa, K., Miyazawa, T. 2007. Conjugated eicosapentaenoic acid inhibits vascular endothelial growth factor-induced angiogenesis by suppressing the migration of human umbilical vein endothelial cells. *J. Nutr.*, 137, 641–646.

Vincent, L., Chen, W., Hong, L., Mirshahi, F., Mishal, Z., Mirshahi-Khorassani, T., Vannier, J.P., Soria, J., Soria, C. 2001. Inhibition of endothelial cell migration by cerivastatin, an HMG-CoA reductase inhibitor: Contribution to its anti-angiogenic effect. *FEBS Lett.*, 495, 159–166.

Yonekura, K., Basaki, Y., Chikahisa, L., Okabe, S., Miyadera, K., Yamada, Y. 1999. UFT and its metabolites inhibit the angiogenesis induced by murine renal cell carcinoma, as determined by a dorsal air sac assay in mice. *Clin. Cancer Res.*, 5, 2185–2191.

7 Chemistry of Tocotrienols

Sanchita P. Ghosh, Martin Hauer-Jensen and K. Sree Kumar

CONTENTS

7.1 INTRODUCTION

Because tocotrienols are the "new kids in the block" of vitamin E, throughout the chapters in this book there will be reference to the chemistry of tocotrienols. In order to avoid redundancy in various chapters, it was thought appropriate to compile the available information on the chemistry of tocotrienols in a separate chapter so that readers can relate to this chapter when they read about the pleiotropic effects of tocotrienols in other chapters.

The natural vitamin E family includes a group of potent, lipid soluble, chain breaking antioxidants—tocopherols (α-, β-, γ-, δ-) and tocotrienols (α-, β-, γ-, δ-). The chapters to follow will review recent data as they relate to the biological and clinical responses of α-, β-, γ- and δ-isoforms of tocotrienol. Evidence is accumulating to indicate that tocotrienols possess cholesterol-reducing (Baliarsingh et al., 2005; Qureshi et al., 1986; Rukmini, 1991), anticancer (Komiyama et al., 1989; Sundram et al., 1989) and neuroprotective properties (Khanna, 2005; Sen et al., 2006; Sen et al., 2004) that are not often exhibited by tocopherols. Whether the differences in the biological responses between tocopherols and tocotrienols (for example, in radioprotection described in Chapter 27) or differences in the biological responses among the various isoforms of tocotrienols (for example, almost 30-fold greater inhibition of hydroxymethyl glutaryl coenzyme A reductase by γ-tocotrienol as compared to α-tocotrienol) are dictated by the dissimilarities in the chemical structures has not been clearly established. Specifically, the role of the isoprenoid side chain of tocotrienols vis-à-vis the phytyl side chain of tocopherols in the differential regulation of biological responses is also unknown. Equally unknown are the roles of methyl groups on the chromanol ring of tocotrienols and tocopherols. The objective of this chapter is to focus more on the chemistry of tocotrienols than tocopherols and to discuss the possible relationship between the chemical structure and biological functions of tocotrienols.

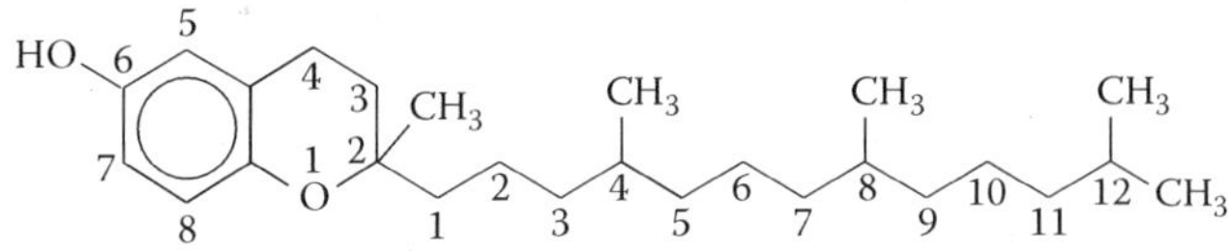

FIGURE 7.1 Structure of tocol.

TABLE 7.1
Structural Terminologies, Molecular Weights and Molecular Formulae of Tocotrienol and Tocopherol Isoforms

Common Name	Structural Terminology	Molecular Formula	Molecular Weight
α-tocotrienol	2,5,7,8-tetramethyl-2-(4,8,12-trimethyltrideca-3,7,11-trienyl)chroman-6-ol	$C_{29}H_{44}O_2$	424.66
β-tocotrienol	2,5,8-trimethyl-2-(4,8,12-trimethyltrideca-3,7,11-trienyl)chroman-6-ol	$C_{28}H_{42}O_2$	410.63
γ-tocotrienol	2,7,8-trimethyl-2-(4,8,12-trimethyltrideca-3,7,11-trienyl) chroman-6-ol	$C_{28}H_{42}O_2$	410.63
δ-tocotrienol	2,8-dimethyl-2-(4,8,12-trimethyltrideca-3,7,11-trienyl) chroman-6-ol	$C_{27}H_{40}O_2$	396.61
α-tocopherol	2,5,7,8-tetramethyl-2-(4,8,12- trimethyltridecyl)chroman-6-ol	$C_{29}H_{50}O_2$	430.71
β-tocopherol	2,5,8-trimethyl-2-(4,8,12-trimethyltridecyl)chroman-6-ol	$C_{28}H_{48}O_2$	416.68
γ-tocopherol	2,7,8-trimethyl-2-(4,8,12-trimethyltridecyl)chromen-6-ol	$C_{28}H_{48}O_2$	416.68
δ-tocopherol	2,8-dimethyl-2-(4,8,12-trimethyltridecyl)chroman-6-ol	$C_{27}H_{46}O_2$	402.65

7.2 CHEMISTRY OF TOCOTRIENOLS

7.2.1 Structures of Isoforms of Tocotrienols and Tocopherols

Structurally, tocotrienols and tocopherols are derived from tocol (Figure 7.1).

The structural terminologies, molecular formulae and molecular weights of all the eight isoforms—α, β, γ and δ of tocotrienols and tocopherols are given in Table 7.1.

Tocotrienols and tocopherols share certain features including a common polar chromanol head (with two rings fused—one phenolic and one heterocyclic) and a phytyl or isoprenoid chain at the C-2 position. Figure 7.2 shows the four isoforms of tocotrienol and Figure 7.3 shows these isoforms for tocopherol.

The names of the four isoforms are based on the substituted methyl groups on the chromanol ring. Tocotrienols differ from tocopherols (Figure 7.3) only by their side chains—both have substituted methyl groups on the chroman ring at identical positions. Tocotrienols have unsaturated isoprenoid side chains with double bonds in the 3', 7' and 11' positions, while tocopherols have saturated phytyl carbon chain.

While tocopherols exist only as free chromanols in nature, tocotrienols can occur naturally in esterified forms (Combs, 1992). Because of the unsaturated bonds in the isoprenoid side chains, tocotrienols are thought to assume a unique conformation. High field (Atkinson, 2006) NMR spectra show a structure of tocotrienols where the side-chain is curved so that it arcs over the chromanol ring. Such curvature shortens the functional length of the tocotrienol molecule, which is thought to make the membrane behavior of tocotrienol different from that of tocopherol (Atkinson, 2006). This arc conformation and easy intercalation may facilitate the use of low concentrations of tocotrienols to exert their physiological functions. For example, nanomolar concentrations of α-tocotrienol uniquely prevent inducible neurodegeneration by regulating specific mediators of cell death (Khanna et al., 2006; Khanna et al., 2003; Sen et al., 2000). Oral supplementation of tocotrienol (Tocomin®, Carotech, Inc.) protects against stroke (Khanna, 2005). Micromolar amounts of tocotrienol inhibit the rate-limiting enzyme of the cholesterol biosynthetic pathway, 3-hydroxy-3-methyl-

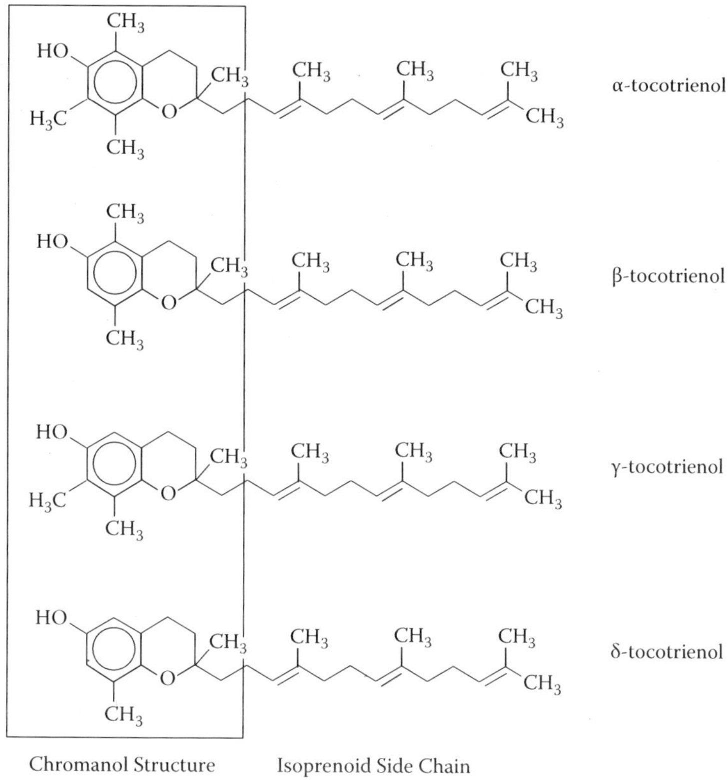

FIGURE 7.2 Chemical structures of the four isoforms of tocotrienols.

glutaryl coenzyme A (HMG-CoA) reductase (Pearce et al., 1992; Pearce et al., 1994). Tocopherols do not share the cholesterol-lowering properties of tocotrienol (Qureshi et al., 2002). γ-Tocotrienol and δ-tocotrienol are significantly more active than α-tocotrienol in suppressing HMG-CoA reductase activity.

The natural tocopherols have three asymmetric carbons at 2, 4' and 8' positions. Biosynthesis of tocopherols in nature yields only one stereoisomer. In contrast, tocopherols produced by chemical synthesis, by condensing isophytol with tri-, di-, or monomethyl hydroquinone, are equimolar racemic mixtures (all-rac) of eight stereoisomers. Thus when tocopherol is synthesized, each tocopherol isoform will have eight stereo isomers and a total of 32 stereo isomers for all the isoforms, whereas in nature there are only four isoforms (Burton and Traber, 1990).

Tocotrienols have only one chiral center at position 2, so they can only have 2D and 2L stereoisomers. However, the presence of the double bonds at positions 3' and 7' of the phytyl tail allows for the existence of four cis/trans geometrical isomers per tocotrienol. Therefore, a total of eight isomers can, at least theoretically be possible for each tocotrienol (Kamal-Eldin, 1996) as well.

In the following two sections we propose that (1) identical metabolic products of tocotrienol and tocopherol with isoprenoid or phytyl side chains accelerate the same *in vivo* reaction and (2) the presence of an –OH group alone does not account for all of the antioxidant function of tocols.

7.2.2 Metabolites of Tocotrienols

Ingested vitamin E (tocotrienols and tocopherols) is converted into chylomicrons together with lipids in the gut absorbed from the intestine, enters the circulation via the lymphatic system and is then transported to the liver with the chylomicrons (Brigelius-Flohe and Traber, 1999). The final metabolic products of excretion of tocotrienols in urine are carboxyethyl hydroxychromans (CEHC)

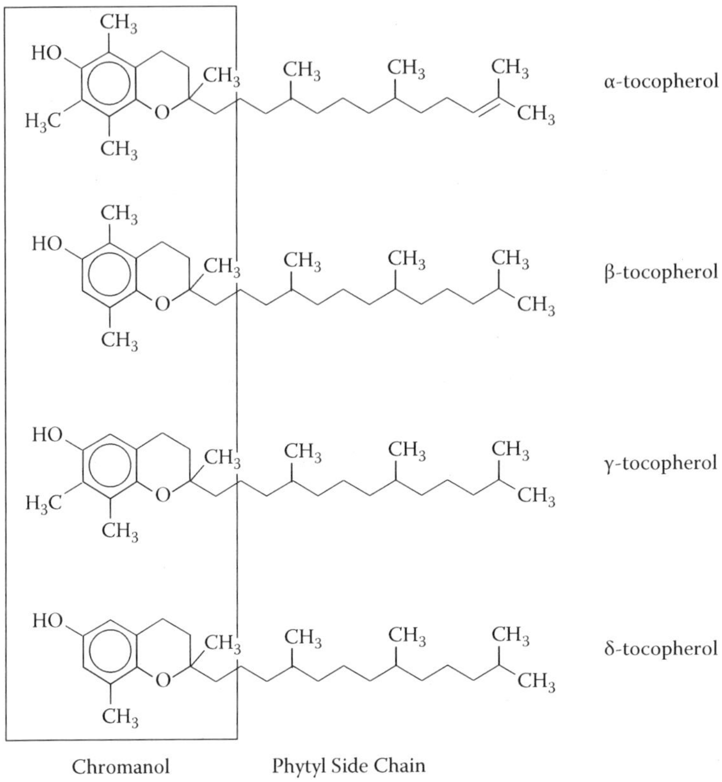

FIGURE 7.3 Chemical structures of the isoforms of tocopherol.

(Lodge et al., 2001). These are formed by the ω-hydroxylation and β-oxidation of the side chain *in vivo* (Kaneko et al., 2000; Swanson et al., 1999). The final products of metabolism of tocopherols are also CEHC (Brigelius-Flohe et al., 2002). Gamma-CEHC is produced and excreted into urine not only after ingestion of γ-tocopherol, but also after oral administration of γ-tocotrienol or other vitamin E analogs in rats as well as after γ-tocotrienol supplementation in humans (Hattori et al., 2000). Gamma-CEHC, produced from the metabolism of γ-tocotrienol or γ-tocopherol, possessed a hormone-like natriuretic function by accelerating sodium secretion and urinary volume in rats given a large sodium intake and therefore may be considered to be a vitamin functioning as a hormone precursor (Saito et al., 2003).

Conversion of α-tocopherol to its quinone, α-tocopheryl quinone increases the activity of α-tocopherol as an anticlotting agent. Alpha-tocopherol has only moderate anticlotting activity by virtue of its mild inhibition of vitamin K-dependent carboxylase, one of the key enzymes that control coagulation. On the other hand, α-tocopheryl quinone is a potent inhibitor of the enzyme and therefore is a potent anticoagulant (Dowd and Zheng, 1995).

7.2.3 Antioxidant Properties of Tocotrienols: Roles of –OH Group and –CH3 Groups?

In vivo defense systems protect aerobic organisms from oxidative stress induced by free radical oxygen or nitrogen species (ROS and RNS). As summarized in Table 7.2 (Noguchi and Etsuo, 1999), each antioxidant has a unique role in these defense systems. Vitamin E has been studied since its discovery in 1922 for its main role as an antioxidant. Due to their lipophilicity, tocopherols and tocotrienols intercalate into the cell membrane where they effectively inhibit lipid peroxidation by scavenging the chain-propagating peroxyl radicals. Cell and organelle membranes, lipoproteins, the

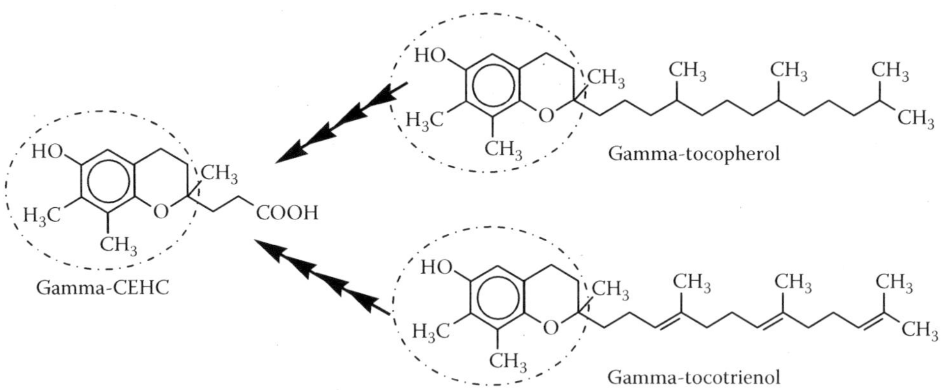

FIGURE 7.4 Formation of γ-CEHC from γ-tocotrienol and γ-tocopherol (Saito et al., 2003).

TABLE 7.2
***In Vivo* Defense Systems Against Reactive Oxygen and Nitrogen Species (ROS, RNS)**

1. Enzymatic Decomposition of ROS	
Catalase	Decomposition of hydrogen peroxide
	$2H_2O_2 \rightarrow 2H_2O + O_2$
Glutathione peroxidase (cellular)	Decomposition of hydrogen peroxide and free fatty acid hydroperoxides
	$H_2O_2 + 2GSH \rightarrow 2H_2O + GSSG$
	$LOOH + 2GSH \rightarrow LOH + H_2O + GSSG$
Glutathione peroxidase (plasma) Phospholipid hydroperoxide Glutathione peroxidase	Decomposition of hydrogen peroxide and phospholipids hydroperoxides
	$PLOOH + 2GSH \rightarrow PLOH + H_2O + GSSG$
Peroxidase	Decomposition of hydrogen peroxide and lipid peroxides
	$LOOH + AH_2 \rightarrow LOH + H_2O + A$
	$H_2O_2 + AH2 \rightarrow 2H_2O + A$
Glutathione S-transferase	Decomposition of lipid hydroperoxides
Superoxide dismutase (SOD)	Disproportionation of superoxide
	$2O_2^{\bullet-} + 2H^+ \rightarrow H_2O_2 + O_2$
2. Non-Enzymatic Scavenging of ROS and RNS	
(a) Sequestration of metal by chelation	
Transferrin, lactoferrin	Sequestration of iron
Heptoglobin	Sequestration of hemoglobin
Hemopexin	Sequestration of heme
Ceruloplasmin, albumin	Sequestration of copper
(b) Quenching of ROS	
Carotenoids, tocols	Quenching singlet oxygen, chain breaking antioxidants
(c) Quenching of RNS	Peroxynitrite (-OONO) quenching by gamma tocotrienol

Source: Adapted from: *Antioxidant Status, Diet, Nutrition and Health*. Andreas M. Papas (Ed) 1999. CRC Press. Boca Raton. Chapter 1. With permission.

adipose tissue, brain and other tissues containing abundant polyunsaturated fatty acids (PUFAs) are particularly vulnerable to lipid peroxidation.

Tocols vary in antioxidant potency. The chromanol structure (Figures 7.2 and 7.3) forms the basis for the antioxidant potency of the tocols. This is accomplished by donating the hydrogen atom from the hydroxyl group of the aromatic ring of the chromanol "head" (Packer et al., 2001). Recently, however, studies have compared the effectiveness of the different isoforms of vitamin E. Some of these studies (Packer et al., 2001; Serbinova et al., 1991; Suzuki et al., 1993) have indicated that α-tocotrienol is a more efficient antioxidant than α-tocopherol because it is recycled more efficiently from its chromanoxyl radical and is more uniformly distributed in the cellular membrane bilayer. Moreover, it has a stronger disordering effect on the membrane lipids, which leads to more efficient interaction between the chromanol "head" and the lipid radicals (Serbinova et al., 1991). The antioxidant activity of tocotrienols, particularly that of γ and δ-tocotrienols, are greater than tocopherols (Watkins et al., 1999).

Vitamin E also plays a critical role in preventing lipid oxidation in lipoproteins. Alpha-tocopherol is the main vitamin E form responsible for this effect in LDL because it is the most abundant (Esterbauer et al., 1991) and the best scavenger of peroxyl radicals. Chylomicrons, however, may carry other tocopherols and tocotrienols in similar or even higher concentration than α-tocopherol, depending on the diet, and they may also play an important role as lipid antioxidants in tissues such as adipose tissue and the liver. Some *in vitro* studies suggested that tocotrienols are significantly more effective than tocopherols in inhibiting LDL oxidation (Serbinova, 1994). In contrast, studies with plasma obtained from rats fed tocotrienol-rich diets indicate approximately similar inhibition by α-tocotrienol and α-tocopherol; γ-tocotrienol and γ-tocopherol had similar effects but lower than α-forms (Suarna et al., 1993).

In addition to peroxyl radicals, tocopherols and tocotrienols trap singlet oxygen (Kaiser et al., 1990) and other reactive species and free radicals. The antioxidant effect of vitamin E on reactive nitrogen species (RNS) has received increasing attention (Christen et al., 1997; Cooney et al., 1993; Kaiser et al., 1990). In biological systems, nitrogen dioxide (NO_2) is produced from the reaction of nitric oxide (NO) with oxygen. Alpha-tocopherol reacts with NO_2 to yield a nitrosating agent, thus acting as a NO_2 scavenger. In contrast, γ-tocopherol reduces NO_2 to NO or reacts with it without generating a nitrosating species (Cooney et al., 1995). The unique ability of γ-tocopherol, probably due to the number and positioning of the methyl groups on the chroman ring, may be particularly important in carcinogenesis, arthritis and neurological diseases, because nitrosating agents can deaminate DNA bases, causing mutations or interfering with important physiological functions. Gamma-tocotrienol may also play an important role in preventing the harmful effects of NO_2. Radiation induces the production of RNS-like NO_2, possibly by stimulating nitric oxide synthase (NOS), using arginine as the substrate. Nitrogen and superoxide formed by radiation can react together to form more toxic peroxynitrite (-OONO). One of the reasons for the superior radioprotection by GT3 may be its action as a peroxynitrite scavenger.

Although it was suggested that the –OH group on the chromanol ring (Figures 7.2 and 7.3) is responsible for the antioxidant activity of tocols (Packer et al., 2001), it alone does not explain the differing antioxidant properties among the various isoforms of tocotrienols and tocopherols. Particularly intriguing is the higher antioxidant properties of tocotrienols as compared with tocopherols (Watkins et al., 1999). The same number of methyl groups and –OH group at identical positions in the chromanol ring indicate that the variations in the antioxidant activities between tocotrienols and tocopherols are due to other structural factors. The higher level of antioxidant activity of γ-tocotrienol can be attributed to its ability to form an "arc" conformation over the chromanol ring (Atkinson, 2006) due to the double bond, which facilitates its intercalation in biomembranes, thereby allowing better antioxidant protection of membrane lipids. If there is a methyl group at position 5 on the chromanol ring, the arc conformation may be difficult due to steric hindrance of the methyl group. Since there is no methyl group at the 5-position on the chromanol ring in γ- and δ-tocotrienol, these two isoforms are biologically more active. This may also explain the higher level of inhibition of HMG-CoA by γ- and δ-tocotrienols as compared with α-tocotrienol (Qureshi et al., 2002), in which the 5-position of chromanol is methylated. Thus it appears that although the –OH group confers the antioxidant property of the tocol, the conformational state of tocotrienol dictated by the double bonds in the isoprenoid side chain and the methyl group at position 5 may determine the net effectiveness of tocotrienols in biological systems. The methyl group at position 5 of the chromanol ring also appears to be associated with a low omega-hydroxylation reaction in the metabolism of tocotrienols and tocopherols by the human microsomal P450 system (Sontag and Parker, 2007).

7.2.4 Role of Isoprenoid Side Chain of Tocotrienols on Biological Activity

Isoprenoids in general are known to affect a variety of biological functions. Isoprenoid modification and its association with the plasma membrane are critical factors for the transforming activity of *ras* protein (Der and Cox, 1991; Kato et al., 1992). Isoprenoid related metabolites are associated with neuropsychiatric disorders (Kurup and Kurup, 2003). The role of isoprenoid groups is not only to help in the anchoring of *ras* protein, but also to function as hydrophobic switches in signaling for specific target structures (Pechlivanis and Kuhlmann, 2006).

As explained in the previous section, the isoprenoid chain of tocotrienols can significantly affect the conformational states and hence their biological properties. It was reported that antioxidant activity may also depend on the length and structure of the side chain rather than on the chromanol methyl groups (Phoenix et al., 1991). The isoprenoid side chain of tocotrienols suppresses the growth of murine B16 melanomas both *in vitro* and *in vivo*. The effectiveness of the isoprenoid chain is influenced by the methyl groups on the chromanol ring of tocotrienols (He et al., 1997). The concentrations of α-, γ- and δ-tocotrienols needed to inhibit the growth of melanoma by 50% (IC50) showed a close relationship with the number of methyl groups on the chromanol ring. Alpha-tocotrienol with three methyl groups was least effective (IC50 = 110 micromole/L). In fact, when all the methyl groups were removed from the chromanol ring, the isoprenoid chain became very potent in suppressing the melanoma growth (IC50 = 0.9 micromole/L).

A significant observation from these studies is that the incorporation of isoprenoid groups into *ras* oncogenes results in the initiation of signaling pathways (Der and Cox, 1991; Kato et al., 1992), but the presence of isoprenoid groups as part of the tocotrienol structure makes tocotrienols inhibitors of malignancy (He et al., 1997). This apparent contradiction in the roles of isoprenoid groups in *ras* and tocotrienols may be explained by the presence of the chromanol ring in the latter. Although both isoprenoid-modified *ras* and tocotrienol are targeted to hydrophobic regions of the membrane, the presence of protein in *ras* and chromanol in tocotrienol may drive them to different microenvironments in the membrane.

7.3 NATURAL SOURCES OF TOCOTRIENOLS

Although tocotrienols are superior to tocopherols in their antioxidant properties, tocotrienols seem to be different as far as their vitamin E equivalent activities are concerned. The National Research Council (NRC) (NRC, 1989) recommended that, for dietary purposes, vitamin E activity be expressed as d-α-tocopherol equivalents (α-TE; 1.0 mg RRR-α-tocopherol = 1.0 α-TE). *All-rac-* α-tocopherol was assigned a value of 0.74 (for 1.0 mg). Biopotency of the esterified forms is computed from the RRR or *all-rac-* α-tocopherol content (Table 7.3) (Acuff et al., 1994; Burton et al., 1998; Kayden and Traber, 1993; Kiyose et al., 1997). This table clearly indicates the sharp distinction between tocopherols and tocotrienols as far as their bioequivalency as vitamin E factors.

Table 7.4 shows the amount of different isoforms of tocotrienols and tocopherols found in a variety of edible oils.

Palm oil and rice bran and its oil represent two good natural sources of tocotrienols. While tocopherols are generally present in common vegetable oils (soy, canola), tocotrienols, on the other hand, are concentrated in cereal grains (oat, rye, barley and rice bran), with the highest level found in crude palm oil. Rice bran, a by-product of the rice milling industry, is a major natural source

TABLE 7.3
Potencies of Tocopherols and Tocotrienols in International Units (IU) or α-Tocopherol Equivalents (α-TE)[a, b]

	IU/mg	α-TE/mg
α-Tocopherols		
Naturally occurring d- or RRR-α-tocopherol and its esters		
d-α-tocopherol	1.49	1.0
d-α-tocopheryl acetate	1.36	0.91
d-α-tocopheryl succinate	1.21	0.81
d-α-tocopheryl polyethylene glycol 1000 succinate (TPGS)	0.39	0.26
Synthetic dl- or all-rac-α- tocopherol and its ester		
dl-α-tocopherol	1.10	0.74
dl-α-tocopheryl acetate	1.0	0.67
dl-α-tocopheryl succinate	0.89	0.60
***Other tocols* (only for diets containing natural form)**		
d-β-tocopherol	0	0.50
d-γ-tocopherol	0	0.10
d-δ-tocopherol	0	0
d-α-tocotrienol	0	0.30
d-β-tocotrienol	0	0
d-γ-tocotrienol	0	0
d-δ-tocotrienol	0	0

[a] United States Pharmacopeia/National Formulary, the International Formulary and International Union of Pure and Applied Chemistry.
[b] National Research Council

Source: *Antioxidant Status, Diet, Nutrition and Health.* Andreas M. Papas (Ed), chapter 10. With permission.

of γ-tocotrienol but a poor source of α-tocotrienol. In addition, rice bran oil provides desmethyl tocotrienols. Two novel tocotrienols were isolated from stabilized and heated rice bran, apart from the known α-, β-, γ- and δ-tocopherols and tocotrienols. These new tocotrienols are known as desmethyl tocotrienol [3, 4-dihydro-2-methyl-2-(4,8,12-trimethyltrideca-3'(E),7'(E), 11'-trienyl)-2H-1-benzopyran-6-ol] and didesmethyl tocotrienol [3, 4-dihydro-2-(4,8,12-trimethyltrideca-3'(E),7'(E), 11'-trienyl)-2H-1-benzopyran-6-ol] (Qureshi et al., 2000). Although scientific evidence is relatively limited, rice bran oil is believed to be a healthy vegetable oil in Asian countries (Sugano et al., 1999). Cereals such as oat, rye and barley contain small amounts of tocotrienol. Alpha-tocotrienol is the predominant form of tocotrienol in oat and barley. Beta-tocotrienol is the major form of tocotrienol found in hulled and dehulled wheats (Panfili et al., 2003). Tocotrienols are synthesized both in edible and inedible plant products. Rubber latex represents a major non-food natural source of tocotrienols (Chow and Draper, 1970; Horvath et al., 2006; Whittle et al., 1966).

7.4 CONCLUSION

Vitamin E (tocopherols and tocotrienols) is a major fat soluble antioxidant, and has significant antioxidant functions. Of the eight isoforms of vitamin E, γ-tocotrienol is receiving greater atten-

TABLE 7.4
Natural Sources of Tocotrienols and Tocopherols

	Tocotrienols (mg/100gms)					Tocopherols (mg/100gms)				
Sources	**alpha**	**beta**	**gamma**	**delta**	**total**	**alpha**	**beta**	**gamma**	**delta**	**total**
Palm oil	20.5	–	43.9	9.4	**73.8**	15.2	–	–	–	**15.2**
Rice bran	23.6	–	34.9	–	**58.5**	32.4	1.8	5.3	–	**39.5**
Wheat germ	2.4	16.5	–	–	**18.9**	117.9	39.8	49.3	11.8	**218.8**
Barley	67	12	12	–	**91**	35	5	5	–	**45**
Oat	18	–	3	–	**21**	18	2	5	5	**30**
Coconut oil	0.5	0.1	1.9	–	**2.5**	0.5			0.6	**1.1**
Palm kernel oil	2.1	–	–	–	**2.1**	1.3	–	–	–	**1.3**
Soya bean oil	–	–	–	–	**0**	10.1	–	59.3	26.4	**95.8**
Safflower oil	–	–	–	–	**0**	38.7	–	38.7	–	**77.4**
Peanut oil	–	–	–	–	**0**	13.0	21.6	2.1	–	**36.7**
Cocoa butter	0.2	–	–	–	**0.2**	1.1	–	17	1.7	**19.8**
Olive oil	–	–	–	–	**0**	5.1	–	–	–	**5.1**
Sunflower oil[a]	–	–	–	–	**0**					**48.7**
Canola oil[a]	–	–	–	–	**0**					**65**

[a] Individual data of the isoforms are not available.

tion due to its better antioxidant activity, superior radioprotective efficacy and potent inhibition of HMG-CoA reductase activity. Different structural components of tocotrienols contribute to their various antioxidant and non-antioxidant functions. Some of these functions are afforded by the conformational states due to the unsaturated bonds in the isoprenoid side chains. Comparison with studies done with *ras* and isoprenoid groups indicate that the chromanol group may have a significant role in the anchoring of tocotrienols at appropriate microenvironments in cell membranes and initiate biological activities. Further structure-activity-relationship (SAR) studies will facilitate the exploitation of the full potential of these tocols in future.

7.5 FUTURE DIRECTIONS

The apparent contradiction in the role of isoprenoids in the modification of *ras* proteins and facilitating carcinogenesis and as part of the molecular structure of tocotrienols in preventing the growth of tumors should be explored further. SAR studies in this direction can lead to significant information not only about the control of carcinogenesis, but also other biological functions where isoprenoid groups are involved.

ACKNOWLEDGMENTS

Financial support: Defense Threat Reduction Agency grants number H.10027_07_AR_R to KSK and HDTRA1-07-C-0028 to MH-J and a University Technology Development Award to KSK by the Maryland Technology Development Corporation (TEDCO). All grants were awarded to The Henry M. Jackson Foundation for the Advancement of Military Medicine Inc., Rockville, MD. KSK was also supported by Armed Forces Radiobiology Research Institute grant RAB2AA.

BIBLIOGRAPHY

Acuff, R. V.; Thedford, S. S.; Hidiroglou, N. N.; Papas, A. M.; Odom, T. A., Jr. 1994. Relative bioavailability of RRR- and all-rac-alpha-tocopheryl acetate in humans: Studies using deuterated compounds. *Am J Clin Nutr*, 60, 397–402.

Atkinson, J., Chemical investigations of tocotrienols: Isotope substitution, fluorophores and a curious curve. *COSTAM*, Nesaretnam, K., Ed. Kuching, Malayasia, 2006; p 22.

Baliarsingh, S.; Beg, Z. H.; Ahmad, J. 2005. The therapeutic impacts of tocotrienols in type 2 diabetic patients with hyperlipidemia. *Atherosclerosis*, 182, 367–74.

Brigelius-Flohe, R.; Kelly, F. J.; Salonen, J. T.; Neuzil, J.; Zingg, J. M.; Azzi, A. 2002. The European perspective on vitamin E: Current knowledge and future research. *Am J Clin Nutr*, 76, 703–16.

Brigelius-Flohe, R.; Traber, M. G. 1999. Vitamin E: Function and metabolism. *Faseb J*, 13, 1145–55.

Burton, G. W.; Traber, M. G. 1990. Vitamin E: Antioxidant Activity, Biokinetics and Bioavailability. *Ann. Rev. Nutr.*, 10, 357–382.

Burton, G. W.; Traber, M. G.; Acuff, R. V.; Walters, D. N.; Kayden, H.; Hughes, L.; Ingold, K. U. 1998. Human plasma and tissue alpha-tocopherol concentrations in response to supplementation with deuterated natural and synthetic vitamin E. *Am J Clin Nutr*, 67, 669–84.

Chow, C. K.; Draper, H. H. 1970. Isolation of gamma-tocotrienol dimers from Hevea latex. *Biochemistry*, 9, 445–50.

Christen, S.; Woodall, A. A.; Shigenaga, M. K.; Southwell-Keely, P. T.; Duncan, M. W.; Ames, B. N. 1997. Gamma-tocopherol traps mutagenic electrophiles such as NO(X) and complements alpha-tocopherol: Physiological implications. *Proc Natl Acad Sci USA*, 94, 3217–22.

Combs, G. F., Jr. 1992. Vitamin E. In *The Vitamins: Fundamental Aspects in Nutrition and Health*. Academic Press: San Diego, p 179–203.

Cooney, R. V.; Franke, A. A.; Harwood, P. J.; Hatch-Pigott, V.; Custer, L. J.; Mordan, L. J. 1993. Gamma-tocopherol detoxification of nitrogen dioxide: Superiority to alpha-tocopherol. *Proc Natl Acad Sci USA*, 90, 1771–5.

Cooney, R. V.; Harwood, P. J.; Franke, A. A.; Narala, K.; Sundstrom, A. K.; Berggren, P. O.; Mordan, L. J. 1995. Products of gamma-tocopherol reaction with NO_2 and their formation in rat insulinoma (RINm5F) cells. *Free Radic Biol Med*, 19, 259–69.

Der, C. J.; Cox, A. D. 1991. Isoprenoid modification and plasma membrane association: Critical factors for ras oncogenicity. *Cancer Cells*, 3, 331–40.

Dowd, P.; Zheng, Z. B. 1995. On the mechanism of the anticlotting action of vitamin E quinone. *Proc Natl Acad Sci U S A*, 92, 8171–5.

Esterbauer, H.; Dieber-Rotheneder, M.; Striegl, G.; Waeg, G. 1991. Role of vitamin E in preventing the oxidation of low-density lipoprotein. *Am J Clin Nutr*, 53, 314S–321S.

Hattori, A.; Fukushima, T.; Yoshimura, H.; Abe, K.; Imai, K. 2000. Production of LLU-alpha following an oral administration of gamma-tocotrienol or gamma-tocopherol to rats. *Biol Pharm Bull*, 23, 1395–7.

He, L.; Mo, H.; Hadisusilo, S.; Qureshi, A. A.; Elson, C. E. 1997. Isoprenoids suppress the growth of murine B16 melanomas *in vitro* and *in vivo*. *J Nutr*, 127, 668–74.

Horvath, G.; Wessjohann, L.; Bigirimana, J.; Jansen, M.; Guisez, Y.; Caubergs, R.; Horemans, N. 2006. Differential distribution of tocopherols and tocotrienols in photosynthetic and non-photosynthetic tissues. *Phytochemistry*, 67, 1185–95.

Kaiser, S.; Di Mascio, P.; Murphy, M. E.; Sies, H. 1990. Physical and chemical scavenging of singlet molecular oxygen by tocopherols. *Arch Biochem Biophys*, 277, 101–8.

Kamal-Eldin, A.; Appelqvist, L. A. 1996. The chemistry and antioxidant properties of tocopherols and tocotrienols. *Lipids*, 31, 671–701.

Kaneko, K.; Kiyose, C.; Ueda, T.; Ichikawa, H.; Igarashi, O. 2000. Studies of the metabolism of alpha-tocopherol stereoisomers in rats using [5-methyl-(14)C]SRR- and RRR-alpha-tocopherol. *J Lipid Res*, 41, 357–67.

Kato, K.; Cox, A. D.; Hisaka, M. M.; Graham, S. M.; Buss, J. E.; Der, C. J. 1992. Isoprenoid addition to Ras protein is the critical modification for its membrane association and transforming activity. *Proc Natl Acad Sci USA*, 89, 6403–7.

Kayden, H. J.; Traber, M. G. 1993. Absorption, lipoprotein transport and regulation of plasma concentrations of vitamin E in humans. *J Lipid Res*, 34, 343–58.

Khanna, S. 2005. Neuroprotective properties of the natural vitamin E alpha-tocotrienol. *Stroke*, 36, 2258–64.

Khanna, S.; Roy, S.; Parinandi, N. L.; Maurer, M.; Sen, C. K. 2006. Characterization of the potent neuroprotective properties of the natural vitamin E alpha-tocotrienol. *J Neurochem*, 98, 1474–86.

Khanna, S.; Roy, S.; Ryu, H.; Bahadduri, P.; Swaan, P. W.; Ratan, R. R.; Sen, C. K. 2003. Molecular basis of vitamin E action: Tocotrienol modulates 12–lipoxygenase, a key mediator of glutamate–induced neurodegeneration. *J Biol Chem*, 278, 43508–15.

Kiyose, C.; Muramatsu, R.; Kameyama, Y.; Ueda, T.; Igarashi, O. 1997. Biodiscrimination of alpha-tocopherol stereoisomers in humans after oral administration. *Am J Clin Nutr*, 65, 785–9.

Komiyama, K.; Iizuka, K.; Yamaoka, M.; Watanabe, H.; Tsuchiya, N.; Umezawa, I. 1989. Studies on the biological activity of tocotrienols. *Chem Pharm Bull (Tokyo)*, 37, 1369–71.

Kurup, R. K.; Kurup, P. A. 2003. Isoprenoid pathway–related membrane dysfunction in neuropsychiatric disorders. *Int J Neurosci*, 113, 1579–91.

Lodge, J. K.; Ridlington, J.; Leonard, S.; Vaule, H.; Traber M. G. 2001. Alpha- and gamma-tocotrienols are metabolized to carboxyethyl-hydroxychroman derivatives and excreted in human urine. *Lipids*, 36, 43–8.

Noguchi, N.; Etsuo, N. 1999. Chemistry of active oxygen species and antioxidants.*Antioxidant Status, Diet, Nutrition and Health*, Papas, A. M., Ed. CRC Press: Boca Raton, Florida, pp 3–20.

NRC, *Recommended Dietary Allowances*. 1989. 10th ed., National Academy Press: Washington D.C.

Packer, L.; Weber, S. U.; Rimbach, G. 2001. Molecular aspects of alpha-tocotrienol antioxidant action and cell signalling. *J Nutr*, 131, 369S–73S.

Panfili, G.; Fratianni, A.; Irano, M. 2003. Normal phase high-performance liquid chromatography method for the determination of tocopherols and tocotrienols in cereals. *J Agric Food Chem*, 51, 3940–4.

Pearce, B. C.; Parker, R. A.; Deason, M. E.; Dischino, D. D.; Gillespie, E.; Qureshi, A. A.; Volk, K.; Wright, J. J. 1994. Inhibitors of cholesterol biosynthesis. 2. Hypocholesterolemic and antioxidant activities of benzopyran and tetrahydronaphthalene analogues of the tocotrienols. *J Med Chem*, 37, 526–41.

Pearce, B. C.; Parker, R. A.; Deason, M. E.; Qureshi, A. A; Wright, J. J. 1992. Hypocholesterolemic activity of synthetic and natural tocotrienols. *J Med Chem*, 35, 3595–606.

Pechlivanis, M.; Kuhlmann, J. 2006. Hydrophobic modifications of Ras proteins by isoprenoid groups and fatty acids—More than just membrane anchoring. *Biochim Biophys Acta*, 1764, 1914–31.

Phoenix, J.; Edwards, R. H.; Jackson, M. J.. The effect of vitamin E analogues and long hydrocarbon chain compounds on calcium-induced muscle damage. A novel role for alpha-tocopherol? *Biochim Biophys Acta* 1991, 1097, 212–218.

Qureshi, A. A.; Burger, W. C.; Peterson, D. M.; Elson, C. E. 1986. The structure of an inhibitor of cholesterol biosynthesis isolated from barley. *J Biol Chem*, 261, 10544–50.

Qureshi, A. A.; Mo, H.; Packer, L.; Peterson, D. M. 2000. Isolation and identification of novel tocotrienols from rice bran with hypocholesterolemic, antioxidant and antitumor properties. *J Agric Food Chem*, 48, 3130–40.

Qureshi, A. A.; Sami, S. A; Salser, W. A.; Khan, F. A. 2002. Dose-dependent suppression of serum cholesterol by tocotrienol-rich fraction (TRF25) of rice bran in hypercholesterolemic humans. *Atherosclerosis*, 161, 199–207.

Rukmini C., Raghuram, R. T. 1991. Nutritional and biochemical aspects of the hypolipidemic action of rice bran oil. *J. Am. Coll. Nutr*, 10, 593–601.

Saito, H.; Kiyose, C.; Yoshimura, H.; Ueda, T.; Kondo, K.; Igarashi, O. 2003. Gamma-tocotrienol, a vitamin E homolog, is a natriuretic hormone precursor. *J Lipid Res*, 44, 1530–5.

Sen, C. K.; Khanna, S.; Roy, S. 2006. Tocotrienols: Vitamin E beyond tocopherols. *Life Sci*, 78, 2088–98.

Sen, C. K.; Khanna, S.; Roy, S.; Packer, L. 2000. Molecular basis of vitamin E action: Tocotrienol potently inhibits glutamate-induced pp60(c-Src) kinase activation and death of HT4 neuronal cells. *J Biol Chem*, 275, 13049–55.

Sen, C. K., Khanna, S., Roy, S. 2004. Tocotrienol: The natural vitamin E to defend the nervous system? *Ann N Y Acad Sci*, 1031, 127–42.

Serbinova, E.; Kagan, V.; Han, D.; Packer, L. 1991. Free radical recycling and intramembrane mobility in the antioxidant properties of alpha-tocopherol and alpha-tocotrienol. *Free Radic Biol Med*, 10, 263–75.

Serbinova, E. L. P. 1994. Antioxidant properties of alpha-tocopherol and alpha-tocotrienol. *Methods Enzymol*, 234, 354–366.

Sontag, T. J.; Parker, R. S. 2007. Influence of major structural features of tocopherols and tocotrienols on their omega-oxidation by tocopherol-omega-hydroxylase. *J Lipid Res*, 48, 1090–8.

Suarna, C.; Hood, R. L.; Dean, R. T.; Stocker, R. 1993. Comparative antioxidant activity of tocotrienols and other natural lipid-soluble antioxidants in a homogeneous system and in rat and human lipoproteins. *Biochim Biophys Acta*, 1166, 163–70.

Sugano, M.; Koba, K.; Tsuji, E. 1999. Health benefits of rice bran oil. *Anticancer Res*, 19, 3651–7.

Sundram, K.; Khor, H. T.; Ong, A. S.; Pathmanathan, R. 1989. Effect of dietary palm oils on mammary carcinogenesis in female rats induced by 7,12–dimethylbenz(a)anthracene. *Cancer Res*, 49, 1447–51.

Suzuki, Y. J.; Tsuchiya, M.; Wassall, S. R.; Choo, Y. M.; Govil, G.; Kagan, V. E.; Packer, L. 1993. Structural and dynamic membrane properties of alpha-tocopherol and alpha-tocotrienol: Implication to the molecular mechanism of their antioxidant potency. *Biochemistry*, 32, 10692–9.

Swanson, J. E.; Ben, R. N.; Burton, G. W.; Parker, R. S. 1999. Urinary excretion of 2,7, 8-trimethyl-2-(beta-carboxyethyl)-6-hydroxychroman is a major route of elimination of gamma-tocopherol in humans. *J Lipid Res*, 40, 665–71.

Watkins, T. R.; Bierenbaum, M. L.; Giampolo, A. 1999. Tocotrienols: Biological and health effects. In *Antioxidant Status, Diet, Nutrition and Health*, Papas, A. M., Ed. CRC Press: Boca Raton, pp 479–496.

Whittle, K. J.; Dunphy, P. J.; Pennock, J. F. 1966. The isolation and properties of delta-tocotrienol from Hevea latex. *Biochem J*, 100, 138–45.

Part D

Mechanisms of Action

8 Antioxidant Activity of Tocotrienols in Cells and Serum

Rossella Simone and Paola Palozza

CONTENTS

8.1 INTRODUCTION

Over the past few decades, free radicals, highly reactive and thereby destructive molecules, have become known increasingly for their importance to human health and disease. Many common and life threatening human diseases, including atherosclerosis, diabetes, cancer and aging, have free radical reactions as an underlying mechanism of injury. Because our bodies are continuously exposed to free radicals and other reactive species of oxygen (ROS) from both external sources (sunlight, other forms of radiation, pollution) and generated endogenously, ROS-mediated tissue injury is a final common pathway for a number of disease processes. Radicals of oxygen (superoxide anion, hydroxyl radicals and peroxy radicals), reactive non-radical oxygen species such as hydrogen peroxide and singlet oxygen, as well as carbon, nitrogen and sulfur radicals make up the variety of reactive molecules that can cause damage to cells. Our conceptual understanding of the interaction of such ROS with living organisms has undergone a remarkable evolution.

Antioxidants are intimately involved in the prevention of cellular damage—the common pathway for cancer, aging and a variety of diseases. These molecules safely interact with free radicals and terminate the chain reaction before vital molecules are damaged. They neutralize free radicals by donating one of their own electrons. The antioxidant nutrients themselves do not become free radicals by donating an electron because they are stable in either form; they act as scavengers, helping to prevent cell and tissue damage that could lead to cellular damage and disease.

α-tocopherol is known to act as a potent antioxidant in biological systems. It is also the most abundant and active form of vitamin E homologues, but recently the role of other forms of vitamin E has received renewed attention. Vitamin E is a generic term that includes eight substances, namely α-, β-, γ- and δ-tocopherol and α-, β-, γ- and δ-tocotrienol. Tocotrienols, formerly known as ζ or η-tocopherols, are similar to tocopherols except that they have an isoprenoid tail with three unsaturation points instead of a saturated phytyl tail. Palm, rice bran and barley oils are particularly rich in tocotrienols. Both tocopherols and tocotrienols are known to possess excellent antioxidant activity, but increasing evidence shows that, at least in *in vitro* studies, tocotrienols suppress ROS production more efficiently than tocopherols. However, compared with tocopherols, tocotrienols have been poorly studied (Traber and Packer 1995; Traber and Sies 1996; Sen et al. 2004, 2006).

This chapter evaluates the available evidence of the antioxidant activity of tocotrienols in cells and serum, focusing on the main factors responsible for the antioxidant activity of these compounds and on their potential as health-maintaining agents.

8.2 ANTIOXIDANT ACTIVITY OF TOCOTRIENOLS IN CELLS

The antioxidant activity of tocotrienols is influenced by several factors. They include: isomeric structure, distribution and mobility within cell membrane, synergistic interactions with other antioxidants, tocotrienol concentration in biological systems. Such factors will be briefly discussed in this section.

8.2.1 Isomeric Structure

Both tocopherols and tocotrienols have four isomers, designated as α-, β-, γ- and δ-, which differ by the number and position of methyl groups on the chroman ring (Machlin, 1991). The antioxidant activities of α-, β-, γ- and δ- tocotrienols have been the subjects of some studies in different biological models, including homogeneous solution, liposomes, isolated membranes and intact cells.

The reactivities toward peroxyl radicals and oxygen radicals generated by metal ions were measured in solution or in sodium dodecyl sulphate (SDS) micelles and found to decrease in the order of α-/β-/γ-/δ-tocotrienols.

In PC liposomes, both α- and γ-tocotrienols were able to inhibit 2,2'-azobis(4-methoxy-2,4-dimethylvaleronitrile) (MeO-AMVN)-induced lipid peroxidation. However, γ-tocotrienol was found to be more effective in prolonging the lag phase as measured by conjugated diene formation when compared with α-tocotrienol (Yoshida et al., 2003).

In rat liver microsomal membranes as well as in rat brain mitochondria, the palm oil fraction, rich in the different tocotrienol isomers, has been reported to be strongly effective in inhibiting lipid peroxidation and protein oxidation induced by different sources of free radicals, including ascorbate-Fe^{2+} and photosensitization agents. When the abilities of the three different isomers of tocotrienol were compared, γ-tocotrienol was the most effective followed by α- and δ-tocotrienol (Kamat et al., 1997).

We recently demonstrated that individual tocotrienols display different antioxidant potencies toward oxidative stress induced *in vitro*, being the order of effectiveness δ-tocotrienol > γ-tocotrienol = α-tocotrienol. δ-tocotrienol exhibited a strong antioxidant activity, as documented by its ability to inhibit lipid peroxidation or free radical generation in isolated rat liver microsomal membranes as well as in RAT-1 immortalized fibroblasts. These effects occurred at micromolar concentrations of the compound and were dose- and time-dependent. Moreover, they were not deeply influenced by the source of free radicals. Whatever the prooxidant used [2,2'-azobis-(2-amidinopropane)dihy drochloride (AAPH) or *tert*- butyl hydroperoxide (*t*-BOOH)], δ-tocotrienol was the best tocotrienol in inhibiting lipid peroxidation. Moreover, it was the most potent tocotrienol, among those tested, in inhibiting reactive oxygen species formation induced by the hydroperoxide as well as by H_2O_2 in cultured fibroblasts. In such cells, the inhibition of ROS generation by tocotrienols paralleled the effect of the compounds in enhancing cell viability, suggesting that the two phenomena are related. Interestingly, in our study, δ-tocotrienol was also the most effective tocotrienol in inhibiting the expression of heat shock proteins (hsps), such as hsp70 and hsp90. (Palozza et al., 2006). ROS have been greatly implicated in the activation of these stress proteins as many oxidizing agents have been shown to result in hsp induction (Martindale and Holbrook, 2002) and treatment of cells with antioxidants prior to stresses attenuates the response (Gorman et al., 1999).

Recently, two novel tocotrienols were isolated from stabilized and heated rice bran, apart from the known α-, β-, γ- and δ-tocopherols and tocotrienols. Their structures were established as desmethyl tocotrienol [3,4-dihydro-2-methyl-2-(4,8,12-trimethyltrideca-3′(E),7′(E),11′-trienyl)-2H-1-benzopyran-6-ol] and didesmethy tocotrienol [3,4-dihydro-2-(4,8,12-trimethyltrideca-3′(E),7′(E),11′-trienyl)-2*H*-1-benzopyran-6-ol]. In an *in vitro* liposome system exposed to AMVN, these tocotrienols had more antioxidant activities than α-tocopherol and known tocotrienols. In particular, the order of activity was *d*-P25-tocotrienol > *d*-P21-tocotrienol > tocotrienol rich fraction (TRF) > δ-tocotrienol > γ-tocotrienol > α-tocotrienol > α-tocopherol. In the same study, these findings were further confirmed by determining the antioxidant activities using a different method, the coupled autoxidation of β-carotene and linoleic acid. The antioxidant activities of known α-, γ- and δ-tocotrienols and TRF (prepared from stabilized and heated rice bran with 6% α-tocopherol) were 22%, 27%, 32% and 24% better than α-tocopherol, respectively (Qureshi et al., 2000).

Although these results collectively indicate that all tocotrienol isomers act as antioxidants in biological systems, from these studies it is not possible to single out the order of their antioxidant potency, probably because of the different models, stressors and concentrations used.

8.2.2 Cell Distribution and Mobility

It is known that the potency of radical-scavenging antioxidants is determined not only by the chemical reactivity toward radicals, but also by other factors, including cell distribution and mobility at the microenvironment.

In many studies, tocotrienols have been reported to have better antioxidant activity than tocopherols (Serbinova et al., 1991; Kamat and Devasagayam, 1995). This could be due to the higher mobility of the polyenoic chain of tocotrienols in the membrane bilayer (Kamat and Devasagayam, 1995). Hence, tocotrienols could be more mobile and less restricted than tocopherols in their interaction with lipid radicals in membranes. According to this, tocotrienols have been reported to exhibit an antioxidant activity similar to tocopherols in homogeneous solutions, but increasing evidence shows that tocotrienols are more potent as antioxidants than tocopherols in isolated membranes and intact cells, as they are shown to be more readily incorporated. It has been emphasized that α-tocotrienol was better incorporated than α-tocopherol in human erythrocytes (Begum and Terao, 2002). Moreover, in HT4 neuron cell cultures, Sen et al. reported a difference in the uptake of these two vitamin E subfamilies: the γ-tocotrienol uptake was more efficient than the α-tocopherol one (Sen et al., 2000). In addition, the exposure of human umbilical vein endothelial cells (HUVECs) to several tocopherol and tocotrienol concentrations show a better incorporation for γ-tocotrienol and α-tocotrienol than the corresponding γ- and α-tocopherol. Interestingly, to achieve the same rate of accumulation as α-tocotrienol, a 10-fold higher concentration of α-tocopherol was needed to be added into the medium (Mutaliba et al., 2003). In a recent study, we reported an increased cellular accumulation of δ-tocotrienol with respect to the α- and γ-isoforms in immortalized fibroblasts (Palozza et al., 2006). Such an observation is not surprising, because it has been reported that a decrease in the level of chromane ring methylation of tocotrienols results in a corresponding decrease in the partition coefficient of these compounds, responsible for a greater cellular uptake. Accordingly, δ-tocotrienol was accumulated to a greater extent than α-tocotrienol in mammary epithelial cells (McIntyre et al., 2000) and α-tocopheryl succinate or hemisuccinate, fewer lipophilic derivatives of α-tocopherol and displayed a significantly greater cellular accumulation than α-tocopherol itself (Tirmenstein et al.,1998; Fariss et al., 1994).

The cellular uptake of tocopherol and tocotrienol isomers was also investigated in Caco2 cell monolayer models (Tsuzuki et al., 2007). The initial accumulation of tocotrienol isomers in Caco2 cells was larger than those of corresponding tocopherol isomers. There was little difference among the cellular accumulations of four tocopherol isomers. These findings suggested that the difference between the molecular structures of the C16 hydrocarbon chain tail in tocopherol and tocotrienol was strongly responsible for the rapid epithelial transport into the Caco2 cells membranes rather than the difference in the molecular structures of their chromanol head groups (Tsuzuki et al., 2007).

On the other hand, no significant difference was observed in the uptake of γ-tocotrienol and α-tocopherol by astrocytes. This could suggest a difference in the mechanism of uptake of vitamin E in astrocytes and other kinds of cells (Mazlan et al., 2006).

8.2.3 Synergistic Interactions with Other Antioxidants

Vitamin E does not work in isolation from other antioxidants; rather it is part of an interlinking set of redox antioxidant cycles (Constantinescu et al., 1993), which has been termed the "antioxidant network." It is hypothesized that vitamin E acts catalytically, i.e., it is efficiently reduced from its free radical (chromanoxyl) form, which arises after quenching lipid radicals, to return back to its reduced native state. This catalysis occurs through the interactions between water- and lipid-soluble substances by both non-enzymatic and enzymatic mechanisms that regenerate vitamin E from its tocotrienoxyl or tocopheroxyl radical back to tocotrienol and tocopherol, respectively. Vitamin C can regenerate vitamin E directly and thiol antioxidants, such as glutathione and lipoic acid, can regenerate vitamin E indirectly via vitamin C. Under conditions in which these systems act synergistically to keep the steady-state concentration of vitamin E radicals low, the loss or consumption of vitamin E is prevented. Such recycling effects can be seen in human low density lipoprotein (LDL) (Kagan et al., 1992) and in membranes enriched with tocopherols or tocotrienols or by feeding animals vitamin E-enriched diets (Suarna et al., 1993; Verlangieri and Bush 1992).

It has been previously reported in isolated membranes that synergistic antioxidant interactions may also occur between α-tocopherol and carotenoids (Palozza and Krinsky, 1992). Recently, similar interactions have also been found in phospholipid liposomes between β-carotene or lycopene and α-tocopherol, α-tocotrienol, or γ-tocotrienol for carotene/phenol ratios of 1:10 and 1:2 but not for 1:1. Because carotenoids were consumed faster than phenolic compounds in such a model, it is possible that they act as protectors of the tocopherols and the tocotrienols through sacrificial oxidation, resulting in antioxidant synergism. Moreover, the synergistic effects in liposomes may also be explained by a sacrificial oxidation of β-carotene or lycopene through reaction with lipid-derived radicals—in effect protecting α-tocopherol and the tocotrienols (Schroeder et al., 2006).

In another study, mixtures of β-carotene and α-tocopherol have been found not to act in a synergistic manner in liposomes, with a β-carotene and α-tocopherol ratio of 1:1 and 1:2 (Roberts and Gordon, 2003). Synergism seems to require that carotenoids are present in concentrations considerably lower than the tocopherol concentration (Wrona et al., 2003). High concentrations of carotenes have been found to act prooxidatively also in other systems (Palozza et al., 2006).

8.3 COMPARATIVE ANTIOXIDANT EFFICIENCY WITH OTHER COMPOUNDS

8.3.1 Tocopherols

Both tocopherols and tocotrienols scavenge the chain-propagating peroxyl radical. When comparing the effectiveness of tocopherols and tocotrienols, at least two factors must be considered, i.e., the substituents on the chromanol nucleus and the properties of the side chain. In homogeneous solutions, the reaction rate constant depends mainly on the number of methyl groups on the nucleus. In membranes, the mobility of the molecule also becomes important and this depends on the structure of the hydrophobic side chain.

No difference in radical-scavenging activity between tocotrienols and tocopherols was found in solution or in SDS micelles. α-, β-, γ- and δ-tocotrienols possess the same chemical reactivities toward oxygen radicals as the corresponding tocopherols. However, the activity of α-tocotrienol in scavenging peroxyl radicals is 1.5-fold higher in liposomes than in α-tocopherol (Serbinova et al., 1991). Moreover, α-tocotrienol exhibited greater peroxyl radical scavenging potency than α-tocopherol in liposomal membranes (Suzuki et al., 1993).

In another study, results by a chemiluminescence assay in a liposome membrane system indicate that α-tocotrienol is at least threefold more efficient as a scavenger of peroxyl radicals than is α-tocopherol (Packer, 1995). These results were confirmed in a recent study, in which α-tocotrienol and α-tocopherol were incorporated in phosphatidyl choline (PC) liposomes. In liposome systems *in vitro*, antioxidant activities of several TRFs extracted from rice bran oil were reported to be between four- and 33-fold higher than α-tocopherol. Moreover, an increase in the antioxidant activity was observed as the proportion of α-tocopherol was decreased in the TRF (Qureshi et al., 2000).

Likewise, the tocotrienol-rich fraction from palm oil was significantly more effective than α-tocopherol in protecting rat brain mitochondria and rat liver microsomes against oxidative damage (Kamat and Devasagayam, 1995; Kamat et al., 1997).

In another study, the efficacy of α-tocotrienol to protect against Fe(II)l NADPH-induced lipid peroxidation in rat liver microsomes was 40 times higher than that of α-tocopherol. Alpha-tocotrienol also was 6.5 times more effective in the protection of cytochrome P-450 against oxidative damage (Serbinova et al., 1991). Moreover, in rat liver mitochondria and microsomes, α-tocotrienol inhibits lipid peroxidation induced by CumOOH/ Fe^{2+} ADP- NADPH system, similar to that of butylated hydroxyl touluene (BHT) and to a greater extent than α-tocopherol (Ghafoorunissa et al., 2004).

In a recent study, the protective effect of α-tocopherol and palm TRF were also compared in both LDL and HUVEC endothelial cells. Human LDL were exposed to the prooxidant action of copper and HUVEC cells were oxidized by arachidonic acid. In this study, greater enhancement of the lag phase for thiobarbituric reactive substances (TBARS) formation in the TRF compared with the α-tocopherol-treated LDL was observed. The effect of TRF on peroxidation of HUVEC cells gave more convincing results regarding the antioxidant potential of TRF than tocopherol. TRF (10 mM) was more effective in reducing TBARS in the cell medium than 25 μM of α-tocopherol and this efficacy was more pronounced with 25 μM TRF (Ghafoorunissa et al., 2004). In contrast, α-tocopherol was observed to behave as a pro-oxidant in these cells when its concentration was increased to 50 μM. The antioxidant potential of TRF was also shown to be higher than α-tocopherol in terms of conjugated diene formation (Ghafoorunissa et al., 2004).

Moreover, treatment of erythrocytes with α-tocopherol and α-tocotrienol suppressed the impairment of erythrocyte deformability as well as membranous lipid peroxidation induced by AAPH and increased erythrocyte deformability even in the absence of the prooxidant (Begum and Terao, 2002). Once again, the protecting effects of α-tocotrienol were significantly higher than those of α-tocopherol. (Begum and Terao, 2002).

Similarly, in *Caenorhabditis elegans* exposed to UV-B light, pre- and postadministration of tocotrienols lowered protein carbonylation and extended mean life span. In contrast, α-tocopherol supplementation had no significant effects (Adachi and Ishii, 2000).

Recently, some studies have been conducted to dissect the antioxidant-independent and -dependent neuroprotective properties of tocotrienols by using different stressors, including H_2O_2, homocysteic acid (HCA), linoleic acid and glutamate and different cell models, including astrocytes (Mazlan et al., 2006), HT4 neuron cells (Sen et al., 2000) and primary neuronal cultures of rat striatum (Khanna et al., 2006). In all these studies, tocotrienols have been reported to exhibit better neuroprotective effects than α-tocopherol. It is hypothesized that these protective effects of tocotrienols are probably independent of their antioxidant activity because they occurred only at multifold higher concentrations (Sen et al., 2000).

Several reasons have been suggested for the increased antioxidant activity of α-tocotrienol vs. α-tocopherol, focusing on the differences in the tail structure. The chromanoxyl radical of α-tocotrienol (α-tocotrienoxyl) has been found to be recycled in membranes and lipoproteins more quickly than the corresponding α-tocopheroxyl radical (Serbinova et al., 1991). Nuclear magnetic resonance studies have indicated that α-tocotrienol is located closer to the membrane surface, which may facilitate recycling. Furthermore, α-tocotrienol has a stronger disordering effect on membranes than α-tocopherol and is distributed more uniformly within the membrane. These properties likely enhance the interaction of chromanols with lipid radicals (Serbinova et al., 1991; Suzuki et al., 1993).

8.4 TOCOTRIENOL CONCENTRATIONS

The hypothesis that the concentration strongly influences the biological activity of tocotrienols has been described by Chandan Sen and his colleagues (Sen et al., 2000; Khanna et al., 2006). They discovered that tocotrienol was effective at two concentrations. At a higher concentration it functioned as an antioxidant, while at lower concentrations its action was independent of its antioxidant properties. To try to discriminate between these two functions, they used two triggers of neurotoxicity: HCA and linoleic acid. Both HCA and linoleic acid cause neurotoxicity with comparable features, such as an increased ratio of oxidized to reduced glutathione GSSG/GSH, raised intracellular calcium concentrations and compromised mitochondrial membrane potential. To observe the activity of tocotrienol, rat neurons were treated with nanomolar concentrations of the vitamin. The results indicated that the neurons were protected from the cell death caused by the HCA by these very low concentrations of tocotrienol. At micromolar concentrations, tocotrienol exhibited antioxidant properties against the oxidative stress caused by linoleic acid (Khanna et al., 2006).

8.4.1 Synthetic Analogues

The antioxidant activity of tocotrienols was also compared with new synthetic compounds. In particular, we found that FeAox-6, a novel synthetic compound which combines, by a stable covalent bond, the chroman head of vitamin E and a polyisoprenyl sequence of four conjugated double bonds into a single molecule (Palozza et al., 2002), showed an antioxidant potency greater than that of tocotrienols (Palozza et al., 2006). The synthetic compound was able to strongly inhibit lipid peroxidation in rat liver microsomal membranes challenged with different free radical sources, including AAPH, *t*-BOOH as well as H_2O_2-induced reactive oxygen species (ROS) production and heat shock protein (hsp) expression in RAT-1 immortalized fibroblasts.

Such an efficiency seems to depend on the concomitant presence of a chromane ring and the phytyl chain in the molecule, which, because of four conjugated double bonds, may induce a greater mobility and a more uniform distribution within cell membrane.

However, when FeAox-6 and α-tocotrienol were compared in their ability to reduce cholesterol accumulation in human macrophages, the extent of the reduction found with α-tocotrienol was greater than that induced by FeAOX-6 and did not correlate with their respective antioxidant capacities (Napolitano et al., 2007).

Pretreatment with vitamin E analogs including α-tocopherol, α -tocotrienol, γ-tocopherol and γ-tocotrienol prevented the cultured cortical neurons from cell death in oxidative stress stimulated by H_2O_2, while Trolox, a cell-permeable analogue of α-tocopherol, did not (Numakawa et al., 2006).

8.4.2 Antioxidant Activity of Tocotrienols in Serum

The antioxidant efficacy of tocotrienols in *in vitro* models is higher than that of tocopherols, although their uptake and distribution *in vivo* are less than that of α-tocopherol. In fact, it is known that only α-tocopherol is selectively and preferentially transferred into plasma lipoproteins by the α-tocopherol transfer protein (Arita et al., 1995). Although this system has a much lower affinity to transport tocotrienols, it has been evident that orally supplemented tocotrienol results in plasma tocotrienol concentration in the range of 1 μM (O'Byrne et al., 2000). It can be hypothesized that if similar tissue levels could be achieved, tocotrienols would be more effective antioxidants than tocopherols. There is some evidence supporting this hypothesis. When supplementation was carried out in a way that allowed comparable tissue concentrations of α-tocopherol and α-tocotrienol to be reached in rat microsomes and mitochondria, tocotrienol-supplemented heart tissues were more resistant to lipid peroxidation *in vitro* than the tocopherol-supplemented counterparts (Serbinova and Packer, 1994). However, it is important to note that tocotrienols belong to a family of plant phenolic compounds, which have a brief and transient nature with respect to their metabolism; i.e., compared with α-tocopherol, they are inferior with regard to tissue retention and half-life.

8.4.3 Animal Studies

Suarna et al. (Suarna et al., 1993) reported that following acute supplementation of rats with a mixed tocotrienols and tocopherol preparation, tocotrienols provided oxidative protection to plasma comparable to that of the corresponding tocopherols.

The supplementation of hyperlipidemic rats with TRF, in addition to lowering cholesterol, inhibited diene conjugated formation in LDL and TBARS production in liver microsomal membranes (Iqbal et al., 2004). Concomitantly, TRF supplementation has been reported to suppress diethylnitrosamine and 2-acetylaminofluorene-induced hepatocarcinogenesis in rats by inhibiting the production of lipid peroxides and conjugated dienes (Iqbal et al., 2004).

The treatment with Ricetrienol®, which contains α-tocopherol, tocotrienol and phytosterol, strongly reduced plasma levels of malondialdehyde (MDA), urinary levels of both isoprostane and 8-hydroxy-deoxy-guanosine (8-OHdG) and increased glutathione peroxidase (GPx) mRNA expression in kidney of diabetic mice. These findings suggest that Ricetrienol® exerts a protective effect against oxidative damage in diabetes mellitus (Kanaya et al., 2004). The antioxidative effects of rice bran extract have been reported in other animal experiments (Qureshi et al., 2000).

The treatment with γ-tocotrienol in spontaneously hypertensive WKY rats normalized nitric oxide synthetase (NOS) activity, reduced lipid peroxide formation and blood pressure. Interestingly, in this study, low doses of γ-tocotrienol (15 mg/kg diet) showed better protection than high doses (30 and 150 mg/kg diet), confirming the possibility that tocotrienols as well as tocopherols may act as pro-oxidants under certain circumstances (Newaz et al., 2003).

When mice were fed on a vitamin E-free diet supplemented with a lipophilic antioxidant (0.04 wt%),α-tocopherol, α-tocotrienol, γ-tocopherol, or 2,3-dihydro-5-hydroxy-4,6-di-tert-butyl-2,2-dipentylbenzofuran (BO-653), a potent synthetic antioxidant, the increases of total hydroxyoctadecadienoic acid (tHODE) and 8-iso-prostaglandin F (2α) in the plasma, erythrocytes, liver and brain were suppressed to levels lower than those of mice fed a standard diet.

A recent study compared the efficiency of tocopherols and tocotrienols in preventing ischemic brain damage induced by the middle cerebral artery occlusion in mice. It is known that free radical-induced lipid peroxidation is recognized as an important factor in the pathogenesis of ischemic brain damage. The results demonstrated that α-tocopherol (2 mM), α-tocotrienol (0.2 and 2 mM) and γ-tocopherol (0.2 and 2 mM), injected via IV immediately before and after the occlusion, could similarly reduce the infarct volume, but α-tocotrienol and γ-tocopherol were 10-fold more efficient than α-tocopherol (Mishima et al., 2003). The antioxidant benefits of tocotrienols supplementation have also been reported in a group of patients with cerebrovascular disease (Tomeo et al., 1995). The supplements used in this clinical intervention study contained both tocopherols and 240 mg of mixed tocotrienols.

8.4.4 Human Studies

O'Byrne et al. conducted the first clinical trial to determine the correlation existing between hypocholesterolemic and antioxidant effects following supplementation with individual purified α-, γ-, or δ-tocotrienyl acetates. Their results indicate that supplements of purified α-, γ-, or δ-tocotrienyl acetates, when given in the dosage of 250 mg/d for 8 weeks, do not provide the dual benefits of cholesterol reduction and antioxidant protection in hyperlipidemic patients, as suggested by other investigators. Contrary to the findings of *in vitro* studies or clinical trials using mixed tocotrienols and tocopherols or γ-T3 supplements (Suarna et al., 1993; Tomeo et al., 1995), they found that supplementation with purified tocotrienyl acetates did not result in significant reductions in serum cholesterol, LDL cholesterol, or apolipoprotein B levels. At the dosage given, only α-tocotrienyl acetate supplements, but not α-tocopheryl acetate or γ-tocotrienyl acetate supplements, provided significant protection to LDL against copper-induced oxidation. Moreover, Wan Nazaimoon et al. reported that non-insulin-dependent diabetes mellitus patients supplemented with Palmvitee, rich in tocotrienols, decreased plasma MDA levels to the same extent as palm-olein, also containing a low amount of vitamin E, suggesting that tocotrienols did not exert further reduction in the peroxide levels (Wan Nazaimoon et al., 1996). In addition, healthy male subjects who took TRE at doses of 80, 160 or 320 mg daily for 2 months, showed significant increase in α,γ, δ-tocotrienol concentrations from baseline to end of treatment with respect to control subjects. However, they did not significantly exhibit differences in arterial compliance and plasma total antioxidant status (TAS) (Rasool et al., 2006). On the contrary, Suarna et al. (1993) reported that following acute supplementation of humans with a mixture of tocotrienol and tocopherol preparations, tocotrienols provided oxidative protection to LDL. Moreover, Tomeo et al. (Tomeo et al., 1995) have provided promising preliminary evidence that supplementation with α-tocotrienol, γ-tocotrienol (total tocotrienols of 240 mg/d) and α-tocopherol (93 mg/ d), led to regression in carotid atherosclerosis in hyperlipidemic patients. The exact mechanism eliciting regression in atherosclerotic plaque is unclear, since serum cholesterol levels were not altered, although significant decreases in serum oxidation products TBARS were noted.

8.5 CONCLUSION

The antioxidant potential of tocotrienols has been the main focus of scientific interest in recent years. *In vitro* experiments showed higher radical scavenging efficiency for tocotrienols compared with tocopherols in biological systems such as isolated membranes and intact cells. However, only a limited number of studies investigated the antioxidant effects of tocotrienols *in vivo* and the results of these studies are controversial. Therefore, these data do not yet provide a sufficient basis for a dietary recommendation of tocotrienols as antioxidants with superior radical scavenging power. More and better-designed *in vivo* studies in animals and especially humans are warranted not only to address the question of the ROS-scavenging potential of tocotrienols compared with other antioxidants, but also to estimate possible synergistic or opposing interactions of tocotrienols with other elements of the antioxidant network.

REFERENCES

Adachi, H., N. Ishii. 2000. Effects of tocotrienols on life span and protein carbonylation in Caenorhabditis elegans. *J. Gerontol A Biol Sci Med Sci*, 55, 280–285.

Arita, M., Y. Sato, A. Miyata, T. Tanabe, E. Takahashi, H.J. Kayden, H. Arai, K. Inoue. 1995. Human α-tocopherol transfer protein-cDNA cloning, expression and chromosomal localization. *Biochem J*, 306, 437–443.

Begum, A.N., J. Terao. 2002. Protective effect of α-tocotrienol against free radical-induced impairment of erytrocytes deformability. *Biosci Biotechnol Biochem*, 66, 398–403.

Constantinescu, A., D. Han, L. Packer. 1993. Vitamin E recycling in human erythrocyte membranes. *J Biol Chem*, 25, 10906–13.

Fariss, M.W., M.B. Fortuna, C.K. Everett, J.D. Smith, D.F. Trent, Z. Djuric. 1994. The selective antiproliferative effects of α-tocopheryl hemisuccinate and cholesteryl hemisuccinate on murine leukemia cells result from the action of the intact compounds. *Cancer Res*, *54*, 3346–3351.

Ghafoorunissa, I.A., S. Hemalatha, M.V. Rao. 2004. Sesame lignans enhance antioxidant activity of vitamin E in lipid peroxidation systems. *Mol Cell Biochem*, 262, 195–202.

Gorman, A.M, B. Heavey, E. Creagh, T.G. Cotter, A. Samali. 1999. Antioxidant mediated inhibition of the heat shock response leads to apoptosis. *FEBS Lett*, 445, 98–102.

Iqbal, J., M. Minhajuddin, Z.H. Beg. 2004. Suppression of diethylnitrosamine and 2-acetylaminofluorene-induced hepatocarcinogenesis in rats by tocotrienol-rich fraction isolated from rice bran oil. *Eur J Cancer Prev*, 13, 515–520.

Kagan, V.E., E.A. Serbinova, T. Forte, G. Scita, L. Packer. 1992. Recycling of vitamin E in human low density lipoproteins. *J Lipid Res*, 33, 385–97.

Kagan, V.E., E.A. Serbinova, L. Packer. 1992. Recycling and antioxidant activity of tocopherol homologues of differing hydrocarbon chain length in liver microsomes. *Arch Biochem Biophys*, 282, 221–225.

Kamat, J.P., H.D. Sarma, T.P. Devasagayam, K. Nesaretnam, Y. Basiron. 1997. Tocotrienols from palm oil as effective inhibitors of protein oxidation and lipid peroxidation in rat liver microsomes. *Mol Cell Biochem*, 170, 131–7.

Kamat, J.P., T.P.A. Devasagayam. 1995. Tocotrienols from palm oil as potent inhibitors of lipid peroxidation and protein peroxidation in rat brain mitochondria. *Neurosci Lett*, 195, 179– 82.

Kanaya, Y., T. Doi, H. Sasaki, A. Fujita, S. Matsuno, K. Okamoto, Y. Nakano et al. 2004. Rice bran extract prevents the elevation of plasma peroxylipid in KKAy diabetic mice *Diabetes Res Clin Pract*, 66, S157–60.

Khanna, S., S.N.L. Roy, M. Parinandi, C.K. Maurer, C. Sen. 2006. Characterization of the potent neuroprotective properties of the natural vitamin E α-tocotrienol. *J Neurochem*, 98, 1474–86.

Machlin, L.J. 1991. *Handbook of Vitamins*, 2nd ed. Marcel Dekker. New York, 99–144.

Martindale, J.L., N.J. Holbrook. 2002. Cellular response to oxidative stress: Signaling for suicide and survival. *J Cell Physiol*, 192, 1–15.

Mazlan, M., T.S. Mian, G.M. Top, W.Z. Wan Ngah. 2006. Comparative effects of α-tocopherol and γ-tocotrienol against hydrogen peroxide induced apoptosis on primary-cultured astrocytes. *J Neurol Sci*, 243, 5–12.

McIntyre, B.S., K.P. Briski, M.A. Tirmenstein, M.W. Fariss, A. Gapor, P.W. Sylvester. 2000. Antiproliferative and apoptotic effects of tocopherols and tocotrienols on normal mouse mammary epithelial cells. *Lipids*, 35, 171–180.

Mishima, K., Tanaka, T., Pu, F., Egashira, N., Iwasaki, K., Hidaka, R. et al. 2003. Vitamin E isoforms alpha-tocotrienol and gamma: Tocopherol prevent cerebral infarction in mice. *Neurosci Lett*, 30, 56–60.

Mutaliba, M.S.A., H. Khaza'aia, W.J.K. 2003. Wahleb. Palm-tocotrienol rich fraction (TRF) is a more effective inhibitor of LDL oxidation and endothelial cell lipid peroxidation than α-tocopherol in vitro. *Food Res Int*, 36, 405–413.

Napolitano M., L. Avanzi, S. Manfredini, E. Bravo. 2007. Effects of new combinative antioxidant FeAOX-6 and α-tocotrienol on macrophage atherogenesis-related functions. *Vascul Pharmacol*, 46, 394–405.

Newaz, M.A, Z. Yousefipour, N. Nawal, N. Adeeb. 2003. Nitric oxide synthase activity in blood vessels of spontaneously hypertensive rats: antioxidant protection by γ-tocotrienol. *J Physiol Pharmacol*, 54, 319–27.

Numakawa, Y., T. Numakawa, T. Matsumoto, Y. Yagasaki, Y., E. Kumamaru, H. Kunugi, T. Taguchi, E. Niki. 2006. Vitamin E protected cultured cortical neurons from oxidative stress–induced cell death through the activation of mitogen-activated protein kinase and phosphatidylinositol 3–kinase. *J Neurochem*, 97, 1191–202.

O'Byrne, D., S. Grundy, L. Packer, S. Devaraj, K. Baldenius, P.P Hoppe, K. Kraemer, K, I. Jialal, M.G. Traber. 2000. Studies of LDL oxidation following α-, γ-, δ-tocotrienyl acetate supplementation of hypercholesterolemic humans. *Free Rad. Biol Med*, 29, 834–845.

Packer, L. 1995. Nutrition and biochemistry of the lipophilic antioxidants, vitamin E and carotenoids. In *Nutrition, Lipids, Health, and Disease*, Ong, A. S. H., Niki, E., Packer, L., Eds., American Oil Chemical Society: Champaign, IL, 8–35.

Palozza, P., N.I. Krinsky. 1992. Beta-carotene and alpha-tocopherol are synergistic antioxidants. *Arch Biochem Biophys*, 297, 184–7.

Palozza, P., E. Piccioni, L. Avanzi, S. Vertuani, G. Calviello, S. Manfredini. 2002. Design, synthesis and antioxidant activity of FeAOX-6, a novel agent deriving from a molecular combination of the chromanyl and polyisoprenyl moieties. *Free Radic Biol Med*, 33, 1724–1735.

Palozza, P., S. Verdecchia, L. Avanzi, S. Vertuani, S. Serini, A. Iannone, S. Manfredini. 2006. Comparative antioxidant activity of tocotrienols and the novel chromanyl-polyisoprenyl molecule FeAox-6 in isolated membranes and intact cells. *Mol Cell Biochem*, 287, 21–32.

Qureshi, A.A., H. Mo, L. Packer, D.M. Peterson. 2000. Isolation and identification of novel tocotrienols from rice bran with hypocholesterolemic, antioxidant and antitumor properties *J. Agric Food Chem*, 483, 130–3140.

Rasool, A.H., K.H. Yuen, K. Yusoff, A.R. Wong, A.R. Rahman. 2006. Dose dependent elevation of plasma tocotrienol levels and its effect on arterial compliance, plasma total antioxidant status and lipid profile in healthy humans supplemented with tocotrienol rich vitamin E. *J Nutr Sci Vitaminol*, 52, 473–8.

Roberts, W.G., M.H. Gordon. 2003. Determination of the total antioxidant activity of fruits and vegetables by a liposome assay. *J Agric Food Chem*, 51, 1486–1493.

Schroeder M.T., E.M. Becker, L.H. Skibsted. 2006. Molecular mechanism of antioxidant synergism of tocotrienols and carotenoids in palm oil. *J Agric Food Chem*, 54, 3445–3453.

Sen C.K., S. Khanna, S. Roy, L. Packer. 2000. Molecular basis of vitamin E action. Tocotrienol potently inhibits glutamate-induced pp60(c-Src) kinase activation and death of HT4 neuronal cells. *J Biol Chem*, 28, 13049–5.

Sen, C.K., S. Khanna,, S. Roy. 2004. Tocotrienol: The natural vitamin E to defend the nervous system? *Ann N Y Acad Sci*, 1031, 127–142.

Sen, C.K., S. Khanna, S. Roy. 2006. Tocotrienols: Vitamin E beyond tocopherols. *Life Sci*, 78, 2088–2098.

Serbinonva, E.A., L. Packer. 1994. Antioxidant properties of tocopherol and tocotrienol, *Meth Enzymol*, 234, 354–367.

Serbinova, E., V. Kagan, D. Han, L. Packer. 1991. Free radical recycling and intramembrane mobility in the antioxidant properties of α-tocopherol and α-tocotrienol. *Free Radic Biol Med*, *10*, 263–75.

Suarna, C., R.L. Hood, R.T. Dean, R. Stocker. 1993. Comparative antioxidant activity of tocotrienols and other natural lipid-soluble antioxidants in a homogeneous system and in rat and human lipoproteins. *Biochim Biophys Acta*, 24, 163–70.

Suzuki, Y.J., M. Tsuchiya, S.R. Wassall, Y.M. Choo, G. Govil, V.E. Kagan, L. Packer. 1993. Structural and dynamic membrane properties of α-tocopherol and α-tocotrienol: Implication to the molecular mechanism of their antioxidant potency. *Biochemistry*, 32, 10692–10699.

Tirmenstein, M.A., B.W. Watson, N.C. Haar, M.W. Fariss. 1998. Sensitive method for measuring tissue α-tocopherol and α-tocopheryloxybutyric acid by high-performance liquid chromatography with fluorometric detection. *J Chromatogr B Biomed Sci Appl*, 707, 308–311.

Tomeo, A.C., M. Geller, T.R. Watkins, A. Gapor, M.L. Bierenbaum. 1995. Antioxidant effects of tocotrienols in patients with hyperlipidemia and carotid stenosis. *Lipids*, 30, 1179–83.

Traber M.G., H. Sies. 1996. Vitamin E in Humans: Demand and delivery. *Annu Rev Nutr*, 16, 321–347.

Traber, M., L. Packer. 1995. Vitamin E—beyond antioxidant function. *Am J Clin Nutr*, 62, 1501–1509.

Tsuzuki, W., R. Yunoki, H. Yoshimura. 2007. Intestinal epithelial cells absorb γ-tocotrienol faster than α-tocopherol. *Lipids*, 42, 163–70.

Verlangieri, A.J., M.J. Bush. 1992. Effects of δ-, α-tocopherol supplementation on experimentally induced primate atherosclerosis. *J Am Coll Nutr*, 11, 131–8.

Wan Nazaimoon W.M., O. 'Sakinah, A. Gapor, B.A.K. Khalid. 1996. Effect of palm olein tocopherol and tocotrienol on lipid peroxidation, lipid profiles and glycemic control in non-insulin diabetes mellitus patients. *Nutr Res*, 16, 1901–1911.

Wrona, M., W. Korytowski, M. Rozanowska, T. Sarna, T.G. Truscott. 2003. Cooperation of antioxidants in protection against photosensitized oxidation. *Free Rad Biol Med*, 35, 1319–1329.

Yoshida, Y., E. Niki, N. Noguchi. 2003. Comparative study on the action of tocopherols and tocotrienols as antioxidants: Chemical and physical effects. *Chem Phys Lipids*, 123, 63–75.

9 Antioxidant Action of Tocotrienols and Tocopherols in Solution and Membranes: Chemical and Physical Effects

Yasukazu Yoshida and Etsuo Niki

CONTENTS

9.1 INTRODUCTION

The action and activity of tocotrienols (T3) as radical-scavenging antioxidants have been studied and compared with those of tocopherols (T) by many investigators. Because the side chain at the 2-position of chromanols exerts small effect on the reactivity of phenolic O-H bond toward free radicals, it is anticipated that the corresponding α-, β-, γ-, and δ-isoforms of T3 and T exert similar antioxidant activity. Some studies show the similar antioxidant activities for T3 and T, while other studies suggest different activities and effects exerted by T3 and T. In this chapter, the chemical and physical effects on the antioxidant action of T3 and T in solution and membranes will be reviewed.

9.2 REACTIVITIES TOWARD FREE RADICALS

There have been several reports concerning the reactivities of T and T3 toward free radicals. As a whole, it has been observed that the corresponding T and T3 exert substantially the same reactivity toward free radicals. Recent studies confirmed this issue by various experimental methods. The relative reactivities of the antioxidants toward peroxyl radicals, chain carrying species in lipid peroxidation, can be clearly and quantitatively assessed by competition methods using appropriate reference compounds. In these methods, it is evaluated how the test compound protects a reference compound from being degraded or consumed by exposure to a controlled free radical flux. The results of typical examples in organic solution using pyrogallosulfonphtalein (Pyrogallol Red) as a reference compound are shown in Figure 9.1 (Yoshida et al., 2003). The peroxyl radicals were generated from the azo initiator at a constant rate (Niki, 1990). The generation of free radicals at a

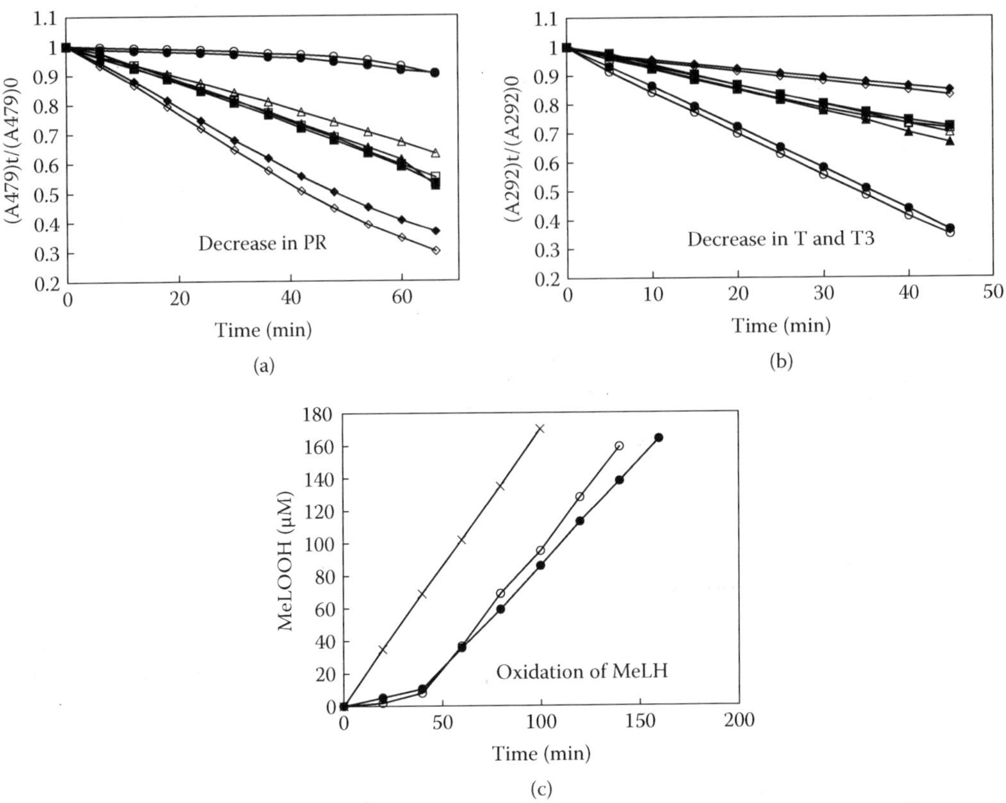

FIGURE 9.1 Reactivities of tocopherols and tocotrienols toward free radicals in solution. (A) Effect of α (circle), β (triangle), γ (square), and δ (diamond) -tocopherols (T) (solid) and -tocotrienols (T3) (open) (15 μM) on the consumption of Pyrogaroll Red (PR) (15 μM) induced by AMVN (2.5 mM) in ethanol at 37°C under air. (A475)t/(A479)0 show the ratio of absorbance at 479 nm due to PR at time t to that of start. (B) Consumption of T and T3 induced by AMVN (10 mM) in acetonitrile at 37°C under air. The symbols are the same as those in (A). (C) Inhibition by αT (solid circle) and αT3 (open circle) (5 μM) of oxidation of methyl linoleate (24.4 mM) induced by AMVN (0.84 mM) in acetonitrile at 37°C. Methyl linoleate hydroperoxide (MeLOOH) was measured in the absence (cross) and presence (circles) of antioxidant.

controlled and constant rate is essential for kinetic study. The results clearly show that the reactivities decrease in the order α > β = γ > δ forms and that the corresponding T and T3 have the same reactivities. It should be noted that T3 and T gave the same induction period (Figure 9.1), suggesting that the stoichiometry number, (the number of free radicals scavenged by each T3 and T molecule) is the same. The measurement of temporal disappearance of T and T3 induced by free radicals also showed the same reactivities of the corresponding T and T3 isoforms in both homogeneous solution and in liposomal membranes (Suarna et al., 1993; Yoshida et al., 2003; Noguchi et al., 2003). These results clearly show that the corresponding isoforms of T3 and T have the same chemical rectivities toward free radicals.

9.3 ANTIOXIDANT ACTIVITIES

The results of *in vitro* studies on the relative antioxidant activities of T and T3 performed in different laboratories are not always consistent. The antioxidant activity against lipid peroxidation has been evaluated by several markers or parameters such as conjugated diene, lipid hydroperoxides, TBARS (thiobarbituric acid reactive substances), oxygen consumption, and induction period (lag phase). It has been observed that the corresponding T and T3 isoforms exert the same antioxidant activities against lipid peroxidation in homogenous solution, that is, they reduced the rate of oxidation to the same level for the same duration (Noguchi et al., 2003; Yoshida et al., 2003). The results shown in Figure 9.1C confirm that αT3 and αT exerted the same antioxidant activities against lipid peroxidation in solution and that γT3 and γT were less potent than α forms. The antioxidant efficacy decreased in the order of $\alpha > \beta = \gamma > \delta$, in agreement with the relative reactivities toward peroxyl radicals. Similar antioxidant activities were reported for αT3 and αT, and also for γT3 and γT against the oxidation of cholesterol in aqueous dispersions containing the polyoxyethylene sorbitol ester Tween 20 initiated by a water-soluble radical initiator, 2,2'-azobis(2-amidinopropane) dihydrochloride (AAPH) (Xu et al., 2001).

On the other hand, the antioxidant activities of T3 and T in the membranes appear to be more complicated. Serbinova et al. (Serbinova et al., 1991) reported that αT3 exerted 40–60 times higher antioxidant activity against iron-ascorbate and iron-NADPH-induced lipid peroxidation in rat liver microsomal membranes and also 6.5 times better protection of cytochrome P-450 by αT3 against oxidative damage than αT. It was also reported that γT3 and αT3 were more effective than αT in inhibiting *in vitro* oxidative damage of both lipids and proteins in rat brain mitochondria induced by iron-ascorbate (Kamat and Devasagayam, 1995). The order of antioxidant effectiveness was reported as δT3 > γT3 = αT3 against the oxidation of isolated rat liver microsomal membranes and immortalized fibroblast cells induced by free radicals and hydroperoxide (Palozza et al., 2006). Furthermore, it was reported that T3 incorporated into human low density lipoprotein (LDL) reacted with peroxyl radicals and suppressed its oxidation as efficiently as the corresponding T isomers (Suarna et al., 1993).

We have compared the antioxidant activities of T and T3 in phosphatidylcholine (PC) liposomal membranes. AlphaT and αT3 suppressed the formation of PC hydroperoxides to the same extent in the oxidation of β-linoleoyl-γ-palmitoyl PC (PLPC) liposomal membranes (Figure 9.2) (Yoshida et al., 2003). The competition between αT3 and αT for scavenging peroxyl radicals in the membranes was studied in two different membranes, one PLPC liposomes and the other dimyristoyl (14:0) PC liposomes. A lipophilic radical initiator 2,2'-azobis(2,4-di-methylvaleronitrile) (AMVN) was incorporated into the same vesicles to generate free radicals within the membranes. It was found that αT3 and αT were consumed at the same rate either in PLPC or 14:0 PC liposomal membranes (Figure 9.2) (Yoshida et al., 2003). These data show that αT3 and αT scavenge peroxyl radicals and suppress lipid peroxidation by substantially the same efficacies in the PC liposomal membranes.

More recently, the action of T3 and T isoforms within the PC liposomal membranes was studied by fluorescence quenching experiments using 2,3-diazabicyclo[2,2,2]-oct-2-ene and fulorazophone L (Sonnen et al., 2005). The quenching of these azoalkanes proceeds by hydrogen atom transfer, as does the scavenging of reactive free radicals by T3 and T. It was found, in agreement with the previous reports, that the rate decreased in the order of $\alpha > \beta - \gamma > \delta$ and the rate constants for the corresponding T3 and T were the same both in solution and in liposomal membranes (Sonnen et al., 2005). Furthermore, the lateral diffusion coefficients were also compared for α and δ-forms of T3 and T and no marked influence of the nature of isoprenoid side chain on diffusion of T3 and T was observed. These results suggest that the difference between T3 and T in the antioxidant action in the membranes is, if any, small.

9.4 PHYSICAL EFFECTS OF T3 AND T ON MEMBRANES

The antioxidant efficacy of T3 and T in the membranes is determined by physical factors such as localization and mobility in the lipophilic domain as well as their chemical reactivity toward free radicals. These issues have been the subject of extensive studies. For example, it was found that the apparent antioxidant activity of αT in the membranes was considerably smaller than that in homogeneous solution (Niki et al., 1986; Kagan et al., 1990) and that the antioxidant activity of αT homologues against lipid peroxidation in natural membranes of liver microsomes and mito-

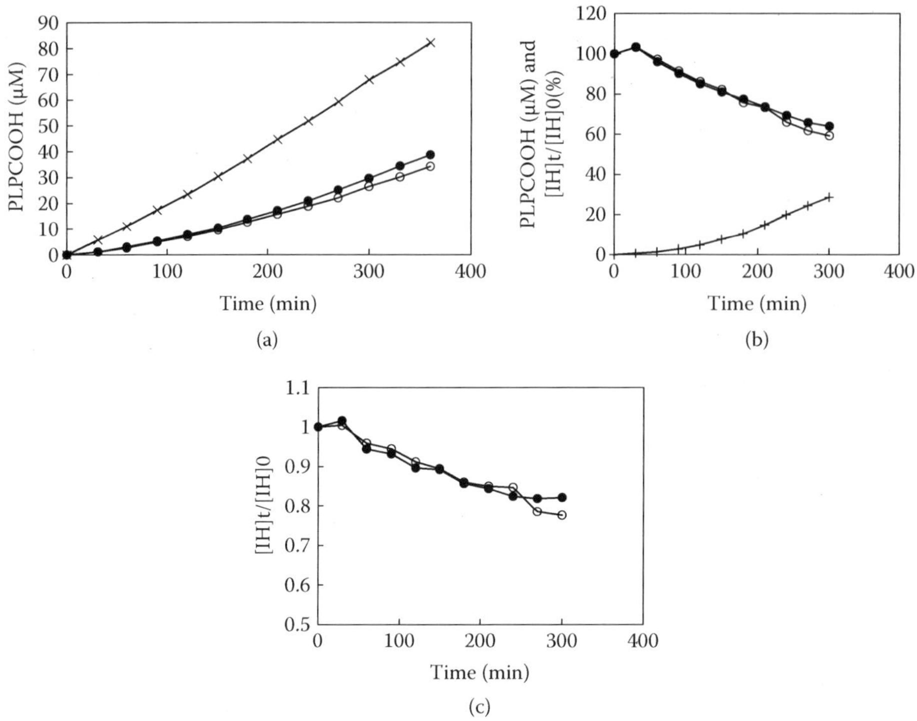

FIGURE 9.2 Inhibition of PC oxidation and scavenging of radicals by αT and αT3 in the membranes. (A) Inhibition by αT (solid circle) or αT3 (open circle) of oxidation of PLPC liposomal membranes. PLPC (2.83 mM) vesicles were oxidized with MeO-AMVN (0.20 mM) in the absence (cross) and presence of antioxidant (5 μM) at 37°C in air. PLPC hydroperoxides (PLPCOOH) were measured with an HPLC as described in the ref. Yoshida et al., 2003. (B, C) Consumption of antioxidant (IH) and accumulation of PLPC hydroperoxides were followed in the oxidation of PLPC (B) and 14:0 PC (C) (2.83 mM) liposomal membranes induced by 0.20 mM MeO-AMVN in the presence of both αT (solid circle) and αT3 (open circle) 37°C.

chondria and brain synaptosomes decreased with increasing length of the side chain (Yamaoka and Carrillo, 1990).

The effects of incorporation of T3 and T on physical properties of membranes have been studied by using chemiluminescence and fluorescence probe (Takahashi et al., 1988; Yoshida et al., 2003; Yamaoka and Carrillo, 1990; Suzuki et al., 1993). AlphaT induces decrease in membrane fluidity (Takahashi et al., 1988).

It was reported that both αT3 and αT affected membrane order to similar effects but that αT3 imposed more motional anisotropy on the membrane (Suzuki et al., 1993). We have also studied the effects of vitamin E homologues in membrane properties by using spin probes, 5-doxylstearic acid (5-NS) and 16-NS (Yoshida et al., 2003). The ESR spectra of the two spin probes, 5-NS and 16-NS, were indistinguishable from each other in homogeneous solution. However, when they were incorporated into the liposomal membranes, they gave different ESR spectra. Table 9.1 summarizes the ESR parameters for the spin probes 5-NS and 16-NS in the multilamellar and unilamellar liposomal membranes containing T3 and T isoforms. The results show that both the correlation times (τc) for 16-NS and order parameters (S) for 5-NS were increased irrespective of isoforms of T3 and T in both multilamellar and unilamellar liposomal membranes. Interestingly, T increased the correlation times of 16-NS and hence, the rigidity of the membranes, more significantly than the corresponding T3. In contrast, T and T3 exerted similar effects for order parameters of 5-NS, which show the fluidity of the liposomal membranes near the water–lipid interface.

TABLE 9.1
ESR Parameters for 16-NS and 5-NS Incorporated into 3 mM Small Unilamellar Vesicles of Dimyristoyl Phosphatidylcholine Liposome in PBS Dispersions at 37°C

		16 NS (τ_c, 10^{-10} s)		5 NS (S)	
Additive	**μ*M***	**Toc**	**Toc-3**	**Toc**	**Toc-3**
None	0	6.85		0.603	
α–	500	8.48	7.77	0.639	0.621
β–	500	7.54	7.33	0.634	0.630
γ–	500	7.10	6.93	0.641	0.632
δ–	500	8.10	7.38	0.641	0.646
cholesterol	500	8.36	0.670		

5-NS: 5-doxyl stearic acid, 16-NS: 16-doxyl stearic acid

Note: ESR spectra were recorded on X-band JEOL JES-TE100 spectrometer.

9.5 INCORPORATION OF T3 AND T INTO MEMBRANES

It was reported previously that αT3 and αT gave the same induction period in the oxidation of PC liposomal membranes induced by AAPH but that, when either αT3 or αT was added to the aqueous suspension of liposomes prepared beforehand, αT3 gave a longer induction period than αT (Yamaoka and Komiyama, 1989).

In order to obtain information on the rate of incorporation of T3 and T into the membranes, they were added into the aqueous suspensions of unilamellar vesicles containing either 5-NS or 16-NS and the change in the ESR parameters was followed. The ESR parameters (S(t) and τ(t)) increased with time and they were compared with those of the membranes into which the spin probe and antioxidant were incorporated simultaneously beforehand (S(∞) and τ(∞)). Figure 9.3 shows the ratio of ESR parameters after 20 min incubation to S(∞) and τ(∞). When all isoforms were incorporated into the membranes, the ratio should be 1.0 and the faster the T3 or T was incorporated into the membrane, the larger the ratio of the ESR parameters. Cholesterol was also studied for comparison. It was found that both the correlation times and order parameters were higher when T3 were added into the aqueous suspensions than T after some specific time of incubation, suggesting that T3 were more readily incorporated into the liposomal membranes than T (Figure 9.3). Cholesterol was less readily incorporated than T.

To elucidate the inter-membrane mobility, the oxidation of multilamellar PLPC liposomes was induced by the lipid-soluble radical initiator AMVN incorporated into PLPC liposomal membranes at 37°C in the presence of either αT3 or αT, which was incorporated into 14:0 PC liposomal membranes separately. The results in Figure 9.5 show that the PLPC hydroperoxides formation was suppressed by 10 μM αT3 and αT localized into the different membranes and that the inhibiting effect by αT3 was more significant than αT. Neither αT3 nor αT at lower concentration (2.5 μM) exerted any appreciable antioxidant effect (Figure 9.4), although they inhibited the oxidation very effectively when they were incorporated into PLPC liposomal membranes. In another experiment, equal concentrations of αT3 and αT were incorporated into 14:0 PC liposomal membranes simultaneously and their effect against the oxidation of PLPC liposomes induced by MeO-AMVN

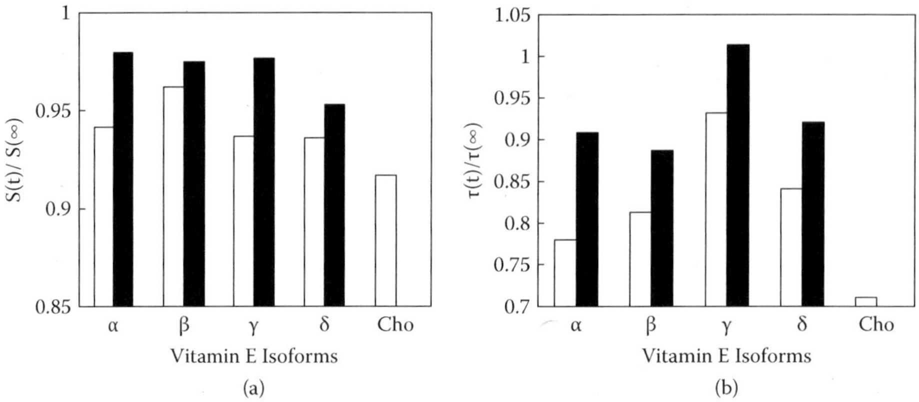

FIGURE 9.3 Incorporation of tocopherols and tocotrienols into membranes as estimated by ESR spin probe technique. T or T3 (0.50 mM) dissolved into methanol (1 vol% of total suspensions) was added into aqueous suspensions of 14:0 PC (2.83 mM) unilamellar liposomal membranes containing either 5-NS (A) or 16-NS (B) (50 μM) and the change in the ESR parameters was followed. Cholesterol was also studied for comparison. The ratios of the ESR parameters after 20 min incubation (except for 5-NS of β-Toc and β-Toc-3, which is 10 min) to those of liposomal membranes prepared by mixing PC, NS and antioxidant beforehand simultaneously are shown. The open and solid bars show the data for αT and αT3, respectively.

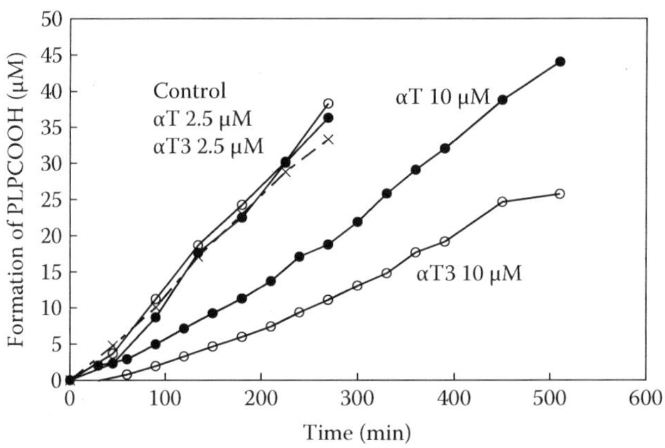

FIGURE 9.4 Oxidation of PLPC liposome (1.42 mM) induced by 1 mM AMVN incorporated into PLPC liposomal vesicles in the absence (cross) and presence of either αT or αT3 incorporated into 14:0 PC liposomal membrane (1.42 mM) at 37°C. Formation of PLPC hydroperoxides in the presence of either αT (solid circle) or αT3 (open circle) was followed as described in the Experimental Section. The concentrations of αT and αT3 were shown in the figure.

incorporated into the same membranes was studied at 37°C (Figure 9.5). It was found that αT3 was consumed faster than αT, suggesting that αT3 migrated faster than αT from 14:0 PC membranes to PLPC membranes. These data given above (Figures 9.2–9.5) show that the difference in the mobilities of αT3 and αT is small within the membranes, but that inter-membrane mobility of αT3 is higher than that of αT. These results are in accordance with the fact that T3 are more readily incorporated into cultured cells, as discussed in other chapters of this book.

9.6 ACTION OF T3 AND T AS REDUCTANT

Metal ions decompose hydrogen peroxide and hydroperoxides to give oxygen radicals, eventually leading to oxidative stress. In general, transition metal ions at higher valency state such as Fe (III)

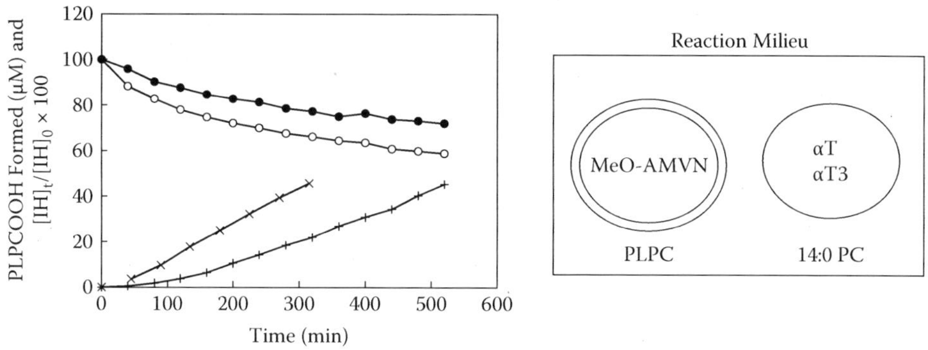

FIGURE 9.5 Formation of hydroperoxides in the oxidation of PLPC liposome (1.42 mM) induced by 0.1 mM MeO–AMVN incorporated into PLPC liposomal membranes in the absence (cross) and presence of both αT and αT3 (plus) incorporated simultaneously into 14:0 PC liposomal membranes (1.42 mM) at 37°C. Consumption of αT (solid circle) and αT3 (open circle) is also shown in the figure.

and Cu (II) decompose peroxides more slowly than those at lower valency state such as Fe (II) and Cu (I). Therefore, a reductant can act as a prooxidant. For example, ascorbate (vitamin C) reduces Fe (III) to yield Fe (II), and the combination of iron-ascorbate has been often used to initiate lipid peroxidation. αT also reduces Fe (III) to Fe (II) (Yamamoto and Niki, 1988) and Cu (II) to Cu (I) (Yoshida et al., 1994). Thus, under certain circumstances, αT may act as a prooxidant (Yamamoto and Niki, 1988; Yoshida et al., 1994; Maiorino et al., 1993; Yamashita et al., 1998). More recently, it was found that αT3 reduces Cu (II) to Cu (I) as rapidly as αT (Yoshida et al., 2003). αT3 and αT are oxidized by Cu (II) to yield α-tocotrienyl quinone (αT3Q) and α-tocopheryl quinone (αTQ), respectively. Under these circumstances, αT3 and αT may act as a prooxidant (Figure 9.7).

$$\alpha\text{T}, \alpha\text{T3} + \text{Cu(II)} \longrightarrow \alpha\text{TQ}, \alpha\text{T3Q} + \text{Cu(I)}$$

$$\text{Cu(II)} + \text{LOOH} \xrightarrow{\text{slow}} \text{Cu(1)} + \text{LOO}^{\cdot} + {}^{+}\text{H}$$

$$\text{Cu(I)} + \text{LOOH} \xrightarrow{\text{fast}} \text{Cu(II)} + \text{LO}^{\cdot} + {}^{-}\text{OH}$$

$$\text{LO}^{\cdot}, \text{LOO}^{\cdot} + \text{lipid} \longrightarrow \text{lipid peroxidation}$$

Interestingly, in contrast to αT3 and αT, β-, γ- and δ-forms of T3 and T did not reduce Cu (II) at appreciable rate. They did not yield the corresponding T3Q or TQ, nor did they exert pro-oxidant effect in the oxidation of methyl linoleate micelles in aqueous dispersions (Figure 9.6) (Yoshida et al., 2003). In support of these observations, it was found that the oxidation potentials of αT3 and αT were significantly lower than those of γT3 and γT (Figure 9.7). The result that T3 and T isoforms have similar oxidation potential also suggests that the corresponding T and T3 isoforms have similar chemical reactivities toward free radicals.

It may be noteworthy that metal ions are sequestered by specific proteins *in vivo*, which makes metal ions stable and difficult to be reduced. Therefore, the pro-oxidant action observed for antioxidants *in vitro* may not be important *in vivo*.

9.7 CONCLUSION

It can be safely concluded that the corresponding isoforms of T3 and T have the same reactivities toward free radicals and the same activities of inhibition of lipid peroxidation in solution, which

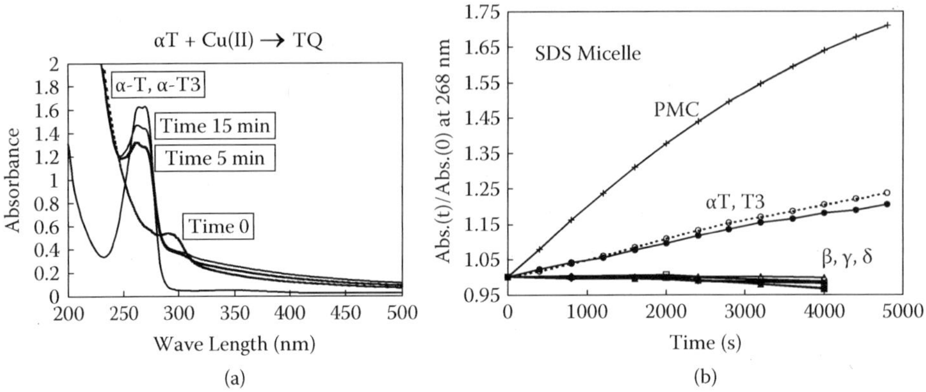

FIGURE 9.6 (A) Absorption spectra of α-tocopheryl quinone (αTQ) formed by the reaction of αT (100 μM) with 300 μM cupric ion (Cu(II)) in acetonitrile and water (1/1, by volume) solution at 37°C under air. Standard spectrum of αTQ(100 μM) is also shown in the figure (A) and the symbol "Time X min" in the figures shows the time after the mixing T with Cu(II). (B) Interaction between vitamin E homologues (100 μM) and cupric ion (100 μM) in methyl linoleate (7.4 mM) micelles containing 0.5 M SDS in aqueous dispersions at 37°C. The increase of absorption at 268 nm is shown as the ratio of absorbance at the time to the initial absorbance (Abs (t)/ Abs (0)). The symbols, circle, triangle, square, diamond, plus, and cross show α-, β-, γ-, δ-tocopherols (solid) and tocotrienols (open), 2,2,5,7,8-pentamethyl-6-chromanol (PMC), and their absence, respectively.

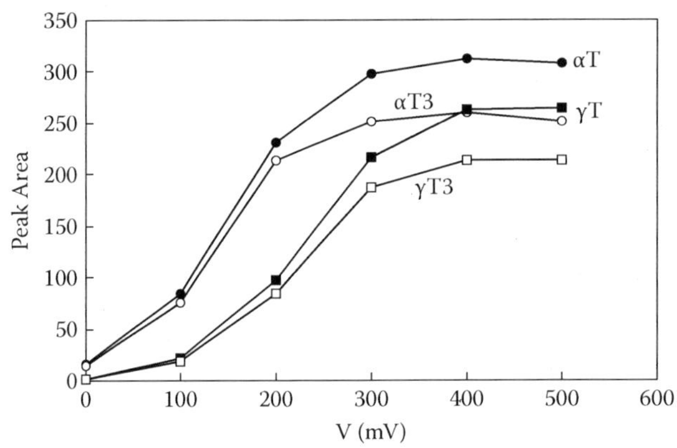

FIGURE 9.7 Oxidation potentials of α– and γ–forms of T and T3 are measured by using an HPLC by an amperometric electrochemical detector (NANOSPACE SI–1, Shiseido, Tokyo, Japan) with an ODS column (LC–18, 5 μm, 250 x 4.6 mm, Supelco, Japan) and methanol/*tert*–butyl alcohol (90/10 by volume) as eluent at 1 ml/min.

decrease in the order of α > β = γ > δ. The mobilities of T3 and T in the membrane are similar. The effects on fluidity of the membrane surface by T3 and T are similar but T reduces fluidity of the membrane interior more significantly than T3, although, unlike cholesterol, the physical effects of T3 and T at physiological concentrations must be small. The mobility of T3 and T within the membranes is similar, but that between the membranes for T3 is larger than T. AlphaT3 and αT are capable of reducing Cu (II) to Cu (I), but β, γ, and δ forms of T3 and T are not.

REFERENCES

Kagan, V. E.; E. A. Serbinova; R. A. Bakalova; Ts. S. Stoytchev; A. N. Erin; L. L. Prilipko; R. P. Evstigneeva. 1990. Mechanisms of stabilization of biomembranes by alpha-tocopherol. *Biochem. Pharmacol.*, 40, 2403–2413.

Kamat, J.P.; T.P. Devasagayam. 1995. Tocotrienols from palm oil as potent inhibitors of lipid–peroxidation and protein oxidation in rat-brain mitochondria. *Neurosci. Lett.*, 195, 179–182.

Maiorino, M.; A. Zamburlini; A. Roveri; F. Urini. 1993. Prooxidant role of vitamin E in copper induced lipid peroxidation. *FEBS Lett.*, 330, 174–176.

Niki, E. 1990. Free radical initiators as source of water- or lipid-soluble peroxyl radicals. *Methods Enzymol.*, 186, 100–108.

Niki, E.; M. Takahashi; E. Komuro. 1986. Antioxidant activity of vitamin E in liposomal membranes. *Chem. Lett.* 6, 1573–1576.

Noguchi, N.; R. Hanyu; A. Nonaka; Y. Okimoto; T. Kodama. 2003. Inhibition of THP–1 cell adhesion to endothelial cells by α-tocopherol and α-tocotrienol is dependent on intracellular concentration of the antioxidants. *Free Rad. Biol. Med.*, 34, 1614–1620.

Palozza, P.; S. Verdecchia; L. Avanzi; S. Vertuani; S. Serini; A. Iannone; S. Manfredini. 2006. Comparative antioxidant activity of tocotrienols and the novel chromanyl-polyisoprenyl molecule FeAox-6 in isolated membranes and intact cells. *Mol. Cell. Biochem.*, 287, 21–32.

Serbinova, E.; V. Kagan; D. Han; L. Packer. 1991. Free radical recycling and intramembrane mobility in the antioxidant properties of α-tocopherol and α-tocotrienol. *Free Rad. Biol. Med.*, 10, 263–275.

Sonnen, A. F.-P.; H. Bakirci; T. Netscher; W. N. Nau. 2005. Effect of temperature, cholesterol content, and antioxidant structure on the mobility of vitamin E constituents in biomembrane models studied by laterally diffusion-controlled fluorescence quenching. *J. Am. Chem. Soc.*, 127, 15575–15584.

Suarna, C.; R. L. Hood; R. T. Dean; R. Stocker. 1993. Comparative antioxidant activity of tocotrienols and other natural lipid-soluble antioxidants in a homogeneous system, and in rat and human lipoproteins. *Biochim. Biophys. Acta*, 1166, 163–170.

Suzuki, Y. J.; M. Tsuchiya; S. R. Wassall; Y. M. Choo; G. Govil; V. E. Kagan; L. Packer. 1993. Structural and dynamic membrane properties of α-tocopherol and α-tocotrienol: implication to the molecular mechanism of their antioxidant potency. *Biochemistry*, 32, 10692–10699.

Takahashi, M.; J. Tsuchiya; E. Niki; S. Urano. 1988. Action of vitamin E as antioxidant in phospholipid liposomal membranes as studied by spin label technique. *J. Nutr. Sci. Vitaminol.*, 34, 25–34.

Yamamoto, K; E. Niki. 1988. Interaction of α-tocopherol with iron: Antioxidant and prooxidant effects of α-tocopherol in the oxidation of lipids in aqueous dispersions in the presence of iron. *Biochim. Biophys. Acta.*, 958, 19–23.

Yamaoka, M.; K. Komiyama. 1989. Antioxidative activities of α-tocotrienol and its derivative in the oxidation of dilinoleoylphosphatidylcholine liposomes. *J Jpn. Oil Chem. Soc.*, 38, 478–485.

Yamaoka, M.; M. J. H. Carrillo. 1990. Effect of tocopherols and tocotrienols on the physicochemical property of the liposomal membrane in relation to their antioxidative activity. *Chem. Phys. Lipids*, 55, 295–300.

Yamashita, N.; M. Murata; S. Inoue; M. J. Burkitt; L. Milne; S. Kawanishi. 1998. Alpha-tocopherol induces oxidative damage to DNA in the presence of copper (II) ions. *Chem. Res. Toxicol.*, 11, 855–862.

Yoshida, Y.; J. Tsuchiya; E. Niki. 1994. Interaction of α-tocopherol with copper and its effect on lipid peroxidation. *Biochim. Biophys. Acta*, 1200, 85–92.

Yoshida, Y.; E. Niki; N. Noguchi. 2003. Comparative study on the action of tocopherols and tocotrienols as antioxidant. *Chem. Phys. Lipids*, 123, 63–75.

Xu, Z.; N. Hua; J. S. Gadber. 2001. Antioxidant activity of tocopherols, tocotrienols, and γ-oryzanol components from rice bran against cholesterol oxidation accelerated by 2,2′-azobis(2-methylpropionamidine) dihydrochloride. *J. Agr. Food Chem.*, 49, 2077–2081.

10 Antiproliferative and Apoptotic Effects of Tocotrienols on Normal and Neoplastic Mammary Epithelial Cells

Paul W. Sylvester

CONTENTS

10.1 CLINICAL SIGNIFICANCE OF THE BREAST CANCER PROBLEM

Worldwide, breast cancer is the most prevalent malignancy in women (Parkin et al. 2001). Although major advances have been made in early detection and treatment, as many women today are unfortunately dying from breast cancer as there were nearly a century ago (Parkin et al. 2001). More alarming is the fact that, until just recently, the incidence of breast cancer had steadily increased for more than 60 years (Parkin et al. 2001). While specific genes such as BRCA1 and BRCA2, which predispose women to breast cancer, have been identified, these genes are estimated to be directly responsible for only 10–15% of all breast cancers (Bishop 1999). The cause for the remaining 85–90% of breast cancers in women is related to yet unknown environmental and nutritional factors. Therefore, it is evident that advances in the area of breast cancer prevention would be of great benefit in significantly reducing breast cancer risk and mortality.

It is well understood that mammary carcinogenesis is a multistage process that involves initiation, promotion and progression (Trosko 2006). Initiation involves those events that occur within a single cell and result in permanent genomic changes. Various chemicals and radiation have been shown to cause genetic mutation and have been implicated as initiators of cancer. In contrast, promotional influences such as nutrition or endocrine history do not necessarily act as mutagens, but enhance the survival and proliferation of initiated cells and thereby allow for the expression of sustained cancerous cell growth (Trosko 2006). Furthermore, hormone and growth factor promotion of cellular growth also enhance the opportunity for mutational events to occur, since elevations in cellular mitotic activity and DNA synthesis are associated with increased susceptibility to carcinogen-induced DNA damage, mutation and subsequent cellular transformation (Sylvester et al. 1983; Sylvester et al. 1986; Trosko 2006).

Finally, progression involves the processes invasiveness and metastasis and is characterized by highly malignant tumor cells invading the surrounding tissue, entering the vascular systems, and traveling to distant organs to settle and grow into secondary tumors. Since conventional therapeutic protocols are primarily directed at primary tumors, metastatic or secondary tumors are mainly responsible for cancer mortality. It has also become apparent that tumor progression is not primarily associated with additional genetic mutations of the transformed tumor cell, but instead results from the silencing or activation of normal genes (Trosko 2006). Since cancer initiation, promotion, and progression can start early in life and long before tumors are detected, understanding the mechanisms by which chemoprotective agents inhibit mammary tumorigenesis would provide essential information necessary not only for basing effective strategies in reducing the risk of breast cancer, but also in clarifying the interactions between genetic and promotional factors in mammary carcinogenesis. Therefore, although genetic mechanisms are essential in breast cancer, promotional factors, such as nutrition and vitamins, can significantly modify the carcinogenesis process. Evidence suggests that the chemoprotective effects of vitamin E, particularly tocotrienols, may occur during the initiation, promotion and progression phases of breast carcinogenesis.

10.2 ANTITUMOR EFFECTS OF DIETARY PALM OIL INTAKE

The initial discovery that tocotrienols acted as potent inhibitors of mammary tumor cell proliferation occurred more than 20 years ago. It was well established that high dietary fat intake significantly enhanced carcinogen-induced mammary tumorigenesis in rats, and studies were being conducted to determine the specific role of fatty acid composition of dietary fat on tumor development (Sylvester et al. 1986a). Dietary fat stimulation of mammary tumor development was found to be associated not only with the level of fat consumed, but also the timing, duration and type of fat consumed (Sylvester et al. 1986a; Sylvester et al. 1986b). High-fat diets containing the polyunsaturated fatty acid linoleic acid (C18:2) were found to be the most potent in stimulating mammary tumor development when given during the promotional phase of carcinogenesis (Sylvester et al. 1986a; Sylvester et al. 1986b). These fats include most liquid vegetable oils, such as corn oil, sunflower oil and safflower oil. In contrast, similar treatments with high-fat diets containing the saturated fatty acid stearic acid (C18:0), such as lard and beef tallow, have little promotional effect on mammary tumor development, but interestingly the opposite trend was observed if these diets are consumed only during the initiation phase of mammary carcinogenesis (Sylvester et al. 1986b). At the time of carcinogen administration, dietary treatment with high lard, and to a lesser extent beef tallow, are found to enhance, while high corn oil diets had little or no effect on subsequent mammary tumorigenesis (Sylvester et al. 1986b). These finding suggest that diets high in stearic acid are stimulatory during the initiation phase, whereas diets high in linoleic acid are stimulatory during the promotional phase of mammary carcinogenesis.

The exceptions to these findings were observed in rats that consumed high palm oil diets, which was found to suppress mammary tumor development when administered during the initiation phase of carcinogenesis in rats (Sylvester et al. 1986b). These findings stimulated additional studies that were designed to determine what was unique to palm oil that was responsible for suppressing mammary tumorigenesis. These studies determined that it was not the macronutrients (fatty acid com-

TABLE 10.1
Vitamin E Levels (mg/L) in Common Dietary Oils

	Tocotrienols			
Dietary Oil	α	γ	δ	**Total Tocotrienol**
Palm	205	439	94	738
Rice Bran	236	349	—	586
Wheat Germ	26	—	—	26
Coconut	5	1	19	25
Palm-Kernel	21	—	—	21
Cocoa Butter	2	—	—	2
Corn	—	—	—	0
Cottonseed	—	—	—	0
Peanut	—	—	—	0
Olive	—	—	—	0
Safflower	—	—	—	0
Soybean	—	—	—	0
Sunflower	—	—	—	0

Source: Information obtained from Cottrell (1991) and Packer et al. (2001).

position), but rather the micronutrients (vitamin E composition) in palm oil that were responsible for mediating its inhibitory effects on mammary tumor development and growth (Sylvester and Theriault 2003; Sylvester and Shah 2005; Sylvester et al. 2005).

All dietary lipids contain variable amounts of vitamin E (Table 10.1). However, vitamin E is a general term used to describe a family of eight different naturally occurring compounds that are very closely related in chemical structure, which is further subdivided into two subgroups called tocopherols and tocotrienols (Figure 10.1). Tocopherols and tocotrienols are both potent antioxidants that regulate peroxidation reactions and control free-radical production within the body (Packer et al. 1999). However, tocotrienols display significantly greater anticancer activity than tocopherols, and the majority of anticancer effects are not dependent on antioxidant activity or potency (Kimmick et al. 1997; Packer et al. 2001). Tocopherols are found in a wide variety of dietary fats, whereas tocotrienols are rare (Table 10.1). The richest natural source of tocotrienols is palm oil (Sylvester and Theriault 2003; Sylvester and Shah 2005; Sylvester et al. 2005). Studies showed that palm oil diets stripped of tocotrienols no longer displayed a protective effect against mammary tumorigenesis in carcinogen-treated rats (Nesaretnam et al. 1992), and provided strong evidence that it was the tocotrienols that were responsible for mediating the antitumor effects resulting from the dietary consumption of palm oil.

10.2.1 Comparative Biopotency of Tocopherols and Tocotrienols

Subsequent studies were then conducted to determine the comparative effects of tocopherols and tocotrienols on normal mammary epithelial cell growth and viability. Direct comparisons between the two vitamin E subclasses show that tocotrienols are significantly more potent than tocopherols (McIntyre et al. 2000a; Sylvester et al. 2001). Furthermore, the biopotency of specific isoforms displayed a consistent relationship corresponding to δ-tocotrienol > γ-tocotrienol > α-tocotrienol >δ-tocopherol > γ- and α-tocopherol. Results showed that chronic treatment with very high doses

Tocopherols

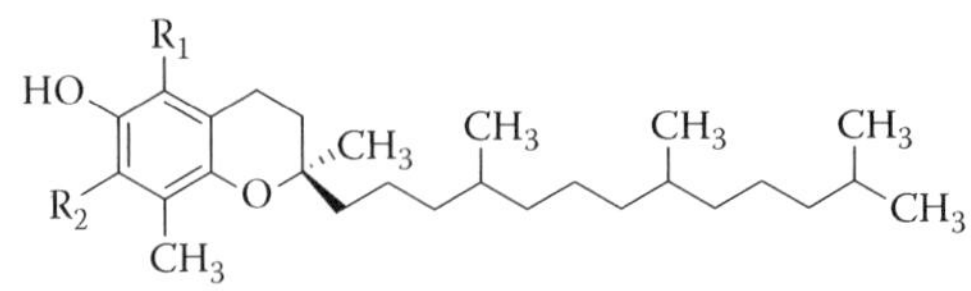

Tocotrienols

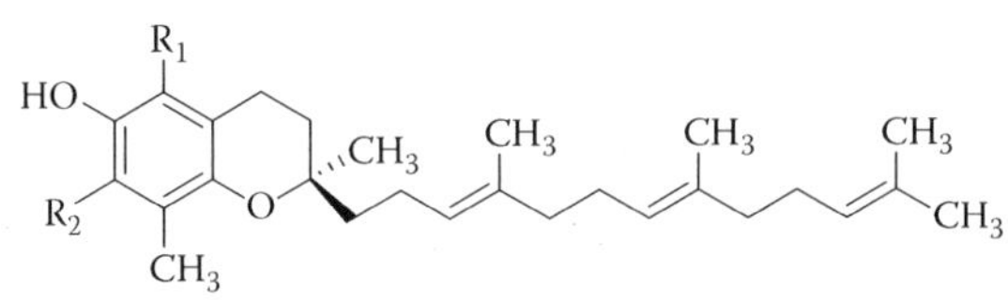

Compound	R_1	R_2	Phytyl Chain
α-tocopherol	CH_3	CH_3	Saturated
β-tocopherol	CH_3	H_3	Saturated
γ-tocopherol	H_3	CH_3	Saturated
δ-tocopherol	H_3	H_3	Saturated
α-tocotrienol	CH_3	CH_3	Unsaturated
β-tocotrienol	CH_3	H_3	Unsaturated
γ-tocotrienol	H_3	CH_3	Unsaturated
δ-tocotrienol	H_3	H_3	Unsaturated

FIGURE 10.1 The generalized structure of vitamin E compounds. Although their chemical structures are very similar, tocopherols have a saturated phytyl tail, whereas tocotrienols have an unsaturated phytyl tail connected at the 1-position of a chromane ring structure. Different isoforms within each subgroup differ from each other based on the degree of chromane ring methylation.

(>250μM) of either α- or γ-tocopherol was not found to have significant effects, whereas treatment with 100–120μM δ-tocopherol significantly inhibited mammary epithelial cell growth as compared with controls (McIntyre et al. 2000a; Sylvester et al. 2001). However, treatment with 50–60 μM α-tocotrienol, 8–14 μM γ-tocotrienol or δ-tocotrienol was also found to significantly inhibit mammary epithelial cell growth as compared with controls (Table 10.2). These findings indicate that both tocopherols and tocotrienols induce antiproliferative and apoptotic effects in normal mouse mammary epithelial cells in primary culture (McIntyre et al. 2000a; Sylvester et al. 2001), but specific tocotrienol isoforms are significantly more potent than corresponding tocopherol isoforms.

Subsequent studies were conducted to determine the comparative effects of tocopherols and tocotrienols on preneoplastic (CL-S1), neoplastic (-SA) and highly malignant (+SA) mouse mammary epithelial cell growth and viability *in vitro* (McIntyre et al. 2000b). The CL-S1 preneoplastic cell line is immortal in culture, but does not grow in soft agarose or form solid tumors upon transplantation back into the mammary gland. The -SA and +SA cell lines were derived from adenocarcinomas that developed spontaneously from the original D1 cell line . The major difference between these neoplastic cell lines is that -SA cells do not grow in soft agarose, whereas +SA cells display anchorage-independent growth when cultured in soft agarose gels. When injected back into the mammary gland fat pad of syngeneic female mice, -SA cells grow to form well-differentiated tumors, while +SA cells form anaplastic adenocarcinomas. In addition, both -SA and +SA cells metastasize to the lung, but +SA tumors are much more aggressive in their growth and metastatic characteristics than -SA tumors. Taken together, these cell lines representing a gradient

TABLE 10.2
Antiproliferative (IC_{50}) and Cytotoxic (LD_{50}) Potencies of Various Tocopherols and Tocotrienols on Normal, Preneoplastic, and Neoplastic Mouse Mammary Epithelial Cells *In Vitro*

Vitamin E Malignant Isoform		Normal (Primary Culture)	Preneoplastic (CL-S1)	Neoplastie (-SA)	Neoplastie (+SA)
TRF	IC_{50}	25 μM	13 μM	7 μM	6 μM
	LD_{50}	110 μM	50 μM	43 μM	38 μM
α-tocopherol	IC_{50}	>120 μM	>120 μM	>120 μM	>120 μM
	LD_{50}	>250 μM	>250 μM	>250 μM	>250 μM
α-tocotrienol	IC_{50}	45 μM	12 μM	7 μM	5 μM
	LD_{50}	238 μM	27 μM	28 μM	23 μM
γ-tocotrienol	IC_{50}	8 μM	8 μM	5 μM	4 μM
	LD_{50}	45 μM	19 μM	17 μM	14 μM
δ-tocotrienol	IC_{50}	7 μM	7 μM	4 μM	3 μM
	LD_{50}	36 μM	16 μM	15 μM	12 μM

Source: Data from McIntyre et al. (2000a and 2000b).

of transformed states provide an ideal experimental model for study of mammary neoplasia and tumor progression.

All tocotrienol isoforms tested were found to decrease preneoplastic (CL-S1), neoplastic (-SA) and highly malignant (+SA) mammary epithelial cell proliferation and viability (McIntyre et al. 2000b). However, the highly malignant +SA cells were found to be the most sensitive, and the preneoplastic CL-S1 cells were found to be the least sensitive to these treatment effects (Table 10.2). These findings were particularly interesting because these effects were observed at treatment doses that had little or no effect on normal mammary epithelial cell growth or viability (McIntyre et al. 2000b). Again, individual tocopherol and tocotrienol isoforms displayed differential antiproliferative and cytotoxic potencies in the preneoplastic, neoplastic and highly malignant mammary epithelial cell lines, but it was clearly evident that normal cells were least sensitive and the highly malignant +SA mammary tumor cells were the most sensitive to the antiproliferative and apoptotic effects of tocotrienols (Table 10.2).

10.3 DIFFERENTIAL CELLULAR UPTAKE OF TOCOPHEROLS AND TOCOTRIENOLS

A possible explanation as to why tocotrienols display significantly higher antiproliferative biopotency than tocopherols is suggested by the findings that tocotrienols are more easily or preferentially taken up by normal, preneoplastic and neoplastic mammary epithelial cells (Figure 10.2). In cell culture studies, tocopherol and tocotrienol levels were undetectable in normal, preneoplastic (CL-S1), neoplastic (-SA) and highly malignant (+SA) mammary tumor cells lines, reflecting the absence of vitamin E in the culture media (McIntyre et al. 2000a; McIntyre et al. 2000b). However, treatment with 120μM α-, γ-, or δ-tocopherol was required to obtain cellular concentrations similar to those obtained with 5μM α-, γ-, and δ-tocotrienol in the preneoplastic and neoplastic mammary epithelial cell lines (McIntyre et al. 2000a; McIntyre et al. 2000b). In summary, the rate uptake of all vitamin E isoforms was found to be significantly greater in the tumor cell lines than in normal mammary epithelial cells grown in primary culture. Furthermore, tocotrienols were found to be selectively taken up at a significantly greater rate than tocopherols in each

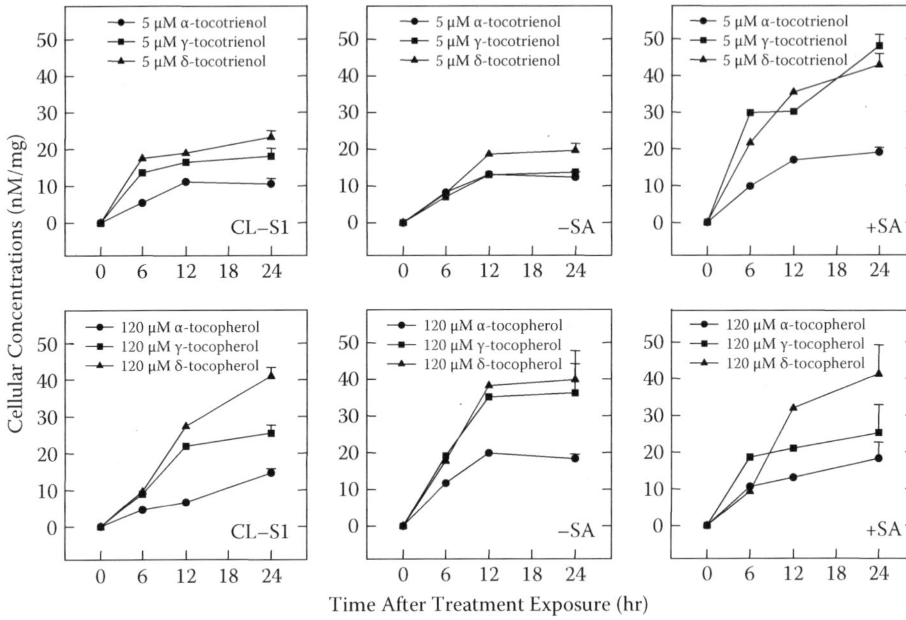

FIGURE 10.2 Cellular accumulation of individual tocopherol and tocotrienol isoforms in preneoplastic (CL-S1), neoplastic (-SA) and highly malignant (+SA) mammary epithelial cells during a 24 hr exposure to 120μM α-, γ-, or δ-tocopherol, or 5μM α-, γ-, or δ-tocotrienol. Data points indicate mean cellular concentration + SEM for 4 replicates in each treatment group containing 1×10^7 cells per each time point.

of these types of normal, preneoplastic, neoplastic and highly malignant mammary epithelial cells (Figure 10.2).

Tocopherols and tocotrienols have the same basic chemical structure characterized by a long phytyl chain attached at the 1-position of a chromane ring structure. However, tocopherols have a saturated phytyl chain, while tocotrienols have an unsaturated phytyl chain, and each subgroup contains several isoforms that differ from each other based on the number of methyl groups bound to their chromane ring (Figure 10.1). The level of phytyl chain saturation or chromane ring methylation appears to be critical in determining the differential biopotency demonstrated by individual vitamin E isoforms (Sylvester and Theriault 2003; Sylvester and Shah 2005; Sylvester et al. 2005). The presence of the three double bonds on the phytyl tail of tocotrienols as compared to tocopherols might result in a less planar molecular conformation that facilitates less restricted transmembrane passage of tocotrienols into the cell. Since cellular accumulation of tocotrienols was greater than that of tocopherols in each cell line, higher concentrations of tocotrienols would occur at intracellular sites of action, thereby inducing a biological response of greater magnitude. However, studies clearly showed that when comparable cellular levels of α-, γ-, or δ-tocopherol and α-, γ-, or δ-tocotrienol were produced in the various mammary tumor cell lines, these treatments did not elicit similar antiproliferative effects. These findings demonstrated that tocotrienols are inherently more potent that tocopherols in suppressing mammary tumor cell growth and tumor cells are much more sensitive to these effects than normal cells.

10.4 ANTIPROLIFERATIVE EFFECTS OF TOCOTRIENOLS

Tocopherols and tocotrienols have been shown to modulate several intracellular signaling pathways involved with mitogenesis in various experimental models (Packer et al. 2001; Sylvester and Theriault 2003; Sylvester et al. 2005). However, cell culture studies utilizing serum-free defined media contain only epidermal growth factor (EGF) as a mitogen have provided convincing evidence as to the mechanism of action by which tocotrienols inhibit EGF-dependent mitogenesis (Packer et al. 2001; Sylvester and Theriault 2003; Sylvester and Shah 2005; Sylvester et al. 2005).

EGF and EGF-like growth factors have been shown to be potent mitogens that stimulate the growth of both normal and neoplastic mammary epithelial cells *in vitro* (Imagawa et al. 1990). The EGF-receptor (ErbB1 or HER1) belongs to the ErbB/HER family of receptor tyrosine kinases that includes four members (ErbB1-4 or HER1-4). Activation of these receptors by their appropriate ligands will induce the formation of homodimers and heterodimers (Bazley and Gullick 2005). Heterodimer formation between different ErbB receptor family members has been shown to provide greater signal duration, diversification and amplification, as compared with their corresponding homodimer receptor complex (Sliwkowski et al. 1994; Karunagaran et al. 1996). This is particularly true for the ErbB2 and the ErbB3 receptors because the ErbB2 receptor has no known ligand (Yarden 2001) and the ErbB3 receptor has no intrinsic tyrosine kinase activity (Olayioye et al. 2000). Heterodimer formation thereby allows ErbB2 and ErbB3 to participate in mitogen-dependent signal transduction. Studies have also shown that the most potent ErbB receptor complex for stimulating cell growth and transformation is composed of ErbB3 with either ErbB1 or ErbB2 (Bazley and Gullick 2005). Following ligand binding and heterodimerization, ErbB3 becomes transphosphorylated by its heterodimer partner, and tyrosine phosphorylated ErbB3 is now able to interact and activate several important intracellular signaling proteins (Sliwkowski et al. 1994; Karunagaran et al. 1996).

10.5 TOCOTRIENOL EFFECTS ON EGF-INDUCED ERBB RECEPTOR FAMILY ACTIVATION

Initial studies were conducted to determine if the antiproliferative effects tocotrienols are associated with a reduction in EGF-receptor mitogenic signaling in normal mammary epithelial cells grown in primary culture and maintained on serum-free defined media containing only EGF as a mitogen. Results showed that tocotrienol inhibition of EGF-dependent normal mouse mammary epithelial cell growth does not result from a decrease in ErbB1-receptor levels or EGF-induced ErbB1-receptor tyrosine kinase activity, indicating that the antiproliferative effects of tocotrienols do not result from suppression in ErbB1-receptor mitogenic responsiveness (Sylvester et al. 2001).

It is well established that EGF stimulation of the EGF-receptor initiates multiple signal transduction pathways associated with cell proliferation, including protein kinase C (PKC) activation (Imagawa et al. 1990; Sylvester et al. 1994; Birkenfeld et al. 1996a, 1996b). Treatment with phorbol ester has been shown to enhance phospholipid-dependent PKC activation and potentiate EGF-dependent mammary epithelial cell growth, whereas treatment with PKC inhibitors induces the opposite results (Imagawa et al. 1990; Sylvester et al. 1994; Birkenfeld et al. 1996, 1996b). PKC consists of a large family of structurally homologous serine/threonine kinases, which display a wide range of tissue and cellular distribution and have distinct sensitivities to lipid activation and regulation (Birkenfeld et al. 1996a, 1996b). Previous studies have shown that PKCα is present in the highest concentrations in normal mammary epithelial cells and the relative levels of this PKC isoform increases throughout the period of log phase growth (Birkenfeld et al. 1996b).

Subsequent studies showed that growth inhibitory doses of tocotrienols were found to have little or no effect on total intracellular levels of PKCα in normal mammary epithelial cells grown in primary culture (Sylvester et al. 2001). However, these same treatments were observed to inhibit EGF-induced PKCα translocation from the cytosolic to membrane fraction. In contrast, treatment with relatively high doses (250 μM) of α- or γ-tocopherol had no effect on EGF-dependent mammary epithelial cell proliferation or PKCα translocation (Sylvester et al. 2001). Previous investigations in vascular smooth muscle cells have shown that α-tocopherol, but not β-tocopherol, indirectly attenuates PKCα activation by stimulating protein phosphatases that act to dephosphorylate and diminish PKCα enzymatic activity (Clement et al. 1997; Ricciarelli et al. 1998). Although α-tocopherol has not been shown to inhibit normal mammary epithelial cell growth, it is possible that similar mechanisms may be involved in mediating the growth inhibitory effects of other tocopherol and tocotrienol isoforms in these cells. Additional studies are still required to determine if specific tocopherol and tocotrienol isoforms stimulate phosphatase activity or alter PKCα phosphorylation levels and enzymatic activity. Nevertheless, these finding suggest that the antiproliferative effects of tocotrienols on EGF-dependent normal mammary epithelial cell mitogenesis are mediated, at least in part, by a reduction in PKC activation.

In order to elucidate the exact intracellular site of action mediating the inhibitory effects of γ-tocotrienol on EGF-dependent neoplastic mammary epithelial cell proliferation, studies were conducted to examine the effects of γ-tocotrienol on EGF-dependent ErbB receptor family activation and tyrosine phosphorylation in these cells. Experimental findings showed that γ-tocotrienol treatment had little or no effect on ErbB1 or ErbB2 tyrosine phosphorylation, but did cause a large reduction in the relative levels of ErbB3 tyrosine phosphorylation (Samant and Sylvester 2006). These finding demonstrated that the antiproliferative effects of γ-tocotrienol on neoplastic mammary epithelial cells are mediated through a reduction in ErbB3 tyrosine phosphorylation and subsequent mitogenic signaling.

10.6 TOCOTRIENOL EFFECTS ON PI3K/PDK/AKT MITOGENIC SIGNALING

PI3Ks represent a family of enzymes that are ubiquitously expressed and activated by most cellular membrane receptors (Jung et al. 2000; Vanhaesebroeck and Aless 2000; Hutchinson et al. 2001). Activation of PI3K results in the 3'-phosphorylation of phosphoinositides within the cell membrane that bind and cause the translocation of Akt (PKB) to the cell membrane, as well as being surrounded by effector proteins that act to transmit PI3K signaling downstream (Vanhaesebroeck and Aless 2000). PI3K-dependent kinases (PDK1 and PDK2) are the best-characterized membrane effector proteins of PI3K, which act to phosphorylate and activate Akt. Activation of Akt subsequently leads to the phosphorylation and regulation of various targets involved in cell survival (IκB, BAD, caspase-9, forkhead and Daf transcription factors), mitogenesis (mTOR), and metabolism (glycogen synthase kinase) (Vanhaesebroeck and Aless 2000). Activated Akt has been shown to phosphorylate various proteins associated with cell survival and proliferation of both normal and neoplastic mammary epithelial cells (Downward 1998; Kandel and Hay 1999; Khwaja 1999; Toker 2000). Akt inactivation is primarily regulated by two phosphatases, phosphatase and tensin homologue deleted from chromosome 10 (PTEN) and protein phosphatase type 2A (PP2A) (Kandel and Hay 1999). PTEN inhibits the activation of PDK-1, whereas PP2A can inhibit PIP_2 mediated phosphorylation of Akt (Kandel and Hay 1999).

Previous studies have shown that treatment with growth inhibitory doses of γ-tocotrienol caused a significant decrease in mitogen-dependent cell cycle progression, as indicated by a nearly 60% decrease in positive PCNA staining in mammary tumor cells (Shah and Sylvester 2005). This same treatment also caused a corresponding large decrease in intracellular levels of phospho-PDK-1 (active) and phospho-Akt (active), as well as Akt kinase activity, as indicated by a relatively large decrease in phospho-GSK-3α/β levels, a downstream substrate of activated Akt (Shah and Sylvester 2005). The inhibitory effects of tocotrienols on the activation of PI3K/PDK/Akt signaling proteins can be seen in Figure 10.3. Tocotrienol inhibition of PI3K/PDK/Akt mitogenic signal was not found to result from increased expression or activity of phosphatases. Studies showed that γ-tocotrienol treatment had no effect on the activity of PTEN and PP2A, phosphatases that are primarily responsible for regulating the dephosphorylation and inactivation of PDK-1 and Akt (Shah and Sylvester 2005).

Additional studies have confirmed that tocotrienol inhibition of mammary tumor cell proliferation was associated with a significant reduction in the phosphatidylinositol 3-kinase (PI3K)/PI3K-dependent kinase (PDK)/Akt mitogenic signaling, but the specific intracellular sites

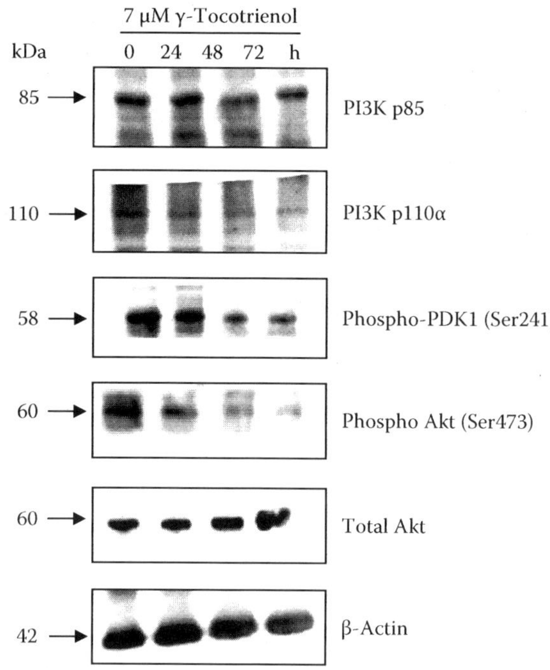

FIGURE 10.3 Western blot analysis of the effects of 7μM γ-tocotrienol on the activation of signaling proteins within the PI3K/PDK/Akt mitogenic pathway. Cells in each treatment group were initially plated at a density of 1×10^6 cells/100mm culture dish. Following treatment exposure, whole cell lysates were prepared for subsequent fractionation by SDS-PAGE (30 μg/lane), followed by western blot analysis.

targeted by γ-tocotrienol in this pathway have not yet been identified (Sylvester and Shah 2005; Sylvester et al. 2005). Subsequent investigations have shown that γ-tocotrienol does not act directly to inhibit PI3K or Akt kinase activity, and had little or no effect on the relative levels of the p85 regulatory subunit or the p110α catalytic subunit of the PI3K, indicating that the inhibitory effects of γ-tocotrienol on PI3K/PDK/Akt mitogenic signaling appear to involve the prevention of ErbB receptor family activation of PI3K (Samant and Sylvester 2006).

Although all ErbB receptor family members share common signaling pathways, individual ErbB receptors preferentially bind specific intracellular substrates based on the presence of defined cytoplasmic domain tyrosine phosphorylation sites (Olayioye et al. 2000; Yarden 2001). This is particularly important for the transphosphorylated ErbB3 heterodimer, which has been shown to be the most efficient activator of PI3K because of specific interactions with the p85 regulatory subunit of this lipid kinase (Bazley and Gullick 2005). Studies have also shown that ErbB3 heterodimers are extremely stable and remain at the cell surface for a prolonged period of time, and suppression of ErbB3 transphosphorylation significantly inhibits PI3K/PDK/Akt signaling and greatly reduce tumor cell proliferation and survival (Holbro et al. 2003; Britten 2004). Excessive Akt signaling promotes oncogenic expression by stimulating tumor cell proliferation, transformation and metastasis, and overexpression of constitutively active Akt has been shown to reverse the proliferative block induced by treatments targeted at inhibiting ErbB receptor mitogenic signaling in neoplastic mammary epithelial cells (Holbro et al. 2003). Since tyrosine phosphorylation of the cytoplasmic domain of ErbB receptors is required for interaction and activation of intracellular substrates, and activated ErbB3 receptor heterodimers are the most potent stimulators of the PI3K/PDK/Akt mitogenic signaling pathway in neoplastic mammary epithelial cells (Fedi et al. 1994; Prigent and Gullick 1994), these data strongly suggest that γ-tocotrienol therapy may be useful for suppressing the growth and survival of breast cancer cells characterized by enhanced expression of ErbB3 receptors.

10.7 TOCOTRIENOLS ON PKA MITOGENIC SIGNALING

Members of the ErbB receptor family have also been shown to be coupled to G proteins that activate adenylyl cyclase, which leads to an elevation in intracellular cAMP levels and activation of cAMP-dependent protein kinases in normal and neoplastic mammary epithelial cells (Imagawa et al. 1990; Bandyopadhyay et al. 1995; Xing and Imagawa 1999). Activation of cAMP-dependent protein kinases is a key event that initiates additional mitogenic cascades (Richards 2001). Experiments were conducted to characterize tocotrienol effects on EGF-induced ErbB1-receptor tyrosine kinase activity, cAMP production and activation of cAMP-dependent protein kinases in preneoplastic mammary epithelial cells grown in culture and maintained on serum-free media containing EGF as a mitogen. Results showed tocotrienol inhibition of EGF-dependent preneoplastic mammary epithelial cell growth does not result from a decrease in either EGF-receptor levels or EGF-induced ErbB1-receptor tyrosine kinase activity (Sylvester et al. 2002). These data indicate that growth inhibitory effects of tocotrienols occur downstream from the EGF-receptor in these cells. In addition, combined treatment with pharmacological agents that either enhanced G protein function (cholera and pertussis toxin) or increased intracellular cAMP levels (forskolin and 8-Br-cAMP) completely reversed the growth inhibitory effects of tocotrienols on these preneoplastic cells (Sylvester et al. 2002). These findings indicate that the antiproliferative effects of tocotrienol are associated with an inhibition of G protein-mediated activation of adenylyl cyclase and cAMP production.

Additional studies showed that tocotrienols specifically inhibit several cAMP-dependent protein kinase mitogenic signaling (Sylvester et al. 2002). Results from these studies clearly show that antiproliferative effects of tocotrienols in preneoplastic mammary epithelial cells do not result from a reduction in EGF-receptor mitogenic responsiveness, but reflect early post-receptor downstream sites of action involved in cAMP production. Further characterization of the intracellular mechanism(s) of action of tocotrienols will increase awareness of the potential value of these vitamin E compounds as chemopreventive agents, as well as provide insights for the potential use of these compounds either alone or in combination with other traditional therapies in the treatment of breast cancer.

10.7.1 Tocotrienol Effects on MAPK Mitogenic Signaling

Another initial event in ErbB receptor tyrosine kinase mitogenic signaling is Ras activation (Denhardt 1996; Kolch 2000). A downstream effector of Ras is c-Raf-1, a serine/threonine kinase, which subsequently phosphorylates and activates the MAPK cascade or MEK/ERK kinase pathway (Denhardt 1996; Kolch 2000). Downstream effectors of ERKs are nuclear transcription factors such as Myc and Elk that ultimately induce various biological responses, including mitogenesis, by directly influencing gene expression (Denhardt 1996; Kolch 2000). Studies showed that treatment with growth inhibiting doses of tocotrienols caused only a slight decrease in total intracellular levels of ERK1 and ERK2 in preneoplastic mammary epithelial cells. However, these treatments did cause a dramatic dose–responsive decrease in phosphorylated (active) ERK1 and ERK2 levels as compared with controls. These findings indicate that tocotrienol inhibition of EGF-dependent preneoplastic mammary epithelial cell proliferation appear to involve downstream post-receptor events that lead to a reduction in ERK1 and ERK2 activation (Sylvester et al. 2002).

10.7.2 Tocotrienol Effects on NFκB Activation

NFκB proteins constitute an inducible family of transcription factors that have been implicated in the regulation of cell proliferation, cell survival, tumor development as well as malignant transformation (Baldwin 1996; Nakshatri et al. 1997; Biswas et al. 2001; Sliva et al. 2002). Furthermore, EGF-induced activation of the PI3K/PDK-1/Akt mitogenic pathway has been shown to enhance NFκB transcriptional activity (Biswas et al. 2000; Biswas et al. 2001). The NFκB family consists of five members (p50, p52, p65 [RelA], c-Rel, and RelB), which can form various homo- or heterodimeric complexes required for binding to DNA and initiating transcription (Baldwin 1996). Classical NFκB is a hetero-dimer composed of the p65 and p50 subunits, and it is the p65 subunit that contains the transcriptional activation domain required for initiating gene transcription (Baldwin 1996). NFκB proteins are sequestered in the cytoplasm in an inactive form when bound to the specific IκB inhibitory proteins, such as IκB-α (Baldwin 1996). A variety of mitogen-dependent kinases, such as PI3K and Akt, can activate the IKK complex to stimulate IκB degradation and NFκB activation (Baldwin 1996; Khwaja 1999; Sakurai et al. 1999; Biswas et al. 2000). Studies have shown that treatment with growth inhibitory doses of γ-tocotrienol resulted in a suppression of NFκB activity in mammary tumor cells (Shah and Sylvester 2005a). This inhibitory effect of γ-tocotrienol on NFκB activation appears to result from the suppression of IKK-α/β activity, an upstream kinase that stimulates NFκB transcriptional activity. Since NFκB play a critical role in development and progression of mammary tumorigenesis, and overexpression of activated NFκB is associated with the development of resistance to chemotherapy in a majority of breast cancer cases (Rohlff and Glazer 1995; Nakshatri et al. 1997; Downward 1998; Biswas et al. 2001; Sliva et al. 2002), these findings provide further evidence that tocotrienols may have potential value as a chemotherapeutic agent for use in the prevention and/or treatment of breast cancer in women.

10.7.3 Synergistic Antiproliferative Effects of Tocotrienols with Other Anticancer Agents

The clinical use of various anticancer agents has been somewhat limited because high-dose therapy is associated with severe toxicity. An example of such anticancer agents is the statins. Statins represent a class of drugs that are widely used to lower high blood cholesterol levels. However, recent evidence suggests that statins may also act as chemoprotective agents against various types of cancers (Graaf et al. 2004). Statins are potent inhibitors of 3-hydroxy-3-methylglutaryl-coenzyme A (HMG-CoA) reductase, an enzyme catalyzing the conversion of HMGCoA to mevalonate, the rate limiting step in cholesterol biosynthesis. Statin-induced inhibition of mevalonate synthesis also reduces the synthesis of downstream non-sterol products such as farnesyl pyrophosphate. These non-sterol products are essential for the isoprenylation of intracellular second messenger mitogenic signaling proteins such as Ras. Early investigations showed that HMGCoA inhibitor blockade of mevalonate synthesis induced cell cycle arrest *in vitro* and inhibited tumor growth *in vivo* (Campbell et al. 2006). Subsequent studies have shown that statins can also inhibit breast, pancreas, liver and prostate tumor cell growth (Thibault et al. 1996; Seeger et al. 2003; Shibata et al. 2004). Nevertheless, the use of statins in cancer trials has been greatly limited by their high-dose toxicity, which is characterized by severe myopathy (Thibault et al. 1996).

Gamma-tocotrienol has also been shown to induce a post-transcriptional down-regulation of HMG-CoA reductase, resulting in a significant reduction in cholesterol synthesis (Parker et al. 1993). Since the mechanism of action by which γ-tocotrienol and statins suppress HMGCoA reductase activity is different from each other, it was hypothesized that combined low-dose treatment with γ-tocotrienol and statins may have synergistic anticancer effects without causing high dose-induced adverse side effects. Studies were recently conducted to investigate the growth inhibitory effects of low-dose treatment of simvastatin, lovastatin, mevastatin and pravastatin alone or in combination with γ-tocotrienol on mammary tumor cells *in vitro*. Results demonstrate that γ-tocotrienol synergistically enhances the antiproliferative effects of statins on the highly malignant +SA mammary epithelial cells *in vitro* (Wali and Sylvester 2007). Combined treatment of subeffective doses of simvastatin, lovastatin, mevastatin or pravastatin with subeffective doses (0.25–2.0 μM) of γ-tocotrienol resulted in nearly an 8–11-fold reduction in the dose of statin required to obtain the same growth inhibitory effects as statin treatment alone. Furthermore, this synergistic growth inhibitory effect of combined treatment of γ-tocotrienol with individual statins was found to be cytostatic, not cytotoxic (Wali and Sylvester 2007).

While treatment with 2–8 μM simvastatin, lovastatin or mevastatin alone was found to significantly inhibit mammary tumor cell growth, it should be pointed out that an oral dose of 25 mg/kg or higher would be required to achieve the same levels of these statins in the blood of humans. However, use of treatment doses of 25mg/kg or higher in humans is associated with severe adverse side effects, particularly myotoxicity (Thibault et al. 1996). As a result, the use of these statins as monotherapy in the prevention or treatment of cancer has been limited in order to avoid potential detrimental effects that would have a negative impact on the health and well-being of the patient. In order to avoid unwanted adverse side effects associated with high-dose statin use, it has been suggested that low-dose statin therapy can be combined with other anticancer agents (Bocci et al. 2005; Duncan et al. 2005; Mantha et al. 2005; McAnally et al. 2007). Therefore, experimental findings may have very important clinical implications in that combined low-dose statin and γ-tocotrienol treatment may be effective in the treatment of breast cancer without the risk of severe myotoxicity that is associated with high-dose statin use (Thibault et al. 1996).

Studies have shown that statins and γ-tocotrienol both inhibit HMGCoA reductase activity and subsequent mevalonate synthesis through independent mechanisms. It has been established that γ-tocotrienol induces a down-regulation in HMGCoA reductase levels through a post-transcriptional acceleration in degradation (Parker et al. 1993), whereas statins act directly to inhibit HMGCoA reductase enzymatic activity (Istvan and Deisenhofer 2001). Since cells treated with statins often display a compensatory up-regulation in HMGCoA reductase expression (Brown et al. 1978), it is possible that combined treatment with γ-tocotrienol counteracts this compensatory response and prevents the restoration of mevalonate synthesis. Since mevalonate is an upstream intermediate in the synthesis of reactive farnesyl residues, synergistic suppression of HMGCoA reductase activity by the combined treatment of statins and γ-tocotrienol might ultimately prevent the farnesylation and anchoring of Ras to the interior of the cell membrane (Casey et al. 1989; Bassa et al. 1999). Once Ras is anchored to the cell membrane, it is able to interact with activated membrane bound receptors, such as the EGF-receptor, and initiate activation of the MAPK and Akt mitogenic signaling pathways (Nakagawa et al. 1998). Therefore, the synergistic antiproliferative effects of combined statin and γ-tocotrienol treatment may result from their independent actions to inhibit HMGCoA reductase activity, mevalonate synthesis and subsequent farnesylation of second messengers involved in mediating EGF-dependent mitogenic signaling. Studies have shown that the synergistic antiproliferative effects of combined treatment of γ-tocotrienol and statins were associated with a suppression in multiple EGF-dependent mitogenic signaling pathways, including a relatively large reduction in the levels of phosphorylated (activated) p44 MAPK and Akt. Taken together, these findings strongly suggest that combined γ-tocotrienol and statin therapy may provide significant health benefits in the prevention or treatment of breast cancer in women, while at the same time avoiding myotoxicity that is associated with high-dose statin treatment.

10.8 APOPTOSIS

Apoptosis or programmed cell death is an important cellular process that is an essential aspect of organ development and remodeling that is initiated at birth and continues throughout life (Kumar et al. 2000). Apoptosis is also a mechanism by which neoplastic cells can be eliminated from the body (Kumar et al. 2000). Apoptosis is characterized by many biochemical and morphological changes occurring in a cell, including the plasma membrane forming small blebs and vesicles, losing contact with the extracellular matrix, and ultimately shrinking and disintegrating without releasing its content into the surrounding area. The deteriorating fragments of cellular debris are then quickly scavenged by the neighboring cells and macrophages in the absence of an inflammatory response (Kumar et al. 2000).

Apoptosis is initiated by the activation of cysteine proteases known as caspases (Cohen 1997; Nicholson 1999). Procaspases are activated by cleavage at a specific site either by themselves or by other caspases (Cohen 1997; Nicholson 1999). Initiator caspases act upstream in the apoptosis cascade and exclusively cleave and activate other caspases called effector caspases, which then cleave other proteins. Initiator procaspases remain in an inactive state through the binding to inhibitory proteins that prevent dimerization and activation. Activation of initiator caspases results from the down-regulation or destruction of these caspase inhibitory proteins. Initiator caspases (caspases-2, -8, -9 and -10) activate effector caspases (caspases 3, 6 and 7), which in turn cleave structural and regulatory proteins (DFF45/ICAD, PARP, lamins, cytokeratins, etc.) and are responsible for most features described above (Cohen 1997; Muzio et al. 1998; Srinivasula et al. 1998; Nicholson 1999). Different caspases have different roles during the initiation and progression of apoptosis, including the destruction of caspase inhibitors, Bcl-2 anti-apoptotic proteins, mitogenic or survival signal transduction pathways, cytoskeleton proteins, and DNA repair and replication enzymes (Ashkenazi and Dixit 1998; Nicholson 1999).

Two of the major mechanisms for caspase activation involve death receptor and mitochondrial stress apoptotic signaling. Death receptors are members of the tumor necrosis factor (TNF) receptor superfamily; they are activated by their corresponding death receptor ligands and include TNF-R1, Fas, TNF-related apoptosis-inducing ligand (TRAIL) receptors, TRAIL-R1 and TRAIL-R2 (Schulze-Osthoff et al. 1998; Walczak and Krammer 2000). Specific ligands to these death receptors include TNFα that activates TNF-R1, FasL that activates Fas, and TRAIL that activates TRAIL-R1 and TRAIL-R2 (Kramer et al. 1997; Schulze-Osthoff et al. 1998; Walczak and Krammer 2000). Following activation, death receptors undergo trimerization and recruit adapter proteins such as FADD through homophilic DD interactions, and initiator procaspases such as procaspase-8 to form the death-inducing signaling complex (DISC) at the membrane that promotes caspase-8 activation (Ashkenazi and Dixit 1998). Within the DISC, procaspase-8 is cleaved to form the active p20 subunit of caspase-8 that subsequently cleave and activate effector caspases such as caspase-3, -6, or -7 and ultimately apoptosis. In contrast, mitochondrial stress-induced caspase activation and apoptosis can be initiated by numerous cellular signals that cause perturbations in the mitochondrial membrane, resulting in the release of pro-apoptotic molecules, such as apoptosis-inducing factor (AIF) and cytochrome c, from the intermembrane space into the cytoplasm (Green and Reed 1998; Susin et al. 1999). Cytochrome c then interacts with Apaf-1, dATP/ATP and procaspase-9 in the cytoplasm to form a complex called the apoptosome, which leads to the activation of caspase-9, which then activates effector caspase-3 or -7, and ultimately leads to apoptosis (Li et al. 1997; Zou et al. 1997; Li et al. 1998). Cytochrome c, required for apoptosome formation, is tightly controlled by the Bcl-2 family of proteins that exits to inhibit (Bcl-2, Bcl-x_L, Bcl-w, Mcl-1 and A1) or promote (Bax, Bak, Bok, Bik, Hrk, Bim and Bad) apoptosis (Oltvai and Korsmeyer 1994; Susin et al. 1999).

10.9 APOPTOTIC EFFECTS OF TOCOTRIENOLS

Initially, studies were conducted to directly compare the apoptotic potency of individual tocopherols and tocotrienols isoforms on normal, preneoplastic, neoplastic and highly malignant mouse mammary epithelial cells *in vitro* (McIntyre et.al., 2000b). Results showed that treatment by very high doses of α- or γ-tocopherol had no effect on viability in any of these types of cells. In contrast, δ-tocopherol and α-, γ- and δ-tocotrienol were found to reduce normal, preneoplastic, neoplastic and malignant mammary epithelial cell viability in a dose-responsive manner, but the tocotrienols were found to be significantly more potent that δ-tocopherol (McIntyre et.al., 2000b). These data also showed that the highly malignant cells were the most sensitive, whereas normal cells were the least sensitive to the apoptotic effects of these individual vitamin E isoforms. These findings were of particular interest because tocotrienol-induced apoptosis was observed in preneoplastic and neoplastic mammary epithelial cells using treatment doses that had no effect on normal cells' viability. The dose-responsive effects of γ-tocotrienol on TUNEL assay positive staining, an indicator of apoptosis, on highly malignant mammary epithelial cells grown in culture are shown in Figure 10.4.

Subsequent studies conducted to determine the intracellular mechanisms mediating tocotrienol-induced apoptosis in neoplastic mammary epithelial cells showed that γ-tocotrienol induced caspase-8 and -3, but not caspase-9 activation, suggesting that tocotrienol-induced apoptosis is

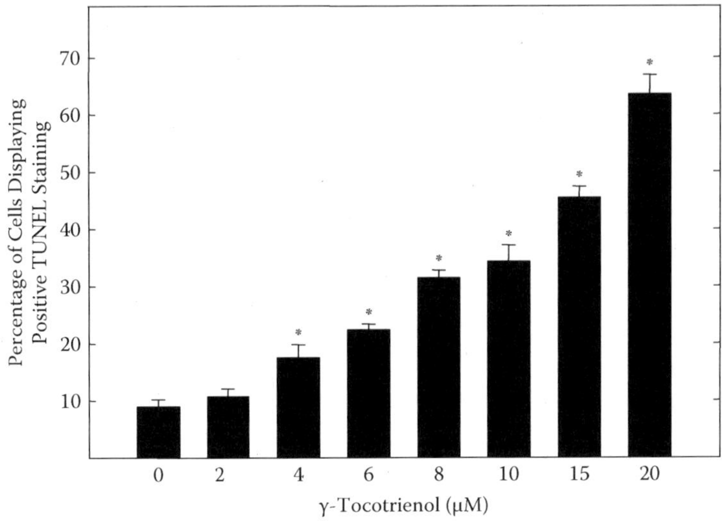

FIGURE 10.4 Effects of 24 hr exposure to 0-20 μM γ-tocotrienol on positive TUNEL staining, an index of active apoptosis, on highly malignant mouse +SA mammary epithelial cells grown in culture. Cells were plated at a density of $1X10^5$ cells/well (6 wells/group) and maintained on serum-free control media for 3 days. Afterward, cells were exposed to treatment media, and 24 hr later, cells were fixed with 4% paraformaldehyde prior to TUNEL assay. Cells were counted in five photomicrographs (80,000 μm^2 area per photomicrograph) for each treatment group. Vertical bars indicate the mean + SEM. *$P < 0.05$, as compared with controls.

mediated through death receptor activation (Shah et al. 2003). In contrast, α-tocopherol had no effect on caspase activation. Furthermore, γ-tocotrienol-induced caspase activation and apoptosis was blocked when treatment was given in combination with specific caspase-8 and -3, but not caspase-9 inhibitors (Shah et al. 2003). These effects of α-tocopherol and γ-tocotrienol treatment on caspase activation are shown in Figure 10.5. Since caspase-8 processing and activation are associated with death receptor-mediated apoptotic signaling, while caspase-9 activation and processing is associated with mitochondrial stress-mediated apoptotic signaling, these findings strongly suggested that tocotrienol-induced apoptosis is mediated by receptor-induced caspase activation and occurs independently of mitochondrial stress-related apoptotic mechanisms in these cells.

The suggestion that tocotrienol-induced cytotoxicity in mouse neoplastic mammary epithelial cells is unrelated to mitochondrial stress apoptotic signaling was later confirmed in another study (Shah and Sylvester 2005b). This study clearly demonstrated that exposure to cytotoxic doses of γ-tocotrienol induced apoptosis, but did not result in a disruption or loss of mitochondrial membrane potential or the release of cytochrome c from the mitochondria into the cytoplasm of neoplastic mammary epithelial cells (Shah and Sylvester 2005b). Furthermore, results also showed that this treatment caused a paradoxical increase in mitochondrial anti-apoptotic and corresponding decrease in mitochondrial pro-apoptotic Bcl-2 family member proteins. The relative intracellular levels of anti- and pro-apoptotic Bcl-2 proteins determine mitochondrial membrane stability and modulate cytochrome c release into the cytoplasm (Hsu et al. 1997; Jaattela 1999; Putcha et al. 1999; Antonsson and Martinou 2000) These findings suggested that mitochondrial membrane stability and integrity might actually be enhanced for a limited period of time following exposure to cytotoxic doses of γ-tocotrienol (Shah and Sylvester 2005b), and that tocotrienols may play a role in suppressing mitochondrial stress-mediated apoptosis (Brigelius-Flohe and Traber 1999). Other investigations have shown γ-tocotrienol-induced apoptosis in human breast cancer cells is associated with a slight disruption in mitochondrial membrane potential and cytochrome c release into the cytoplasm, but tocotrienols failed to alter Bcl-2 protein levels and did not induce caspase-9 activation (Takahashi and Loo 2004), whereas others have reported that tocotrienols altered the ratio of Bax/Bcl-2 to

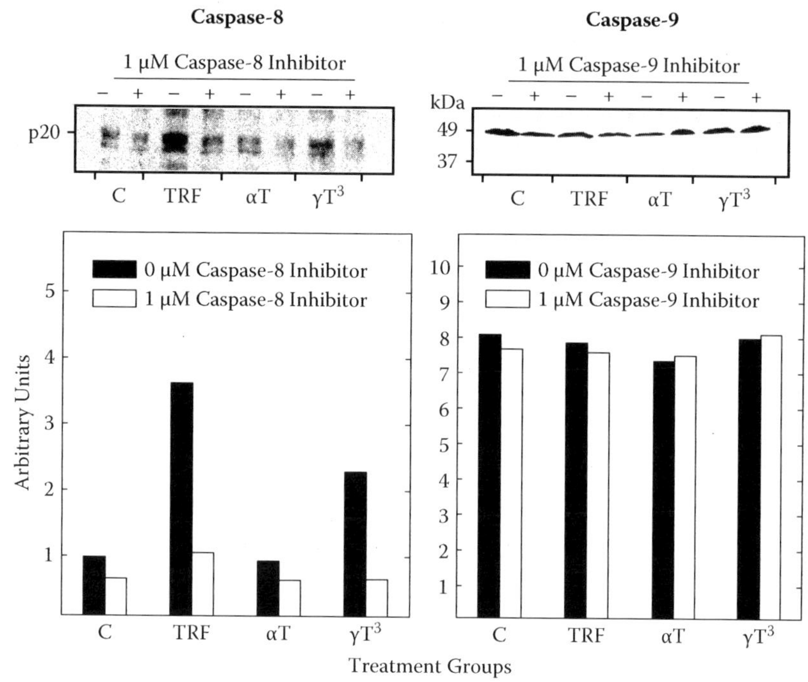

FIGURE 10.5 Western blot analysis and scanning densitometric analysis of the relative levels of active p20 processed form of caspase-8 (death receptor activated), inactive (49 kDa) and active processed (37 kDa) forms of caspase-9 (mitochondrial stress activated) in malignant +SA mammary epithelial cells treated for 24 hours with 0-50 μM TRF, 0-200 μM α-tocopherol (αT), or 0-20 μM γ-tocotrienol (γT^3) treatment media. Prior to treatment exposure, cells in each treatment group were grown in control media for 3 days. Following treatment, whole cell lysates (100 μg/lane) from the different treatment groups were fractionated by SDS-PAGE and then subjected to western blot analysis for caspase-8, and -9 levels. Vertical bars in the densitometric graphs indicate the integrated optical density of bands visualized in each lane.

induce mitochondrial disruption, cytochrome c release and caspase-9 activation in human colon carcinoma cells (Agarwal et al. 2004). At present, it is not understood why different intracellular signaling mechanisms appear to be involved in mediating the apoptotic effects of tocotrienols in different types of cancer cells. Additional studies are required to determine the specific intracellular sites of action that these different vitamin E compounds target in order to fully understand the specific mechanisms of action mediating their anticancer and apoptotic effects, as well as to further clarify the potential value of these compounds as chemotherapeutic agents in the prevention and treatment of breast cancer.

Since previous studies showed that tocotrienol-induced apoptosis was mediated through the activation of caspase-8 and -3 in neoplastic mammary epithelial cells and caspase-8 activation is associated with death receptors apoptotic signaling (Shah et al. 2003;), additional studies were conducted to determine the exact death receptor/ligand involved in tocotrienol-induced apoptosis. Treatment with high doses of TNFα, FasL, TRAIL, or apoptosis-inducing Fas antibody failed to induce death in +SA mouse neoplastic mammary epithelial cells, indicating that this particular mammary tumor cell line is resistant to death receptor-induced apoptosis (Shah and Sylvester 2004). Furthermore, treatment with a cytotoxic dose of γ-tocotrienol had no effect on total, membrane or cytosolic levels of Fas, FasL or FADD, and did not induce translocation of Fas, FasL or FADD from the cytosolic to the membrane fraction (Shah and Sylvester 2004). However, it was also shown that tocotrienol treatment induced a large decrease in phosphatidylinositol 3-kinase (PI3K)/PI3K-dependent kinase (PDK-1)/Akt mitogenic signaling and the subsequent downregulation of FLIP, an endogenous inhibitor of caspase-8 processing and activation (Shah and Sylvester 2004). Since stimulation of the PI3K/PDK/Akt mitogenic pathway is associated with increased FLIP expression, and enhanced cellular proliferation and survival, it was concluded that tocotrienol-induced caspase-8 activation and apoptosis in malignant +SA mammary epithelial cells is associated with suppression in PI3K/PDK-1/Akt mitogenic signaling and subsequent reduction in intracellular FLIP levels. These findings are significant in light of knowledge that resistance to death receptor-induced apoptosis is associated with enhanced tumorigenesis, multi-drug resistance, and enhanced survival in a number of tumor cell types of cancers (Hughes et al. 1997; Reed 1999; Yu et al. 1999). A reduction in the expression of death receptors or their ligands, as well as mutations within genes encoding for death receptors, is associated with insensitive or nonfunctional death receptors in various types of tumor cells (Watanabe-Fukunaga et al. 1992; Fisher et al. 1995; Hughes et al. 1997; Reed 1999). In addition, resistance to apoptotic stimuli can be acquired through up-regulation and enhanced activity of various mitogen-dependent signaling pathways, particularly the PI3K/PDK/Akt mitogenic signaling pathway (Watanabe-Fukunaga et al. 1992; Fisher et al. 1995; Hughes et al. 1997; Downward 1998; Kandel and Hay 1999; Reed 1999; Vanhaesebroeck and Waterfield 1999; Varadhachary et al. 2001; Neve et al. 2002). Studies have also shown that nonfunctional death receptors are associated with cancer cell escape and survival from normal immunosurveillance mechanisms (Hughes et al. 1997; Reed 1999; Yu et al. 1999). Furthermore, tocotrienols have been found to significantly inhibit human breast cancer cell growth and viability regardless of estrogen receptor status (Nesaretnam et al. 1995; Guthrie et al. 1997; Nesaretnam et al. 1998; Nesaretnam et al. 2000). Therefore, tocotrienols have a unique property of inducing apoptosis in a wide variety of tumor cells that possess insensitive or nonfunctional death receptors or display multi-drug-resistance to traditional chemotherapeutic agents.

10.10 CONCLUSIONS

An abundance of experimental evidence has demonstrated that α-tocopherol treatment has no significant antiproliferative or apoptotic activity, whereas tocotrienols display potent antitumor activity against a wide variety of cancer cell types in animal and cell culture studies (Neuzil et al. 2002; Sylvester and Theriault 2003; Kline et al. 2004; Sylvester et al. 2005). Furthermore, clinical and epidemiological studies have shown consistent results demonstrating a protective effect of α-tocopherol against the development and progression of cancer (Bostick et al. 1993; Sung et al. 2003; Virtamo et al. 2003). However, experimental data primarily obtained in cell culture and, to a lesser extent, animal studies, has provided strong evidence indicating that natural tocotrienols display very potent antiproliferative and apoptotic activity against a variety to tumor cell types, and may provide significant value as therapeutic agents in the prevention and treatment of cancer in humans. However, tocotrienol therapy has not yet been rigorously tested in clinical trials. Furthermore, very little is presently understood regarding the biokinetics of tocotrienols in humans and additional studies in this area are required to optimize the effectiveness of tocotrienol therapy. Additional pharmaceutics research is clearly needed, particularly in the areas of vitamin E kinetics, formulation and drug delivery. Important information obtained from these pharmaceutics studies could then be used to conduct meaningful and highly controlled long-term intervention studies in humans. Finally, one of the most intriguing aspects of tocotrienols is their characteristic selectivity to induce apoptosis in cancer but not normal cells. Likewise, tocotrienols also display the unique ability to induce apoptosis in tumor cells containing nonfunctional death receptors. Taken together, these findings strongly suggest that the tocotrienol forms of vitamin E may provide significant benefit in the prevention and treatment of cancer when used either alone as monotherapy or in combination with other anticancer agents.

ACKNOWLEDGMENTS

This work was performed at the College of Pharmacy, University of Louisiana at Monroe, Monroe, LA 71209-0470 and supported by a grant from the NIH (Grant CA86833). The author would also like to thank Dr. Abdul Gapor of the Malaysian Palm Oil Board for generously providing purified tocotrienols for use in experimental studies.

REFERENCES

Agarwal, M.K., M.L. Agarwal, M. Athar and S. Gupta. 2004. Tocotrienol-rich fraction of palm oil activates p53, modulates Bax/Bcl2 ratio and induces apoptosis independent of cell cycle association. *Cell Cycle,* 3, 205–211.

Antonsson, B. and J.D. Martinou. 2000. The Bcl-2 protein family. *Exp. Cell Res.*, 256, 50–57.

Ashkenazi, A. and V.M. Dixit. 1998. Death receptors: Signaling and modulation. *Science*, 281, 1305–1308.

Baldwin, A.S., Jr. 1996. The NF–kappa B and I kappa B proteins: New discoveries and insights. *Annu Rev Immunol,* 14, 649–683.

Bandyopadhyay, G.K., W. Imagawa and S. Nandi. 1995. Role of GTP-binding proteins in the polyunsaturated fatty acid stimulated proliferation of mouse mammary epithelial cells. *Prostaglandins Leukot Essent Fatty Acids,* 52, 151–158.

Bassa, B.V., D.D. Roh, N.D. Vaziri, M.A. Kirschenbaum and V.S. Kamanna. 1999. Effect of inhibition of cholesterol synthetic pathway on the activation of Ras and MAP kinase in mesangial cells. *Biochim Biophys Acta,* 1449, 137–149.

Bazley, L.A. and W.J. Gullick. 2005. The epidermal growth factor receptor family. *Endocr Relat Cancer,* 12 Suppl 1, S17–27.

Birkenfeld, H.P., B.S. McInntyre, K.P. Briski and P.W. Sylvester. 1996a. Role of protein kinase C in modulating epidermal growth factor- and phorbol ester-induced mammary epithelial cell growth in vitro. *Exp Cell Res,* 223, 183–191.

Birkenfeld, H.P., B.S. McIntyre, K.P. Briski and P.W. Sylvester. 1996b. Protein kinase C isoenzyme expression in normal mouse mammary epithelial cells grown in primary culture. *Proc Soc Exp Biol Med,* 213, 65–70.

Bishop, D.T. 1999. BRCA1 and BRCA2 and breast cancer incidence: A review. *Ann Oncol,* 10 Suppl 6, 113–119.

Biswas, D.K., A.P. Cruz, E. Gansberger and A.B. Pardee. 2000. Epidermal growth factor-induced nuclear factor kappa B activation: A major pathway of cell–cycle progression in estrogen-receptor negative breast cancer cells. *Proc Natl Acad Sci USA,* 97, 8542–8547.

Biswas, D.K., S.C. Dai, A. Cruz, B. Weiser, E. Graner and A.B. Pardee. 2001. The nuclear factor kappa B (NF-kappa B): A potential therapeutic target for estrogen receptor negative breast cancers. *Proc Natl Acad Sci USA,* 98, 10386–10391.

Bocci, G., A. Fioravanti, P. Orlandi, N. Bernardini, P. Collecchi, M. Del Tacca and R. Danesi. 2005. Fluvastatin synergistically enhances the antiproliferative effect of gemcitabine in human pancreatic cancer MIAPaCa-2 cells. *Br J Cancer,* 93, 319–330.

Bostick, R.M., J.D. Potter, D.R. McKenzie, T.A. Sellers, L.H. Kushi, K.A. Steinmetz and A.R. Folsom. 1993. Reduced risk of colon cancer with high intake of vitamin E: The Iowa Women's Health Study. *Cancer Res,* 53, 4230–4237.

Brigelius-Flohe, R. and M.G. Traber. 1999. Vitamin E: Function and metabolism. *Faseb J,* 13, 1145–1155.

Britten, C.D. 2004. Targeting ErbB receptor signaling: A pan ErbB approach to cancer. *Mol Cancer Ther,* 3, 1335–1342.

Brown, M.S., J.R. Faust, J.L. Goldstein, I. Kaneko and A. Endo. 1978. Induction of 3-hydroxy-3-methylglutaryl coenzyme A reductase activity in human fibroblasts incubated with compactin (ML-236B), a competitive inhibitor of the reductase. *J Biol Chem,* 253, 1121–1128.

Campbell, M.J., L.J. Esserman, Y. Zhou, M. Shoemaker, M. Lobo, E. Borman, F. Baehner, A.S. Kumar, K. Adduci, C. Marx, E.F. Petricoin, L.A. Liotta, M. Winters, S. Benz and C.C. Benz. 2006. Breast cancer growth prevention by statins. *Cancer Res,* 66, 8707–8714.

Casey, P.J., P.A. Solski, C.J. Der and J.E. Buss. p21ras is modified by a farnesyl isoprenoid. *Proc Natl Acad Sci USA 1989,* 86, 8323–8327.

Clement, S., A. Tasinato, D. Boscoboinik and A. Azzi. 1997. The effect of alpha-tocopherol on the synthesis, phosphorylation and activity of protein kinase C in smooth muscle cells after phorbol 12-myristate 13-acetate down-regulation. *Eur J Biochem,* 246, 745–749.

Cohen, G.M. Caspases: The executioners of apoptosis. *Biochem J* 1997, 326, 1–16.

Cottrell, R.C. 1991. Introduction: Nutritional aspects of palm oil. *Am J Clin Nutr,* 53, 989S–1009S.

Denhardt, D.T. 1996. Signal-transducting protein phosphorylation cascades mediated by Ras/Rho protein in the mammalian cell: the potential for multiplex signaling. *Biochem J,* 318, 729–747.

Downward, J. 1998. Mechanisms and consequences of activation of protein kinase B/Akt. *Curr Opin Cell Biol,* 10, 262–267.

Duncan, R.E., A. El-Sohemy and M.C. Archer. 2005. Regulation of HMG-CoA reductase in MCF-7 cells by genistein, EPA, and DHA, alone and in combination with mevastatin. *Cancer Lett,* 224, 221–228.

Fedi, P., J.H. Pierce, P.P. di Fiore and M.H. Kraus. 1994. Efficient coupling with phosphatidylinositol 3-kinase, but not phospholipase C gamma or GTPase-activating protein, distinguishes ErbB-3 signaling from that of other ErbB/EGFR family members. *Mol Cell Biol,* 14, 492–500.

Fisher, G.H., F.J. Rosenberg, S.E. Straus, J.K. Dale, L.A. Middleton, A.Y. Lin, W. Strober, M.J. Lenardo and J.M. Puck. 1995. Dominant interfering Fas gene mutations impair apoptosis in a human autoimmune lymphoproliferative syndrome. *Cell,* 81, 935–946.

Graaf, M.R., D.J. Richel, C.J. van Noorden and H.J. Guchelaar. 2004. Effects of statins and farnesyltransferase inhibitors on the development and progression of cancer. *Cancer Treat Rev,* 30, 609–641.

Green, D.R. and J.C. Reed. 1998. Mitochondria and apoptosis. *Science,* 281, 1309–1312.

Guthrie, N., A. Gapor, A.F. Chambers and K.K. Carroll. 1997. Inhibition of proliferation of estrogen receptor-negative MDA-MB-435 and -positive MCF-7 human breast cancer cells by palm oil tocotrienols and tamoxifen, alone and in combination. *J Nutr,* 127, 544S–548S.

Holbro, T., R.R. Beerli, F. Maurer, M. Koziczak, C.F. Barbas, 3rd and N.E. Hynes. 2003. The ErbB2/ErbB3 heterodimer functions as an oncogenic unit: ErbB2 requires ErbB3 to drive breast tumor cell proliferation. *Proc Natl Acad Sci USA,* 100, 8933–8938.

Hsu, Y.T., K.G. Wolter and R.J. Youle. 1997. Cytosol-to-membrane redistribution of Bax and Bcl-X(L) during apoptosis. *Proc Natl Acad Sci USA,* 94, 3668–3672.

Hughes, S.J., Y. Nambu, O.S. Soldes, D. Hamstra, A. Rehemtulla, M.D. Iannettoni, M.B. Orringer and D.G. Beer. 1997. Fas/APO–1 (CD95) is not translocated to the cell membrane in esophageal adenocarcinoma. *Cancer Res,* 57, 5571–5578.

Hutchinson, J., J. Jin, R.D. Cardiff, J.R. Woodgett and W.J. Muller. 2001. Activation of Akt (protein kinase B) in mammary epithelium provides a critical cell survival signal required for tumor progression. *Mol Cell Biol,* 21, 2203–2212.

Imagawa, W., G.K. Bandyopadhyay and S. Nandi. 1990. Regulation of mammary epithelial cell growth in mice and rats. *Endocr Rev,* 11, 494–523.

Istvan, E.S. and J. Deisenhofer. 2001. Structural mechanism for statin inhibition of HMG-CoA reductase. *Science,* 292, 1160–1164.

Jaattela, M. 1999. Escaping cell death: Survival proteins in cancer. *Exp Cell Res,* 248, 30–43.

Jung, F., J. Haendeler, C. Goebel, A.M. Zeiher and S. Dimmeler. 2000. Growth factor-induced phosphoinositide 3-OH kinase/Akt phosphorylation in smoth muscle cells: Induction of cell prolifertion and inhibition of cell death. *Cardiovascular Res,* 48, 148–157.

Kandel, E.S. and N. Hay. 1999. The regulation and activities of the multifunctional serine/threonine kinase Akt/PKB. *Exp Cell Res,* 253, 210–229.

Karunagaran, D., E. Tzahar, R.R. Beerli, X. Chen, D. Graus-Porta, B.J. Ratzkin, R. Seger, N.E. Hynes and Y. Yarden. 1996. ErbB-2 is a common auxiliary subunit of NDF and EGF receptors: Implications for breast cancer. *Embo J,* 15, 254–264.

Khwaja, A. 1999. Akt is more than just a Bad kinase. *Nature,* 401, 33–34.

Kimmick, G.G., R.A. Bell and R.M. Bostick. 1997. Vitamin E and breast cancer: A review. *Nutr Cancer,* 27, 109–117.

Kline, K., W. Yu and B.G. Sanders. 2004. Vitamin E and breast cancer. *J Nutr,* 134, 3458S–3462S.

Kolch, W. 2000. Meaningful relationships: The regulation of the Ras/Raf/Mek/Erk pathway by protein interactions. *Biochem J,* 351, 289–305.

Kramer, J.K., L. Blais, R.C. Fouchard, R.A. Melnyk and K.M. Kallury. A rapid method for the determination of vitamin E forms in tissues and diet by high-performance liquid chromatography using a normal-phase diol column. *Lipids* 1997, 32, 323–330.

Kumar, R., R.K. Vadlamudi and L. Adam. 2000. Apoptosis in mammary gland and cancer. *Endocr Relat Cancer,* 7, 257–269.

Li, H., H. Zhu, C.J. Xu and J. Yuan. 1998. Cleavage of BID by caspase 8 mediates the mitochondrial damage in the Fas pathway of apoptosis. *Cell,* 94, 491–501.

Li, P., D. Nijhawan, I. Budihardjo, S.M. Srinivasula, M. Ahmad, E.S. Alnemri and X. Wang. 1997. Cytochrome c and dATP-dependent formation of Apaf-1/caspase-9 complex initiates an apoptotic protease cascade. *Cell,* 91, 479–489.

Mantha, A.J., J.E. Hanson, G. Goss, A.E. Lagarde, I.A. Lorimer and J. Dimitroulakos. 2005. Targeting the mevalonate pathway inhibits the function of the epidermal growth factor receptor. *Clin Cancer Res,* 11, 2398–2407.

McAnally, J.A., J. Gupta, S. Sodhani, L. Bravo and H. Mo. 2007. Tocotrienols potentiate lovastatin–mediated growth suppression in vitro and in vivo. *Exp Biol Med* (Maywood), 232, 523–531.

McIntyre, B.S., K.P. Briski, M.A. Tirmenstein, M.W. Fariss, A. Gapor and P.W. Sylvester. 2000a. Antiproliferative and apoptotic effects of tocopherols and tocotrienols on normal mouse mammary epithelial cells. *Lipids*, 35, 171–180.

McIntyre, B.S., K.P. Briski, A. Gapor and P.W. Sylvester. 2000b. Antiproliferative and apoptotic effects of tocopherols and tocotrienols on preneoplastic and neoplastic mouse mammary epithelial cells. *Proc Soc Exp Biol Med.* 224, 292–301.

Muzio, M., B.R. Stockwell, H.R. Stennicke, G.S. Salvesen and V.M. Dixit. 1998. An induced proximity model for caspase–8 activation. *J Biol Chem,* 273, 2926–2930.

Nakagawa, H., T. Mutoh, T. Kumano and M. Kuriyama. 1998. HMG-CoA reductase inhibitor–induced L6 myoblast cell death: involvement of the phosphatidylinositol 3-kinase pathway. *FEBS Lett,* 438, 289–292.

Nakshatri, H., P. Bhat-Nakshatri, D.A. Martin, R.J. Goulet, Jr. and G.W. Sledge, Jr. 1997. Constitutive activation of NF-kappaB during progression of breast cancer to hormone-independent growth. *Mol Cell Biol,* 17, 3629–3639.

Nesaretnam, K., S. Dorasamy and P.D. Darbre. 2000. Tocotrienols inhibit growth of ZR-75-1 breast cancer cells. *Int J Food Sci Nutr,* 51 Suppl, S95–103.

Nesaretnam, K., N. Guthrie, A.F. Chambers and K.K. Carroll. 1995. Effect of tocotrienols on the growth of a human breast cancer cell line in culture. *Lipids*, 30, 1139–1143.

Nesaretnam, K., H.T. Khor, J. Ganeson, Y.H. Chong, K. Sundram, and A. Gapor. 1992. The effects of vitamin E tocotrienols from palm oil on chemically induced mammary carcingenesis in female rats. *Nutr. Res,* 12, 879–892.

Nesaretnam, K., R. Stephen, R. Dils and P. Darbre. 1998. Tocotrienols inhibit the growth of human breast cancer cells irrespective of estrogen receptor status. *Lipids*, 33, 461–469.

Neuzil, J., K. Kagedal, L. Andera, C. Weber and U.T. Brunk. 2002. Vitamin E analogs: A new class of multiple action agents with anti-neoplastic and anti-atherogenic activity. *Apoptosis*, 7, 179–187.

Neve, R.M., T. Holbro and N.E. Hynes. 2002. Distinct roles for phosphoinositide 3-kinase, mitogen-activated protein kinase and p38 MAPK in mediating cell cycle progression of breast cancer cells. *Oncogene*, 21, 4567–4576.

Nicholson, D.W. 1999. Caspase structure, proteolytic substrates, and function during apoptotic cell death. *Cell Death Differ,* 6, 1028–1042.

Olayioye, M.A., R.M. Neve, H.A. Lane and N.E. Hynes. 2000. The ErbB signaling network: Receptor heterodimerization in development and cancer. *Embo J,* 19, 3159–3167.

Oltvai, Z.N. and S.J. Korsmeyer. 1994. Checkpoints of dueling dimers foil death wishes [comment]. *Cell*, 79, 189–192.

Packer, L., G. Rimbach and F. Virgili. 1999. Antioxidant activity and biologic properties of a procyanidin-rich extract from pine (Pinus maritima) bark, pycnogenol. *Free Radic Biol Med,* 27, 704–724.

Packer, L., S.U. Weber and G. Rimbach. 2001. Molecular aspects of α-tocotrienol antioxidant action and cell signaling. *J. Nutr,* 131, 369S–373S.

Parker, R.A., B.C. Pearce, R.W. Clark, D.A. Gordon and J.J. Wright. 1993. Tocotrienols regulate cholesterol production in mammalian cells by post-transcriptional suppression of 3-hydroxy-3-methylglutaryl-coenzyme A reductase. *J Biol Chem,* 268, 11230–11238.

Parkin, D.M., F. Bray, J. Ferlay and P. Pisani. 2001. Estimating the world cancer burden: Globocan 2000. *Int J Cancer,* 94, 153–156.

Prigent, S.A. and W.J. Gullick. 1994. Identification of c-erbB-3 binding sites for phosphatidylinositol 3'-kinase and SHC using an EGF receptor/c-erbB-3 chimera. *Embo J,* 13, 2831–2841.

Putcha, G.V., M. Deshmukh and E.M. Johnson, Jr. 1999. BAX translocation is a critical event in neuronal apoptosis: Regulation by neuroprotectants, BCL-2, and caspases. *J Neurosci,* 19, 7476–7485.

Reed, J.C. 1999. Dysregulation of apoptosis in cancer. *J Clin Oncol,* 17, 2941–2953.

Ricciarelli, R., A. Tasinato, S. Clement, N.K. Ozer, D. Boscoboinik and A. Azzi. 1998. Alpha-tocopherol specifically inactivates cellular protein kinase C alpha by changing its phosphorylation state. *Biochem J,* 334, 243–249.

Richards, J.S. 2001. New signaling pathways for hormones and cyclic adenosine 3',5'-monophosphate action in endocrine cells. *Mol Endocrinol,* 15, 209–218.

Rohlff, C. and R.I. Glazer. 1995. Regulation of multidrug resistance through the cAMP and EGF signalling pathways. *Cell Signal,* 7, 431–443.

Sakurai, H., H. Chiba, H. Miyoshi, T. Sugita and W. Toriumi. 1999. IkappaB kinases phosphorylate NF-kappaB p65 subunit on serine 536 in the transactivation domain. *J Biol Chem,* 274, 30353–30356.

Samant, G.V. and P.W. Sylvester. 2006. Gamma-tocotrienol inhibits ErbB3-dependent PI3K/Akt mitogenic signalling in neoplastic mammary epithelial cells. *Cell Prolif,* 39, 563–574.

Schulze-Osthoff, K., D. Ferrari, M. Los, S. Wesselborg and M.E. Peter. 1998. Apoptosis signaling by death receptors. *Eur J Biochem,* 254, 439–459.

Seeger, H., D. Wallwiener and A.O. Mueck. 2003. Statins can inhibit proliferation of human breast cancer cells in vitro. *Exp Clin Endocrinol Diabetes,* 111, 47–48.

Shah, S., A. Gapor and P.W. Sylvester. 2003. Role of caspase-8 activation in mediating vitamin E-induced apoptosis in murine mammary cancer cells. *Nutr Cancer,* 45, 236–246.

Shah, S. and P.W. Sylvester. 2004. Tocotrienol-induced caspase-8 activation is unrelated to death receptor apoptotic signaling in neoplastic mammary epithelial cells. *Exp Biol Med,* 229, 745–755.

Shah, S.J. and P.W. Sylvester. 2005a. Gamma-tocotrienol inhibits neoplastic mammary epithelial cell proliferation by decreasing Akt and nuclear factor kappaB activity. *Exp Biol Med,* 230, 235–241.

Shah, S.J. and P.W. Sylvester. 2005b. Tocotrienol-induced cytotoxicity is unrelated to mitochondrial stress apoptotic signaling in neoplastic mammary epithelial cells. *Biochem Cell Biol,* 83, 86–95.

Shibata, M.A., Y. Ito, J. Morimoto and Y. Otsuki. 2004. Lovastatin inhibits tumor growth and lung metastasis in mouse mammary carcinoma model: A p53-independent mitochondrial-mediated apoptotic mechanism. *Carcinogenesis,* 25, 1887–1898.

Sliva, D., M.T. Rizzo and D. English. 2002. Phosphatidylinositol 3-kinase and NF-kappaB regulate motility of invasive MDA-MB-231 human breast cancer cells by the secretion of urokinase-type plasminogen activator. *J Biol Chem,* 277, 3150–3157.

Sliwkowski, M.X., G. Schaefer, R.W. Akita, J.A. Lofgren, V.D. Fitzpatrick, A. Nuijens, B.M. Fendly, R.A. Cerione, R.L. Vandlen and K.L. Carraway, 3rd. 1994. Coexpression of erbB2 and erbB3 proteins reconstitutes a high affinity receptor for heregulin. *J Biol Chem,* 269, 14661–14665.

Srinivasula, S.M., M. Ahmad, T. Fernandes-Alnemri and E.S. Alnemri. 1998. Autoactivation of procaspase-9 by Apaf-1-mediated oligomerization. *Mol Cell,* 1, 949–957.

Sung, L., M.L. Greenberg, G. Koren, G.A. Tomlinson, A. Tong, D. Malkin and B.M. Feldman. 2003. Vitamin E: The evidence for multiple roles in cancer. *Nutr Cancer,* 46, 1–14.

Susin, S.A., H.K. Lorenzo, N. Zamzami, I. Marzo, B.E. Snow, G.M. Brothers, J. Mangion, E. Jacotot, P. Costantini, M. Loeffler, N. Larochette, D.R. Goodlett, R. Aebersold, D.P. Siderovski, J.M. Penninger and G. Kroemer. 1999. Molecular characterization of mitochondrial apoptosis–inducing factor. *Nature,* 397, 441–446.

Sylvester, P.W., C.F. Aylsworth, D.A. Van Vugt and J. Meites. 1983. Effects of alterations in early hormonal environment on development and hormone dependency of carcinogen–induced mammary tumors in rats. *Cancer Res,* 43, 5342–5346.

Sylvester, P.W., C. Ip and M.M. Ip. 1986a. Effects of high dietary fat on the growth and development of ovarian-independent carcinogen-induced mammary tumors in rats. *Cancer Res,* 46, 763–769.

Sylvester, P.W., M. Russell, M.M. Ip and C. Ip. 1986b. Comparative effects of different animal and vegetable fats fed before and during carcinogen administration on mammary tumorigenesis, sexual maturation, and endocrine function in rats. *Cancer Res,* 46, 757–762.

Sylvester, P.W., H.P. Birkenfeld, H.L. Hosick and K.P. Briski. 1994. Fatty acid modulation of epidermal growth factor-induced mouse mammary epithelial cell proliferation in vitro. *Exp Cell Res,* 214, 145–153.

Sylvester, P.W., B.S. McIntyre, A. Gapor and K.P. Briski. 2001. Vitamin E inhibition of normal mammary epithelial cell growth is associated with a reduction in protein kinase C(alpha) activation. *Cell Prolif,* 34, 347–357.

Sylvester, P.W., A. Nachnani, S. Shah and K.P. Briski. 2002. Role of GTP-binding proteins in reversing the antiproliferative effects of tocotrienols in preneoplastic mammary epithelial cells. *Asia Pacific J Clin Nutr,* 11, S452–S459.

Sylvester, P.W. and A. Theriault. 2003. Role of tocotrienols in the prevention of cardiovascular disease and breast cancer. *Curr Top Nutraceutical Res,* 1, 121–136.

Sylvester, P.W. and S.J. Shah. 2005. Mechanisms mediating the antiproliferative and apoptotic effects of vitamin E in mammary cancer cells. *Front Biosci,* 10, 699–709.

Sylvester, P.W., S.J. Shah and G.V. Samant. 2005. Intracellular signaling mechanisms mediating the antiproliferative and apoptotic effects of gamma-tocotrienol in neoplastic mammary epithelial cells. *J Plant Physiol,* 162, 803–810.

Takahashi, K. and G. Loo. 2004. Disruption of mitochondria during tocotrienol-induced apoptosis in MDA-MB-231 human breast cancer cells. *Biochem Pharmacol,* 67, 315–324.

Thibault, A., D. Samid, A.C. Tompkins, W.D. Figg, M.R. Cooper, R.J. Hohl, J. Trepel, B. Liang, N. Patronas, D.J. Venzon, E. Reed and C.E. Myers. 1996. Phase I study of lovastatin, an inhibitor of the mevalonate pathway, in patients with cancer. *Clin Cancer Res,* 2, 483–491.

Toker, A. 2000. Protein kinases as mediators of phosphoinositide 3-kinase signaling. *Mol Pharmacol,* 57, 652–658.

Trosko, J.E. 2006. Dietary modulation of the multistage, multimechanisms of human carcinogenesis: Effects on initiated stem cells and cell–cell communication. *Nutr Cancer,* 54, 102–110.

Vanhaesebroeck, B. and D.R. Aless. 2000. The PI3K-PDK1 connection: More than just a road to PKB. *Biochem J,* 346, 561–576.

Vanhaesebroeck, B. and M.D. Waterfield. 1999. Signaling by distinct classes of phosphoinositide 3-kinases. *Exp Cell Res,* 253, 239–254.

Varadhachary, A.S., M. Edidin, A.M. Hanlon, M.E. Peter, P.H. Krammer and P. Salgame. 2001. Phosphatidylinositol 3'-kinase blocks CD95 aggregation and caspase-8 cleavage at the death-inducing signaling complex by modulating lateral diffusion of CD95. *J Immunol,* 166, 6564–6569.

Virtamo, J., P. Pietinen, J.K. Huttunen, P. Korhonen, N. Malila, M.J. Virtanen, D. Albanes, P.R. Taylor and P. Albert. 2003. Incidence of cancer and mortality following alpha-tocopherol and beta-carotene supplementation: A postintervention follow-up. *JAMA*, 290, 476–485.

Walczak, H. and P.H. Krammer. 2000. The CD95 (APO-1/Fas) and the TRAIL (APO-2L) apoptosis systems. *Exp Cell Res,* 256, 58–66.

Wali, V.B. and P.W. Sylvester. 2007. Synergistic antiproliferative effects of gamma-tocotrienol and statin treatment on mammary tumor cells. *Lipids* (in press).

Watanabe-Fukunaga, R., C.I. Brannan, N.G. Copeland, N.A. Jenkins and S. Nagata. 1992. Lymphoproliferation disorder in mice explained by defects in Fas antigen that mediates apoptosis. *Nature*, 356, 314–317.

Xing, C. and W. Imagawa. 1999. Altered MAP kinase (ERK1,2) regulation in primary cultures of mammary tumor cells: Elevated basal activity and sustained response to EGF. *Carcinogenesis*, 20, 1201–1208.

Yarden, Y. 2001. The EGFR family and its ligands in human cancer: Signalling mechanisms and therapeutic opportunities. *Eur J Cancer,* 37 Suppl 4, S3–8.

Yu, W., M. Simmons-Menchaca, A. Gapor, B.G. Sanders and K. Kline. 1999. Induction of apoptosis in human breast cancer cells by tocopherols and tocotrienols. *Nutr Cancer,* 33, 26–32.

Zou, H., W.J. Henzel, X. Liu, A. Lutschg and X. Wang. 1997. Apaf-1, a human protein homologous to C. elegans CED-4, participates in cytochrome c-dependent activation of caspase-3. *Cell*, 90, 405–413.

11 DNA Polymerase Inhibition

Yoshiyuki Mizushina, Hiromi Yoshida and Teruo Miyazawa

CONTENTS

11.1 INTRODUCTION

DNA polymerase (pol, i.e., DNA-dependent DNA polymerase, E.C.2.7.7.7) catalyzes the addition of deoxyribonucleotides to the 3'-hydroxyl terminus of a primed double-stranded DNA molecule (Bebenek and Kunkel, 2004). The human genome encodes at least 13 pols that conduct cellular DNA synthesis (Friedberg et al., 2000). As shown in Table 11.1, eukaryotic cells reportedly contain three replicative types: pols α, δ and ε, mitochondrial pol γ and at least 11 repair types: pols β, δ, ε, ζ, η, θ, ι, κ, λ, μ and REV 1. Pols can be classified into six main groups based on their phylogenetic relationships with *Escherichia coli* (*E. coli*) pol I (family A), *E. coli* pol II (family B), *E. coli* pol III (family C), eukaryarchaeotic pol II (family D), human pol β (family X) and *E. coli* UmuC/DinB and eukaryotic RAD30/xeroderma pigmentosum variant (family Y) (Friedberg et al., 2000). All known eukaryotic enzymes are either family A, family B, family X, or family Y enzymes (Table 11.1). No eukaryotic homologues of family C or family D pols were detected (www.ncbi.nlm.nih.gov/) despite detailed sequence searches using the PSI-BLAST program.

Although the function of each pol is shown in Table 11.1, the detailed molecular mechanism and the *in vivo* function of pol species are not clear. If inhibitors of each pol were available, the biological and *in vivo* functions of these enzymes could be elucidated more precisely and these inhibitors are useful tools and molecular probes to distinguish pols. Moreover, pol inhibitors could also be employed as anticancer chemotherapy agents, because they inhibit cell proliferation. We therefore established an assay to detect pol inhibitors and have searched natural materials including foods for more than 10 years. We previously found that retinoic acid, which is a vitamin A-related compound (Murakami et al., 2002), and vitamins D2 and D3 (Mizushina et al., 2003) inhibited the activities of replicative pols such as pol α. Therefore, we investigated the inhibitory effect of vitamin E, which is a water-insoluble (i.e., lipid-soluble) vitamin the same as vitamins A and D.

TABLE 11.1
Eukaryotic DNA Polymerases

Name	Human Chromosomal Location	Pol Family	Function
Pol α	Xp22.1–p21.3	B	Primer function in DNA replication
Pol β	8p12–11	X	Base excision repair
Pol γ	15q24	A	Mitochondrial DNA replication and repair
Pol δ	19q13.3	B	DNA replication, nucleotide and base excision repair
Pol ε	12q24.3	B	DNA replication, nucleotide and base excision repair
Pol ζ	6q21–22.2	B	Translesion synthesis
Pol η	6p12–21	Y	Accurate translesion synthesis
Pol θ	3q13.3	A	? (DNA repair of crosslinks)
Pol ι	18q21.1	Y	Translesion synthesis
Pol κ	5q13	Y	Translesion synthesis
Pol λ	10	X	? (Meiosis-associated DNA repair)
Pol μ	7p13	X	? (Somatic hypermutation)
REV 1	2q11	Y	Translesion synthesis

Modified from Friedberg et al. (2000).

11.2 EFFECT OF VITAMIN E COMPOUNDS ON MAMMALIAN DNA POLYMERASES

The assay method for pol activity was described previously (Mizushina et al., 1996; Mizushina et al., 1997). The substrates of the pols were poly(dA)/oligo(dT)$_{12-18}$ and 2'-deoxythymidine 5'-triphosphate (dTTP) as the DNA template-primer and nucleotide substrate (i.e., 2'-deoxynucleoside 5'-triphosphate (dNTP)), respectively. One unit of pol activity was defined as the amount of enzyme that catalyzed the incorporation of 1 nmol of dNTP (i.e., dTTP) into the synthetic DNA template-primers (i.e. poly(dA)/oligo(dT)$_{12-18}$, A/T = 2/1) in 60 min at 37°C under normal reaction conditions for each enzyme (Mizushina et al., 1996; Mizushina et al., 1997).

First, the inhibition of the activities of calf pol α, rat pol β and human pol λ by 100 μM of vitamin E compounds was investigated (Figure 11.1). α-, β-, γ- and δ-tocopherols were purchased from Sigma (St. Louis, MO, USA). α- to δ-tocotrienols were provided by Fuji Chemical Industry Co. Ltd. (Toyama, Japan). These compounds were of analytical grade. Pol α and pols β and λ were used as representative replicative pol and repair-related pols, respectively (Friedberg et al., 2000). The four tocopherols did not influence the activities of mammalian pols at all, whereas α- to δ-tocotrienols inhibited pol λ activity, but did not suppress the activities of pols α and β.

11.3 INHIBITORY EFFECTS OF TOCOTRIENOLS ON THE ACTIVITIES OF DNA POLYMERASES AND OTHER DNA METABOLIC ENZYMES

As shown in Table 11.2, four tocotrienols inhibited the activity of human pol λ to the same extent as they inhibited plant (i.e., rice) pol λ. δ-tocotrienol had the strongest inhibitory effect among the tocotrienols and in order of their effect, the tocotrienols ranked as follows: δ- > β- > γ- > α-tocotrienol. These results suggest that methyl groups at positions C1 and C3 of the benzene ring in tocotrienol weaken the inhibitory effect on pol λ. These compounds had no influence at all on the activities of nuclear pols such as pols α, β, δ, ε, η, ι and κ, or mitochondrial replicative pol γ. α- to δ-tocotri-

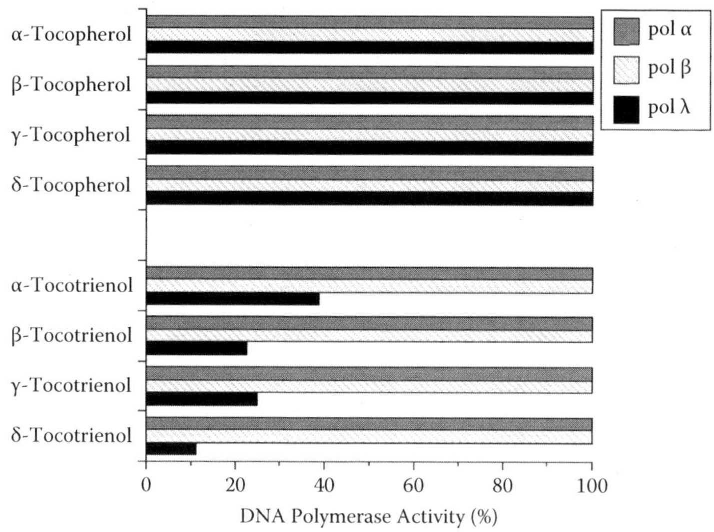

FIGURE 11.1 Effect of vitamin E compounds on the activities of mammalian pols α, β and λ. Each vitamin E compound (100 μM) was incubated with each pol (0.05 units). Pol activities were measured as described previously (Mizushina et al., 1996; Mizushina et al., 1997). Enzymatic activity in the absence of compound was taken as 100%.

enols had no inhibitory effect on fish pols α and δ, insect pols α, δ and ε, plant pols I (α-like) and II (β-like), or prokaryotic pols such as the Klenow fragment of *E. coli* pol I, *Taq* pol and T4 pol.

These compounds also did not inhibit the activities of other DNA-metabolic enzymes such as calf primase of pol α, HIV-1 reverse transcriptase, T7 RNA polymerase, T4 polynucleotide kinase and bovine deoxyribonuclease I. These results suggest that α- to δ-tocotrienols can selectively inhibit the activity of eukaryotic pol λ. On the other hand, α- to δ-tocopherols did not influence the activities of any enzymes tested (data not shown). The three double bonds in the unsaturated side chain of tocotrienols may be important for the inhibition of eukaryotic pol λ. The fact that tocotrienols, which are vitamin E compounds in plants, are inhibitors of a pol species, pol λ, is of great interest.

11.4 INHIBITION BY δ-TOCOTRIENOL OF FULL-LENGTH OR FRAGMENTS OF HUMAN DNA POLYMERASE λ

Pol λ is a recently described eukaryotic pol, whose main member is pol β (Garcia-Diaz et al., 2000) comprising enzymes involved in DNA repair processes. Human pol λ (63.4 kDa, residues 1-575) consists of a nuclear localization signal (NLS) (residues 1-35), a BRCA1 C-terminus (BRCT) domain (residues 36-132), a proline-rich region (residues 133-244) and a pol β-like region containing two helix-hairpin-helixes (HhHs) and a pol X motif (residues 245-575) (Shimazaki et al., 2002). The C-terminal part of pol λ (residues 244-575) is composed of a catalytic core which is similar to pol β (Garcia-Diaz et al., 2000). A truncated pol λ, in which the BRCT motif was deleted from the N-terminal region (i.e., the C-terminal region including the pol β-like region), has pol activity.

Because, in this report, δ-tocotrienol was the most potent inhibitor of pol λ among the vitamin E isomers, we then investigated the dose–response curves of the inhibition by δ-tocotrienol of intact or truncated human pol λ (Figure 11.2). Full-length pol λ and the N-terminal deleted versions, del-1 pol λ (residues 133-575) and del-2 pol λ (residues 245-575), were prepared. The inhibition of intact pol λ and del-1 pol λ was dose-dependent, with 50% inhibition observed at doses of 18.4 and 90.1 μM, respectively. The inhibitory effect of δ-tocotrienol on full-length pol λ was approximately 5-fold stronger than that on del-1 pol λ. On the other hand, δ-tocotrienol did

TABLE 11.2
IC_{50} Values of α- to δ-Tocotrienols on the Activities of Various DNA Polymerases and Other DNA Metabolic Enzymes

Enzyme	IC_{50} Values of Tocotrienols (μ*M*)			
	α-	β-	γ-	δ-
Mammalian DNA Polymerases				
Calf DNA polymerase α	>200	>200	>200	>200
Rat DNA polymerase β	>200	>200	>200	>200
Human DNA polymerase γ	>200	>200	>200	>200
Human DNA polymerase δ	>200	>200	>200	>200
Human DNA polymerase ε	>200	>200	>200	>200
Human DNA polymerase η	>200	>200	>200	>200
Human DNA polymerase ι	>200	>200	>200	>200
Human DNA polymerase κ	>200	>200	>200	>200
Human DNA polymerase λ	80.6	27.5	38.7	18.4
Fish DNA Polymerases				
Cherry salmon DNA polymerase α	>200	>200	>200	>200
Cherry salmon DNA polymerase δ	>200	>200	>200	>200
Insect DNA Polymerases				
Fruit fly DNA polymerase α	>200	>200	>200	>200
Fruit fly DNA polymerase δ	>200	>200	>200	>200
Fruit fly DNA polymerase ε	>200	>200	>200	>200
Plant DNA Polymerases				
Cauliflower DNA polymerase I (α-like)	>200	>200	>200	>200
Cauliflower DNA polymerase II (β-like)	>200	>200	>200	>200
Rice DNA polymerase λ	84.0	30.2	41.3	20.5
Prokaryotic DNA Polymerases				
E. coli DNA polymerase I (Klenow fragment)	>200	>200	>200	>200
Taq DNA polymerase	>200	>200	>200	>200
T4 DNA polymerase	>200	>200	>200	>200
Other DNA Metabolic Enzymes				
Calf primase of DNA polymerase α	>200	>200	>200	>200
HIV-1 reverse transcriptase	>200	>200	>200	>200
T7 RNA polymerase	>200	>200	>200	>200
T4 Polynucleotide kinase	>200	>200	>200	>200
Bovine deoxyribonuclease I	>200	>200	>200	>200

Note: These compounds were incubated with each pol (0.05 units) and other DNA metabolic enzymes. One unit of pol activity was defined as the amount of enzyme that catalyzed the incorporation of 1 nmol of dNTP (i.e., dTTP) into synthetic DNA template-primers (i.e., poly(dA)/oligo$(dT)_{12\text{-}18}$, A/T = 2/1) in 60 min at 37°C under normal reaction conditions for each enzyme (Mizushina et al., 1996; Mizushina et al., 1997). Enzyme activity in the absence of the compounds was taken as 100%.

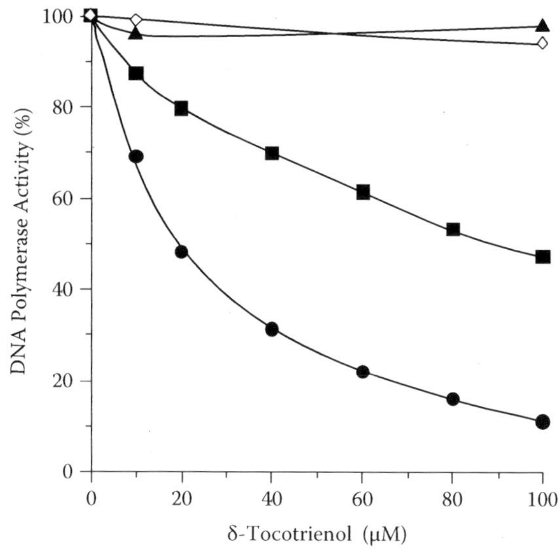

FIGURE 11.2 Dose–response curves of δ-tocotrienol (0 to 100 μM). The enzymes used (0.05 units each) were rat pol β (open diamond), full-length human pol λ (residues 1-575, closed circle), del-1 of human pol λ (residues 133-575, closed square) and del-2 of human pol λ (residues 245-575, closed triangle).

not influence the activity of del-2 pol λ lacking a NLS, BRCT domain and proline-rich region, nor did it suppress pol β activity.

11.5 INTERACTION OF δ-TOCOTRIENOL WITH THE DOMAIN REGION OF DNA POLYMERASE λ

Pol λ belongs to the pol X family, which includes pols β, μ and λ, terminal deoxynucleotidyltransferase, yeast pol IV, mitochondrial pol β, nuclear pol β from protozoans and 20-kDa African swine fever virus pol X (Friedberg et al., 2000; Burgers et al., 2001). Family X pols are composed of an NLS, a BRCT domain, a proline-rich region and a pol β-like region containing two HhHs and a pol X motif (Figure 11.3); however, pol β (residues 1-335) lacks a NLS, a BRCT domain and a proline-rich region. Human pol λ shares 54, 47 and 30 % homology with human pols β and μ and yeast pol IV, respectively. Interestingly, δ-tocotrienol inhibited only the activities of full-length pol λ and del-1 pol λ among the eukaryotic pols, although it did not influence the activities of del-2 pol λ (245-575) or pol β (Figure 11.3). The δ-tocotrienol-induced inhibition of full-length pol λ was non-competitive with respect to both the DNA template-primer and the dNTP substrate (data not shown), indicating that δ-tocotrienol did not directly bind to either the DNA template-binding site or the dNTP substrate-binding site of pol λ. Since both the DNA template-primer and dNTP substrate-binding sites are present in the pol β-like region of pol λ (Garcia-Daiz et al., 2000), δ-tocotrienol may not directly bind to the pol β-like core. These results suggest that δ-tocotrienol binds to or interacts with the N-terminal region containing the NLS, BRCT domain and proline-rich region of pol λ directly and subsequently inhibits enzymes having the pol β-like region of pol λ (Figure 11.3).

11.6 CONCLUSION

Since angiogenesis is essential for tumor growth, its inhibition is likely to prevent a cancer from becoming metastatic (Folkman and Klagsbrun, 1987). Several studies have reported that dietary exposure to vitamin E has potential health benefits in preventing cancer (Theriault et al., 1999), but the actual mechanisms involved are not understood. This review indicated that the inhibitory

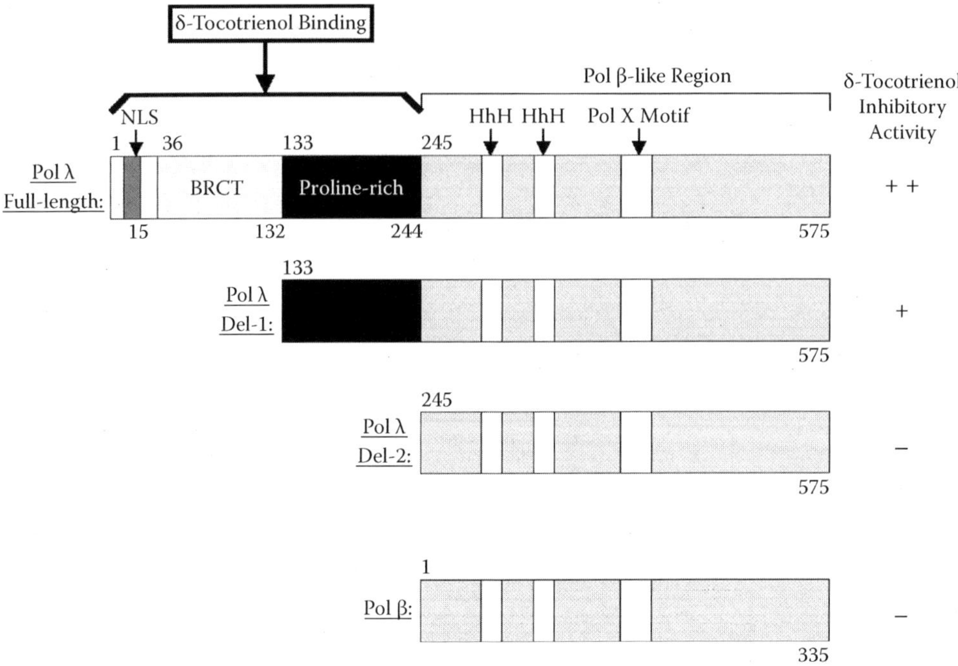

FIGURE 11.3 Schematic representation of pols λ and β of the pol X family. The NLS, BRCT domain, proline-rich region, HhH and pol X motif are indicated. The pol β-like region includes two HhHs and a pol X motif. The inhibitory activity of δ-tocotrienol against these pols is indicated below, "++" IC_{50} value = <50 μM, "+" IC_{50} value = 50 to 200 μM and "-" IC_{50} value = >200 μM.

effect on pol λ by α- to δ-tocotrienols, which are unsaturated vitamin E compounds, is the same as that on the proliferation of and formation of tubes by BAEC (i.e., δ- > β- > γ- > α-tocotrienol, Table 11.2) (Inokuchi et al., 2003). These results led us to hypothesize that the inhibition of tumor growth by vitamin E is mediated in part by its pol λ inhibitory activity and antiangiogenic activity. Angiogenesis is involved in tumor growth and metastasis, atherosclerosis and diabetic retinopathy (Folkman, 1995). Our recent study revealed that a polyphenolic pol λ-selective inhibitor, petasiphenol (Mizushina et al., 2002), is a potent antiangiogenic inhibitor and that petasiphenol affects endothelial cell functions involved in angiogenesis (Matsubara et al., 2004). Pols and angiogenesis are very import targets for anticancer agents (Holden, 1997); thus, it is of interest whether pol λ inhibitors have antiangiogenic activity.

ACKNOWLEDGMENTS

We are grateful for the donations of calf pol α by Dr. M. Takemura of Tokyo University of Science (Tokyo, Japan), rat pol β by Dr. A. Matsukage of Japan Women's University (Tokyo, Japan), human pol γ by Dr. M. Suzuki of Nagoya University School of Medicine (Nagoya, Japan), human pols δ and ε by Dr. K. Sakaguchi of Tokyo University of Science (Chiba, Japan), human pols η and ι by Dr. F. Hanaoka and Dr. C. Masutani of Osaka University (Osaka, Japan), human pol κ by Dr. H. Ohmori and Dr. E. Ohashi of Kyoto University (Kyoto, Japan) and human pol λ by Dr. O. Koiwai and Dr. N. Shimazaki of Tokyo University of Science (Chiba, Japan).

This work was supported in part by a Grant-in-Aid for Kobe-Gakuin University Joint Research (A) and "Academic Frontier" Project for Private Universities: matching fund subsidy from the Ministry of Education, Science, Sports and Culture of Japan (MEXT), 2006-2010, (Y. M. and H. Y.). Y. M. acknowledges Grant-in-Aid for Young Scientists (A) (No. 19680031) from MEXT and Grant-in-aid from the Nakashima Foundation (Japan), Foundation of Oil and Fat Industry Kaikan (Japan), and the Salt Science Research Foundation, No. 08S3 (Japan).

REFERENCES

Bebenek, K., T.A. Kunkel. 2004. *DNA Repair and Replication: Advances in Protein Chemistry*; W. Yang (Ed.), Elsevier: San Diego, vol. 69, pp. 137–165.

Burgers, P.M., E.V. Koonin, E. Bruford, L. Blanco, K.C. Burtis, M.F. Christman, W.C. Copeland, E.C. Friedberg, F. Hanaoka, D.C. Hinkle, C.W. Lawrence, M. Nakanishi, H. Ohmori, L. Prakash, S. Prakash, C.A. Reynaud, A. Sugino, T. Todo, Z. Wang, J.C. Weill, R. Woodgate. Eukaryotic DNA polymerases: Proposal for a revised nomenclature. *J. Biol. Chem.* 2001, *276*, 43487–43490.

Folkman, J., M. Klagsbrun. 1987. Angiogenic factors. *Science*, *235*, 442–447.

Folkman, J. 1995. Angiogenesis in cancer, vascular, rheumatoid and other disease. *Nat. Med.*, *1*, 27–31.

Friedberg, E.C., W.J. Feaver, V.L. Gerlach. 2000. The many faces of DNA polymerases: Strategies for mutagenesis and for mutational avoidance. *Proc. Natl. Acad. Sci. USA*, *97*, 5681–5683.

Garcia-Diaz, M., O. Dominguez, L.A. Lopez-Fernandez, L.T. de Lera, M.L. Saniger, J.F. Ruiz, M. Parraga, M.J. Garcia-Ortiz, T. Kirchhoff, J. del Mazo, A. Bernad, L. Blanco. 2000. DNA polymerase λ (Pol λ), a novel eukaryotic DNA polymerase with a potential role in meiosis. *J. Mol. Biol.*, *301*, 851–867.

Holden, J.A. 1997. Human deoxyribonucleic acid topoisomerase: Molecular targets of anticancer drugs. *Ann. Clin. Lab. Sci.*, *27*, 402–412.

Inokuchi, H., H. Hirokane, T. Tsuzuki, K. Nakagawa, M. Igarashi, T. Miyazawa. 2003. Anti-angiogenic activity of tocotrienol. *Biosci. Biotechnol. Biochem.*, *67*, 1623–1627.

Matsubara, K., K. Mori, Y. Mizushina. 2004. Petasiphenol which inhibits DNA polymerase λ is an inhibitor of *in vitro* angiogenesis. *Oncol. Rep.*, *11*, 447–451.

Mizushina, Y., N. Tanaka, H. Yagi, T. Kurosawa, M. Onoue, H. Seto, T. Horie, N. Aoyagi, M. Yamaoka, A. Matsukage, S. Yoshida, K. Sakaguchi. 1996. Fatty acids selectively inhibit eukaryotic DNA polymerase activities *in vitro*. *Biochim. Biophys. Acta*, *1308*, 256–262.

Mizushina, Y., S. Yoshida, A. Matsukage, K. Sakaguchi. 1997. The inhibitory action of fatty acids on DNA polymerase β. *Biochim. Biophys. Acta*, *1336*, 509–521.

Mizushina, Y., S. Kamisuki, N. Kasai, T. Ishidoh, N. Shimazaki, M. Takemura, H. Asahara, S. Linn, S. Yoshida, O. Koiwai, F. Sugawara, H. Yoshida, K. Sakaguchi. 2002. Petasiphenol: A DNA polymerase λ inhibitor. *Biochemistry*, *41*, 14463–14471.

Mizushina, Y., X. Xu, C. Murakami, T. Okano, M. Takemura, H. Yoshida, K. Sakaguchi. 2003. Selective inhibition of mammalian DNA polymerase α by vitamin D2 and D3, *J. Pharmacol. Sci.*, *92*, 283–290.

Murakami, C., M. Takemura, Y. Sugiyama, S. Kamisuki, H. Asahara, M. Kawasaki, T. Ishidoh, S. Linn, S. Yoshida, F. Sugawara, H. Yoshida, K. Sakaguchi, Y. Mizushina. 2002. Vitamin A-related compounds, all-trans retinal and retinoic acids, selectively inhibit activities of mammalian replicative DNA polymerases, *Biochim. Biophys. Acta*, *1574*, 85–92.

Shimazaki, N., K. Yoshida, T. Kobayashi, S. Toji, T. Tamai, O. Koiwai. 2002. Over-expression of human DNA polymerase λ in *E. coli* and characterization of the recombinant enzyme. *Genes Cells*, *7*, 639–651.

Theriault, A., J.T. Chao, Q. Wang, A. Gapor, K. Adeli. 1999. Tocotrienol: A review of its therapeutic potential. *Clin. Biochem.*, *32*, 309–319.

12 Tocotrienols in Altering the Expression of Adhesion Molecules

Yuji Naito and Toshikazu Yoshikawa

CONTENTS

12.1 INTRODUCTION

We have demonstrated that α-tocopherol inhibits the expression of mRNA and protein for adhesion molecules by human umbilical vein endothelial cells (HUVEC) in response to stimulation with oxidized low-density lipoprotein (oxLDL) or interleukin (IL)-1 (Yoshikawa et al. 1998). In addition, we have shown in both *in vitro* and *ex vivo* studies that α-tocopherol decreases the expression of CD11b/CD18 on human monocytes induced by oxLDL (Yoshikawa et al. 1998; Terasawa et al. 2000; Yoshida et al. 2000). These data support the hypothesis that vitamin E supplementation may reduce the extent of the oxLDL-induced monocyte-endothelial interaction and, thus, be protective against atherosclerosis. This hypothesis may be supported by studies in murine models of atherosclerosis. In contrast, clinical trials using this vitamin have given a more confused picture than expected, with results ranging from a significant protective action to the absence of any effect. A recent VEAPS study has demonstrated that α-tocopherol supplementation (dl-α-tocopherol 400 IU/day) significantly raises plasma vitamin E levels, reduces circulating oxLDL and reduces LDL oxidative susceptibility, the progression of the intima-media thickness of the common carotid artery, however, is not reduced by the treatment (Hodis et al. 2002).

Recently, the role of tocotrienols, another form of vitamin E, has received renewed attention. It has been demonstrated that tocotrienol has a potent action in the inhibition of lipid peroxidation (Serbinova et al. 1991), inhibition of monocyte adherence (Theriault et al. 2002; Noguchi et al. 2003; Naito et al. 2005) and neuroprotection (Khanna et al. 2003) compared with tocopherol. This review focuses on recent advances that have revealed the mechanisms by which tocotrienol may exert its protection against atherosclerosis.

12.2 ADHESION MOLECULES IN ATHEROSCLEROSIS

Increased adherence of monocytes to the endothelium constitutes one of the early visible changes in atherosclerosis. Monocytes are initially attracted to lesion-prone sites by cell-adhesion mole-

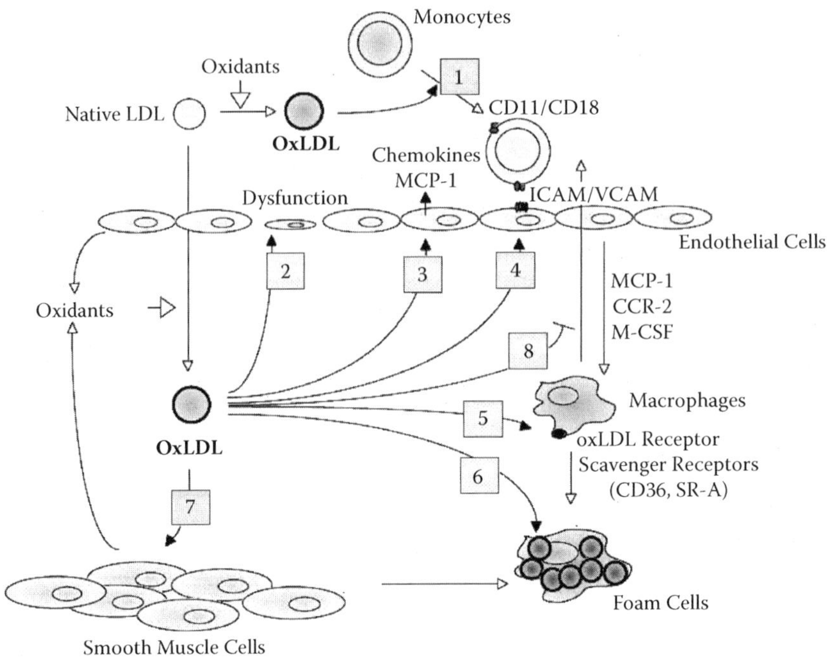

FIGURE 12.1 Role of oxidized LDL in atherogenesis. Oxidized LDL (oxLDL) in the blood stream stimulates the up-regulation of CD11b/CD18 adhesion molecule expression on monocytes (1). The entry of LDL into the subendothelial space is followed by its oxidation by reactive oxygen species generated from smooth muscle cells and endothelial cells. OxLDL can induce endothelial dysfunction (2) and expression of cytokines (3), growth factors and several cell-surface adhesion molecules (4) that are capable of recruiting circulating monocytes and T lymphocytes into the intima. OxLDL activates the development of monocytes into macrophages where the uptake of oxLDL via the scavenger receptor is rapid (5, 6) and inhibits the migration of macrophages (8). OxLDL stimulates cell proliferation and transmigration of smooth muscle cells (7).

cules expressed on activated endothelial cells. The initial tethering and rolling are mediated by the selectin family of adhesion proteins (L-selectin expressed constitutively on almost all leukocytes, P-selectin and E-selectin expressed on the surface of activated endothelium). The interaction of the selectins with their ligands does not support the firm adhesion that is required for subsequent monocyte extravasation unless the initial attachment is followed by a second event that leads to the engagement of integrins. Monocytes express both the β1 integrin CD49d/CD29 and β2 integrins CD11a/CD18, CD11b/CD18 and CD11c/CD18. The strong attachment of the monocytes to the endothelium is mediated by the interaction of the integrins with a class of ligands that belong to the immunoglobulin superfamily, most notably vascular cell-adhesion molecule 1 (VCAM-1) and intracellular cell-adhesion molecule 1 (ICAM-1) (Figure 12.1). Both selectins and integrins are highly expressed by the activated endothelium in proximity to atherosclerotic lesions but to a much lesser extent by normal endothelium (Cybulsky and Gimbrone 1991; Poston et al. 1992; Li et al. 1993; Nakashima et al. 1998). Furthermore, the presence of VCAM-1 and ICAM-1 on the vasculature is associated with increased intimal leukocyte accumulation.

Recently, several useful models of atherosclerosis have been created by the genetic alteration of lipid metabolism. The most widely used of these models involves a gene disruption of apolipoprotein E. The advantages of this model include the fact that the lesions develop at a much earlier age, exhibit more of the features observed in humans and can be induced by both low- and high-fat diets. Similar to human and rabbit lesions, oxidized lipoprotein epitopes are found in lesions of apoE-deficient mice and sera from these mice contain high titers of autoantibodies that recognize oxidized lipoproteins and can stain lesions in rabbits (O'Neill 1997). In apoE$^{-/-}$ mice, ICAM-1 is constitutively increased at the lesion-prone site and VCAM-1 is also present at the same site as ICAM-1. Thus, the adherence of monocytes may occur after an increase in one or more of the adhesion molecules, which may act in concert with chemotactic molecules such as monocyte chemotactic protein-1 (MCP-1), interleukin-8 (IL-8) and oxLDL. In these mice, it has been shown that additional knockout of the gene for vascular adhesion molecules such as ICAM-1, platelet-endothelial cell adhesion molecule-1 (PECAM-1) and VCAM-1 results in significantly less atherosclerosis in the proximal aorta (Collins et al. 2000; Zibara et al. 2000). These results indicate that the inflammatory response, including the expression of adhesion molecules, plays a crucial role in the initial development of atherosclerosis.

In addition to basic evidence that endothelial adhesion molecules play a crucial role in the development of atherosclerosis, recent clinical investigations show that soluble forms of these molecules may be a biomarker of atherosclerosis. Consumption of 30 g ethanol per day for 28 days has reduced the serum concentrations of hs-CRP and soluble forms of VCAM-1 and ICAM-1 in male healthy volunteers (Estruch et al. 2004). A conbination of diet and exercise has reduced the elevated concentrations of soluble forms of ICAM-1 and E-selectin in diabetic men (Roberts et al. 2006). These data suggest that intensive lifestyle modification including diet may improve novel cardiovascular risk factors in human.

In resting monocytes, most of CD11b/CD18 and CD11c/CD18 is stored in intracellular granules. Stimulation of monocytes with inflammatory mediators rapidly mobilized these integrins to the cell surface, where they become accessible for chemokine-dependent activation to mediate firm adhesion. It has been reported that monocytes from patients with hypercholesterolemia display increased CD11b-dependent adhesion to endothelial cells (Weber et al. 1997). Recently, Han et al. (Han et al. 2003) demonstrated a causal link between plasma levels of LDL and integrin expression and showed that monocytes from LDL receptor-deficient mice on a high-fat diet have increased CD11b expression as well as CD11b-dependent adhesion to endothelial cells. These findings suggest that in addition to the effects on endothelial cells, lipoproteins may also induce phenotypic changes of circulating monocytes that may be pertinent to the recruitment process.

12.3 OXIDIZED LDL HYPOTHESIS

There is considerable evidence that the inflammatory response induced by oxLDL contributes to the development of atherosclerosis (Steinberg 1997). OxLDL or their metabolites have been found in atherosclerotic lesions in both human and animal models (Yla-Herttuala 1999) and are known to contain several lipid-derived bioactive molecules such as oxysterols (hydroxycholesterols and ketocholesterols), phospholipids and fatty acid peroxides. OxLDL exhibits a wide variety of potentially atherogenic properties, including the stimulation of monocyte migration, promotion of the adhesion of monocytes to cultured endothelial cells and inhibition of endothelium-dependent vasodilatation (Figure 12.1). OxLDL is avidly taken up by macrophages, resulting in foam cell formation (Parthasarathy et al. 1986). In particular, oxLDLs have been shown to stimulate endothelial cells to express several proteins that contribute to the early stage of atherosclerosis, including MCP-1, macrophage-colony-stimulating factor (M-CSF), VCAM-1 and ICAM-1 (Liao et al. 1997; Steinberg 1997).

It is well known that several cytokines such as Il-1β and TNF-α induce the surface expression of ICAM-1 and VCAM-1 on endothelial cells through the activation of a redox-sensitive transcriptional factor, nuclear factor-κB. In our experiments, ICAM-1 and VCAM-1 expression on oxLDL- or oxysterol-stimulated HUVEC or HAEC was found to occur in the same fashion as after stimulation with IL-1β (Yoshikawa et al. 1998). However, native LDL had no effect on the expression of endothelial adhesion molecules. Yoshida et al. (Yoshida et al. 2000) have demonstrated that adherence of mononuclear leukocytes to oxLDL-activated human umbilical vascular endothelial cells (HUVEC) is much increased compared with unstimulated HUVEC. In addition, treatment of HUVEC with monoclonal antibody to ICAM-1 or VCAM-1 inhibits adherence of monocytes in a dose dependent manner. These results suggest that oxLDL may induce almost the same signal transduction pathway

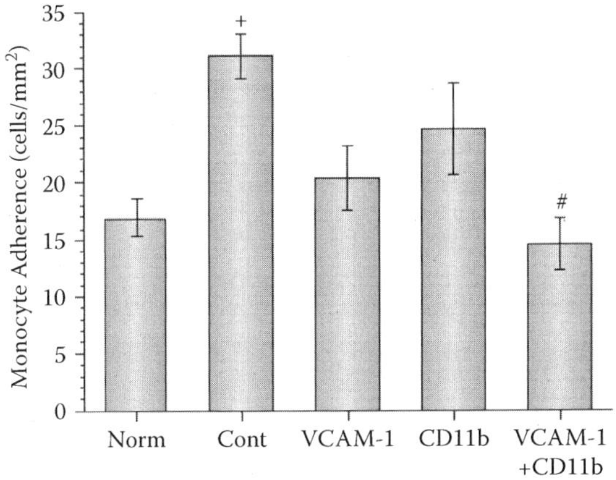

FIGURE 12.2 Effects of monoclonal antibodies for CD11b and VCAM-1 on 25-hydroxycholesterol-stimulated adhesiveness of HAECs to U937 monocytic cells. Human aortic endothelial cells (HAECs) were pretreated for 18 hours with 25-hydroxycholesterol (20 μM). Binding between U937 and HAECs was measured. The results are given as the number of adherence cells per high-power field and are the mean + SE of experiments performed in triplicate on three separate occasions. $^{+}p<0.05$ compared with unstimulated HAECs (norm) and $^{\#}p<0.05$ compared with 25-hydroxycholestrol-stimulated HAECs (cont). (Naito et al. 2005. Tocotrienols reduce 25-hydroxycholesterol-induced monocyte–endothelial cell interaction by inhibiting the surface expression of adhesion molecules. *Atherosclerosis, 180.* With permission.)

for the synthesis of ICAM-1 and VCAM-1 as that stimulated by IL-1β, but the precise mechanism involved still needs to be investigated.

The cytotoxicity or biological activity of oxLDL has been alternatively linked to the formation of various aldehydes and to the conversion of phospholipids to lysophospholipids, as well as to the oxidation of cholesterol to oxysterol. More specifically, a number of *in vivo* and *in vitro* studies have suggested the determinant role of oxysterols in inducing cytotoxicity in endothelial cells (Peng et al. 1985; Boissonneault et al. 1991). Oxysterols such as 7-, 25- and 27-hydroxycholesterol have a wide range of biological activities similar to those of oxLDL (Brown and Jessup 1999). Among these oxysterols, 7-ketocholesterol and 25-hydroxycholesterol enhance the expression of adhesion molecules on human aortic endothelial cells (HAECs) by increasing the production of reactive oxygen species (Shimozawa et al. 2004; Naito et al. 2005). As shown in Figure 12.2, the combination treatment with anti-VCAM-1 and anti-CD11b monoclonal antibodies significantly reduces the monocyte adherence to 25-hydroxycholesterol-stimulated HAECs (Naito et al. 2005), indicating that the interaction between monocytes and 25-hydroxycholesterol-stimulated endothelial cells involves a CD11b/VCAM-1-dependent pathway. These data are consistent with our previous studies using modified LDL oxidized by $CuSO_4$ *in vitro* instead of 25-hydroxycholesterol (Yoshida et al. 2000).

12.4 TOCOTRIENOLS AND ENDOTHELIAL FUNCTION

It has recently been reported that α-tocotrienol is a potent and effective agent in the reduction of cellular adhesion molecule expression and monocytic cell adherence (Theriault et al. 2002). Pretreatment of HUVEC with various concentrations of α-tocotrienol (5–25 μM) for 20 h followed by tumor necrosis factor (TNF) -α stimulation is found to produce an inhibitory effect on VCAM-1 cell surface expression as well as monocytic cell adhesion to HUVEC. Compared to α-tocopherol and α-tocophetyl succinate, α-tocotrienol displays a more profound inhibitory effect on adhesion molecule expression and monocytic cell adherence. This inhibitory action by α-tocotrienol on TNF-α-induced monocyte adhesion is shown to be NF-κB-dependent and is interestingly reversed with co-incubation with farnesol and geranylgeraniol, suggesting a role for prenylated proteins in

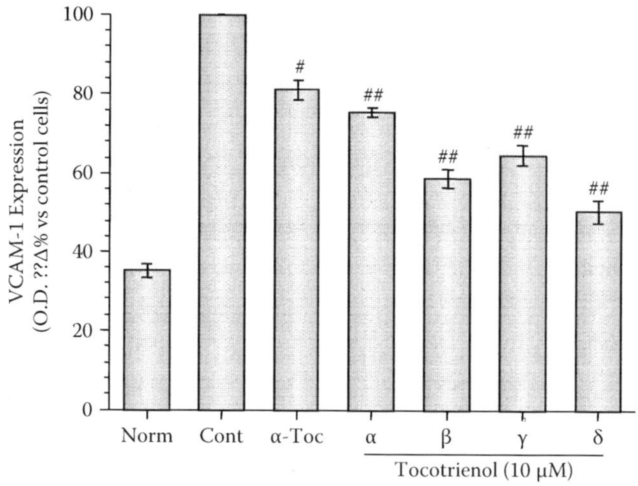

FIGURE 12.3 Effects of a-tocopherol and tocotrienols on 25-hydroxycholesterol-induced surface expression of VCAM-1 on HAECs pretreated for 18 hours with α-tocopherol and tocotrienols (10 μM) followed by 25-hydroxycholesterol (20 μM for 18 hours). The expression of VCAM-1 was determined by ELISA. The results are given as percentage variation of O.D. versus 25-hydroxycholesterol-induced VCAM-1 expression in non-pretreated HAECs and are the mean + SE of experiments performed in triplicate on three separate occasions. #p<0.05 and ##p<0.01 compared with 25-hydroxycholesterol-stimulated VCAM-1 expression in non-pretreated HAECs (cont). (Naito et al. 2005. Tocotrienols reduce 25-hydroxycholesterol-induced monocyte–endothelial cell interaction by inhibiting the surface expression of adhesion molecules. *Atherosclerosis, 180.* With permission.)

the regulation of adhesion molecule expression. In addition, it has been found that δ-tocotrienol is a potent and effective agent for the reduction of cellular VCAM-1 and E-selectin expression and monocytic cell adherence compared to α-tocotrienol and γ-tocotrienol (Chao et al. 2002).

We have recently compared the effects of α-tocopherol and four isoforms of tocotrienol on the adherence of monocytes to endothelial cells. In our study, human aortic endothelial cells (HAEC) in confluent monolayers prepared in 48-well plates were stimulated with 7-ketocholestrol or 25-hydroxycholesterol. Subsequently, HAEC were washed with HBSS and U937 monocytic cells were added to each well and incubated at 37°C for 30 min. The plates were washed three times with HBSS and fixed in 1% paraformaldehyde in PBS. The number of adherent cells was counted in 20 microscopic fields defined by an eyepiece and VCAM-1 expression was determined by ELISA. α-Tocopherol (10 μM) did not affect the number of adherent monocytic cells and VCAM-1 expression; in contrast, pretreatment of HAEC with either 10 μM α-tocotrienol, β-tocotrienol, γ-tocotrienol, or δ-tocotrienol for 18 hours prior to stimulation with oxysterol all resulted in significant inhibitory effects on monocytic cell adherence and VCAM-1 expression (Naito et al. 2005) (Figure 12.3, Figure 12.4). These results suggest that the reduction of monocyte adhesion by tocotrienol can be attributed to decreased adhesion molecule expression. Notably, δ-tocotrienol exerted a more profound inhibitory action on monocytic cell adherence than α-tocotrienol and α-tocopherol.

Recently, Noguchi et al. (2003) have clearly explained the differences among these tocotrienols with regard to their inhibitory effects on monocyte–endothelial interactions. They have shown that a-tocotrienol accumulates in human umbilical endothelial cells to levels approximately 10-fold greater than those of α-tocopherol and that the efficacy of tocotrienol in the reduction of VCAM-1 expression and the adhesion of monocytic cells to endothelial cells is also 10-fold higher than that of tocopherol. To confirm the data from Noguchi et al. (2003), we have measured the intracellular concentration of each vitamin E analog after the incubation for 18 hours in our study. We have shown that tocotrienol accumulates in HAECs to levels approximately 25–95-fold greater than that of α-tocopherol (Naito et al. 2005) (Figure 12.5). These results indicate that the inhibitory

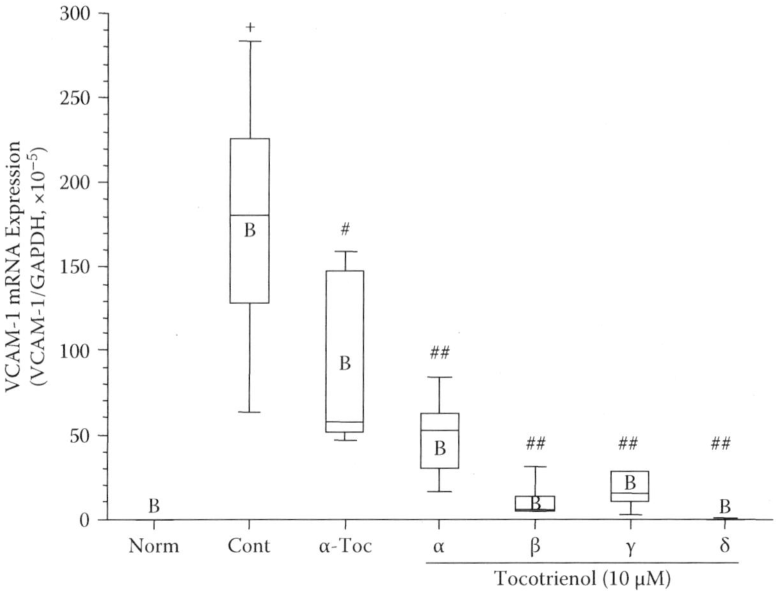

FIGURE 12.4 RT-PCR showing the effect of α-tocopherol and tocotrienols on VCAM-1 mRNA expression in HAECs exposed to 25-hydroxycholesterol. HAECs were pretreated for 18 hours with α-tocopherol and tocotrienols (10 μM) followed by 25-hydroxycholesterol (20 μM for 2 hours). RT-PCR analysis of total RNA extracts was performed. Nonstimulated (lane 1), 25-hydroxycholesterol-stimulated nonpretreated HAECs (lane 2), pretreated with α-tocopherol (lane 3), α-tocotrienol (lane 4), β-tocotrienol (lane 5), γ-tocotrienol (lane 6), δ-tocotrienol (lane 7). Three independent experiments gave similar results and data shown are representative of these experiments. (Naito et al. 2005. Tocotrienols reduce 25-hydroxycholesterol-induced monocyte–endothelial cell interaction by inhibiting the surface expression of adhesion molecules. *Atherosclerosis, 180.* With permission.)

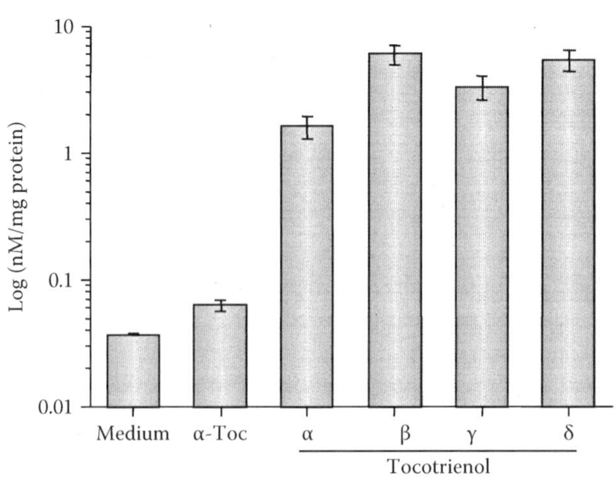

FIGURE 12.5 Intracellular concentration of tocopherols and tocotrienols in HAECs exposed to 10 μM α-tocopherol, α-tocotrienol, β-tocotrienol, γ-tocotrienol, or δ-tocotrienol for 18 h and the intracellular concentrations of these analogs were analyzed by the HPLC. Values represent the mean + SE of three independent experiments. (Naito et al. 2005. Tocotrienols reduce 25-hydroxycholesterol-induced monocyte–endothelial cell interaction by inhibiting the surface expression of adhesion molecules. *Atherosclerosis, 180.* With permission.)

effects of vitamin E analogs on the adhesiveness of endothelial cells correlate with their intracellular concentrations.

Our data derived from cultured cells is recently confirmed by an *in vitro* experiment performed by Yoshida et al. (2003), who compared the antioxidant properties for these 8 vitamin E homologues and obtained the following results: (1) the corresponding tocopherols and tocotrienols exert the same reactivity toward radicals and the same antioxidant activities against lipid peroxidation in solution and liposomal membranes; (2) tocopherols have a more significant physical effect than tocotrienols on the increase in rigidity at the membrane interior; and (3) tocotrienols are more readily transferred between the membrane and incorporated into the membrane than tocopherols. These data indicate that the superior antioxidant activity of tocotrienols in membranes depends on the structure of the hydrophobic side chain, which is important for the mobility of the molecule and that, in homogenous solutions, the reaction rate constant between vitamin E and the peroxyl radical depends primarily on the number of methyl groups on the chromanol nucleus (Yoshida et al. 2003).

Although the exact molecular mechanism for inhibition of the endothelial inflammatory response by tocotrienols has not been elucidated, recent reports suggest that tocotrienols affect the mRNA expression of several genes and activate/regulate the targeted proteins (Anderson et al. 2003; Khanna et al. 2003; Landes et al. 2003). Recent advances in genomics and proteomics should provide addition information regarding the novel mechanism for the inhibition of atherosclerosis by tocotrienols.

12.5 INHIBITION OF ATHEROSCLEROSIS IN A MURINE MODEL BY TOCOTRIENOL

In addition to the regulation of the inflammatory response of endothelial cells, it has been reported by cell-culture studies that tocotrienols influence cholesterol synthesis by directly regulating the expression of 3-hydroxy-3-methylglutaryl-coenzyme A reductase (HMG-CoA reductase), principally through a post-transcriptional process involving accelerated degradation of the reductase protein (Parker et al. 1993). This effect was ascribed to the side chain's unique ability to increase cellular farnesol, which in turn has been shown to downregulate HMG-CoA reductase activity (Theriault et al. 1999). Among the four isomers, δ-tocotrienol is the most potent HMG-CoA reductase inhibitor (Qureshi et al. 2000).

Black et al. (2000) firstly evaluated the effects of palm-vitamin E, α-tocopherol and palm-carotenoids on apoE$^{+/-}$ female mice, which develop atherosclerosis when fed diets high in triglycerides and cholesterol. With supplements of 0.5 g/100 g or 1.5 g/100 g palm-vitamin E, the size of the lesions was 92 or 98% smaller, respectively. In contrast, the 0.5 g/100 g α-tocopherol and palm carotenoid supplements had no effect. These results indicate that these antiatherogenic effects of palm-vitamin E are probably due to the content of tocotrienols in the supplement. Qureshi et al. have recently shown that the tocotrienol-rich fraction (TRF_{25}) and didesmethyl tocotrienol (*d*-P_{25}-T3 with no methyl groups on the chromanol ring) of rice bran inhibit atherosclerotic lesions in C57BL/6 apoE-deficient mice (Qureshi et al. 2001a) and cholesterogenesis in hereditary hypercholesterolemic swine (Qureshi et al. 2001b) and have demonstrated a superior efficacy of tocotrienols compared with α-tocopherol. In their experiments, mice were fed the tested diet with or without 100 μg d-α-tocopherol, TRF_{25}, or d-P_{25}-T3/g. They have demonstrated that the novel tocotrienol d-P_{25}-T3 can substantially reduce the growth of atherosclerotic plaques in all three of the tested mouse genotypes (apoE$^{+/+}$, apoE$^{+/-}$ and apoE$^{-/-}$) and diet combinations that produce plaque.

Recently, we investigated the effect of a tocotrienol-rich diet (0.02%) on the development of atherosclerotic lesion in apoE$^{-/-}$ mice. The composition of various vitamin E analogues was 33.9% α-tocotrienol, 4.0% β-tocotrienol, 47.1% γ-tocotrienol, 11.0% d-tocotrienol and 0.1% γ-tocopherol. Atherosclerotic lesion analyses followed the standard protocol in our laboratory. Frozen sections of

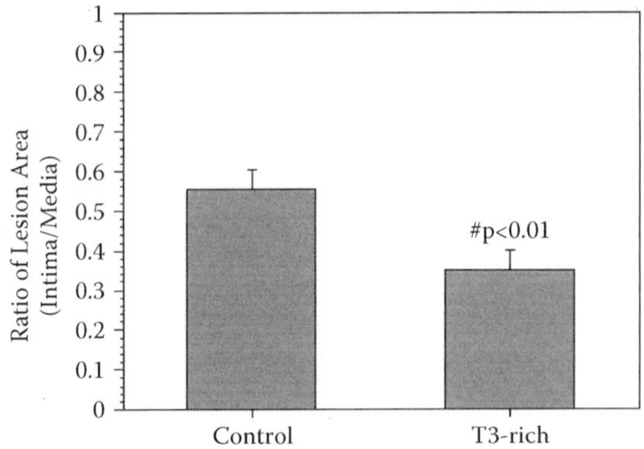

FIGURE 12.6 Effect of tocotrienol-rich diet on atherosclerotic lesion in apolipoprotein E-deficient mice. Each datum represents the mean+SE of the lesion size of three sections measured in each mouse.

the proximal aorta were stained with Sudan IV and counterstained with hematoxylin. The areas of atherosclerotic lesions were measured, using National Institutes of Health 1.59 Imaging Software. The average of lesion areas in sections from three anatomically defined positions was taken as the lesion size of each animal. As shown in Figure 12.6, the long-term treatment with tocotrienol-rich diet for 31 weeks significantly reduced the ratio of the atherosclerotic lesion area compared to the control diet.

Tocotrienol shows a tissue-specific accumulation in rats, mice and hamsters, although α-tocopherol accumulates in the various tissues and plasma. Ikeda et al. (2000; 2001) have shown that α- and γ-tocotrienols are present in the adipose tissue and skin of rats, nude mice and hairless mice fed a diet containing the tocotrienol-rich fraction extracted from palm oil containing α-tocopherol and α- and γ-tocotrienols. In our study, we examined the distribution of α- and γ-tocotrienols in apoE$^{-/-}$ mice fed a tocotrienol-rich (0.02%) diet for 5 weeks. As shown in Figure 12.7, α- and γ-tocotrienols preferentially accumulate in the aorta and heart tissues. The concentrations of these tocotrienols are either not detected or <2.0 nmol/g in the liver and kidney by the HPLC method using a Develosil 60-5 colum (The measurement was performed by Dr. Ikeda S., Sugiyama Jogakuin University). Although α-tocotrienol is detected in plasma of mice fed a diet containing α-tocotrinol, γ-tocotrienol is not detected in plasma, liver, or kidney of the mice fed γ-tocotrienol. This discrepancy was also reported by the previous study using the rat (Ikeda et al. 2003). To confirm the superior anti-atherogenicity of tocotrienol compared with tocopherol, the bioavailability after its oral administration in rodents as well as humans should be further clarified.

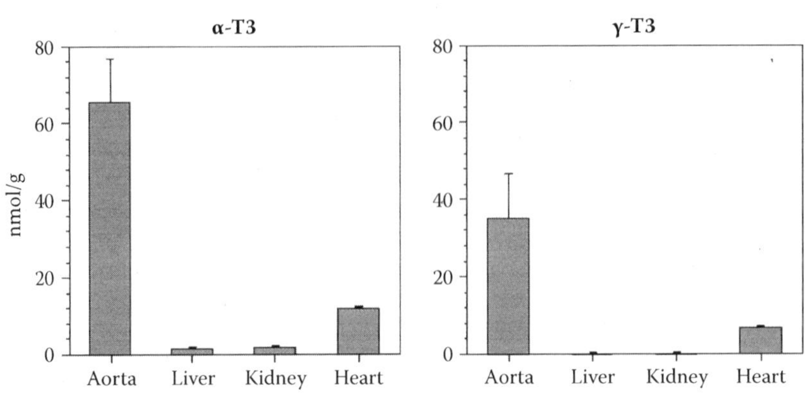

FIGURE 12.7 α-tocotrienol (α-T3) and γ-tocotrienol (γ-T3) concentrations in the tissues of apolipoprotein E-deficient mice fed tocotrienol-rich diet.

12.6 CONCLUSION

Although the exact mechanism for the inhibition of atherosclerotic lesions by tocotrienols has not been elucidated, evidence suggests that tocotrienols affect several distinct steps in the pathways leading to the formation of complex atherosclerotic lesions, especially the inhibition of cholesterol synthesis and the regulation of the inflammatory response of endothelial cells. In this chapter, we focused on their action in altering the expression of adhesion molecules, which are involved in the pathogenesis of atherosclerosis as a first step.

REFERENCES

Anderson, S.L., J. Qiu and B.Y. Rubin. 2003. Tocotrienols induce IKBKAP expression: A possible therapy for familial dysautonomia. *Biochem Biophys Res Commun*, *306*, 303–309.

Black, T.M., P. Wang, N. Maeda and R.A. Coleman. 2000. Palm tocotrienols protect ApoE +/– mice from diet-induced atheroma formation. *J Nutr*, *130*, 2420–2426.

Boissonneault, G.A., B. Hennig and C.M. Ouyang. 1991. Oxysterols, cholesterol biosynthesis and vascular endothelial cell monolayer barrier function. *Proc Soc Exp Biol Med*, *196*, 338–343.

Brown, A.J. and W. Jessup. 1999. Oxysterols and atherosclerosis. *Atherosclerosis*, *142*, 1–28.

Chao, J.T., A. Gapor and A. Theriault. 2002. Inhibitory effect of delta-tocotrienol, a HMG CoA reductase inhibitor, on monocyte-endothelial cell adhesion. *J Nutr Sci Vitaminol (Tokyo)*, *48*, 332–337.

Collins, R.G., R. Velji, N.V. Guevara, M.J. Hicks, L. Chan and A.L. Beaudet. 2000. P-Selectin or intercellular adhesion molecule (ICAM)-1 deficiency substantially protects against atherosclerosis in apolipoprotein E-deficient mice. *J Exp Med*, *191*, 189–194.

Cybulsky, M.I. and M.A. Gimbrone, Jr. 1991. Endothelial expression of a mononuclear leukocyte adhesion molecule during atherogenesis. *Science*, *251*, 788–791.

Estruch, R., E. Sacanella, E. Badia, E. Antunez, J.M. Nicolas, J. Fernandez-Sola, D. Rotilio, G. de Gaetano, E. Rubin and A. Urbano-Marquez. 2004. Different effects of red wine and gin consumption on inflammatory biomarkers of atherosclerosis: A prospective randomized crossover trial. Effects of wine on inflammatory markers. *Atherosclerosis*, *175*, 117–123.

Han, K.H., Y. Chen, M.K. Chang, Y.C. Han, J.H. Park, S.R. Green, A. Boullier and O. Quehenberger. 2003. LDL activates signaling pathways leading to an increase in cytosolic free calcium and stimulation of CD11b expression in monocytes. *J Lipid Res*, *44*, 1332–1340.

Hodis, H.N., W.J. Mack, L. LaBree, P.R. Mahrer, A. Sevanian, C.R. Liu, C.H. Liu, J. Hwang, R.H. Selzer and S.P. Azen. 2002. Alpha-tocopherol supplementation in healthy individuals reduces low-density lipoprotein oxidation but not atherosclerosis: The Vitamin E Atherosclerosis Prevention Study (VEAPS). *Circulation*, *106*, 1453–1459.

Ikeda, S., T. Niwa and K. Yamashita. 2000. Selective uptake of dietary tocotrienols into rat skin. *J Nutr Sci Vitaminol (Tokyo)*, *46*, 141–143.

Ikeda, S., T. Tohyama, H. Yoshimura, K. Hamamura, K. Abe and K. Yamashita. 2003. Dietary alpha-tocopherol decreases alpha-tocotrienol but not gamma-tocotrienol concentration in rats. *J Nutr*, *133*, 428–434.

Ikeda, S., K. Toyoshima and K. Yamashita. 2001. Dietary sesame seeds elevate alpha- and gamma-tocotrienol concentrations in skin and adipose tissue of rats fed the tocotrienol-rich fraction extracted from palm oil. *J Nutr*, *131*, 2892–2897.

Khanna, S., S. Roy, H. Ryu, P. Bahadduri, P.W. Swaan, R.R. Ratan and C.K. Sen. 2003. Molecular basis of vitamin E action. Tocotrienol modulates 12-lipoxygenase, a key mediator of glutamate-induced neurodegeneration. *J Biol Chem*, 278, 43508–43515.

Landes, N., P. Pfluger, D. Kluth, M. Birringer, R. Ruhl, G.F. Bol, H. Glatt and R. Brigelius-Flohe. 2003. Vitamin E activates gene expression via the pregnane X receptor. *Biochem Pharmacol*, *65*, 269–273.

Li, H., M.I. Cybulsky, M.J. Gimbrone and P. Libby. 1993. Inducible expression of vascular cell adhesion molecule-1 by vascular smooth muscle cells *in vitro* and within rabbit atheroma. *Am J Pathol*, *143*, 1551–1559.

Liao, L., R.M. Starzyk and D.N. Granger. 1997. Molecular determinants of oxidized low-density lipoprotein-induced leukocyte adhesion and microvascular dysfunction. *Arterioscler Thromb Vasc Biol*, *17*, 437–444.

Naito, Y., M. Shimozawa, M. Kuroda, N. Nakabe, H. Manabe, K. Katada, S. Kokura, H. Ichikawa, N. Yoshida, N. Noguchi and T. Yoshikawa. 2005. Tocotrienols reduce 25-hydroxycholesterol-induced monocyte–endothelial cell interaction by inhibiting the surface expression of adhesion molecules. *Atherosclerosis*, *180*, 19–25.

Nakashima, Y., E.W. Raines, A.S. Plump, J.L. Breslow and R. Ross. 1998. Upregulation of VCAM-1 and ICAM-1 at atherosclerosis-prone sites on the endothelium in the ApoE-deficient mouse. *Arterioscler Thromb Vasc Biol*, *18*, 842–851.

Noguchi, N., R. Hanyu, A. Nonaka, Y. Okimoto and T. Kodama. 2003. Inhibition of THP-1 cell adhesion to endothelial cells by alpha-tocopherol and alpha-tocotrienol is dependent on intracellular concentration of the antioxidants. *Free Radic Biol Med*, *34*, 1614–1620.

O'Neill, T.P. 1997. Apolipoprotein E-deficient mouse model of human atherosclerosis. *Toxicol Pathol*, *25*, 20–21.

Parker, R.A., B.C. Pearce, R.W. Clark, D.A. Gordon and J.J. Wright. 1993. Tocotrienols regulate cholesterol production in mammalian cells by post-transcriptional suppression of 3-hydroxy-3-methylglutaryl-coenzyme A reductase. *J Biol Chem*, *268*, 11230–11238.

Parthasarathy, S., S.G. Young, J.L. Witztum, R.C. Pittman and D. Steinberg. 1986. Probucol inhibits oxidative modification of low density lipoprotein. *J. Clin. Invest.*, *77*, 641–644.

Peng, S.K., C.B. Taylor, J.C. Hill and R.J. Morin. 1985. Cholesterol oxidation derivatives and arterial endothelial damage. *Atherosclerosis*, *54*, 121–133.

Poston, R.N., D.O. Haskard, J.R. Coucher, N.P. Gall and R.R. Johnson-Tidey. 1992. Expression of intercellular adhesion molecule-1 in atherosclerotic plaques. *Am J Pathol*, *140*, 665–673.

Qureshi, A.A., H. Mo, L. Packer and D.M. Peterson. 2000. Isolation and identification of novel tocotrienols from rice bran with hypocholesterolemic, antioxidant and antitumor properties. *J Agric Food Chem*, *48*, 3130–3140.

Qureshi, A.A., D.M. Peterson, J.O. Hasler-Rapacz and J. Rapacz. 2001a. Novel tocotrienols of rice bran suppress cholesterogenesis in hereditary hypercholesterolemic swine. *J Nutr*, *131*, 223–230.

Qureshi, A.A., W.A. Salser, R. Parmar and E.E. Emeson. 2001b. Novel tocotrienols of rice bran inhibit atherosclerotic lesions in C57BL/6 ApoE-deficient mice. *J Nutr*, *131*, 2606–2618.

Roberts, C.K., D. Won, S. Pruthi, S.S. Lin and R.J. Barnard. 2006. Effect of a diet and exercise intervention on oxidative stress, inflammation and monocyte adhesion in diabetic men. *Diabetes Res Clin Pract*, *73*, 249–259.

Serbinova, E., V. Kagan, D. Han and L. Packer. 1991. Free radical recycling and intramembrane mobility in the antioxidant properties of alpha-tocopherol and alpha-tocotrienol. *Free Radic Biol Med*, *10*, 263–275.

Shimozawa, M., Y. Naito, H. Manabe, K. Uchiyama, M. Kuroda, K. Katada, N. Yoshida and T. Yoshikawa. 2004. 7-Ketocholesterol enhances the expression of adhesion molecules on human aortic endothelial cells by increasing the production of reactive oxygen species. *Redox Rep*, *9*, 370–375.

Steinberg, D. 1997. Low density lipoprotein oxidation and its pathobiological significance. *J Biol Chem*, *272*, 20963–20966.

Terasawa, Y., H. Manabe, N. Yoshida, M. Uemura, N. Sugimoto, Y. Naito, T. Yoshikawa and M. Kondo. 2000. Alpha-tocopherol protects against monocyte Mac-1 (CD11b/CD18) expression and Mac-1-dependent adhesion to endothelial cells induced by oxidized low-density lipoprotein. *Biofactors*, *11*, 221–233.

Theriault, A., J.T. Chao and A. Gapor. Tocotrienol is the most effective vitamin E for reducing endothelial expression of adhesion molecules and adhesion to monocytes. *Atherosclerosis* 2002, *160*, 21–30.

Theriault, A., J.T. Chao, Q. Wang, A. Gapor and K. Adeli. 1999. Tocotrienol: A review of its therapeutic potential. *Clin Biochem*, *32*, 309–319.

Weber, C., W. Erl, K.S. Weber and P.C. Weber. 1997. HMG-CoA reductase inhibitors decrease CD11b expression and CD11b-dependent adhesion of monocytes to endothelium and reduce increased adhesiveness of monocytes isolated from patients with hypercholesterolemia. *J Am Coll Cardiol*, *30*, 1212–1217.

Yla-Herttuala, S. 1999. Oxidized LDL and atherogenesis. *Ann N Y Acad Sci*, *874*, 134–137.

Yoshida, N., H. Manabe, Y. Terasawa, H. Nishimura, F. Enjo, H. Nishino and T. Yoshikawa. 2000. Inhibitory effects of vitamin E on endothelial-dependent adhesive interactions with leukocytes induced by oxidized low density lipoprotein. *Biofactors*, *13*, 279–288.

Yoshida, Y., E. Niki and N. Noguchi. 2003. Comparative study on the action of tocopherols and tocotrienols as antioxidant: Chemical and physical effects. *Chem Phys Lipids*, *123*, 63–75.

Yoshikawa, T., N. Yoshida, H. Manabe, Y. Terasawa, T. Takemura and M. Kondo. 1998. Alpha-tocopherol protects against expression of adhesion molecules on neutrophils and endothelial cells. *BioFactors*, *7*, 15–19.

Zibara, K., E. Chignier, C. Covacho, R. Poston, G. Canard, P. Hardy and J. McGregor. 2000. Modulation of expression of endothelial intercellular adhesion molecule-1, platelet-endothelial cell adhesion molecule-1 and vascular cell adhesion molecule-1 in aortic arch lesions of apolipoprotein E-deficient compared with wild-type mice. *Arterioscler Thromb Vasc Biol*, *20*, 2288–2296.

13 Uptake, Distribution and Protective Action of Tocotrienols in Cultured Cells

Noriko Noguchi, Yoshiro Saito and Etsuo Niki

CONTENTS

13.1 INTRODUCTION

Cultured cells have often been used for the study of oxidative stress and its inhibition in order to bridge the gap between *in vitro* and *in vivo* systems. The protective effects of various antioxidants against cytotoxicity induced by different types of oxidative insult have been studied extensively. In general, the test antioxidant is added into the cell culture medium to mimic the physiological conditions. The efficacy of antioxidant depends on the uptake and localization in the culture medium as well as its inherent activity. Therefore, the uptake and distribution of antioxidants into the cells are important determining factor for antioxidant effects. In this chapter, these issues for tocotrienols (T3) are reviewed and discussed in comparison with tocopherols (T).

13.2 PROTECTIVE ACTIVITY AND UPTAKE OF T3 AND T INTO CULTURED CELLS

In 2000, Sen and his colleagues found that αT3 and γT3 were more effective than αT in preventing glutamate-induced death of HT4 hippocampal neuronal cells. They also found that the uptake of T3 from the culture medium into cells was more efficient than that of T. It was also found that T3 were more effective than the corresponding isoforms of T in preventing the cytotoxicity induced by selenium deficiency in Jurkat cells, in which oxidative stress played a causative role (Saito et al., 2003). Table 13.1 summarizes the median effective dose (ED50), the concentration required for antioxidant to inhibit 50% cell death. The effects of αT3 and αT are compared in Figure 13.1 (Saito et al., 2003). They show that the T3 was more potent than T and the activity decreased in the order of $\alpha > \beta = \gamma > \delta$, which is the same order as that for radical scavenging. It may be noteworthy that the ED50 for 2,2,5,7,8-pentamethyl-6-chromanol (PMC) and Trolox was 65 and 630 nM respectively, much higher than those for T3 and T.

Table 13.1 also shows that the ED50 concentrations for T3 and T are below 100 nM, which is much lower than that in human plasma. It may be noteworthy that the concentration in the lipophilic domain where vitamin E functions is important, not in the culture medium. The concentrations

TABLE 13.1
Protective Effects of Vitamin E Isoforms on Cell Death Induced by Selenium Deficiency

	ED50 (nM)	
Isoform	T3	T
α	13 ± 6.5	36 ± 8.1
β	24 ± 2.9	31 ± 2.3
γ	23 ± 5.0	40 ± 17
δ	39 ± 10	46 ± 9.3

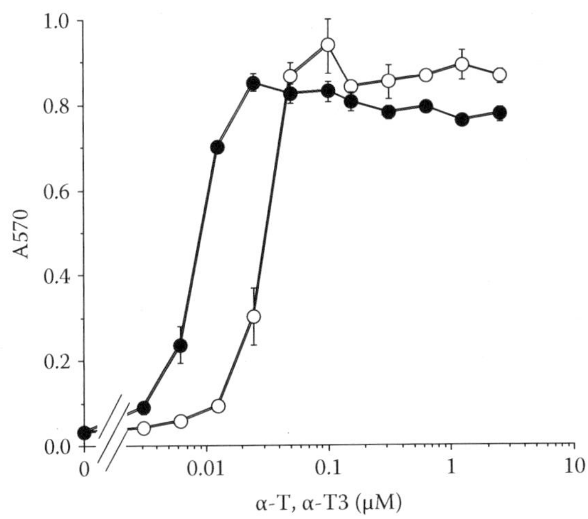

FIGURE 13.1 Effect of the addition of αT3 and αT on the viability of cells in a Se-deficient serum-free medium. In the presence of variable amounts of αT3 (closed circle) and αT (open circle), Jurkat cells were cultured for 3 days in a Se-deficient medium (ITA-RPMI: RPMI-1640 medium containing 5 μg/ml human insulin, 5 μg/ml human transferrin, 92 nM $FeCl_3$ and 2.5 mg/ml bovine serum albumin). After this time, the viability was measured by 3-[4, 5-dimethylthiazol-2-yl]-2, 5-di-phenyltetrazolium bromide (MTT) assay and the mean ± SE of three experiments are shown.

of vitamin E and lipids in the human plasma are roughly 20–30 μM and 20 mM, respectively, the molecular ratio of vitamin E to lipids being 1/1000 to 1.5/1000. The concentrations of lipids in the cultured cells are typically in the order of 10 μM and hence 100 nM of vitamin E is not surprisingly low, although the important concentration is obviously the one actually taken up into cells from the culture medium.

The uptake of T3 and T into cultured cells was measured using Jurkat cells (Saito et al., 2004). As shown in Figure 13.2, the content of αT3 increased with incubation time and reached a plateau after 6 h of incubation time. On the other hand, the cellular content of αT increased linearly with incubation time up to 72 h. Interestingly, the initial rate of cellular uptake of αT3 was 70-fold higher than that of αT. The cellular content of αT3 and αT increased with increasing initial concentration in the culture medium. The cellular content of αT3 was 6.5 and 2.2-fold higher than that of αT after incubation for 24 h and 72 h, respectively.

The protective effects of αT3 and αT against the cytotoxicity induced by cumene hydroperoxide were compared under similar conditions (Saito et al., 2004). The Jurkat cells were treated with 1 μM αT3 or 6 μM αT for 24 h to obtain the cells containing the same amounts of antioxidants. It was

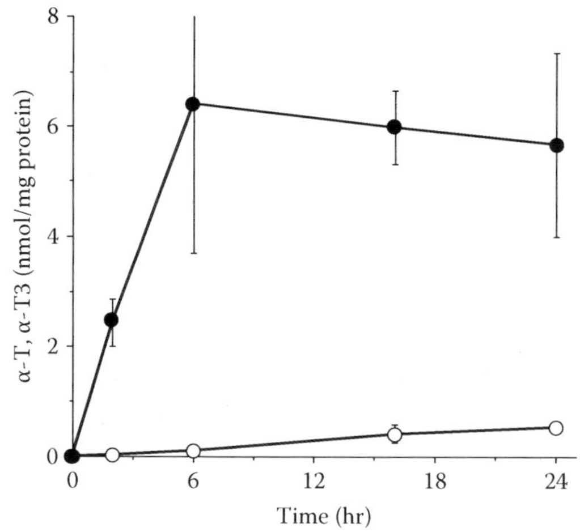

FIGURE 13.2 Cellular uptake of αT3 and αT into Jurkat cells. Jurkat cells were cultured in serum-free RPMI-1640 medium (ITSA-RPMI: ITA-RPMI medium containing 100 nM sodium selenite) with 1 μM αT3 or 1 μM αT for the indicated times and the cellular vitamin E content was measured using an HPLC system with an electrochemical detector. Mean values of cellular vitamin E content are shown with SE (n = 3).

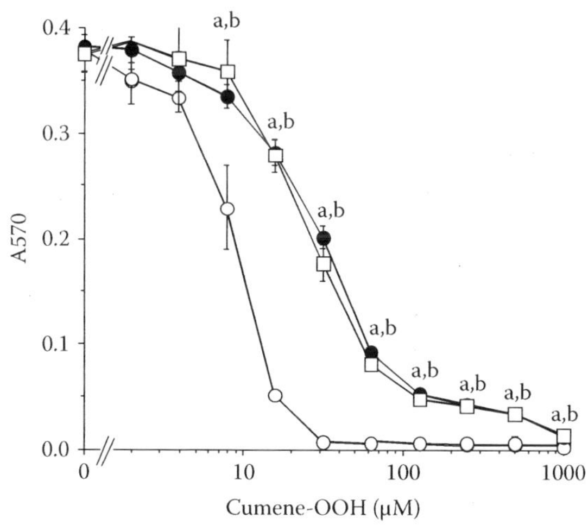

FIGURE 13.3 Effect of αT3 on the cell death caused by cumene hydroperoxides. Jurkat cells were cultured in ITSA-RPMI without (open circle) and with 1μM αT3 (open square) or 6 μM αT (closed circle) for 24 hr and then cells were washed and treated with variable amounts of cumene hydroperoxide for 6 hr. The cell viability was measured by MTT assay and the means ± SE of the three experiments are shown. a; $p < 0.05$ when compared with αT3 fortified cells and control cells. b; $p < 0.05$ when compared with αT fortified cells and control cells.

found in fact that the cells thus obtained contained 6.2 ± 2.6 and 5.9 ± 3.6 nmol/mg protein of αT3 and αT, respectively. When these cells were challenged by cumene hydroperoxide, αT3 and αT exerted the same protective effects (Figure 13.3) (Saito et al., 2004). These results further confirm that αT3 and αT exert similar antioxidant effects in the cells against oxidative stress.

13.3 EFFECT OF T3 ON EXPRESSION OF ADHESION MOLECULES

Endothelial vascular cell adhesion molecule-1 (VCAM-1), intercellular adhesion molecule-1(ICAM-1) and endothelial leukocyte adhesion molecule-1 (E-selectin) have received much attention in con-

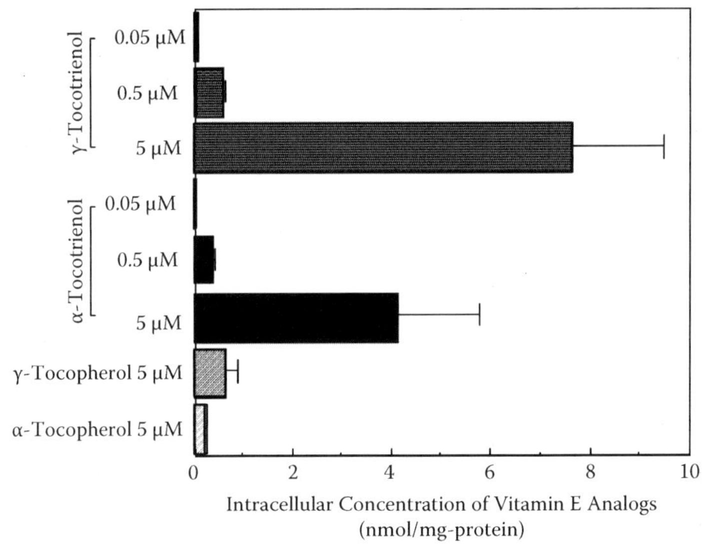

FIGURE 13.4 Accumulation of vitamin E analogs in HUVEC, which were exposed to 0.05, 0.5 or 5 μM αT3, γT3, αT, or γT for 24 h and the intracellular concentrations of these analogs were analyzed. Values represent mean ± SD of three independent experiments in triplicate.

nection with atherosclerosis. The effects of αT on monocyte adhesion have been studied extensively (Chan 1998, Theriault et al., 1999). Several reports show that T3 isoforms are more effective than T in reducing the endothelial expression of adhesion molecules and also adhesion of monocytes (Theriault et al., 2002, Chao et al., 2002, Noguchi et al., 2003, Naito et al., 2005). Theriault and his colleagues examined the relative inhibitory effects of αT3 and other vitamin E homologues on cell surface adhesion molecule using human umbilical vein endothelial cells (HUVEC). They found that αT3 exerted a more profound inhibitory effect on adhesion molecule expression and monocyte cell adherence (Theriault et al., 2002). They also found that δT3 displayed a more profound inhibitory effect than αT3 on the surface expression of adhesion molecules in TNF-α activated HUVEC (Chao et al., 2002). In these studies, however, the uptake and content of T3 and T in the cells were not measured.

The accumulation of vitamin E analogs in endothelial cells was measured after exposure of 0.05μM, 0.5 μM or 5 μM vitamin E analogs to HUVEC for 24 h. The concentrations of αT, γT, αT3 and γT3 in the cells were quite different, the relative concentration being αT = 1, γT = 3, αT3 = 17 and γT3 = 33 (Figure 13.4). The expression of VCAM-1 induced by stimulation with TNF-α was measured by flow cytometry using a monoclonal antibody against VCAM-1. The expression of VCAM-1 was reduced by αT3 and αT in a concentration-dependent manner (Figure 13.5A). αT3 appeared to exert stronger effect than αT. However, αT3 at a 10 times lower concentration than that of αT showed a similar inhibitory effect on the expression of VCAM-1 compared with that of αT.

The effect of T3 and T on the adhesion of monocytic cells to HUVEC was also studied (Noguchi et al., 2003). Incubation of HUVEC with TNF-α for 4 h induced about a 10-fold increase in adhesion of THP-1 cells compared with that to unstimulated HUVEC (Figure 13.5B). This increase in HUVEC adhesiveness was significantly reduced by αT3 and αT in a concentration-dependent manner. Again, αT3 was more effective than αT at the same concentration added into the medium. However, when the adherent cell numbers were plotted against the intracellular concentrations of αT3 and αT, a good reverse correlation ($R^2 = 0.903$) was observed. These results clearly show that T3 and T exert the same inhibitory effects on the expression of adhesion molecules and adhesion of monocytic cells.

Naito and his colleagues (Naito et al., 2005) also studied the effect of T3 and T on the inhibition of VCAM-1 expression on human aortic endothelial cells (HAEC) induced by 25-hydroxycholes-

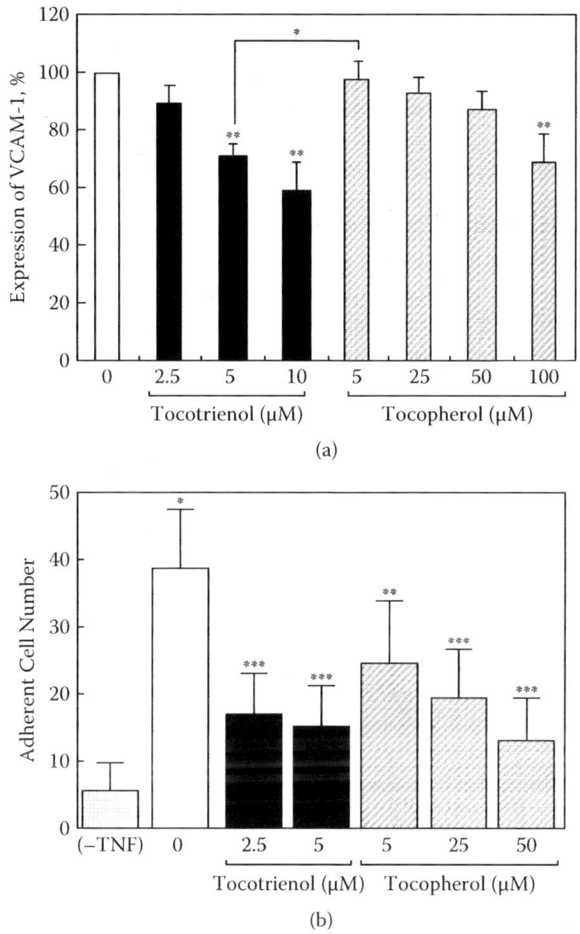

FIGURE 13.5 Concentration dependent inhibition of VCAM-1 expression and adhesion of THP-1 cell by vitamin E analogs. After treatment of HUVEC with several concentrations of αT3 or αT for 20 h, the cells were stimulated with 5 ng/ml TNF-α for 4 h. (A) VCAM-1 was measured using an antibody which was labeled with phycoerythrin. Values represent mean ± SD of three independent experiments in triplicate. $^{*}p < 0.005$, $^{**}p < 0.01$ vs. TNF-treated (0). (B) After stimulation of HUVECs with TNF-α, the cells were washed and THP-1 cells were overlaid on the cells. After 30 min incubation, the adherent cells were counted. Values represent mean ± SD of three independent experiments in more than triplicate. $^{*}p < 0.005$ vs. untreated with TNF (–TNF), $^{**}p < .01$ vs. TNF-treated, $^{***}p < 0.005$ vs. TNF-treated.

terol (25-OHCh). It was observed that the pretreatment of HAEC with T3 and T at a concentration of 10 μM significantly suppressed the surface expression of VCAM-1; the inhibition extent being 38, 63, 54, 77 and 29% for αT3, βT3, γT3, δT3 and αT, respectively. When the effects of T3 and T on the adhesion of monocytes to HAEC stimulated by 25-OHCh were also examined, it was found they suppressed it by the same relative potency as that observed for VCAM-1 expression. This order correlated fairly well with the intracellular concentrations of T3 and T measured under the same experimental conditions.

13.4 CELLULAR DISTRIBUTION OF T3 AND T

In order to analyze the cellular distribution of αT3 and αT, Jurkat cells were incubated with 1 μM αT3 or αT for 24 h and then fractionated by differential centrifugation (Saito et al., 2004). The cells were homogenized by nitrogen decompression using Parr Cell Disruption Bombs. The nuclear fractions were prepared by centrifugation at 500 x g for 10 min and suspended in a homogenizing buffer. Mitochondrial fraction was obtained from postnuclear fractions by centrifugation at 5,000 x g for 10 min and the microsomal and cytosolic fractions were obtained by centrifugation at 105,000 x g for 60 min. The distribution of each subcellular fraction was judged by standard enzymatic measurements, cytochrome c oxidase (mitochondrial marker), NADPH-cytochrome c reductase (microsomal marker) and lactate dehydrogenase (cytosolic marker). The cell constituents were extracted with chloroform and methanol (2:1 by volume) and lipids in the chloroform layer were analyzed by using a thin-layer chromatography equipped with a flame ionization detection system.

Intracellular vitamin E was detected using HPLC systems with electrochemical detection. Cell samples in PBS were mixed with chloroform/methanol (2:1) and then cellular vitamin E in the lower chloroform layer was analyzed with an HPLC using a postcolumn amperometric electrochemical detector.

It was found that the subcellular distribution was similar for αT3 and αT (Figure 13.6) and that, interestingly, their contents were directly correlated with lipid contents (Figure 13.7). The mechanism by which vitamin E is distributed within the cell and reaches mitochondria and the nucleus has not been well elucidated. The vitamin E-regulating proteins such as α-tocopherol transfer protein (α-TTP), cytosolic tocopherol-associated protein (TAP) and tocopherol binding protein (TBP) may function as cellular transporter of vitamin E (Brigelius-Flohe and Traber, 1999, Blatt et al., 2001). The results shown in Figure 13.7 suggest that the cellular distribution of αT3 and αT is determined similarly by the lipid distribution.

13.5 CONCLUSION

There have been many reports, other than those referred to above, on the effects of T3 on cultured cells in relation to apoptosis (Rickmann et al., 2007, Mazlan et al., 2006, Sakai et al., 2006, Shah and Sylvester, 2005, Shun et al., 2004, Sakai et al., 2004), down-regulation of telomerase activity (Eitsuka et al., 2006), protection from oxidative damage of neuronal cells (Numakawa et al., 2006, Palozza et al., 2006, Osakada et al., 2004) and anti-proliferative effect (Samant and Sylvester, 2006). In general, T3 are added to the culture medium, but considering the total content of lipids in the medium, the amount usually added can be quite excessive and physiologically irrelevant. It has been known, for example,that excess vitamin A induces membrane modification and hemolysis (Murphy, 1973, Urano et al., 1992). It should be emphasized that the incorporation of T3 should be measured in order to examine the protective and/or prooxidative action and function of T3 in the cultured cells. The bioavailability and physiological concentrations of vitamin E analogues are determined primarily by α-TTP. The affinity of αT3 relative to αT is only 12.4% (Hosomi et al., 1997) and T3 is metabolized faster than T (Brigelius-Flohe and Traber, 1999). A higher antioxidant activity of T3 than T and/or specific function of T3 have been proposed (Packer et al., 2001, Sen et al., 2006). In order to raise the physiological concentrations, a topical administration such as to skin (Ikeda et al., 2000) and eyes (Tanito et al., 2004) or other efficient delivery system may be promising.

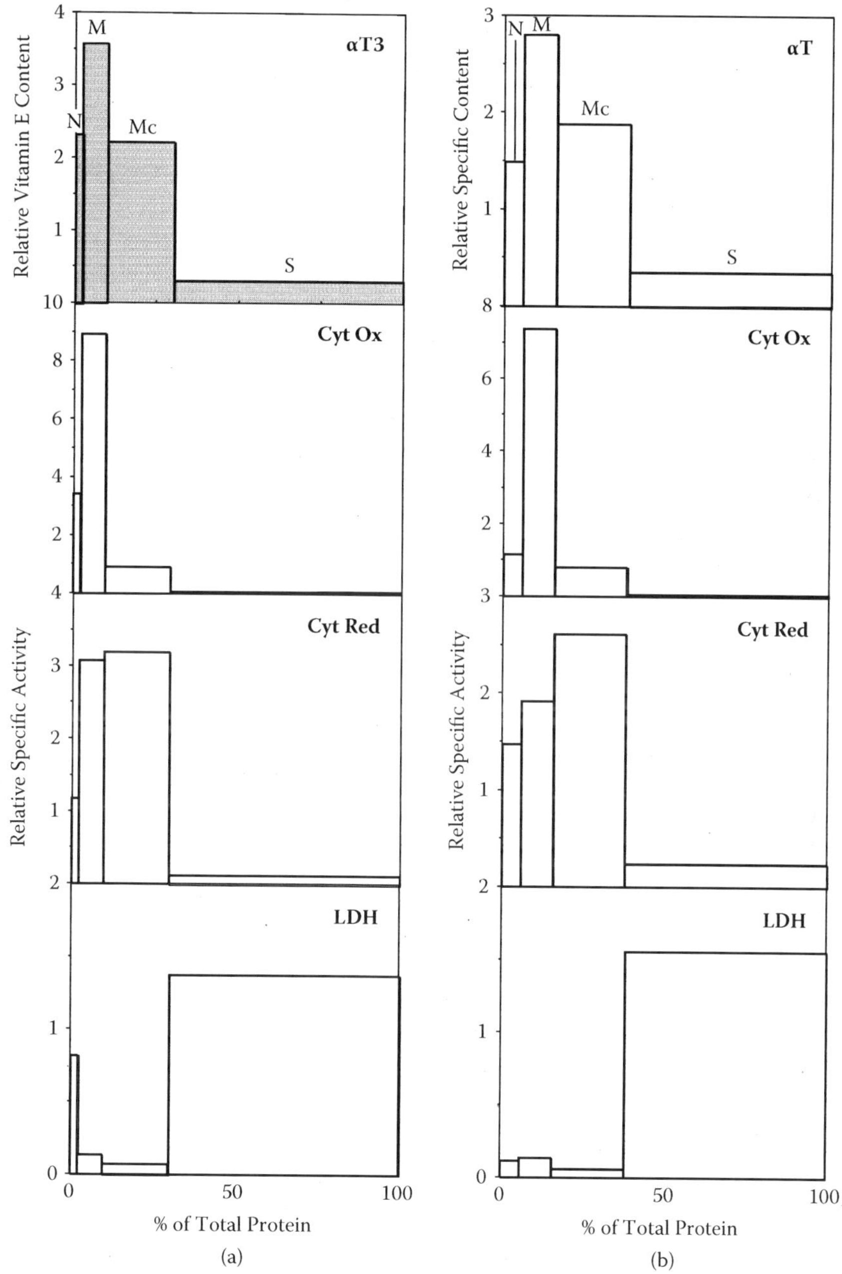

FIGURE 13.6 Subcellular localization of α-tocotrienol and α-tocopherol. Jurkat cells were cultured in ITSA-RPMI containing 1 μM αT3 (a) or αT (b) for 24 hr. These cells were fractionated by differential centrifugation into nuclear fraction (N), mitochondrial fraction (M), microsomal fraction (Mc) and cytosolic fraction (S) and the contents of vitamin E and protein were measured. The distribution of marker proteins was determined by enzymatic activity. Cytochrome c oxidase (Cyt Ox), NADPH-cytochrome c reductase (Cyt Red) and lactate dehydrogenase (LDH) were measured as marker enzymes of mitochondria, microsome and cytosol, respectively.

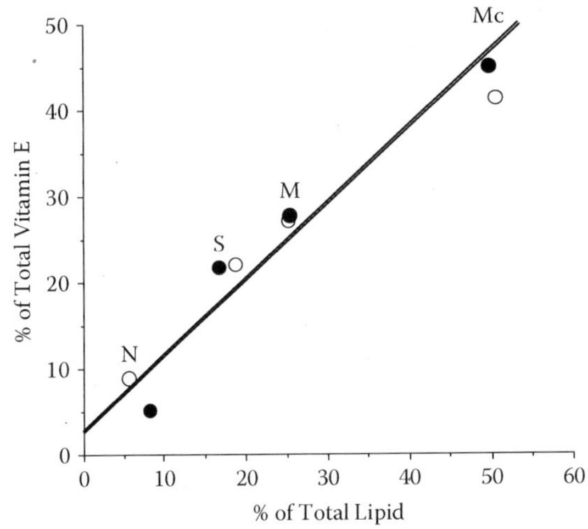

FIGURE 13.7 Correlation between vitamin E (αT3, closed circle; αT, open circle) and lipid contents in subcellular fractions. The experimental conditions are the same as in Figure 13.6

REFERENCES

Blatt, D. H., Leonard, S. W., Traber, M. G. 2001. Vitamin E kinetics and the function of tocopherol regulatory proteins. *Nutrition*, 17, 799–805.

Brigelius-Flohe, R., Traber, M. G. 1999. Vitamin E: Function and metabolism. *FASEB J.*, 13, 1145–1155.

Chan, A. C. 1998. Vitamin E and atherosclerosis. *J. Nutr.*, 128, 1593–1596.

Chao, J.-T., Gapor, A., Theriault, A. 2002. Inhibitory effect of δ-tocotrienol, a HMG CoA reductase inhibitor, on monocyte-endothelial cell adhesion. *J. Nutr. Sci. Vitaminol.*, 48, 332–337.

Eitsuka, T., Nakagawa, K., Miyazawa, T. 2006. Down-regulation of telomerase activity in DLD-1 human colorectal adenocarcinoma cells by tocotrienol., *Biochem. Biophys. Res. Commun.*, 348, 170–175.

Hosomi, A., Arita, M., Sato, Y., Kiyose, C., Ueda, T., Igarashi, O., Arai, H., Inoue, K. 1997. Affinity for α-tocopherol transfer protein as a determination of the biological activities of vitamin E analogs. *FEBS Lett.*, 409, 105–108.

Ikeda, S., Niwa, T., Yamashita, K. 2000. Selective uptake of dietary tocotrienols into rat skin. *J. Nutr. Sci. Vitaminol.*, 46, 141–143.

Mazlan, M., Mian, T. S., Top, G. M., Ngah, W. Z. W. 2006. Comparative effects of α-tocopherol and γ-tocotrienol against hydrogen peroxide-induced apoptosis on primary-cultured astrocytes. *J. Neurol. Sci.*, 243, 5–12.

Murphy, M. J. Jr. 1973. Effects of vitamin A on the erythrocyte membrane surface. *Blood*, 41, 893–899

Naito, Y., Shimozawa, M., Kuroda, M., Nakabe, N., Manabe, H., Katada, K., Kokura, S., Ichikawa, H., Yoshida, N., Noguchi, N., Yoshikawa, T. 2005. Tocotrienols reduce 25-hydroxycholesterol-induced monocyte-endothelial cell interaction by inhibiting the surface expression of adhesion molecules. *Atherosclerosis*, 180, 19–25.

Noguchi, N., Hanyu, R., Nonaka, A., Okimoto, Y., Kodama, T. 2003. Inhibition of THP-1 cell adhesion to endothelial cells by α-tocopherol and α-tocotrienol is dependent on intracellular concentration of the antioxidants. *Free Rad. Biol. Med.*, 34, 1614–1620.

Numakawa, Y., Numakawa, T., Matsumoto, T., Yagasaki, Y., Kumamaru, E., Kunugi, H., Taguchi, T., Niki, E. 2006. Vitamin E protected cultured cortical neurons from oxidative stress-induced cell death through the activation of mitogen-activated protein kinase and phosphatidylinositol 3-kinase. *J. Neurochem.*, 97, 1191–1202.

Osakada, F., Hashino, A., Kume, T., Katsuki, H., Kaneko, S., Akaike, A. 2004. α–tocotrienol provides the most potent neuroprotection among vitamin E analogs on cultured striatal neurons. *Neuropharmacology*, 47, 904–915.

Packer, L., Weber, S. U., Rimbach, G. 2001. Molecular aspects of α-tocotrienol antioxidant action and cell signaling. *J. Nutr.*, 131, 369S–373S.

Palozza, P., Verdecchia, S., Avanzi, L., Vertuani, S., Serini, S., Iannone, A., Manfredini, S. 2006. Comparative antioxidant activity of tocotrienols and the novel chromanyl-polyisoprenyl molecule FeAox-6 in isolated membranes and intact cells. *Mol. Cell. Biochem.*, 287, 21–32.

Rickmann, M., Vaquero, E. C., Malagelada, J. R., Molero, X. 2007. Tocotreinols induce apoptosis and autophagy in rat pancreatic stellate cells through the mitochondrial death pathway. *Gastroenterology*, 132, 2518–2532.

Saito, Y., Yoshida, Y., Akazawa, T., Takahashi, K., Niki, E. 2003. Cell death caused by selenium deficiency and protective effect of antioxidants. *J. Biol. Chem.*, 278, 39428–39434.

Saito, Y., Yoshida, Y., Nishio, K., Hayakawa, M., Niki, E. 2004. Characterization of cellular uptake and distribution of vitamin E. *Ann. N. Y. Acad. Sci.*, 1031, 368–375.

Sakai, M., Okabe, M., Tachibana, H., Yamada, K. 2006. Apoptosis induction by γ-tocotrienol in human hetatoma Hep3B cells. *J. Nutr. Biochem.*, 17, 672–676.

Sakai, M., Okabe, M., Yamaskai, M., Tachibana, H., Yamada, K. 2004 .Induction of apoptosis by tocotrienol in rat hepatoma dRLh-84 cells. *Anticancer Res.*, 24, 1683–1688.

Samant, G. V., Sylvester, P. W. 2006. Gamma-tocotrienol inhibits ErbB3-dependent PI3K/Akt mitogenic signalling in neoplastic mammary epithelial cells. *Cell Prolif.*, 39, 563–574.

Sen, C. K., Khanna, S., Roy, S., Packer, L. 2000. Molecular basis of vitamin E action. *J. Biol. Chem.*, 275, 13049–13055.

Sen, C. K., Khanna, S., Roy, S. 2006. Tocotrienols: Vitamin E beyond tocopherols. *Life Sci.*, 78, 2088–2098.

Shah, S. J., Sylvester, P. W. 2005. Tocotrienol-induced cytotoxicity is unrelated to mitochondrial stress apoptotic signaling in neoplastic mammary epithelial cells. *Biochem. Cell Biol.*, 83, 86–95.

Shun, M. C., Yu, W., Gapor, A., Parsons, R., Atkinson, J., Sanders, B. G., Kline, K. 2004. Pro-apoptotic mechanisms of action of a novel vitamin E analog (alpha-TEA) and a naturally occurring form of vitamin E (delta-tocotrienol) in MDA-MB-435 human breast cancer cells. *Nutr. Cancer*, 48, 95–105.

Tanito, M., Itoh, N., Yoshida, Y., Hayakawa, M., Ohira, A., Niki, E. 2004. Distribution of tocopherols and tocotrienols to rat ocular tissues after topical ophthalmic administration. *Lipids*, 39, 469–474.

Theriault, A., Chao, J.-T., Wang, Q., Gapor, A., Adeli, K. 1999. Tocotrienol: A review of its therapeutic potential. *Clin. Biochem.*, 32, 309–319.

Theriault, A., Chao, J.-T., Gapor, A. 2002. Tocotrienol is the most effective vitamin E for reducing endothelial expression of adhesion molecules and adhesion to monocytes. *Atherosclerosis*, 160, 21–30.

Tsuzuki, W., Yunoki, R., Yoshimura, H. 2007. Intestinal epithelial cells absorb γ-tocotrienol faster than α-tocopherol. *Lipids*, 42, 163–170.

Urano, S., Inomori, Y., Sugawara, T., Kato, Y., Kitahara, M., Hasegawa, Y., Matsuo, M., Mukai, K. 1992. Vitamin E: Inhibition of retinol-induced hemolysis and membrane-stabilizing behavior. *J. Biol. Chem.*, 267, 18365–18370.

Wada, S., Satomi, Y., Murakoshi, M., Noguchi, N., Yoshikawa, T., Nishino, H. 2005. Tumor suppressive effects of tocotrienol *in vivo* and *in vitro*. *Cancer Lett.*, 229, 181–191.

Part E

Cancer Prevention and Treatment

14 Anticancer Effects of Tocotrienols and Tocopherols Irrespective of Antioxidative Properties

Tomohiro Yano and Nantiga Virgona

CONTENTS

14.1 INTRODUCTION

Vitamin E is a generic term referring to an entire class of compounds that is further divided into two groups called tocopherols and tocotrienols. There are at least eight different isoforms of vitamin E: alpha-, beta-, gamma- and delta-tocopherols and alpha-, beta-, gamma- and delta-tocotrienols. Each tocotrienol molecule differs from the corresponding tocopherol molecule only in the side chain. Tocopherols have a saturated side chain, a phytyl group attached to their chromanol ring, while the side chain of tocotrienols is unsaturated and forms an isoprenoid group. The isoforms of tocotrienols differ in their methyl substituents on the chromanol ring. The alpha-form involves three methyl groups, while the beta- and gamma- have two and delta-form only one methyl group. Each of these forms has a reportedly different biopotency (Azzi and Stocker 2000; Brigelius-Flohe and Traber 1999).

Vitamin E localizes cellular membranes in which it effectively blocks lipid peroxidation. Both tocopherols and tocotrienols shut down the chain reaction of lipid peroxidation. Comparing the efficacy of each vitamin E isoform, two factors are important, i.e., the substituents on the chromanol ring and the properties of the side chain. In homogeneous systems, the reaction rate constant depends mainly on the number of methyl groups on the chromanol ring. In membranes, the mobility of the molecule is also rate-limiting, and this depends on the structure of the hydrophobic side chain. The scavenging activity of alpha-tocotrienol against peroxyl radicals in liposomes is higher than that of alpha-tocopherol (Packer et al. 2001). The efficacy of alpha-tocotrienol to protect against $Fe(II)^+$ NADPH-induced lipid peroxidation in rat liver microsomes was 40 times higher than that of alpha-tocopherol.

Several reasons have been suggested for the increased antioxidant activity of alpha-tocotrienol vs. alpha-tocopherol, focusing on the differences in the tail structure. The chromanoxyl radical of alpha-tocotrienol (alpha-tocotrienoxyl) has been found to be recycled in membranes and lipoproteins more quickly than the corresponding alpha-tocopheroxyl radical (Packer et al. 2001). Furthermore, alpha-tocotrienol has a stronger disordering effect on membranes than alpha-tocopherol and is distributed more uniformly within the membrane. These properties likely enhance the interaction of chromanols with lipid radicals (Packer et al. 2001). Overall, it seems that tocotrienols as radical scavengers are more effective in biomembranes than the corresponding tocopherols. The potential antioxidant properties of tocopherols and tocotrienols exactly contribute to a part of their antitumorigenic effect, while recent reports indicate that the antitumorigenic effect of vitamin E mainly depends on their redox-silent property irrespective of antioxidant effect (Neuzil et al. 2007). In this chapter, we refer to redox-silent analogues of alpha-tocotrienol and alpha-tocopherol as new promising agents for cancer therapy and prevention.

14.2 CANCER THERAPY AND PREVENTION BASED ON NONANTIOXIDATIVE EFFECTS OF ALPHA-TOCOPHEROL

14.2.1 Regulation of Signal Transduction Related to Growth of Tumor Cells By Alpha-Tocopherol Independent of Antioxidant Effects

The vitamin E molecule is divided into three different domains (Neuzil et al. 2007). The functional domain (I) has the substitution pattern at position C6 of the chromanol ring. The phenolic OH group status determines whether the molecule behaves as redox-active or redox-silent. The well-documented antioxidant properties of alpha-, beta-, gamma- and delta-tocopherols resulted in their application in cancer clinical trials. However, there was no positive outcome concerning the use of free tocopherols in cancer prevention (Pham and Plakogiannis, 2005). On the other hand, chemical modifications at C6 lead to redox-silent derivatives (ethers, esters, and amides) that prove to be potent anti-tumorigenic agents (Birringer et al. 2003; Tomic-Vatic et al. 2005; Yano et al. 2000). The signaling domain (II) exhibits several activities that are independent of the antioxidant nature of tocopherols and are given by the methylation pattern of the aromatic ring. For instance, protein kinase C is best inhibited by alpha-tocopherol, while the other tocopherols are less potent despite having equal antioxidant activity, indicating that PKC is inhibited by non-antioxidant molecule mechanisms of vitamin E.

The inhibitory effect of alpha-tocopherol contributes to the reduction of cell proliferation in many different cells types (several cancer cells, vascular smooth muscular cells, macrophages, fibroblasts, and mesangial cells among others) (Neuzil et al. 2001; Sylvester et al. 2001; Tada et al. 1997). In addition to the inhibition of PKC, alpha-tocopherol has direct and indirect effects on several enzymes involved in signal transduction, such as diacylglycerol kinase, cyclooxygenase-2, phospholipase A_2, mitogen activated protein kinase signal transduction pathway (Table 14.1) (Azzi et al. 2002; Rimbach et al. 2002; Zingg and Azzi, 2004) irrespective of antioxidant property. The hydrophobic domain (III) is involved with docking of vitamin E analogues in biological membranes

TABLE 14.1
Modulation Effect of Alpha-Tocotrienol on Several Enzymes Involved in Signal Transduction

Enzyme Inhibition	Enzyme Activation
Protein kinase C alpha and delta	Phospho-serine/threonine phosphatase 2A
Protein kinase B	Phospho-tyrosineprotein phosphatase
Phosphopholipase A2	Diacylglycerol kinase alpha
Cyclooxygenase-2	
5-, 12-, and 15-Lipoxygenases	
Mitogenactivated protein kinases	

and lipoproteins, and is determined by modification of the aliphatic side chain. The multi-modulating effects of several enzymes by alpha-tocopherol in a nonantioxidant manner directly and indirectly contribute to the growth suppression in several types of tumor cells (Azzi et al. 2002). Thus tumor regulation based on the nonantioxidant property of alpha-tocopherol is a promising strategy to establish a new cancer preventive and therapeutic procedure.

14.2.2 Anti-Proliferative Activity of Redox-Silent Tocopherol Analogues

As mentioned in the introduction, OH group at position C6 of the chromanol ring involved in tocopherol is a redox-active site. In order to block the antioxidant property, several types of redox-silent tocopherol derivatives have been synthesized and evaluated for their cytotoxic activity against tumor cells (Arya et al. 1998; Birringer et al. 2003; Galli et al. 2004; Kogure et al. 2005; Nuezil et al. 2001; Shun et al. 2004; Shiau et al. 2006; Tomic-Vatic et al. 2005; Vraka et al. 2006; Yano et al. 2000). Alpha-tocopheryl succinate (TOS) bearing a succinyl ester at position C6 of the chromanol ring is the most representative analogue. The structure–activity relationship of cytotoxic activity against tumor cells has been extensively studied using dicarboxylic esters of tocopherols (Birringer et al. 2003; Kogure et al. 2005), because methylation of the free carboxyl group leads to noncharged derivatives without proapoptogenic activity. Of these compounds, unsaturated dicarboxylic esters, such as alpha-tocopheryl oxalate and malonate have greater cytotoxic activity than alpha-TOS, but the former two induced nonselective cytotoxicity in tumor-bearing mice (Kogure et al. 2005). On the other hand, alpha-TOS is a potent inducer of cell death in a multitude of malignant cells though the compound is largely nontoxic toward normal cells (Birringer et al. 2003). Since agents having apoptogenic activity, which are weak acids, are selectively taken up by malignant cells due to the acidic interstitium of the tumor compared to normal cells (Kozin et al. 2001), an addition of a chargeable group to the chromanol ring contributes to the selectivity of alpha-TOS against cancer cells. In other dicarboxylic esters of tocopherols, increasing the chain length of the dicarboxylic acid leads to decreased apoptogenic activity as shown for glutaric acid, methylated glutaric acid, and pimelic acid (Birringer et al. 2003; Kogure et al. 2004). Comparing apoptogenic activity among succinyl esters of the tocopherol isomers (alpha-, beta-, gamma- and delta-form), alpha-TOS posseses the highest apoptogenic activity, followed by beta-TOS, gamma-TOS, and delta-TOS (Birringer et al. 2003). These reports lead us to a conclusion that alpha-TOS is the most effective redox-silent analogue of tocopherols toward cancer cells of dicarboxylic esters of tocopherols.

However, oral administration of alpha-TOS is not as effective as its apoptogenic activity would suggest because the ester bond in alpha-TOS is cleaved by intestinal esterase (Wu et al. 2004). To overcome the problem of ester bond cleavage, 6-*O*-carboxypropyl-alpha-tocopherol (TE), an ether derivative of alpha-tocopherol, has been synthesized. By replacing the ester bond with an ether bond (Figure 14.1), the TE is resistant to hydrolysis (Yano et al. 2000; Shiau et al. 2006). The other

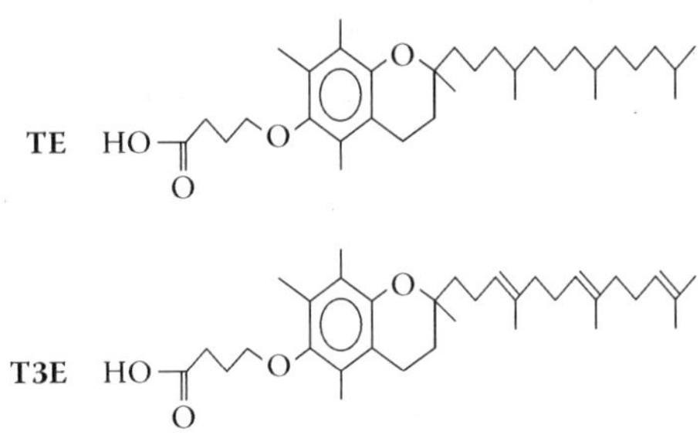

FIGURE 14.1 Structure of TE and T3E.

effective alternative strategy to enhance pro-apoptotic activity of alpha-TOS is by replacement of the ester bond by an amide bond (Tomic-Vatic et al. 2005). Due to the well established fact that anilinic amides are much less prone to hydrolysis than the corresponding phenolic esters, introducing an amide bond in place of the ester bond is reasonable. Furthermore, several nonspecific esterases exist in the intestinal mucosal cells and in the blood, whereas peptidase exhibit a much narrower specificity, thus the replacement by an amide bond is rational to enhance bioavailability of alpha-tocopherol analogues (Neuzil et al. 2007). This rationale is further evidenced by pro-drugs with an amide linkage, which are more stable in the intestine and blood than their corresponding ester derivatives (Sugawara et al. 2000).

14.2.3 Molecular Mechanism of Negative Growth Control in Tumor Cells by Alpha-TOS and TE

Mitochondria are organelles essential for life and death (Newmeyer and Ferguson, 2003). They are major sources of cellular energy in the form of ATP as well as being involved in a number of intricate and regulated processes leading to apoptosis. The precise mechanisms whereby mitochondria provide several signal molecules and mediators provoking the transition of cancer cells to apoptogenic stages are not known in detail. Even so, an increasing number of anticancer drugs are being discovered that induce apoptosis by targeting mitochondria. Such agents, called mitocans, destabilize mitochondria, thereby causing the cytosolic release of apoptogenic factors (Neuzil et al. 2006; Green and Reed, 1998). Mitochondria provide beneficial targets by which one can selectively kill cancer cells, with the advantage of limited side effects on normal cells. This is because the predominant mechanism of the selective effect whereby mitochondria-targeted anticancer drugs kill cancer cells relies on the ability of the drugs (mitocans) to disrupt the energy-producing systems (mitochondria) of cancer cells and the activation of the mitochondria-dependent death signaling pathways (Neuzil et al. 2006). Compounds that are classed as mitocans include those that affect mitochondria-associated activities such as hexokinase inhibition, activation of the mitochondrial permeability transition pore, inhibition of Bcl-2 anti-apoptotic proteins, and blocking of the electron transport/respiratory chain.

One group of mitocans includes redox-silent analogues of vitamin E, epitomized by alpha-TOS (Neuzil et al. 2004). This agent has been shown to selectively kill malignant cells at concentrations nontoxic to normal cells and tissues (Neuzil et al. 2001) and regardless of whether the cells contain mutations in key tumor suppressor genes, such as p53 (Weber et al. 2002). The generally higher levels of esterases in normal cells such as hepatocytes cleaves alpha-TOS to produce tocopherol (Don and Hogg, 2004), leading to less toxicity of this analogue on normal cells.

Another reason for the cancer cell-specific toxicity of alpha-TOS is the accumulation of reactive oxygen species (ROS) in cancer cells compared with normal cells (Wang et al. 2005), mainly due to fewer antioxidant defenses in cancer cells than in normal cells (Neuzil et al. 2006). The accumulation of ROS in cancer cells by alpha-TOS triggers a mitochondria-induced cascade of apoptotic procedure (Neuzil et al. 2006). Complex II (succinate-ubiquinone oxidoreductase) of the mitochondrial redox chain, in particular the ubiquinone (UbQ)-binding site, has been determined as an important molecular target of alpha-TOS (Neuzil et al. 2006). Thus, blocking electron transfer along the mitochondrial redox chain by alpha-TOS displacing UbQ, leads to electrons recombining with molecular oxygen to yield ROS. In the occurrence of mitochondria-triggered apoptosis, ROS most likely play two major roles in mitochondrial translocation of Bax and cytosolic mobilization of Cytochrome (Cyt) c.

In normal cells, monomeric Bax is located predominantly in the cytoplasm, with the C-terminal mitochondrial docking motif hidden due to its conformation. ROS production causes dimerization of Bax in the cytosol by generating disulfide bridges between critical cysteine residues as a product of the initial mitochondrial events in intrinsic apoptogenic signaling (D'Alessio et al. 2005). Then, Bax moves to the mitochondrial outer membrane (MOM), where Bax dimers aggregate to form a transmembrane channel. (Degli-Esposti and Dive, 2003). Several domains within the Bax molecule are critical for Bax oligomerization and movement to the MOM, where Bax dimers associate into tetramers and octamers and form a trans-membrane channel to pass through larger molecules, such as Cyt c (Antonsson et al. 2001). Cyt c is anchored to the mitochondrial inner membrane by its affinity for the mitochondria-specific phospholipids cardiolipin (CL), and the binding is disrupted upon oxidation of CL by ROS derived from oxidative phosphorylation complexes in mitochondria (Petrosillo et al. 2001). That is, alpha-TOS-generated ROS lead to CL oxidation and subsequent Cyt c detachment from the phospholipid, followed by cytoplasmic re-localization of Cyt c via Bax channels (Zha et al. 1996). This cytosolic mobilization of Cyt c is a trigger for mitochondria-dependent apoptosis (Ottonello et al. 2002).

In addition to these events, inactivation of Bcl-2 and Bcl-xL-dependent antiapoptotic effects is required for mitochondria-initiated apoptosis by alpha-TOS. Since Bcl-2 and Bcl-xL contain BH3 binding domains and bind Bax via the Bax BH3 domain (Perier et al. 2005), they exert their anti-apoptotic activity by diverting Bax and preventing it from forming MOM channels. Alpha-TOS can bind to the BH3 domains of Bcl-2 and Bcl-xL (Shiau et al. 2006), and this binding allows for the free Bax pool to be increased. As a result, Bax dimerization increases, promoting formation of MOM channels and mitochondria-initiated apoptosis (Figure 14.2).

In addition to the mitochondria-induced cell death pathway, alpha-TOS suppresses the activity of the extrinsic cell death pathway based on the activation of cell surface death receptors (DRs) (Yu et al. 1999). DRs such as Fas (tumor necrosis factor receptor) are constitutively expressed on the surface of mammalian cells, and impairing the receptor systems endows some of malignant cells with resistance to DRs-induced apoptosis (Strivastava, 2001). On the other hand, alpha-TOS changes

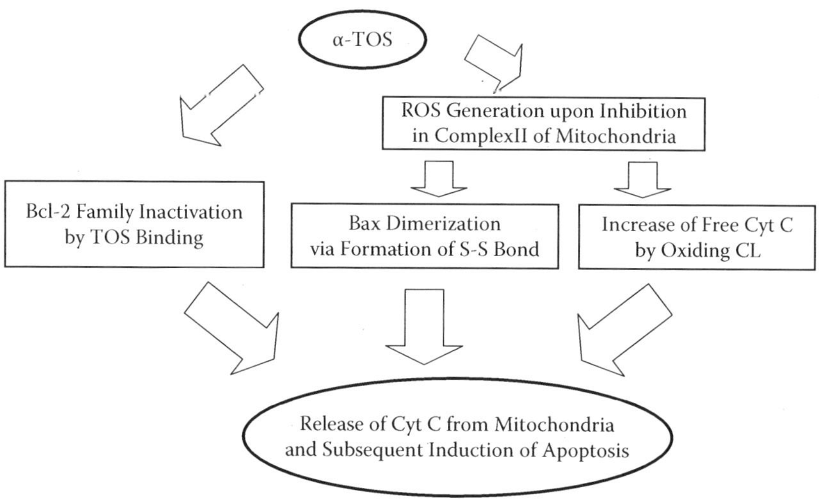

FIGURE 14.2 Molecular mechanism of mitochondria-dependent apoptosis by α-TOS.

Fas-resistant type to sensitive type in breast cancer cells via mobilization of the cytosolic Fas protein to the cell surface (Turley et al. 1997b). In a similar study, alpha-TOS enhances expression of Fas, the Fas-associated death domain, and caspase-8 in gastric cancer cells, whereas Fas antisense oligonucleotide inhibits expression of the Fas-associated death domain protein and decreases caspase-8 activity (Wu et al. 2002). Other than Fas, TNF-related apoptosis-inducing ligand (TRAIL) is a key molecule in the extrinsic cell death pathway. TRAIL is largely selective for malignant cells, whereas the Fas ligand is toxic to normal cells (French and Tschopp, 1999). Additionally, cancer cells escape from TRAIL-dependent cell death by altering the balance between TRAIL receptors and the nonapoptogenic decoy receptors (Buchsbaum et al. 2006). Thus, TRAIL-dependent cell death signaling has emerged as a potential antitumor therapeutic target. Alpha-TOS sensitizes the resistant mesothelioma (MM) and osteosarcoma cells to TRAIL (Tomasetti et al. 2004). On the contrary, alpha-TOS has antagonistic effect on TRAIL-induced cell death in non-malignant MM cells (Tomasetti et al. 2004).

This selective cytotoxic effect of alpha-TOS depends on several related events. Alpha-TOS induces expression and activation of p53, which in turn induces expression of TRAIL receptor 1 (DR4) and TRAIL receptor 2 (DR5) without modulation of expression of the decoy receptors in MM cells (Tomasetti et al. 2004; Tomasetti et al. 2006). Since MM cells have the overexpression of caspase-8 inhibitor FLIP, exogenous TRAIL is ineffective to induce apoptosis in the MM cells irrespective of expression of DR4 and DR5 (Rippo et al. 2004). Alpha-TOS also inhibits the induction of FLIP via the suppression of NF-kappabeta-dependent trans-activation (Kreuz et al. 2001). As a result, the alteration by alpha-TOS contributes to a shift in the balance between anti-apoptotic and pro-apoptotic signals in favor of the latter, triggering apoptotic signaling. Overall, combination of activation in the mitochondria-induced cell death pathway and the extrinsic cell death pathway is associated with potential apoptotic effect of alpha-TOS in cancer cells.

Cell cycle progression is largely regulated by signal pathways that link the cell cycle machinery to the transcription apparatus. Of these factors, E2F, particularly E2F-1, functions to enhance cell growth by advancing quiescence cells through G1 into S phase (Pietenpol et al. 2002). Typically, E2F-1 activity is inhibited during G1 by binding with the dephosphorylated RB susceptibility gene product (Dyson, 1998). Alpha-TOS induces growth suppression and G1 arrest of cancer cells via negative regulation of E2F-1 transcription activity, and this negative effect depends on reduction of E2F-1 protein level as well as the protein phosphorylated level (Turley et al. 1997a). E2F-1 acts as a central transcription factor required for the expression of Myc and thymidylate synthase, which are necessary for transition from G1 to S phase in cell cycle (Turley et al. 1997a). Thus, the anti-proliferation effect of alpha-TOS is mainly due to the suppression of the E2F-1-dependent transcription activity. TE, another redox-silent analogue of alpha-tocopherol, suppresses abnormal cell proliferation at the promotion stage of lung tumorigenesis in mice, in a similar manner (Yano et al. 2001). In this report, TE significantly inhibits induction of ornithine decarboxylase (ODC), a rate-limiting enzyme of polyamine biosynthesis and subsequent cell proliferation at the promotion stage of lung tumorigenesis in mice treated with carcinogen, and the suppression of ODC depends on the inhibition of Myc-dependent transcription activity via the regulation of E2F-1 activity. Also, other studies have demonstrated that TE has a similar anti-carcinogenic effect with alpha-TOS (Akazawa et al. 2002; Nishikawa et al. 2003; Chang et al. 2007). These reports suggest that TE acts as a potential anticarcinogenic agent *in vivo* as well as *in vitro*, based on similar mechanisms to that of alpha-TOS.

14.3 CANCER THERAPY AND PREVENTION BASED ON NONANTIOXIDATIVE EFFECTS OF TOCOTORIENOLS

14.3.1 Multi-Physiological Effects of Tocotrienols

Structurally, tocotrienols differ from tocopherols by the presence of three transbonds in the hydrocarbon tail. The unsaturated side chain of tocotrienol allows for more efficient penetration into tissues that have saturated fatty layers, such as brain. Comparing the antioxidant efficacy of tocopherols and tocotrienols, the free radical scavenging effects of tocotrienols appear superior due to the better distribution into the fatty layers of the cell membrane (Packer et al. 2001). Indeed, tocotrienols, not tocopherols, administration reduces oxidative damages and extends the mean life span of *Caenorhabditis elegans* (Adachi and Ishii, 2000). Also, based on these unsaturations in the isoprenoid side-chain, tocotrienols have a unique conformation (Sen et al. 2007). Alpha-tocotrienol is very likely much more flexible in the side chain and it puts a greater curvature stress on phospholipids membranes. In fact, tocotrienols possess numerous functions that are not shared by tocopherols (Sen et al. 2006). For example, nanomolar levels of alpha-tocotrienol specifically prevent inducible neurogeneration and protect against stroke by regulating specific mediators of cell death (Sen et al. 2000; Khanna et al. 2005). Micromolar levels of tocotrienols suppress the activity of 3-hydroxy-3-methylglutaryl coenzyme A (HMG-CoA) reductase, the hepatic enzyme responsible for cholesterol synthesis (Chen and Cheng, 2006). Tocopherols do not share the cholesterol-lowering properties of tocotrienols (Qureshi et al. 2002). Furthermore, tocotrienols, but not tocopherols, inhibit both proliferation and tube formation of bovine aortic endothelial cells, indicating that tocotrienols have anti-angiogenic properties (Inokuchi et al. 2003).

14.3.2 Negative Growth Control of Tumor Cells by Tocotrienols

Unlike in the case of the neuroprotection where alpha-tocotrienol is the most potent isoform, there is a consensus that gamma- and delta-tocotrienols are the most potent anticancer agent of all natural existing tocotrienols (Sen et al. 2006). Breast cancer has been most extensively studied in cell culture and rodent *in vivo* models for efficacy of tocotrienols. For example, tocotrienols inhibit the proliferation of estrogen receptor-positive MCF-7 human breast cancer cells, and the IC50 for tocotrienol mixture (TRF), alpha-, gamma- and delta-tocotrienols have been estimated to be 4,6, 2 and 2 (microg/ml), respectively (Guthrie et al. 1997). In contrast, the efficiency of α-tocopherol under the same condition is 20–50 time slower with an IC50 of 125 microg/ml. In addition to estrogen receptor-responsive MCF-7 cells, the difference of sensitivity among tocotrienol isoforms has been observed in estrogen receptor-nonresponsive human breast cancer cells (MDA-MB-435) (Yu et al. 1999). Alpha-, gamma- and delta-tocotrienols induce MDA-MB-435 cells to undergo apoptosis, with concentrations for half-maximal response of 176, 28, and 13 microg/ml, respectively.

14.3.3 Molecular Mechanism of Negative Growth Control in Tumor Cells by Tocotrienols

As mentioned, tocotrienols decrease the level of serum total cholesterol and LDL cholesterol and control the risk of coronary heart disease in hypercholesterolemic humans (Qureshi et al. 2002). Mechanistic evidence on the cholesterol-lowering effect of tocotrienols is becoming clear, and one main mechanism is based on the effect that tocotrienols influence mevalonate pathway in mammalian cells by posttranscriptional suppression of HMG-CoA reductase, mainly due to regulation of degradation of the reductase protein (Song and DeBose-Boyd, 2006). Additionally, HMG-CoA reductase plays a key role in controlling cell proliferation by generating prenyl intermediates, particularly farnesyl and geranyl-geranyl moieties, so the up-regulation of the enzyme in tumors finally stimulates cell proliferation via the increase of prenylation in Ras family molecules (Singh et al. 2003). In normal liver, HMG-CoA reductase has resistance to sterol feedback regulation, whereas the reductase in tumor tissues retains sensitivity to the posttranscriptional regulation (Sen et al. 2007). As a consequence, tocotrienols are effective in suppressing mevalonate synthesis, leading to depletion of farnesyl pyrophosphate and geranylgeranyl pyrophosphate, which are incorporated posttranslationally into growth control-associated proteins such as Ras. Thus, in addition to their effects in lowering cholesterol, tocotrienols are also effective therapeutic agents for treating tumors having activation of Ras family molecule-dependent signal pathways.

Molecular mechanisms by which tocotrienols selectively kill breast cancer cells are also being studied characterized. TRF or gamma-tocotrienol treatment increases intracellular activity and levels of caspase-8 and -3 but not caspase-9, and treatment with specific caspase-8 or -3 inhibitors, but not caspase-9 inhibitor, completely blocked the tocotrienol-induced apoptosis in mammary cancer cells, indicating that the tocotrienol-triggered apoptosis depends on the activation of caspase-8 signal pathway but not that of caspase-9 pathway (Shah et al. 2003). However, the tocotrienol-induced apoptosis dose not relate to death receptor apoptotic signaling in mammary cancer cells (Shah and Sylvester, 2004). In this study, gamma-tocotrienol significantly suppresses the activity of phosphatidylinositol 3-kinase (PI3K)-dependent kinase 1(PKD1) and Akt. Moreover, tocotrienol reduces the level of FLIP, an antiapoptotic protein that inhibits caspase-8 activation. Because stimulation of PI3K/PKD/Akt pathway is associated with increased FLIP expression and cell survival, the tocotrienol-induced caspase-8 activation and apoptosis in the cancer cells appears to result from the suppression of the PI3K/PKD/Akt signal pathway, and subsequent reduction in FLIP expression (Sylvester and Shah, 2005). Alternatively, another molecular mechanism on the induction of apoptosis by gamma-tocotrienol, NF-kappabeta pathway has been proposed (Ahn et al. 2007). Gamma-tocotrienol actually abolishes NF-kappabeta activation by several agonist-induced factors, and down-regulates the expressions of NF-kappabeta-regulated gene products associated with molecules such as antiapoptosis (IAP1, IAP2, Bcl-xL, Bcl-2, FLIP, XIAP, Bfl-1/A1, TRAF1, and Survivin), proliferation (cyclin D1, Cox2, and Myc), invasion (MMP-9 and ICAM-1) and angiogenesis (vascular endothelial growth factor). This inhibitory event by gamma-tocotrienol finally leads to potentiation of apoptosis (Ahn et al. 2007). On the other hand, there is still conflicting evidence as to whether mitochondria-initiated cell death signal pathway contributes to the tocotrienol-induced apoptosis in cancer cells (Shah et al. 2003; Takahashi and Loo, 2004).

14.3.4 Antiproliferative Activity of Redox-Silent Tocotrienol Analogue

As mentioned, tocotrienols and tocopherols have the same basic chemical structure characterized by a long phytyl chain attached at position C6 of the chromanol ring, however the phytyl chain in tocopherols is saturated, whereas in tocotrienols it is unsaturated (Kamal-Eldin and Appelqvist, 1996). Tocotrienols posses more potential anticancer properties than tocopherols, possibly due to the difference of the side chain between tocotreinols and tocopherols (Theriault et al. 1999). Moreover, compared with tocopherols, tocotrienols are more quickly taken up by the cancer cells, suggesting that this can be one reason that tocotrienols are so effective in selectively killing them (Sakai et al. 2004). These reports strongly indicate that redox-silent tocotrienol analogues have more potential activity than tocopherol ones as anticarcinogenic agents. However, there are still few reports on this aspect of tocotrienols.

A recent report clearly demonstrated that a redox-silent derivative of alpha-tocotrienol, 6-*O*-carboxypropyl-alpha-tocotreinol (T3E; Figure 14.1) shows a potent cytotoxic effect against human lung cancer cells, compared with alpha-tocotrienol and TE (Yano et al. 2005). This report shows beneficial aspects of T3E as an anticarcinogenic agent. Lung cancer cell (A549) used in this study has constitutive activation of Ras protein based on a mutation in K-*ras* gene, and the up-regulation of Ras-dependent signaling caused by the constitutive activation contributes to cell proliferation and survival in the cancer cells (Kato-Stankiewicz et al. 2002). As expected, T3E suppresses the activation of Ras family molecules (Ras and Rho) via the inhibition of prenylation in the molecules, leading to G1 arrest in cell cycle via the inhibition of cyclin D and subsequently induced cell death based on the reduction of Bcl-xL level and disruption of actin cytoskeleton (Yano et al. 2005). Additionally, T3E has strong cytotoxic effect against the lung cancer cells but no toxic effect against non-tumorigenic cells (Yano et al. 2005). Because the ether bond in T3E is not subjected to enzymatic hydrolysis *in vivo*, the anticancer property of T3E seems to be effective in clinical applications. Overall, T3E is a better redox-silent analogue of vitamin E than other redox-silent analogues of vitamin E such as TE.

14.3.5 A New Aspect of Tocotrienol-Dependent Anticancer Property

The activation of c-Src activation is absolutely required for occurrence of a neurodegenerative patho-physiological condition, and tocotrienols, especially alpha-tocotrienol, effectively protect against the occurrence of the neurodegenerative condition (Sen et al. 2000). Alpha-tocotrienol suppresses the activation of c-Src in the process of the neurodegeneration at nanomolar levels at which the agent shows no antioxidant property, suggesting that this inhibitory effect is independent of antioxidant property. Src activity in cancers increases several fold compared with that in normal tissues, and the elevation in the Src activity is associated with tumor progression (Lutz et al. 1998; Yonezawa et al. 2005). Furthermore, tumor cells undergo genetic and adaptive changes that allow them to survive and proliferate in hypoxic environments, leading to aggressive tumor behavior, and a key event necessary for the adaptation of the tumor cells is to induce the activation of Src (Harris, 2002). Thus, redox-silent analogues of alpha-tocotrienol such as T3E can be a promising anticancer agent to target Src.

14.4 SUMMARY

We have attempted in this chapter to focus on the current status of redox-silent analogues of alpha-tocopherol and alpha-tocotrienol as promising anticancer agents. Of the redox-silent analogues of vitamin E, alpha-TOS has been extensively studied regarding its characters as an anticancer agent, including the molecular mechanisms. Through these extensive studies, it has been clear that alpha-TOS has some beneficial aspects as an anticancer agent. For instance, alpha-TOS shows selective cytotoxicity against several tumor cells without any influence on nontumorigenic cells and effectively kills malignant tumor cells having severe chemo-resistance against conventional chemotherapeutic agents. However, the ester bond in alpha-TOS is easily cleaved by intestinal esterase, so we cannot expect the anticancer effect of alpha-TOS *in vivo*. To overcome the demerit of the ester bond cleavage, an ether redox-silent analogue of alpha-tocopherol, TE, has been synthesized. Indeed, TE acts as a chemopreventive agent in a mouse carcinogenic model. However, the anticarcinogenic effect of TE is ineffective in malignant tumor cells such as A549 cells. In contrast, an ether redox-silent analogue of alpha-tocotrienol, T3E, kills such malignant tumor cells with much less toxic effect against non-tumorigenic cells. Collectively, redox-silent analogues of tocotrienols such as T3E are promising as new potential anticancer agents compared with redox-silent analogues of tocopherols.

REFERENCES

Adachi, H., N. Ishii. 2000. Effects of tocotrienols on life span and protein carbonylation in Caenorhabditis elegans. *J. Gerontol. A Biol .Sci. Med. 55*, B280–B285.

Ahn, K.S., G. Sethi, K. Krishnan, B.B. 2007. Aggarwal. Gamma-tocotrienol inhibits nuclear factor–kappa-beta signaling pathway through inhibition of receptor-interacting protein and TAK1 leading to suppression of antiapoptotic gene products and potentiation of apoptosis. *J. Biol. Chem. 282*, 809–820.

Akazawa, A., K. Nishikawa, K. Suzuki, R. Asano, I. Kumadaki, H. Satoh, K. Hagiwara, S.J. Shin, T. Yano. Induction of apoptosis in a human breast cancer cell overexpressing ErbB–2 receptor by alpha-tocopheryloxybutyric acid. *Jpn. J. Pharmacol.* 2002, *89*, 417–421.

Antonsson, B., S. Montessuit, B. Sanchez, J.C. Martinou. 2001. Bax is present as a high molecular weight oligomer/complex in the mitochondrial membrane of apoptotic cells. *J. Biol. Chem., 276*,11615–11623.

Arya, P., N. Alibhai, H. Qin, G.W. Burton, G. Batist, S.X. You, M.A. Alaoui-Jamali. 1998. Design and synthesis of analogs of vitamin E: Antiproliferative activity against human breast adenocarcinoma cells. *Bioorg. Med. Chem. Lett., 8*, 2433–2438.

Azzi, A., A. Stocker. 2000. Vitamin E: Non-antioxidant roles. *Prog. Lipid Res., 39*, 231–255.

Azzi, A., R. Ricciarelli, J.M. Zingg. 2002. Non-antioxidant molecular functions of alpha-tocopherol (vitamin E). *FEBS Lett., 519*, 8–10.

Birringer, M., J.H. EyTina, B.A. Salvatore, J. Neuzil. 2003. Vitamin E analogues as inducers of apoptosis: Structure–function relationship. *Br. J. Cancer, 88*, 1948–1955.

Brigelius-Flohé, R., M.G. Traber. 1999. Vitamin E: Function and metabolism. *FASEB J.*, *13*, 1145–1155.

Buchsbaum, D.J., T. Zhou, A.F. Lobuglio. 2006. TRAIL receptor-targeted therapy. *Future Oncol.*, *2*, 493–508.

Chang, E., J. Ni, Y. Yin, C.C. Lin, P. Chang, N.S. James, S.R. Chemler, S. Yeh. 2007. Alpha-vitamin E derivative, RRR-alpha-tocopheryloybutyric acid inhibits the proliferation of prostate cancer cells. *Asia. J. Androl.*, *9*, 31–139.

Chen, C.W., H.H. Cheng. 2006. Rice bran oil diet increases LDL-receptor and HMG-CoA reductase mRNA expressions and insulin sensitivity in rats with streptozotocin/nicotinamide-induced type 2 diabetes. *J. Nutr.*, *136*, 1472–1476.

D'Alessio, M., M. De Nicola, S. Coppola, G. Gualandi, L. Pugliese, C. Cerella, S. Cristofanon, P. Civitareale, M.R. Ciriolo, A. Bergamaschi, A. Magrini, L. Ghibelli. 2005. Oxidative Bax dimerization promotes its translocation to mitochondria independently of apoptosis. *FASEB J.*, *19*, 1504–1506.

Degli-Esposti, M., C. Dive. 2003. Mitochondrial membrane permeabilisation by Bax/Bak. *Biochem. Biophys. Res. Commun.*, *304*, 455–461.

Don, A.S., P.J. Hogg. 2004. Mitochondria as cancer drug targets. *Trends Mol. Med.*, *10*, 372–378.

Dyson, N. 1998. The regulation of E2F by pRB-family proteins. *Genes Dev.*, *12*, 2245–2262.

French, L.E., J. Tschopp. 1999. The TRAIL to selective tumor death. *Nat. Med.*, *5*, 146–147.

Galli, F., A.M. Stabile, M. Betti, C. Conte, A. Pistilli, M. Rende, A. Floridi, A. Azzi. 2004. The effect of alpha- and gamma-tocopherol and their carboxyethyl hydroxychroman metabolites on prostate cancer cell proliferation. *Arch. Biochem. Biophys.*, *423*, 97–102.

Green, D.R., J.C. Reed. 1998. Mitochondria and apoptosis. *Science*, *28*, 11309–11312.

Guthrie, N., A. Gapor, A.F. Chambers, K.K. Carroll. 1997. Inhibition of proliferation of estrogen receptor-negative MDA-MB-435 and -positive MCF-7 human breast cancer cells by palm oil tocotrienols and tamoxifen, alone and in combination. *J Nutr.*, *127*, 544S–548S.

Harris, A.L. 2002. Hypoxia: A key regulatory factor in tumour growth. *Nat. Rev. Cancer*, *2*, 38–47.

Inokuchi, H., H. Hirokane, T. Tsuzuki, K. Nakagawa, M. Igarashi, T. Miyazawa. 2003. Anti-angiogenic activity of tocotrienol. *Biosci. Biotechnol. Biochem.*, *67*, 1623–7.

Kamal-Eldin, A., A.A. Appelqvist. 1996. The chemistry and antioxidant properties of tocopherols and tocotrienols. *Lipids*, *31*, 671–701.

Kato-Stankiewicz, J., I. Hakimi, G. Zhi, J. Zhang, I. Serebriiskii, E. Guo, H. Edamatsu, H. Koide, S. Menon, R. Eckl, S. Sakamuri, Y. Lu, Q.Z. Chen, S. Agarwal, W.R. Baumbach, E.A. Golemis, F. Tamanoi, V. Khazak. 2002. Inhibitors of Ras/Raf-1 interaction identified by two-hybrid screening revert Ras-dependent transformation phenotypes in human cancer cells. *Proc. Natl. Acad. Sci. USA*, *994*, 398–403.

Khanna, S., S. Roy, A. Slivka, T.K. Craft, S. Chaki, C. Rink C, M.A. Notestine, A.C. DeVries, N.L. Parinandi, C.K. Sen. 2005. Neuroprotective properties of the natural vitamin E alpha-tocotrienol. *Stroke* *36*, 2258–2264.

Kogure, K., S. Hama, M. Kisaki, H. Takemasa, A. Tokumura, I. Suzuki, K. Fukuzawa. 2004. Structural characteristic of terminal dicarboxylic moiety required for apoptogenic activity of alpha-tocopheryl esters. *Biochim. Biophys, Acta*, *1672*, 93–99.

Kogure, K., S. Manabe, I. Suzuki, A. Tokumura, K. Fukuzawa. 2005. Cytotoxicity of alpha-tocopheryl succinate, malonate and oxalate in normal and cancer cells *in vitro* and their anticancer effects on mouse melanoma *in vivo*. *J. Nutr. Sci, Vitaminol (Tokyo)*, *51*, 392–397.

Kozin, S.V., P. Shkarin, L.E. Gerweck. 2001. The cell transmembrane pH gradient in tumors enhances cytotoxicity of specific weak acid chemotherapeutics. *Cancer Res.*, *61*, 4740–4743.

Kreuz, S., D. Siegmund, P. Scheurich, H. Wajant. 2001. NF-kappabeta inducers upregulate cFLIP, a cycloheximide-sensitive inhibitor of death receptor signaling. *Mol. Cell Biol.*, *21*, 3964–3973.

Lutz, M.P., I.B. Esser, B.B. Flossmann-Kast, R. Vogelmann, H. Luhrs, H. Friess, M.W. Buchler, G. Adler. 1998. Overexpression and activation of the tyrosine kinase Src in human pancreatic carcinoma. *Biochem. Biophys. Res, Commun.*, *243*, 503–508.

Neuzil, J., T. Weber, A. Schroder, M. Lu, G. Ostermann, N. Gellert, G.C. Maybe, B. Olejnicka, A. Nègre-Salvayre, M. Stícha, R.J. Coffey, C. Weber. 2001. Induction of cancer cell apoptosis by alpha-tocopheryl succinate: Molecular pathways and structural requirements. *FASEB J.*, *15*, 403–415.

Neuzil, J., M. Tomasetti, A.S. Mellick, R. Alleva, B.A. Salvatore, M. Birringer, M.W. Fariss. 2004. Vitamin E analogues: A new class of inducers of apoptosis with selective anticancer effects. *Curr. Cancer Drug Targets*, *4*, 355–372.

Neuzil, J., X.F. Wang, L.F. Dong, P. Low, S.J. Ralph. 2006. Molecular mechanism of "mitocan"-induced apoptosis in cancer cells epitomizes the multiple roles of reactive oxygen species and Bcl-2 family proteins. *FEBS Lett.*, *580*, 5125–5129.

Neuzil, J., M. Tomasetti, Y. Zhao, L.F. Dong, M. Birringer, X.F. Wang, P. Low, K. Wu, B.A. Salvatore, S.J. Ralph. 2007. Vitamin E analogs, a novel group of "mitocans," as anticancer agents: The importance of being redox silent. *Mol. Pharmacol.*, *71*, 1185–99.

Newmeyer, D.D., S. Ferguson-Miller. 2003. Mitochondria: Releasing power for life and unleashing the machineries of death. *Cell*, *112*, 481–490.

Nishikawa, K., H. Satoh, A. Hirai, K. Suzuzki, R. Asano, I. Kumadaki, K. Hagiwara, T. Yano. 2003. Alpha-Tocopheryloxybutyric acid enhances necrotic cell death in breast cancer cells treated with chemotherapy agent. *Cancer Lett.*, *201*, 51–56.

Ottonello, L., G. Frumento, N. Arduino, M. Bertolotto, P. Dapino, M. Mancini, F. Dallegri. 2002. Differential regulation of spontaneous and immune complex-induced neutrophil apoptosis by proinflammatory cytokines. Role of oxidants, Bax and caspase-3. *J. Leukoc. Biol.*, *72*, 125–132.

Packer, L., S.U. Weber, Rimbach, G. 2001. Molecular aspects of alpha-tocotrienol antixoidantaction and cell signaling. *J.Nutr.*, *131*, 369S–373S.

Perier, C., K. Tieu, C. Guegan, C. Caspersen, V. Jackson-Lewis, V. Carelli, A. Martinuzzi, M. Hirano, S. Przedborski, M. Vila. 2005. Complex I deficiency primes Bax-dependent neuronal apoptosis through mitochondrial oxidative damage. *Proc. Natl. Acad. Sci. USA*, *102*, 19126–19131.

Petrosillo, G., F.M. Ruggiero, M. Pistolese, G. Paradies. 2001. Reactive oxygen species generated from the mitochondrial electron transport chain induce cytochrome c dissociation from beef-heart submitochondrial particles via cardiolipin peroxidation. Possible role in the apoptosis. *FEBS Lett.*, *509*, 435–438.

Pham, D.Q., R. Plakogiannis. 2005. Vitamin E supplementation in cardiovascular disease and cancer prevention: Part 1. *Ann. Pharmacother.*, *39*, 1870–1878.

Pietenpol, J.A., Z.A. Stewart. 2002. Cell cycle checkpoint signaling: Cell cycle arrest versus apoptosis. *Toxicology*, *181–182*, 475–481.

Qureshi, A.A., S.A. Sami, W.A. Salser, F.A. Khan. 2002. Dose-dependent suppression of serum cholesterol by tocotrienol-rich fraction (TRF25) of rice bran in hypercholesterolemic humans. *Atherosclerosis*, *161*, 199–207.

Rimbach, G., A.M. Minihane, J. Majewicz, A. Fischer, J. Pallauf, F. Virgli, P.D. Weinberg. 2002. Regulation of cell signaling by vitamin E. *Proc. Nutr. Soc.*, *61*, 415–425.

Rippo, M.R., S. Moretti, S. Vescovi, M. Tomasetti, S. Orecchia, G. Amici, A. Catalano, A. Procopio. 2004. FLIP overexpression inhibits death receptor-induced apoptosis in malignant mesothelial cells. *Oncogene*, *23*, 7753–7760.

Sakai, M., M. Okabe, M. Yamasaki, H. Tachibana, K. 2004. Yamada. Induction of apoptosis by tocotrienol in rat hepatoma dRLh-84 cells. *Anticancer Res.*, *24*, 1683–1688.

Sen, C.K., S. Khanna, S. Roy, L. Packer. 2000. Molecular basis of vitamin E action: Tocotrienol potently inhibits glutamate-induced pp60(c-Src) kinase activation and death of HT4 neuronal cells. *J. Biol. Chem.*, *275*, 13049S–13055S.

Sen, C.K., S. Khanna, S. Roy. 2006. Tocotrienols: Vitamin E beyond tocopherols. *Life Sci.*, *78*, 2088–2098.

Sen, C.K., S. Khanna, S. Roy. 2007. Tocotrienols in health and disease: The other half of the natural vitamin E family. *Mol. Aspects Med.*, *28*, 692–728.

Shah, S., A. Gapor, P.W. Sylvester. 2003. Role of caspase-8 activation in mediating vitamin E-induced apoptosis in murine mammary cancer cells. *Nutr. Cancer*, *45*, 236–246.

Shah, S., P.W. Sylvester. 2004. Tocotrienol-induced caspase-8 activation is unrelated to death receptor apoptotic signaling in neoplastic mammary epithelial cells. *Exp. Biol. Med. (Maywood)*, *229*, 745–755.

Shiau, C.W., J.W. Huang, D.S. Wang, J.R. Weng, C.C. Yang, C.H. Lin, C. Li, C.S. Chen. 2006. Alpha-tocopheryl succinate induces apoptosis in prostate cancer cells in part through inhibition of Bcl-xL/Bcl-2 function. J. *Biol. Chem.*, *281*, 11819–11825.

Shun, M.C., W. Yu, A. Gapor, R. Parsons, J. Atkinson, B.G. Sanders, K. Kline. 2004. Pro-apoptotic mechanisms of action of a novel vitamin E analog (alpha-TEA) and a naturally occurring form of vitamin E (delta-tocotrienol) in MDA-MB-435 human breast cancer cells. *Nutr. Cancer*, *48*, 95–105.

Singh, R.P., R. Kumar, N. Kapur. 2003. Molecular regulation of cholesterol biosynthesis: Implications in carcinogenesis. *J. Environ. Pathol. Toxicol. Oncol.*, *22*, 75–92.

Song, B.L., R.A. DeBose-Boyd. 2006. Insig-dependent ubiquitination and degradation of 3-hydroxy-3-methylglutaryl coenzyme a reductase stimulated by delta- and gamma-tocotrienols. *J. Biol. Chem.*, *281*, 25054–25061.

Srivastava, R.K. 2001. TRAIL/Apo-2L: Mechanisms and clinical applications in cancer. *Neoplasia*, *3*, 535–546.

Sugawara, M., W. Huang, Y.J. Fei, F.H. Leibach, V. Ganapathy, M.E. Ganapathy. 2000. Transport of valganciclovir, a ganciclovir prodrug, via peptide transporters PEPT1 and PEPT2. *J. Pharm. Sci.*, *89*, 781–789.

Sylvester, P.W., B.S. McIntyre, A. Gapor, K.P. Briski. 2001. Vitamin E inhibition of normal mammary epithelial cell growth is associated with a reduction in protein kinase C(alpha) activation. *Cell Prolif.*, *34*, 347–357.

Sylvester, P.W., S. Shah. 2005. Intracellular mechanisms mediating tocotrienol-induced apoptosis in neoplastic mammary epithelial cells. *Asia Pac. J. Clin. Nutr.*, *14*, 366–373.

Tada, H, H. Ishii, S. Isogai. 1997. Protective effect of D-alpha-tocopherol on the function of human mesangial cells exposed to high glucose concentrations. *Metabolism*, *46*, 779–784.

Takahashi, K., G. Loo. 2004. Disruption of mitochondria during tocotrienol-induced apoptosis in MDA-MB-231 human breast cancer cells. *Biochem. Pharmacol.*, *67*, 315–324.

Theriault, A., J.T. Chao, Q. Wang, A. Gapor, K. Adeli. 1999. Tocotrienol: A review of its therapeutic potential. *Clin. Biochem.*, *32*, 309–319.

Tomasetti, M., M.R. Rippo, R. Alleva, S. Moretti, L. Andera, J. Neuzil, A. Procopio. 2004. Alpha-tocopheryl succinate and TRAIL selectively synergise in induction of apoptosis in human malignant mesothelioma cells. *Br. J. Cancer*, *90*, 1644–1653.

Tomasetti, M., L. Andera, R. Alleva, B. Borghi, J. Neuzil, A. Procopio. 2006. Alpha-tocopheryl succinate induces DR4 and DR5 expression by a p53–dependent route: Implication for sensitisation of resistant cancer cells to TRAIL apoptosis. *FEBS Lett.*, *580*, 1925–31.

Tomic-Vatic, A., J.H. EyTina, J.M. Chapmann, E. Mahdavian, J. Neuzil, B.A. Salvatore. 2005. Vitamin E amides, a new class of vitamin E analogues with enhanced pro–apoptotic activity. *Int. J. Cancer*, *117*, 181–193.

Turley, J.M., T. Fu, F.W. Ruscetti, J.A. Mikovits, D.C. Bertolette. M.C. Birchenall-Roberts. 1997a. Vitamin E succinate induces Fas–mediated apoptosis in estrogen receptor-negative human breast cancer cells. *Cancer Res.*, *57*, 881–890.

Turley, J.M., F.W. Ruscetti, S.J. Kim, T. Fu, F.V. Gou, M.C. Birchenall-Roberts. 1997b. Vitamin E succinate inhibits proliferation of BT-20 human breast cancer cells: Increased binding of cyclin A negatively regulates E2F transactivation activity. *Cancer Res.*, *57*, 2668–2675.

Vraka, P.S., C. Drouza, M.P. Rikkou, A.D. Odysseos, A.D. Keramidas. 2006. Synthesis and study of the cancer cell growth inhibitory properties of alpha-, gamma-tocopheryl and gamma-tocotrienyl 2-phenylselenyl succinates. *Bioorg. Med. Chem.*, *14*, 2684–2696.

Wang, X.F., P.K. Witting, B.A. Salvatore, J. Neuzil. 2005. Vitamin E analogs trigger apoptosis in HER2/erbB2-overexpressing breast cancer cells by signaling via the mitochondrial pathway. *Biochem. Biophys. Res. Commun.*, *326*, 282–289.

Weber, T., M. Lu, L. Andera, H. Lahm, N. Gellert, M.W. Fariss, V. Korinek, W. Sattler, D.S. Ucker, A. Terman, A. Schroder, W. Erl, U.T. Brunk, R.J. Coffey, C. Weber, J. Neuzil. 2002. Vitamin E succinate is a potent novel antineoplastic agent with high selectivity and cooperativity with tumor necrosis factor-related apoptosis-inducing ligand (Apo2 ligand) *in vivo*. *Clin. Cancer Res.*, *8*, 863–89.

Wu, K., Y. Zhao, B.H. Liu, Y. Li, F. Liu, J. Guo, W.P. Yu. 2002. RRR-alpha-tocopheryl succinate inhibits human gastric cancer SGC-7901 cell growth by inducing apoptosis and DNA synthesis arrest. *World J. Gastroenterol.*, *8*, 26–30.

Wu, Y., K. Zu, J. Ni, S. Yeh, D. Kasi, N.S. James, S. Chemler, C. Ip. 2004. Cellular and molecular effects of alpha-tocopheryloxybutyrate: Lessons for the design of vitamin E analog for cancer prevention. *Anticancer Res.*, *24*, 3795–3802.

Yano, T., S. Yajima, K. Hagiwara, I. Kumadaki, Y. Yano, S. Otani, M. Uchida, T. Ichikawa. 2000. Vitamin E inhibits cell proliferation and the activation of extracellular signal-regulated kinase during the promotion phase of lung tumorigenesis irrespective of antioxidant effect. *Carcinogenesis*, *21*, 2129–2133.

Yano, T., Y. Yano, S. Yajima, I. Kumadaki, T. Ichikawa, S. Otani, K. Hagiwara. 2001. The suppression of ornithine decarboxylase expression and cell proliferation at the promotion stage of lung tumorigenesis in mice by alpha-tocopheryloxybutyric acid. *Biochem. Pharmacol.*, *61*, 1177–1181.

Yano, Y., H. Satoh, K. Fukumoto, I. Kumadaki, T. Ichikawa, K. Yamada, K. Hagiwara, T. Yano. 2005. Induction of cytotoxicity in human lung adenocarcinoma cells by 6-O-carboxypropyl–alpha-tocotrienol, a redox-silent derivative of alpha-tocotrienol. *Int. J. Cancer.*, *115*, 839–846.

Yonezawa, Y., Y. Nagashima, H. Sato, N. Virgona, K. Fukumoto, S. Shirai, H. Hagiwara, T. Seki, T. Ariga, H.Senba, K. Suzuki, R. Asano, K. Hagiwara, T. Yano. 2005. Contribution of the Src family of kinases to the appearance of malignant phenotypes in renal cancer cells. *Mol Carcinog.*, *43*, 188–197.

Yu, W., K. Israel, Q.Y. Liao, C.M. Aldaz, B.G. Sanders, K. Kline. 1999. Vitamin E succinate (VES) induces Fas sensitivity in human breast cancer cells: Role for Mr 43,000 Fas in VES-triggered apoptosis. *Cancer Res.*, *59*, 953–961.

Zha, H., C. Aime–Sempe, T. Sato, J.C. Reed. 1996. Proapoptotic protein Bax heterodimerizes with Bcl-2 and homodimerizes with Bax via a novel domain (BH3) distinct from BH1 and BH2. *J. Biol. Chem.*, *271*, 7440–7444.

Zingg, J.M, A. Azzi. 2004. Non-antioxidant activities of vitamin E. *Cur. Med. Chem.*, *11*, 1113–1133.

15 Role of the Mevalonate Pathway in Tocotrienol-Mediated Tumor Suppression

Huanbiao Mo and Charles E. Elson

CONTENTS

15.1 INTRODUCTION

The tocotrienols, at physiologically attainable concentrations, arrest the *in vitro* growth of cell lines derived from broadly diverse human and animal tumors and, at several fold higher concentrations, the growth of physiologically normal cells. Preclinical studies demonstrate the suppression of the growth of implanted tumors, absent an impact on the growth of the host and of carcinogenesis initiated by diverse carcinogens. The tocotrienol-mediated suppression of cell growth, an action involving both the accumulation of cells in the G1 phase of the cell cycle and the initiation of apoptosis, is reversed by supplemental mevalonate or specific mevalonate-derived products. It therefore appears reasonable to attribute the chemoprotective actions of the tocotrienols to the suppression of 3-hydroxy-3-methylglutaryl coenzyme A reductase activity, a dysregulated activity in tumor cells that retains sensitivity to the posttranscriptional down regulation triggered by the tocotrienols. In support of this reasoning, parallels are drawn between the impacts of statins and tocotrienols on components of signaling networks that modulate cell cycle, anti-apoptotic and apoptotic activities.

15.2 TOCOTRIENOLS SUPPRESS THE GROWTH OF TUMOR CELLS

Stemming from the seminal findings of Komiyama et al.. (Komiyama et al., 1989) the efficacy of the tocotrienols in suppressing the growth of cultured cells has been demonstrated in cells isolated from breast (Birringer et al., 2003; Guthrie et al., 1997a; Guthrie et al., 1997b; McIntyre et al., 2000a; Mo and Elson, 1999; Nesaretnam et al., 1995; Nesaretnam et al., 1998; Nesaretnam et al., 2000; Shah et al., 2003; Shah and Sylvester, 2004; Shah and Sylvester, 2005a; Shah and Sylvester, 2005b; Shun et al., 2004; Sylvester et al., 2005; Sylvester and Shah, 2005a, Sylvester and Shah, 2005b; Takahashi and, Loo, 2004; Yu et al., 1999), liver (Har and Keong, 2005; Sakai et al., 2004; Sakai et al., 2006; Wada et al., 2005), prostate (Conte et al., 2004; McAnally et al., 2007; Mo and Elson, 2004; Odysseos et al., 2002; Srivastava et al., 2006), skin (He et al.,1997; McAnally et al., 2007; Mo and Elson,1999), colon (Eitsuka et al., 2006; Mo and Elson,1999), blood (Ahn et al., 2007; Mo and Elson,1999), lung (Komiyama et al., 1989; McAnally et al., 2007), lymph gland (Birringer et al., 2003), cervix (Komiyama et al.,1989) and nerve (Birringer et al., 2003) tumors. Further studies revealed the potencies of γ- and δ-tocotrienol relative to that of the less potent α-tocotrienol (Conte et al., 2004; Guthrie et al., 1997b; Inokuchi et al., 2003; McIntyre et al., 2000a; McIntyre et al., 2000b; Yu et al., 1999). The tocopherols on the other hand have little impact on the growth of tumor cells (Birringer et al., 2003; Har and Keong 2005; Jiang et al., 2004; Komiyama et al., 1989; McIntyre et al., 2000a; Sylvester and Shah, 2005b). Findings pointing to the lack of impact of α-tocopherol on the growth of tumor cells suggest that an action other than an antioxidant activity underlies the tumor-suppressive action of the tocotrienols (Neuzil et al., 2007; Yano et al., 2005). When evaluated using estrogen receptor positive MCF7 human breast cancer cells, the 50% inhibitory concentrations (IC50s) of α-tocotrienol, γ-tocotrienol and δ-tocotrienol were 14, 5 and 5 μ mol/L respectively (Guthrie et al., 1997b). Similar degrees of potency were reported for neoplastic –SA and highly malignant +SA mouse mammary epithelial cells. IC50 values for α-tocotrienol, γ-tocotrienol and δ-tocotrienol for the neoplastic cells are 7, 5 and 4 μ mol/L respectively and for highly malignant cells, 5, 4 and 3 μ mol/L respectively (McIntyre et al., 2000a). In highly malignant B16F10 melanoma cells, the IC50 values for α-tocotrienol, γ-tocotrienol and δ-tocotrienol were 110, 20 and 10 μ mol/L (He et al., 1997). The IC50 values for γ- and δ-tocotrienol in HepG2 cells were 27.4 and 9.6 μ mol/L (Wada et al., 2005). The tocotrienols suppressed the growth of human colorectal carcinoma cells in the order α- < γ- < β- < δ- with the IC50 values for the latter pair estimated to fall around 47 and 24 μ mol/L (Eitsuka et al., 2006). Studies evaluating the potency of γ-tocotrienol found substantially different IC50 values depending on the human cell line examined. The IC50 values reported for human tumor cell lines (Mo and Elson, 1999; Nesaretnam et al., 1998; Takahashi and, Loo, 2004) fall between 4 [HL-60 (Mo and Elson, 1999)] and 100 [PC-3, LNCAP (Odysseos et al., 2002)] μ mol/L. Values for MCF7 (Mo and Elson, 1999; Nesaretnam et al., 1998; Yu et al., 1999), DU145 (McAnally et al., 2007; Odysseos et al., 2002), PC3 (Odysseos et al., 2002), MDA-MB-23 (Nesaretnam et al., 1998), MDA-MB-435 (Guthrie et al., 1997b) and HepG2 (Wada et al., 2005) cells fall between 6.6 and 75 μ mol/L.

Of critical importance are findings that normal cells have far lower sensitivity than equivalent malignant cells to the growth-suppressive action of the tocotrienols (Goh et al., 1994; Har and Keong, 2005; McIntyre et al., 2000a; McIntyre et al., 2000b; Sakai et al., 2004; Shah and Sylvester, 2005a; Shun et al., 2004; Srivastava and Gupta, 2006; Sylvester et al., 2005; Sylvester and Shah, 2005a; Sylvester and Shah, 2005b). For example, significant reductions in the growth of normal mouse mammary epithelial cells were attained with 50–60 and 8–14 μ mol/L α-tocotrienol and δ-tocotrienol, respectively (McIntyre et al., 2000b) whereas the IC50 values determined for highly malignant mammary epithelial cells were several fold lower (McIntyre et al., 2000a).

The lower end of the aforementioned IC50 values (4-6.6 μ mol/L) for tocotrienols in suppressing tumor cell proliferation is physiologically attainable. The attainment of similar levels in human plasma has been reported. Human subjects consuming a tocol blend consisting of 15–20% α-tocopherol, 12–15% α-tocotrienol, 35–40% γ-tocotrienol and 25–30% δ-tocotrienol (200 mg/d, 4 weeks) had plasma levels of the respective tocols at 13.21±0.76, 8.14±0.68, 7.46±0.73 and 5.91±0.67 μ mol/L (Quershi et al., 1991), results confirmed by Yap et al. (2001). In a later study, subjects were given 400 mg of a tocol blend consisting of 19% α-tocopherol, 29% γ-tocopherol, 23% α-tocotrienol, 29% δ-tocotrienol and 1% γ-tocotrienol, plasma levels of the tocols peaked at 4 hr with 7.51±0.28 μ mol/L α-tocopherol, 3.83±0.58 μ mol/L γ-tocopherol, 2.94±0.68 μ mol/L α-tocotrienol, 3.16±0.96 μ mol/L δ-tocotrienol and 1.41±0.39 μ mol/L γ-tocotrienol (Khosla et al., 2006). Tocotrienols are more enriched in lymph, adipose tissues and skin (Hayes et al., 1993; Traber et al., 1998; Ikeda et al., 2000; Podda et al., 1996).

Similar blood levels were attained in animal studies. Following intragastric perfusion of a 200 mg tocol blend consisting of 21% α-tocopherol, 1% β-tocopherol, 1% γ-tocopherol, 1% δ-tocopherol, 21% α-tocotrienol, 4% β-tocotrienol, 37% γ-tocotrienol and 9% δ-tocotrienol, the levels of α- and γ-tocotrienol in the serum of Sprague-Dawley rats peaked at 1.2 and 0.6 μ mol/L respectively (Okabe et al., 2002). The tocotrienol isomers were concentrated in the adipose tissues and mesenteric lymph nodes, the latter reported to have concentrations of each in excess of 80 μ mol/kg. Plasma concentrations of γ-tocotrienol in hamsters fed diets providing 23, 58 and 263 mg γ-tocotrienol/kg body weight for 4 weeks were <0.2, 0.5 and 14 μ mol/L respectively (Raederstorff et al., 2002). These studies demonstrate the achievement of plasma tocotrienol levels sufficient to support the anticancer activities recorded in the following studies.

15.3 TOCOTRIENOLS SUPPRESS CHEMICALLY INITIATED CARCINOGENESIS

Tocol extracts of palm oil (Gould et al., 1991; Nesaretnam et al., 1992; Wada et al., 2005) and rice bran oil (Iqbal et al., 2003) suppress 7,12-dimethylbenz [α] anthracene-initiated mammary carcinogenesis (Iqbal et al., 2003; Nesaretnam et al., 1992), 4-nitroquinoline-1-oxide initiated lung carcinogenesis (Wada et al., 2005) and diethylnitrosamine- (Rahmat et al., 1993a; Rahmat et al., 1993b) and 2-acetylaminofluorine- (Ngah et al., 1991; Rahmat et al., 1993a; Rahmat et al., 1993b; Shamaan et al., 1993) initiated liver carcinogenesis as well as the development of spontaneous liver tumors in male C3H/He mice (Wada et al., 2005). A-tocopherol, on the other hand, did not suppress MNU-initiated mammary carcinogenesis (Beth et al., 1987). Given the variations in the proportions of the primary tocols, α-tocopherol and α- and γ-tocotrienols in the various extracts estimates of the levels of the individual tocotrienol isomers required to have a significant impact are not calculated.

An *in vitro* study suggests that the tocotrienols suppress chemical carcinogenesis during the promotion phase. Assays of 12-O-tetradecanoylphorbol-13-acetate-activated Epstein-Barr virus early antigen expression in EBV-genome-carrying human lymphoblastoid cells showed that γ- and δ-tocotrienol but not α-tocopherol inhibit expression (Goh et al., 1994).

In an early study the tocols extracted from palm oil had no impact on 7,12-dimethylbenz anthracene- and N-methylnitrosourea-initiated mammary carcinogensis (Gould et al., 1991). Subsequent findings suggested that the presence of α-tocopherol in the tocol extract attenuated the impact of the tocotrienol constituents (Qureshi et al., 1996). Two reports suggest that dietary α-tocopherol has an equal if not slightly greater impact than γ-tocotrienol on 2-acetylaminofluorine-initiated liver carcinogensis (Makpol et al., 1997; Rahmat et al., 1993a).

15.4 TOCOTRIENOLS SUPPRESS THE GROWTH OF IMPLANTED TUMORS

When evaluated in transplant models the tocotrienols have significantly suppressed the growth of implanted sarcoma 180 (Komiyama et al., 1989), Ehrlich carcinoma (Komiyama et al., 1989), IMC carcinoma (Komiyama et al., 1989), meth A fibrosarcoma (Komiyama et al.,1989), B16 melanoma (He et al., 1997; McAnally et al., 2007), PC-3 prostate (Kumar et al., 2006) and MCF-7 mammary (Nesaretnam et al., 2004) cells. Intraperitoneal injections of γ-tocotrienol 20 mg (about 0.05 μ mol)/kg body weight/d extended the life span of mice following implants of sarcoma 180, Erlich carcinoma, IMC carcinoma and meth A fibrosarcoma by 78%, 117%, 63% and 35% respectively (Komiyama et al., 1989). A diet providing an estimated 0.4 μ mol γ-tocotrienol for 10 days prior to and following the implantation of B16 melanoma cells in the flanks of C57BL female mice yielded a significant increase (17%) in the time to detection of a solid tumor and a decrease (50%) in the weight of tumors excised 28 d post implant (He et al., 1997). In a more rigorous study, a diet providing 7 μ mol γ-tocotrienol per day was fed after solid B16 melanomas were detected in the flanks of C57BL mice; this treatment yielded a 35% increase in the mean survival time (He et al., 1997). More recently, a diet providing 3 μ mol δ-tocotrienol per day was fed to C57/BL mice beginning 2 days following the implantation of melanoma B16 cells; at 24 d post implant tumors excised from treated mice weighed significantly less (50%) than those from the controls (McAnally et al., 2007).

Γ-tocotrienol augmented the impact of radiation on the growth of prostate tumors. Human PC3 prostate tumor cells were implanted in groups of nude BALB/c mice and grown to 5 mm diameter. One group of experimental mice received by subcutaneous injection 400 mg γ-tocotrienol/kg body weight before the tumor site was irradiated (12 Gy ^{60}Cobalt). Twenty-four days following radiation, the size of tumors from the mice receiving the tocotrienol injection was reduced by 40% compared with those in mice subjected only to radiation (Kumar et al., 2006).

A blend of tocotrienols (38% γ-, 22% α-, 12% δ-) emulsified in drinking water at a final concentration of 0.05% through a 40-week period significantly reduced (80%) the number of tumors in the livers of C3H/He mice, a strain with a high incidence of spontaneous liver tumors (Wada et al., 2005). A similar blend was fed (1 mg/d) to athymic nude mice bearing MCF7 human mammary tumor cell implants. At 22 weeks the size of the tumors was significantly reduced (Nesaretnam et al., 2004).

In summary, diets supplemented with tocol blends enriched in tocotrienols or specific tocotrienol significantly suppressed mammary, lung and liver carcinogenesis initiated by 7,12-dimethylbenz [α] anthracene, N-methylnitrosourea, 4-nitroquinoline-1-oxide, diethylnitrosamine, 2-acetylaminofluorine and 12-0-tetradecanoylphorbol-13-acetate, the development of spontaneous liver tumors and the growth of implanted melanoma, prostate and mammary tumors. In light of this broad demonstration of the tumor-suppressive efficacy of the tocotrienols it is surprising that there is a lack of consensus regarding the mode of the anti-tumor action consisting of both an increase in apoptotic activity and a cell cycle arrest.

15.5 SIGNALING ACTIONS THAT CONTROL THE FATE OF CELLS

Now we turn to the signaling aspects impacted by the tocotrienols. Outlines of the multiple signaling networks that control the fate of cells, be it proliferation, differentiation, or apoptosis are presented on various websites such as http://www.cellsignal.com/. Ras (Lee and McCubrey, 2002; Sears and Nevins, 2002), RhoA (Fritz and Kaina, 2006), Raf/MEK/ERK (Hayden et al., 2006; Lee and McCubrey, 2002; Meric-Bernstam and Hung, 2006; Teicher, 2006), mitogen-activated protein kinases (MAPK) (Jakowlew, 2006; Meric-Bernstam and Hung, 2006), c-Jun (Lee and McCubrey, 2002; Meric-Bernstam and Hung 2006), c-myc (Dang et al., 2006; Jakowlew, 2006; Meric-Bernstam and Hung 2006; Sears and Nevins, 2002; Takada et al., 2005), cyclin D/cdk4/6 (Guttridge et al., 1999; Hinz et al., 1999; Jakowlew, 2006; Schumm et al., 2006; Sears and Nevins, 2002; Sutherland and Musgrove, 2004; Takada et al., 2005; Takebayashi et al., 2003; Viallard et al., 2001), protein kinase C (PKC) (Hayden et al., 2006; Lee and McCubrey, 2002; Meric-Bernstam and Hung 2006; Teicher, 2006), phosphatidylinositol 3-kinase (PI3K) (Hayden et al., 2006; Meric-Bernstam and Hung, 2006), Akt (Lee and McCubrey, 2002; Meric-Bernstam and Hung, 2006), I κ B kinase (IKK) (Hayden et al., 2006; Meric-Bernstam and Hung, 2006; Takada et al., 2004; Takada et al., 2005; Teicher, 2006), I κ B (Hayden et al., 2006; Meric-Bernstam and Hung, 2006; Takada et al., 2005; Teicher, 2006), NF κ B (Meric-Bernstam and Hung, 2006; Feng et al., 2004; Guttridge et al., 1999; Hayden et al., 2006; Hinz et al., 1999; Lee and McCubrey, 2002; Montaner et al., 1998; Perona et al.,

1997; Schumm et al., 2006; Takada et al., 2004; Takada et al., 2005; Takebayashi et al., 2003; Yin et al., 2000), c-Jun N-terminal kinase (JNK) (Lee and McCubrey, 2002; Montaner et al., 1998), Bcl-2 (Adams and Cory, 2007; Budihardjo et al., 1999; Jakowlew, 2006; Takada et al., 2005; Yin et al., 2006), Bcl-xL (Adams and Cory, 2007; Budihardjo et al., 1999; Feng et al., 2004; Jakowlew, 2006; Meric-Bernstam and Hung, 2006; Takada et al., 2005), FLICE-Like Inhibitory Protein (FLIP) (Lamkanfi et al., 2007), COX-2 (Meric-Bernstam and Hung, 2006; Takada et al., 2004; Takada et al., 2005; Teicher, 2006), matrix metalloproteinases (MMP) (Fingleton, 2007), vascular endothelial growth factor (VEGF) (Feleszko et al., 1999; Herbst, 2006) and telomerase (Stewart and Weinberg, 2006; Yin et al., 2000) serve networks comprising growth stimulatory and anti-apoptotic activities. Growth arrest and apoptotic functions are manifested via p21^{Cip1} (Schumm et al., 2006; Sherr, 2004; Sutherland and Musgrove, 2004; Viallard et al., 2001), transforming growth factor-β (TGF-β) (Jakowlew, 2006; Sherr, 2004), p53 (Jakowlew, 2006; Schumm et al., 2006; Sherr, 2004; Stewart and Weinberg, 2006), Fas (Roos and Kaina, 2006), Bad (Jakowlew, 2006; Meric-Bernstam and Hung, 2006; Yin, 2006), Bax (Budihardjo et al., 1999; Jakowlew, 2006; Yin, 2006), Bid (Fabregat et al., 2007), apoptotic protease-activating factor-1 (Apaf-1) (Herr and Debatin, 2001) and caspase (Budihardjo et al., 1999; Meric-Bernstam and Hung, 2006; Yin et al., 2000). Inhibition of the former and activation of the latter have been deemed to be the actions responsible for the antitumor activity of the tocotrienols resulting in G1 arrest (Crowell and Elson, 2001; Mo and Elson, 1999; Srivastava and Gupta, 2006; Yano et al., 2005) and apoptosis (Agarwal et al., 2004; Ahn et al., 2007; Har and Keong, 2005; McIntyre et al., 2000a; McIntyre et al., 2000b; Mo and Elson, 1999; Sakai et al., 2004; Sakai et al., 2006; Shah et al., 2003; Shah and Sylvester, 2004; Shah and Sylvester, 2005b; Shun et al., 2004; Srivastava and Gupta, 2006; Takahashi and Loo, 2004; Wada et al., 2005; Yu et al., 1999).

15.6 TOCOTRIENOLS SUPPRESS ACTIVITIES ASSOCIATED WITH GROWTH AND SURVIVAL

Tocotrienols suppress network activities associated with growth and anti-apoptosis comprised of Ras (Yano et al., 2005), RhoA (Yano et al., 2005), Raf/MEK/ERK (Sen et al., 2000; Sylvester et al., 2002; Yano et al., 2005), MAPK (Sylvester et al., 2002), c-Jun (Shun et al., 2004), c-myc (Ahn et al., 2007; Eitsuka et al., 2006; Nakagawa et al., 2004; Nesaretnam et al., 2004), cyclin D/cdk4 (Ahn et al., 2007; Yano et al., 2005), PKC (Eitsuka et al., 2006; Nakagawa et al., 2004; Sylvester et al., 2001), PI3K (Samant and Sylvester, 2006; Sylvester et al., 2002), Akt (Shah and Sylvester, 2004; Shah and Sylvester, 2005a; Sylvester et al., 2002; Sylvester et al., 2005), IKK (Ahn et al., 2007; Shah and Sylvester, 2005a; Sylvester et al., 2005), I [κ] B (Ahn et al., 2007; Shah and Sylvester, 2005a; Sylvester et al., 2005), NF κ B (Ahn et al., 2007; Shah and Sylvester, 2005a; Sylvester et al., 2005), JNK (Shun et al., 2004), Bcl-2 (Agarwal et al., 2004; Ahn et al., 2007), Bcl-xL (Ahn et al., 2007; Yano et al., 2005), COX-2 (Ahn et al., 2007), (MMP) (Ahn et al., 2007), VEGF (Ahn et al., 2007), FLIP (Ahn et al., 2007) and telomerase (Eitsuka et al., 2006; Nakagawa et al., 2004).

15.7 TOCOTRIENOLS ACTIVATE ACTIVITIES SUPPORTING GROWTH ARREST AND APOPTOSIS

Tocotrienols activate network activities supporting growth arrest and apoptosis: p21$^{Cip1/WAF1}$ (Agarwal et al., 2004), TGF- β (Shun et al., 2004), p53 (Agarwal et al., 2004), Fas (Shun et al., 2004), Bax (Agarwal et al., 2004; Sakai et al., 2006), Apaf-1 (Agarwal et al., 2004), caspase (Agarwal et al., 2004; Odysseos et al., 2002; Sakai et al., 2004; Sakai et al., 2006; Shah et al., 2003; Shah and Sylvester, 2004; Sylvester et al., 2005; Sylvester and Shah, 2005a; Sylvester and Shah, 2005b) and Bid fragmentation (Sakai et al., 2006). Additionally tocotrienols suppress angiogenesis (Ahn et al., 2007; Inokuchi et al., 2003; Miyazawa et al., 2004; Mizushina et al., 2006; Nakagawa et al., 2004) and it is suggested, by limiting the posttranslational processing, suppress the nuclear location of lamin B (Mo and Elson, 1999).

As noted above, tumor cell lines differ in sensitivity to the tocotrienols. Following are results of studies employing diverse tumor cell lines that examined the impact of tocotrienols on aspects of signaling pathways. Differences in the impact on diverse signaling pathways might explain the differences in sensitivity.

Incubation of human colon carcinoma RKO cells with a blend of tocotrienols (tocotrienol rich fraction [TRF] of palm oil) yielded a dose-dependent (15-180 μ mol/L, the rationale for calculating these values is not provided) increase in apoptotic cell death independent of an effect on the cell cycle (Agarwal et al., 2004). Apoptotic signals were composed of dose-dependent induction of p53 and concomitantly $p21^{WAF1}$, and a time-dependent induction of apoptotic protease-activating factor-1 (Apaf-1) and decrease in Bcl-2 expression coupled with a stabilization of Bax protein. As a consequence of the shift in the Bax/Bcl-2, cytochrome c is released from the mitochondria; the interaction of cytochrome c with Apaf-1 activates caspase-9, the resulting protease cascade activates caspase-3, the major effector of apoptosis. Although induced, $p21^{WAF1}$ did not result in an arrest of the cell cycle (Agarwal et al., 2004).

Mitochondria were disrupted in estrogen-non-responsive MDA-MB-231 human breast cancer cells incubated with approximately 30 μ mol/L γ-tocotrienol; the disruption was attributed to a collapse of the mitochondrial membrane potential resulting in a mitochondrial permeability transition resulting in the release of cytochrome c (Takahashi and Loo, 2004). Contrary to other findings described herein, the apoptotic activity triggered by γ-tocotrienol was not traceable to enhanced caspase and poly (ADP-ribose) polymerase (PARP) activities (Ahn et al., 2007; Sakai et al., 2006) or a change in the pro-/anti-apoptotic (Bax/Bcl-2) ratio (Takahashi and Loo, 2004). Δ-tocotrienol induced estrogen-non-responsive MDA-MB-435 and estrogen-responsive MCF-7 human breast cancer cells, but not in normal human mammary epithelial cells and immortalized but non-tumorigenic human MCF-10A cells, to undergo high levels of apoptosis in a concentration- and time-dependent fashion (Shun et al., 2004). The δ-tocotrienol-induced apoptosis involved up-regulation of TGF-β receptor II expression and the restoration of both the TGF-β and Fas signaling pathways that contribute to the activation of JNK-mediated apoptosis (Shun et al., 2004).

When HepB3 cells were incubated with 25 and 50 μ mol/L γ-tocotrienol, the latter treatment yielded an increased PARP cleavage by caspase-3, an indicator of apoptosis. Caspase-8 and caspase-9 activation occurred earlier than caspase-3 activation. Also, the levels of pro-apoptotic Bax protein and caspase-8 mediated, pro-apoptotic Bid fragmentation were increased, the latter enhancing cyctochrome c release from the mitochondria. Since Bcl-2 expression was not affected, the Bax/Bcl-2 ratio tilted toward apoptosis (Sakai et al., 2006). Caspase-8 and caspase-3 activities and DNA fragmentation were elevated in rat hepatoma dRLh-84 cells but not in normal rat hepatocyte RLN-10 cells following incubation with tocotrienol (Sakai et al., 2004).

Incubation of highly malignant +SA mammary cells with 0-20 μ mol/L γ-tocotrienol resulted in a dose-dependent decrease in cell viability with 20 μ mol/L γ-tocotrienol causing approximately 80% cell death (Shah and Sylvester, 2004); the IC50 value fell around 15 μ mol/L γ-tocotrienol. Concomitant with the increase in caspase-8 and caspase-3 activities, but not in caspase-9 activity (Shah et al., 2003; Shah and Sylvester, 2004) as observed in RKO cells (Agarwal et al., 2004), during a 24-hr incubation with 20 μ mol/L γ-tocotrienol was a decrease in the level of an anti-apoptotic protein that inhibits the activation of caspase-8 (FLIP). Consistent with the reduced level of FLIP was the down-regulation of the PI3K/PI3K-dependent kinase (PDK)/serine/threonine protein kinase (Akt) mitogenic signaling pathway, the pathway that increases the expression of FLIP. Cell viability in the presence of 20 μ mol/L γ-tocotrienol was restored with the addition of caspase-8 and caspase-3 inhibitors. In a second study, a dose-responsive decrease in the viability of +SA cells was attained with 1–8 μ mol/L γ-tocotrienol; a 60% reduction in growth was achieved with 4 μ mol/L γ-tocotrienol. This reduction in growth attributed to both apoptosis and cell cycle arrest was associated with reductions in epidermal growth factor-dependent PI3K/PDK-1/Akt and Nuclear Factor κ

B (NF κ B) mitogenic signaling. Reduced phosphorylation of Bad, a consequence of reduced Akt activity, prevents its dissociation from the Bcl-2/Bcl-xL complex thereby promoting its pro-apoptotic function. In the cytosol NF κ B is complexed with inhibitory protein (I κ B); phosphorylation of I κ B catalyzed by Akt-activated IKK causes the dissociation of the complex. Activated NF κ B is translocated to the nucleus and binds to DNA to initiate genes that enhance cell proliferation and survival. The inhibitory effects of γ-tocotrienol on cell growth may be attributed to the direct inhibition of Akt or of an upstream kinase, PI3K, PDK-1, or both (Samant and Sylvester, 2006; Shah and Sylvester, 2005a; Sylvester et al., 2002; Sylvester et al., 2005). In +SA cells incubated with α-tocotrienol (20 μ mol/L) caspase-8 and caspase-3, but not caspase-9, were activated and levels of activated PDK-1 and Akt were decreased with a subsequent reduction in FLIP expression (Sylvester and Shah, 2005a).

Findings that caspase-9 is not activated in +SA mammary cells incubated with levels of γ-tocotrienol sufficient to initiate apoptosis and the paradoxical decrease in pro-apoptotic proteins and increase in anti-apoptotic proteins provide evidence that it is the suppression of the PI3K/PDK-1/Atk mitogenic signaling rather than mitochondrial stress signaling that triggers apoptosis (Sylvester and Shah, 2005a).

Γ-tocotrienol (25 μ mol/L) blocked the TNF-induced activation of NF κ B in human myeloid KBM-5 cells, human adenocarcinoma H1299 lung cells, human embryonic (A293) kidney cells and human MCF-7 breast cancer cells and constitutive NF κ B in human myeloma (U266) and squamous carcinoma (SCC4) cells (Ahn et al., 2007). Consistent with earlier findings (Shah and Sylvester, 2005a) the tocotrienol-mediated suppression of NF κ B-dependent reporter gene expression in KBM-5 cells traces to the inhibition of PI3K/PDK/Akt signaling, Akt-activated IKK, I κ B phosphorylation and degradation (Ahn et al., 2007). As a consequence, γ-tocotrienol suppressed the expression of genes supporting proliferation (cyclin D1 and c-myc) and invasion (COX-2, MMP, VEGF) and anti-apoptotic activities (Bcl-xL, Bcl-2, FLIP). As a consequence of the reduced level of FLIP caspase activities were elevated.

Findings that supplemental L-mevalonate reversed the γ-tocotrienol-mediated suppression of NF κ B activity in KBM-5 cells (Ahn et al., 2007) argues against the view that the tocotrienols directly inhibit Akt or an upstream kinase (Samant and Sylvester, 2006; Shah and Sylvester, 2005a; Sylvester et al., 2002; Sylvester et al., 2005).

Inhibition of telomerase, an activity that maintains telomere length, offers an alternative rationale for explaining the tocotrienol-mediated impact on the growth of tumor cells (Eitsuka et al., 2006). The dose-dependent decrease in cell viability, determined in DLD-1 human colorectal adenocarcinoma cells incubated with 5-20 μ mol/L δ-tocotrienol, was traced to parallel decreases in telomerase activity, human telomerase reverse transcriptase (hTERT) expression, c-myc expression and cellular protein kinase C (PKC) activity. These observations suggest that tocotrienols reduce telomerase activity by down regulating hTERT and c-myc expression, previously noted in MCF7 cells (Nesaretnam et al., 2004), through inhibition of PKC activity (Eitsuka et al., 2006), the latter action previously noted in mammary epithelial cells (Sylvester et al., 2001).

α-tocotrienol, a less potent isomer, very modestly suppressed the growth of A549 human lung adenocarcinoma cells (Yano et al., 2005). A redox-silent derivative, 6-*O*-carboxypropyl-α-tocotrienol, proved to be a very potent inhibitor of growth, impacts tracing both to cell cycle arrest and apoptotic activity. The derivative was first shown to block the activation (membrane localization) of K-Ras presumably by attenuating HMG CoA reductase activity, a presumption supported by findings that supplemental farnesol (20 μ mol/L) reversed the block. The subsequent inhibition of a downstream activity (MEK) reduced the level of cyclin D, therein blocking the progression of cells from the G1 to the S phase of the cell cycle. Although the expression of anti-apoptotic Bcl-2 was not suppressed, expression of anti-apoptotic Bcl-xL was blocked. Pro-apoptotic Bax was stabilized; the resulting shift in the pro-/anti-apoptotic ratio favors the stimulation of the caspase cascade (Yano et al., 2005). Also supporting apoptotic events was the suppression of RhoA prenylation and membrane localization, an effect reversed by a supplement of geranyl-geranyl pyrophosphate (10–20 μ mol/L) and concomitant disruption of the actin cytoskeleton (Yano et al., 2005).

In summary, tocotrienols induced the expression of p53 (RKO) and supported a pro-apoptotic shift in the (Bad or Bax)/(Bcl-2 or Bcl-xL) ratio in human colon carcinoma (RKO), human hepatoma (HepB3), human malignant mammary (+SA) and human myeloid (KBM-5) cells but not in human mammary MDA-MB-231 cells. Caspase-activating functions consistent with the change in the pro-apoptotic ratio, e.g. cytochrome c release (RKO), decreased mitochondrial membrane potential (MDA-MB-231), decreased FLIP expression (+SA and KBM-5) and Apaf-1 release (RKO) in cells were recorded. Caspase-8 and caspase-3 activities were increased in human colon carcinoma (RKO), human hepatoma (HepB3), rat hepatoma (dRLh-84), human myeloid (KBM-5) and human malignant mammary (+SA) cells. Caspase-9 activity was increased in human colon carcinoma (RKO), human hepatoma (HepB3) cells but not in human malignant mammary (+SA) cells. PARP activity was elevated in HepB3 and dRLh-84 cells but not in MDA-MB-231 cells. TGF-β receptor expression and restoration of TGF-β, Fas signaling and activation of JNK-mediated apoptosis occurred in MCF-7 and MDA-MB-231 cells. Telomerase activity (DLD-1) and telomerase reverse transcriptase expression (DLD-1) and c-myc expression (DLD-1, KBM-5, MCF7) were decreased in cells incubated with tocotrienol.

Tocotrienol-mediated inhibition of PI3K/PDK-1/Akt (+SA, KBM-5), inhibition of IKK activity and I κ B degradation (+SA, KBM-5), inhibited NF κ B (+SA, KBM-5, H1299, A293, MCF-7, U266, SCC4), which precedes the suppressed expression of genes supporting proliferative (cyclin D, c-myc), invasive (COX-2, MMP, VEGF) and anti-apoptotic (Bcl-xL, Bcl-2, FLIP) activities recorded in KBM-5 cells; $p21^{WAF1}$ is induced in RKO cells.

Where evaluated, co-incubation with L-mevalonate (Agarwal et al., 2004; Ahn et al., 2007) or intermediate products of mevalonate metabolism (Yano et al., 2005) reversed the growth-suppressive impact of tocotrienol. Recent findings reveal that the total arrest of the growth of MIA PaCa-2 and PANC-1 pancreatic carcinoma cells imposed by 50 μ mol/L δ-tocotrienol is reversed with the concomitant addition of 0.5 mmol/L mevalonolactone to the incubation media (Mo et al., unpublished).

15.8 CENTRAL ROLE OF 3-HYDROXY-3-METHYLGLUTARYL COENZYME A REDUCTASE

Findings that supplemental mevalonate and mevalonate-derived products reverse the impact of the tocotrienols point to a central role of 3-hydroxy-3-methylglutaryl coenzyme A (HMG CoA) reductase, an activity suppressed by the tocotrienols (Khor et al., 1995; Khor and Ng, 2000; Parker et al., 1993; Qureshi et al., 1986; Song and DeBose-Boyd, 2006; Theriault et al., 1999). Competitive inhibitors of HMG CoA reductase, collectively the statins, similarly suppress the synthesis of mevalonate and downstream products. As a class, the statins may have potential as chemotherapeutic agents (Jakobisiak and Golab, 2003; Wong et al., 2002). Analyses of statin-treated cells reveal the concentration-dependent inhibition of cell growth and G1 arrest (Brown and Goldstein, 1980; Denoyelle et al., 2001; Gray-Bablin et al., 1997; Jakobisiak et al., 1991; Keyomarsi et al., 1991; Muller et al., 1998; Park et al., 2001; Rao et al., 1998; Shibata et al., 2003; Shibata et al., 2004; Sivaprasad et al., 2006; Soma et al., 1995; Ukomadu et al., 2003a; Ukomadu et al., 2003b; van de Donk et al., 2003; Wachtershauser et al., 2001) and apoptotic cell death (Agarwal et al., 2002; Bansal et al., 1989; Borner et al., 1995; Chapman-Shimshoni et al., 2003; Choi and Jung, 1999; Denoyelle et al., 2001; Dimitroulakos et al., 1999; Dimitroulakos et al., 2001; Horiguchi et al., 2004; Jones et al., 1994; Macaulay et al., 1999; Miquel et al., 1996; Muller et al., 1998; Nishida et al., 2005; Notarnicola et al., 2004; Padayatty et al., 1997; Park et al., 2001; Perez-Sala et al., 1995; Perez-Sala and Mollinedo 1994; Rubins et al., 1998; Satoh et al., 1996; Shellman et al., 2005; Shibata et al., 2003; Shibata et al., 2004; van de Donk et al., 2003; Wong et al., 2001; Wu et al., 2004). Parallel to the tocotrienol-mediated growth suppression, statins suppress the proliferation of tumor cells originated from breast (Alonso et al., 1998; Denoyelle et al., 2001; Dimitroulakos et al., 2001; Gray-Bablin et al., 1997; Keyomarsi et al., 1991; Shibata et al., 2003; Shibata et al., 2004; Wejde et al., 1992), liver (Morris et al., 1995), prostate (Borner et al., 1995; Dimitroulakos et al., 2001; McAnally et al., 2007; Padayatty et al., 1997; Park et al., 2001; Shibata et al., 2003), skin (Carlberg et al., 1996; Feleszko et al., 1998; McAnally et al., 2007; Shellman et al., 2005; Sora et al., 1994), colon (Mehta et al., 1998; Notarnicola et al., 2004; Ukomadu et al., 2003a), blood (Bansal et al., 1989; Chapman-Shimshoni et al., 2003; Dimitroulakos et al., 1999; Dimitroulakos et al., 2001; Mo and Elson 1999; Newman et al., 1994; Newman et al., 1997; Perez-Sala et al., 1995; Perez-Sala and Mollinedo 1994; Wong et al., 2001), lung (Andela et al., 2003; McAnally et al., 2007), lymph gland (Issat et al., 2004; Rozados et al., 2005; van de Donk et al., 2003), cervix (Dimitroulakos et al., 2001) and nerve (Castellano et al., 1994; Dimitroulakos and Yeger, 1996; Dimitroulakos et al., 2001; Jones et al., 1994; Macaulay et al., 1999; Prasanna et al., 1996) tissues.

15.9 STATINS SUPPRESS ACTIVITIES ASSOCIATED WITH GROWTH AND ANTI-APOPTOSIS

Statins suppress network activities associated with growth and anti-apoptosis composed of Ras (Bouterfa et al., 2000; Denoyelle et al., 2001; Rao et al., 1998), RhoA (Denoyelle et al., 2001; Denoyelle et al., 2003; Garcia-Roman et al., 2001; Ghosh et al., 1999; Li et al., 2002), Raf/MEK/ERK (Choi et al., 2003; Wu et al., 2004), MAPK (Bouterfa et al., 2000; Choi et al., 2003; Wu et al., 2004), c-Jun (Cerezo-Guisado et al., 2007), c-myc (Denoyelle et al., 2003; Park et al., 2001), cyclin D/cdk4 (Ahn et al., 2007, Denoyelle et al., 2003; Park et al., 1999; Park et al., 2001; Rao et al., 1998; Wachtershauser et al., 2001), PKC (Soma et al., 1994), PI3K (McGuire et al., 1994), Akt (Denoyelle et al., 2003; McGuire et al., 1994), IKK (Ahn et al., 2007), I κ B (Ahn et al., 2007; Feleszko et al., 1999), NF κ B (Ahn et al., 2007; Denoyelle et al., 2001; Feleszko et al., 1999; Zelvyte et al., 2002), JNK (Feleszko et al., 1999), Bcl-2 (Ahn et al., 2007; Garcia-Roman et al., 2001; Park et al., 1999), Bcl-xL (Ahn et al., 2007; Garcia-Roman et al., 2001), COX-2 (Ahn et al., 2007), MMP (Denoyelle et al., 2003; Taras et al., 2007; Zelvyte et al., 2002) and VEGF (Feleszko et al., 1999).

15.10 STATINS ACTIVATE ACTIVITIES SUPPORTING GROWTH ARREST AND APOPTOSIS

Statins activate network activities supporting growth arrest and apoptosis: $p21^{Cip1/WAF1}$ (Denoyelle et al., 2001; Denoyelle et al., 2003; Ghosh et al., 1999; Lee et al., 1998; Li et al., 2002; Shibata et al., 2003; Wachtershauser et al., 2001), TGF- β (Baccante et al., 2004), p53 (Gudas et al., 1994), Bax (Shibata et al., 2004), caspase and PARP cleavage (Chapman-Shimshoni et al., 2003; Denoyelle et al., 2001; DiMatola et al., 2001; Marcelli et al., 1998; Zhong et al., 2003) and Fas (Gniadecki, 2004). Additionally, statins suppress angiogenesis (Ahn et al., 2007; Feleszko et al., 1999) and the nuclear location of lamin B (DiMatola et al., 2001).

15.11 PARALLEL IMPACTS OF TOCOTRIENOLS AND STATINS

The parallel impacts of the tocotrienols and statins on signaling networks that control the fate of cells may be traced to the inhibition of HMG CoA reductase activity and the resultant limitations on the pools of essential mevalonate-derived products required for the posttranslational modification of the cysteine residue in the conserved carboxyl terminal sequence of diverse proteins, e.g. RhoA (Agarwal et al., 2002; Denoyelle et al., 2003), Ras (Bouterfa et al., 2000; Cuthbert and Lipsky, 1997) which have roles in signal transduction (Mo and Elson, 2004), roles upstream of NF κ B, Akt and caspase activities.

15.12 MULTIVALENT REGULATION OF HMG COA REDUCTASE ACTIVITY

HMG CoA reductase is under multivalent feedback regulation (Brown and Goldstein, 1980) incorporating factors modulating transcription, translation and degradation of the enzyme (Goldstein et al., 2006; Goldstein and Brown 1990; Nakanishi et al., 1988). Transcription of reductase is initiated by the binding of sterol regulatory element binding proteins (SREBPs) (Brown and Goldstein 1997; Horton et al., 2002), membrane proteins located in the endoplasmic reticulum (ER), to the octameric nucleotide sequence, GTGCGGTG, known as the sterol regulatory element (Goldstein and Brown 1990) in the reductase promoter region. Nascent SREBPs are bound to a second ER protein named SREBP cleavage activating protein (SCAP) (Brown and Goldstein 1999; Hua et al., 1996). Cholesterol, the bulk end product of the mevalonate pathway, of which the reductase is a rate-limiting enzyme, exerts a feedback control on reductase expression at the transcriptional level. Cholesterol buildup in the ER membrane leads to a conformational change of SCAP that results in the binding of SCAP with yet other ER proteins, Insigs (Yang et al., 2002), forming a SCAP/SREBP/Insig complex that prevents the entry of the active fragment of SREBP into nucleus (Sun et al., 2005) and the consequent activation of HMG CoA reductase transcription. Cholesterol depletion leads to the rapid ubiquitination and degradation of Insig-1 (Gong et al., 2006) which liberates SCAP/SREBP and releases the catalytic fragment of SREBPs into the nucleus for the activation of reductase transcription. 25-Hydroxycholesterol also down-regulates the stability of HMGR mRNA (Choi et al., 1993), a process mediated by the 3'-untranslated sequences of HMGR mRNA (Choi and Peffley, 1995).

The three isoforms of SREBPs, SREBP-1a, SREBP-1c and SREBP-2, encoded by two SREBP genes, have distinctive yet overlapping functions in regulating lipid synthesis (Horton et al., 2002). SREBP-1c predominates in the liver for controlling fatty acid synthesis, but lacks any direct significant roles in cholesterol biosynthesis other than regulating the expression of enzymes generating NADPH that is required for cholesterol synthesis (Shimano et al., 1997). SREBP-1a is predominantly found in cultured cells; it is expressed at constitutively low levels in the liver. SREBP-2 has a wider presence in cultured cells, liver and other tissues (Shimomura et al., 1997). Both SREBP-2 and SREBP-1a regulate the expression of genes whose protein products are involved in cholesterol biosynthesis. Elevated SREBP-2 is able to compensate partially for the loss of functions of SREBP-1s in knockout mice (Shimano et al., 1997), but *srebp2* knockout is embryonically lethal. In proliferating cells such as human embryonic kidney HEK-293 cells (Hannah et al., 2001) and human Caco-2 colon adenocarcinoma cells (Field et al., 2001), sterols suppress the processing of SREBP-2, but not that of SREBP-1a.

Sterol-mediated transcriptional down-regulation is complemented by repression of the translation of reductase mRNA mediated by mevalonate-derived nonsterols and acceleration of reductase degradation mediated by both sterols and nonsterols (Nakanishi et al., 1988). Nonsterols alone (Bradfute and Simoni, 1994; Peffley and Gayen, 1997; Peffley and Gayen, 1998) or in association with an oxysterol (Nakanishi et al., 1988; Peffley, 1992; Peffley and Sinensky, 1985) may modulate the translational efficiency of reductase mRNA. The degradation of reductase is dependent on the abundance of sterol and non-sterol products (Straka and Panini, 1995). The half-life of reductase in sterol- and isoprenoid-rich cells is at least 10-fold shorter than that in sterol-deprived cells (Gil et al., 1985). Interestingly, reductase degradation is also mediated by Insigs, which also participate in the regulation of the reductase transcription. The cholesterol precursor, lanosterol, triggers the binding of reductase to Insig (Sever et al., 2003b; Song et al., 2005a), which is a part of a larger four-protein complex that ubiquitinates reductase (Sever et al., 2003a; Song et al., 2005b). The ubiquitinated reductase is then transported to proteosome for degradation (Song et al., 2005b). *Trans, trans*-Farnesol (farnesol), a sesquiterpene derived from the mevalonate pathway, was shown to be the triggering molecule for reductase degradation (Correll et al., 1994; Correll and Edwards, 1994). More recently, a diterpene geranylgeraniol was postulated to stimulate the degradation of reductase (Sever et al., 2003a; Song and DeBose-Boyd 2006). Tocotrienols with a farnesol moiety suppress

Tocopherol

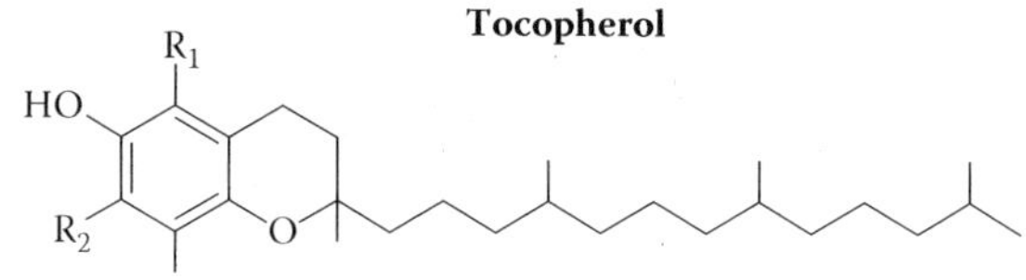

Tocotrienol

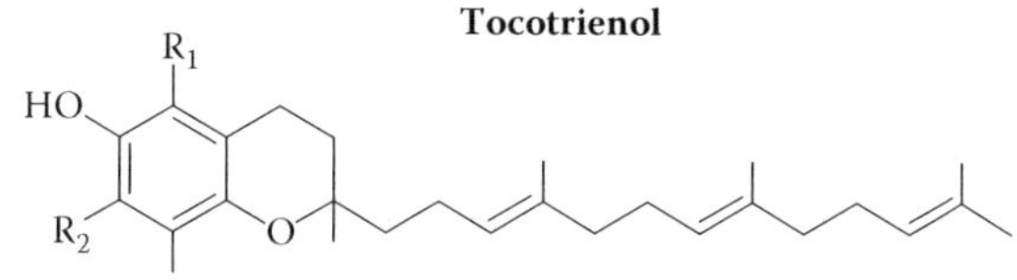

	Tocopherols/Tocotrienols			
	α–	β–	γ–	δ–
R_1	CH_3	CH_3	H	H
R_2	CH_3	H	CH_3	H

FIGURE 15.1 Structures of tocopherols and tocotrienols, which contain saturated phytyl tail and unsaturated isoprenoid side chain, respectively. Alpha-, β-, gamma- and δ-isomers of tocols differ in the number and/or location of the methyl groups on the chromanol ring. The growth-suppressive activities of the tocopherols are negligible in comparison with those of the tocotrienols, of which the isomers with fewer methyl groups have higher anti-proliferation, cell cycle-arresting and apoptosis-inducing properties.

reductase activity (Khor et al., 1995; Khor and Ng, 2000; Parker et al., 1993; Qureshi et al., 1986; Song and DeBose-Boyd, 2006; Theriault et al., 1999). The more prominent γ- and δ-isomers (Figure 15.1) were found to enhance ubiquitination and degradation of reductase. In addition, δ-tocotrienol blocks the processing of SREBPs and may therefore have transcriptional control of reductase activity (Song and DeBose-Boyd, 2006). The relative impacts of the tocotrienol isomers on HMG CoA reductase activity parallels their impacts on tumor cell proliferation.

15.13 DYSREGULATED HMG COA REDUCTASE ACTIVITY IN TUMORS

In 1958 Potter advanced the deletion hypothesis, namely that a fundamental lesion of malignant cells is a feedback control defect allowing the uninhibited synthesis of key growth intermediates. Shortly thereafter, Siperstein and Fagan (1964) reported the dysregulation of cholesterol synthesis in tumors and tumor-bearing animals. Subsequently, the elevated (Azrolan and Coleman, 1989; Barnard et al., 1984; Bennis et al., 1993; Broitman et al., 1993; Brown et al., 1973; Bruscalalupi et al., 1985; Caruso et al., 2002; Cerda et al., 1995; Chen et al., 1978; Coni et al., 1992; Engstrom and Schofield, 1987; Erickson et al., 1988; Feingold et al., 1983; George and Goldfarb, 1980; Goldfarb and Pitot, 1971; Gregg et al., 1982; Hentosh et al., 2001; Lehoux et al., 1984; Mitchell et al., 1978; Notarnicola et al., 2004; Philippot et al., 1977; Rossiello et al., 1994; Singh et al., 2003; Siperstein et al., 1971; Vitols et al., 1994; Yachnin et al., 1984) and sterol-feedback resistant (Azrolan and Coleman, 1989; Barnard et al., 1984; Bennis et al., 1993; Broitman et al., 1993; Caruso et al., 2002; Cerda et al., 1995; Feingold et al., 1983; Gregg et al., 1982; Hentosh et al., 2001; Mitchell, et al., 1978; Philppott et al., 1977; Rossiello et al., 1994; Singh et al., 2003; Tabacik et al., 1987) HMG CoA reductase activity was reported to occur in diverse tumors as well as in embryonic and differentiating tissues and in carcinogen-treated and regenerating liver. The dysregulated reductase activity has been traced to a decrease in LDL cholesterol binding (Barnard et al., 1984; Broitman et al., 1993; Caruso et al., 2002), an increase in the activation state (Feingold et al., 1983) and the hypomethylation pattern on the reductase gene, a pattern also noted for genes coding c-myc and H-ras (Rossiello et al., 1994). Investigations by other researchers have not identified differences in activation state of the enzyme (Bennis et al., 1993) and methylation pattern of the gene (Hentosh et al., 2001). The over-expression (Brown and Goldstein, 1997; Hannah et al., 2001; Hentosh et al., 2001; Osborne et al., 2000; Shimomura et al., 1997) of the SREBP-1a, a transcription factor modulating the transcription of the HMG CoA reductase gene, has been demonstrated in rapidly proliferating cells. Human colon tumor (Caco2) and leukemic (CEM) cells have seven-fold higher copies of HMG CoA reductase mRNA than normal colon cells (CCD-18) and human lymphocytes (Hentosh et al., 2001). Furthermore, the mature SREBP-1s are stabilized during mitotsis by Cdk1/cyclin B-mediated phosphorylation (Bengoechea-Alonso and Ericsson, 2006).

Differing from SREBP-1c, the closely related transcription factor prominent in liver (Shimano et al., 1997), the more potent SREBP-1a (Brown and Goldstein, 1997) does not respond to sterol-mediated down-regulation (Field et al., 2001; Hannah et al., 2001; Shimano et al., 1996). However, the elevated sterol feedback-resistant HMG CoA reductase activity in tumors retains sensitivity to secondary feedback regulation (Bennis et al., 1993). Whereas the statins suppress HMG CoA reductase activity and cause concomittant mevalonate-reversible suppression of cell growth in normal and tumor cells, the latter cells are uniquely sensitive to the impact of the mevalonate-reversible, posttranscriptional suppression of reductase activity imposed by the tocotrienols. Imposition of limiting pools of mevalonate-derived products, e.g. farnesyl pyrophosphate, geranylgeranyl pyrophosphate and dolichol phosphate, attenuates the initial regulatory activities delineated in figures available at http://www.cellsignal.com/.

15.14 ATTENUATION OF HMG COA REDUCTASE ACTIVITY OFFERS A NOVEL APPROACH TO CHEMOTHERAPY

Phase I and II clinical trials demonstrate that clinically significant tumor responses are achieved with high (25 mg/kg body wt/day) doses of statins (Kim et al., 2001; Thibault et al., 1996). Attendant toxicities preclude the widespread application of such protocols. *In vitro* studies demonstrated the synergistic advantage of a treatment consisting of a sub-effective dose of a statin in combination with a tocotrienol (McAnally et al., 2007; Mo et al., 2005; Mo and Elson, 1999, 2004; Wali and Sylvester, 2006). Concentrations of the agents that yielded non-significant impacts on the 48-h growth of B16 melanoma cells (1 μ mol/L lovastatin, 5 μ mol/L δ-tocotrienol) yielded a 70% suppression growth (McAnally et al., 2007). Treatment of highly malignant +SA mammary epithelial cells with 2–8 μ mol/L lovastatin yielded a concentration-dependent suppression of 96-h growth; blends of sub-effective doses of lovastatin (0.25 μ mol/L) and γ-tocotrienol (0.25-2.0 μ mol/L) resulted in significant suppressions of growth (Wali and Sylvester, 2006). An early preclinical study demonstrated a similar synergistic impact. The growth of B16 melanoma tumors implanted in flanks of mice was not significantly influenced by diets providing 11.5 mg lovastatin or 6.8 mg δ-tocotrienol/kg body wt/day; a diet providing a blend of the agents yielded a significant 60% suppression of tumor growth (McAnally et al., 2007). The level of lovastatin administered in this preliminary study is about one half the minimum level required to achieve a significant response in early clinical trials.

15.15 SUMMARY

Pools of mevalonate-derived products are essential for the posttranslational processing and biological function of Ras, Rho and growth factor receptors (Mo and Elson, 2004), proteins that have early roles in diverse signaling networks that control the fate of cells. As a consequence, competitive inhibitors of HMG CoA reductase activity, the rate-limiting step in the mevalonate pathway, impose a mevalonate-reversable arrest of cells in the G1 phase of the cell cycle and initiate apoptosis. The tocotrienols trigger posttranscriptional actions that modestly down-regulate HMG CoA reductase activity in sterol-responsive cells. The dysregulated sterol feedback-resistant reductase activity in tumor cells and tumors exhibits high sensitivity to the posttranscriptional actions triggered by the tocotrienols. As a consequence, the impact of the tocotrienols on the growth of normal cells and tissues is nonexistent, whereas the growth of tumor cells and tumors responds to tocotrienols in a dose-dependent, mevalonate-reversible manner. A novel approach to the control of tumor growth absent an effect on the host combines the unique sensitivity of the dysregulated tumor HMG CoA reductase activity to the posttranscriptional actions of the tocotrienols with the inhibitory action of low-dose statins.

REFERENCES

Adams, J., S. Cory. 2007. The Bcl-2 apoptotic switch in cancer development and therapy. *Oncogene, 26*, 1324–1337.

Agarwal, B., B. Halmos, A. Feokistov, P. Protiva, W. Ramey, M. Cheen, C. Pothoulakis, J. LaMont, P. Holt. 2002. Mechanism of lovastatin-induced apoptosis in intestinal epithelial cells. *Carcinogenesis, 23*, 521–528.

Agarwal, M., M. Agarwal, M. Athar, S. Gupta. 2004. Tocotrienol-rich fraction of palm oil activates p53, modulates Bax/Bcl2 ratio and induces apoptosis independent of cell cycle association. *Cell Cycle, 3*, 205–211.

Ahn, K., G. Sethi, K. Krishnan, B. Aggarwal. 2007. Gamma-tocotrienol inhibits nuclear factor-kappaB signaling pathway through inhibition of receptor-interacting protein and TAK1 leading to suppression of antiapoptotic gene products and potentiation of apoptosis. *J. Biol. Chem., 282*, 809–820.

Alonso, D., H. Farina, G. Skilton, M. Gabri, M. De Lorenzo, D. Gomez. 1998. Reduction of mouse mammary tumor formation and metastasis by lovastatin, an inhibitor of the mevalonate pathway of cholesterol synthesis. *Breast Can. Res. Treat., 50*, 83–93.

Andela, V., M. Pirri, E. Schwarz, E. Puzas, R. O'Keefe, J. Rosenblatt, R. Rosier. 2003. The mevalonate synthesis pathway as a therapeutic target in cancer. *Clin. Orthop.*, S59–66.

Azrolan, N., P. Coleman. 1989. A discoordinant increase in the cellular amount of 3-hydroxy-3-methylglutaryl-CoA reductase results in the loss of rate-limiting control over cholesterogenesis in a tumor cell-free system. *Biochem. J., 258*, 421–425.

Baccante, G., G. Minicione, M. Di Marcantonio, A. Piccirelli, F. Cuccurullo, E. Porreca. 2004. Pravastatin up-regulates transforming growth factor-b1 in THP-1 human macrophages effect on scavenger receptor class A expression. *Biochem. Biophys. Res. Commun., 314*, 704–710.

Bansal, N., A. Houle, G. Melnykovych. 1989. Comparison of dexamethasone and lovastatin (mevinolin) as growth inhibitors in cultures of T-cell derived human acute leukemia lines (CEM). *Leuk. Res., 13*, 875–882.

Barnard, G., S. Erickson, C. Cooper. 1984. Lipoprotein metabolism by rat hepatomas. Studies on the etiology of defective dietary feedback inhibition of cholesterol synthesis. *J. Clin. Invest., 74*, 173–184.

Bengoechea-Alonso, M., J. Ericsson. 2006. Cdk1/cyclin B-mediated phosphorylation stabilizes SREBP-1 during mitosis. *Cell Cycle, 5*, 1708–1718.

Bennis, F., G. Favre, F. Le Gaillard, G. Soula. 1993. Importance of mevalonate-derived products in the control of HMG-CoA reductase activity and growth of human lung adenocarcinoma cell line A549. *Int. J. Cancer, 55*, 640–645.

Beth, M., M. Berger, Y. Aksoy, D. Schmahl. 1987. Effects of vitamin A and E supplementation to diets containing two different fat levels on methylnitrosourea-induced mammary carcinogenesis in female SD-rats. *Br. J. Cancer, 56*, 445–449.

Birringer, M., J. EyTina, B. Salvatore, J. Neuzil. 2003. Vitamin E analogues as inducers of apoptosis: Structure–function relation. *Br. J. Cancer, 88*, 1948–1955.

Borner, M., C. Myers, O. Sartor, Y. Sei, T. Toko, J. Trepel, E. Schneider. 1995. Drug-induced apoptosis is not necessarily dependent on macromolecular synthesis or proliferation in the p53-negative human prostate cancer cell line PC-3. *Cancer Res., 55*, 2122–2128.

Bouterfa, H., V. Sattelmeyer, S. Czub, D. Vordermark, K. Roosen, J. Tonn. 2000. Inhibition of Ras farnesylation by lovastatin leads to downregulation of proliferation and migration in primary cultured human glioblastoma cells. *Anticancer Res., 20*, 2761–2772.

Bradfute, D.L., R.D. Simoni. 1994. Non-sterol compounds that regulate cholesterogenesis. Analogues of farnesyl pyrophosphate reduce 3-hydroxy-3-methylglutaryl-coenzyme A reductase levels. *J. Biol. Chem., 269*, 6645–6650.

Broitman, S., S. Cerda, J. Wilkinson. 1993. Cholesterol metabolism and colon cancer. *Prog. Food Nutr. Sci.*, *17*, 1–40.

Brown, M.S., J.L. Goldstein. 1980. Multivalent feedback regulation of HMG CoA reductase, a control mechanism coordinating isoprenoid synthesis and cell growth. *J. Lipid Res.*, *21*, 505–517.

Brown, M.S., J.L. Goldstein. 1997. The SREBP pathway: Regulation of cholesterol metabolism by proteolysis of a membrane–bound transcription factor. *Cell*, *89*, 331–340.

Brown, M.S., J.L. Goldstein. 1999. A proteolytic pathway that controls the cholesterol content of membranes, cells and blood. *Proc. Natl. Acad. Sci. USA*, *96*, 11041–11048.

Brown, M.S., J.L. Goldstein, M. Siperstein. 1973. Regulation of cholesterol synthesis in normal and malignant tissue. *Fed. Proc.*, *32*, 2168–2173.

Bruscalalupi, G., S. Leoni, M. Mangiantini, M. Minieri, S. Spagnuolo, A. Trentlanc. 1985. True uncoupling between cholesterol synthesis and 3-hydroxy-3-methylglutaryl coenzyme A reductase in an early stage of liver generation. *Cell. Mol. Biol.*, *31*, 365–368.

Budihardjo, I., H. Oliver, M. Lutter, X. Luo, X. Wang. 1999. Biochemical pathways of caspase activation during apoptosis. *Ann. Rev. Cell Develop. Biol.*, *15*, 269–290.

Carlberg, M., A. Dricu, H. Blegen, M. Wang, M. Hjertman, P. Zickert, A. Hoog, O. Larsson. 1996. Mevalonic acid is limiting for N-linked glycosylation and translocation of the insulin-like growth factor-1 receptor to the cell surface. Evidence for a new link between 3-hydroxy-3-methylglutaryl-coenzymel a reductase and cell growth. *J. Biol. Chem.*, *271*, 17453–17462.

Caruso, M., M. Notarnicola, A. Cavallini, A. Di Leo. 2002. 3-hydroxy-3-methylglutaryl coenzyme A reductase activity and low–density lipoprotein receptor expression in diffuse-type and intestinal-type human gastric cancer. *J. Gastroenterol.*, *37*, 504–508.

Castellano, F., G. Bruscallaupi, S. Columba, L. Di Croce, A. Trentalance, G. Augusti-Tocco. 1994. Characterization of the response of growth and differentiation to lipoproteins and agents affecting cholesterol metabolism in murine neuroblastoma cells. *Int. J. Dev. Neurosci.*, *12*, 77–84.

Cerda, S., J. Wilkinson, S. Broitman. 1995. Regulation of cholesterol synthesis in four colonic adenocarcinoma cell lines. *Lipids.*, *30*, 1083–1092.

Cerezo-Guisado, M., A. Alvarez-Barrientos, R. Argent, L. Garcia-Marin, M. Bragado, M. Lorenzo. 2007. C-Jun N-terminal protein kinase signalling pathway mediates lovastatin-induced rat brain neuroblast apoptosis. *Biochim. Biophys. Acta.*, *1771*, 164–176.

Chapman-Shimshoni, D., M. Yuklea, J. Radnay, H. Shapiro, M. Lishner. 2003. Simvastatin induces apoptosis of B-CLL cells by activation of mitochondrial caspase 9. *Exp. Hematol.*, *31*, 779–783.

Chen, H., A. Kandutsch, H. Heineiger. 1978. The role of cholesterol in malignancy. *Prog. Exp. Tumour Res.*, *22*, 275–316.

Choi, J.W., S.E. Jung. 1999. Lovastatin-induced proliferation inhibition and apoptosis in C6 glial cells. *J. Pharmacol. Exp. Ther.*, *289*, 572–579.

Choi, J.W., E.N. Lundquist, D.M. Peffley. 1993. Inhibition of protein synthesis in baby-hamster kidney cells blocks oxysterol-mediated suppression of 3-hydroxy-3-methylglutaryl-CoA reductase mRNA at a post-transcriptional level. *Biochem. J.*, *296*, 859–866.

Choi, J.W., D.M. Peffley. 1995. 3'-untranslated sequences mediate post-transcriptional regulation of 3-hydroxy-3-methylglutaryl-CoA reductase mRNA by 25-hydroxycholesterol. *Biochem. J.*, *307*, 233–238.

Choi, M., S. Rolle, M. Rane, H. Haller, F. Luft, R. Kettritz. 2003. Extracellular signal-related kinase inhibition by statins inhibit neutrophil activation by ANCA. *Kidney Internat.*, *63*, 96–106.

Coni, P., J. Pang, G. Pichiri-Coni, S. Hsu, P. Rao, S. Rakalakshmi, D. Sarma. 1992. Hypomethylation of β-hydroxy-β-methylglutaryl coenzyme A reductase gene and its expression during hepatocarcinogenesis in the rat. *Carcinogenesis*, *13*, 497–499.

Conte, C., A. Floridi, C. Aisa, M. Piroddi, F. Galli. 2004. Gamma-tocotrienol metabolism and antiproliferative effect in prostate cancer cells. *Ann. NY Acad. Sci.*, *1031*, 391–394.

Correll, C.C., P.A. Edwards. 1994. Mevalonic acid-dependent degradation of 3-hydroxy-3-methylglutaryl-coenzymel A reductase *in vivo* and *in vitro*. *J. Biol. Chem.*, *269*, 633–638.

Correll, C.C., L. Ng, P.A. Edwards. 1994. Identification of farnesol as the non-sterol derivative of mevalonic acid required for the accelerated degradation of 3-hydroxy-3-methylglutaryl-coenzymel A reductase. *J. Biol. Chem.*, *269*, 17390-17393.

Crowell, P., C. Elson. 2001. Isoprenoids, health and disease. In *Handbook of Nutraceuticals and Functional Foods*, CRC Series in Modern Nutrition. R. Wildman, Ed. CRC Press: Boca Raton, 31–53.

Cuthbert, J., P.E. Lipsky. 1997. Regulation of proliferation and Ras localization in transformed cells by products of mevalonate metabolism. *Cancer Res.*, *57*, 3498–3505.

Dang, C.V., K.A. O'Donnell, K.I. Zeller, T. Nguyen, R.C. Osthus, F. Li. 2006. The c-Myc target gene network. *Semin. Cancer Biol.*, *16*, 253–264.

Denoyelle, C., P. Albanese, G. Uzan, L. Hong, J.P. Vannier, J. Siria, C. Soria. 2003. Molecular mechanism of the anti-cancer activity of cerivastatin, an inhibitor of HMG-CoA reductase, on aggressive human breast cancer cells. *Cell Signal.*, *15*, 327–338.

Denoyelle, C., M. Vasse, M. Korner, Z. Mishall, F. Ganne, J.P. Vannier, J. Soria, C. Soria. 2001. Cerivastatin, an inhibitor of HMG-CoA reductase, inhibits the signaling pathways involved in the invasiveness and metastatic properties of highly invasive breast cancer cell lines: An *in vitro* study. *Carcinogenesis*, *22*, 1139–1148.

Di Matola, T., F. D'Ascoli, C. Luongo, M. Bifulco, G. Rossi, G. Fenzi, M. Vitale. 2001. Lovastatin-induced apoptosis in thyroid cells: Involvement of cytochrome c and lamin B. *Eur. J. Endocrinol.*, *145*, 645–50.

Dimitroulakos, J., D. Nohynek, K.L. Backway, D.W. Hedley, H. Yeger, M.H. Freedman, M.D. Minden, L.Z. Penn. 1999. Increased sensitivity of acute myeloid leukemias to lovastatin-induced apoptosis: A potential therapeutic approach. *Blood*, *93*, 1308–1318.

Dimitroulakos, J., L.Y. Ye, M. Benzaquen, M.J. Moore, S. Kamel-Reid, M.H. Freedman, H. Yeger, L.Z. Penn. 2001. Differential sensitivity of various pediatric cancers and squamous cell carcinomas to lovastatin-induced apoptosis: Therapeutic implications. *Clin. Cancer Res.*, *7*, 158–167.

Dimitroulakos, J, H. Yeger. 1996. HMG-CoA reductase mediates the biological effects of retinoic acid on human neuroblastoma cells: Lovastatin specifically targets P-glycoprotein-expressing cells. *Nat. Med.*, *2*, 326–333.

Eitsuka, T., K. Nakagawa, T. Miyazawa. 2006. Down-regulation of telomerase activity in DLD-1 human colorectal adenocarcinoma cells by tocotrienol. *Biochem. Biophys. Res. Commun.*, *348*, 170–175.

Engstrom, W., P.N. Schofield. 1987. Expression of the 3-hydroxy-3-methyl-glutaryl coenzyme A-reductase and LDL-receptor genes in human embryonic tumors and in normal fetal tissues. *Anticancer Res.*, *7*, 337–342.

Erickson, S.K., A.D. Cooper, G.F. Barnard, C.M. Havel, J.A. Watson, K.R. Feingold, A.H. Moser, M. Hughes-Fulford, M.D. Siperstein. 1988. Regulation of cholesterol metabolism in a slow–growing hepatoma *in vivo*. *Biochim. Biophys. Acta*, *960*, 131-138.

Fabregat, I., C. Roncero, M. Fernandez. 2007. Survival and apoptosis: A dysregulated balance in liver cancer. *Liver Int.*, *27*, 155-162.

Feingold, K.R., M.H. Wiley, A.H. Moser, M.D. Siperstein. 1983. Altered activation state of hydroxymethylglutaryl-coenzymel A reductase in liver tumors. *Arch. Biochem. Biophys.*, *226*, 231–241.

Feleszko, W., E.Z. Balkowiec, E. Sieberth, M.A. Marczak, A. Giermasz, A. Czajka, M. Jakobisiak. 1999. Lovastatin and tumor necrosis factor-α exhibit potentiated antitumor effects against Ha-ras-transformed murine tumor via inhibition of tumor-induced angiogenesis. *Int. J. Cancer*, *81*, 560–567.

Feleszko, W., R. Zagozdzon, J. Golab, M. Jakobisiak. 1998. Potentiated antitumour effects of cisplatin and lovastatin against MmB16 melanoma in mice. *Eur. J. Cancer*, *34*, 406–411.

Feng, B., S. Cheng, C.Y. Hsia, L.B. King, J.G. Monroe, H.C. Liou. 2004. NF-kappaB inducible genes BCL-X and cyclin E promote immature B-cell proliferation and survival. *Cell. Immunol.*, *232*, 9–20.

Field, E.J., E. Born, S. Murthy, S.N. Mathur. 2001. Regulation of sterol regulatory element-binding proteins by cholesterol flux in CaCo-2 cells. *J. Lipid Res.*, *42*, 1687–1698.

Fingleton, B. 2007. Matrix metalloproteinases as valid clinical targets. *Curr. Pharm. Des.*, *13*, 333–346.

Fritz, G., B. Kaina. 2006. Rho GTPases: Promising cellular targets for novel anticancer drugs. *Curr. Cancer Drug Targets*, *6*, 1–14.

Garcia-Roman, N., A.M. Alvarez, M.J. Toro, A. Montes, M.J. Lorenzo. 2001. Lovastatin induces apoptosis of spontaneously immortalized rat brain neuroblasts: Involvement of nonsterol isoprenoid biosynthesis inhibition. *Mol. Cell. Neurosci.*, *17*, 329–341.

George, R., S. Goldfarb. 1980. Inhibition of 3-hydroxy-3-methylglutaryl coenzyme A reductase activity in Morris hepatoma 7800 after intravenous injection of mevalonic acid. *Cancer Res.*, *40*, 4717–4721.

Ghosh, P.M., M.L. Moyer, G.E. Mott, J.I. Kreisberg. 1999. Effect of cyclin E overexpression on lovastatin-induced G1 arrest and RhoA inactivation in NIH3T3 cells. *J. Cell. Biochem.*, *74*, 532–543.

Gil, G., J.R. Faust, D.J. Chin, J.L. Goldstein, M.S. Brown. 1985. Membrane-bound domain of HMG CoA reductase is required for sterol-enhanced degradation of the enzyme. *Cell*, *41*, 249–258.

Gniadecki, R. 2004. Depletion of membrane cholesterol causes ligand-independent activation of Fas and apoptosis. *Biochem. Biophys. Res. Commun.*, *320*, 165–169.

Goh, S.H., N.F. Hew, A.W. Norhanom, M. Yadav. 1994. Inhibition of tumour promotion by various palm-oil tocotrienols. *Int. J. Cancer*, *57*, 529–531.

Goldfarb, S., H.C. Pitot. 1971. The regulation of β-hydroxy–β-methylglutaryl coenzyme A reductase in Morris hepatomas 5123C, 7800 and 9618A. *Cancer Res.*, *31*, 1879–1882.

Goldstein, J.L., M.S. Brown. 1990. Regulation of the mevalonate pathway. *Nature*, *343*, 425–430.

Goldstein, J.L., R.A. DeBose-Boyd, M.S. Brown. 2006. Protein sensors for membrane sterols. *Cell*, *124*, 35–46.

Gong, Y., J.N. Lee, P.C. Lee, J.L. Goldstein, M.S. Brown, J. Ye. 2006. Sterol-regulated ubiquitination and degradation of Insig-1 creates a convergent mechanism for feedback control of cholesterol synthesis and uptake. *Cell Metab.*, *3*, 15–24.

Gould, M.N., J.D. Haag, W.S. Kennan, M.A. Tanner, C.E. Elson. 1991. A comparison of tocopherol and tocotrienol for the chemoprevention of chemically induced rat mammary tumors. *Am. J. Clin. Nutr.*, *53*, 1068S–1070S.

Gray-Bablin, J., S. Rao, K. Keyomarsi. 1997. Lovastatin induction of cyclin-dependent kinase inhibitors in human breast cells occurs in a cell cycle-independent fashion. *Cancer Res.*, *57*, 604–609.

Gregg, R.G., J.R. Sabine, P.A. Wilce. 1982. Regulation of 3-hydroxy-3-methylglutaryl coenzyme A reductase in rat liver and Morris hepatomas 5123C, 9618A and 5123tc. *Biochem. J.*, *204*, 457–462.

Gudas, J.M., M. Oka, F. Diella, J. Trepel, K.H. Cowan. 1994. Expression of wild-type p53 during the cell cycle in normal human mammary epithelial cells. *Cell Growth Differ.*, *5*, 295–304.

Guthrie, N., A. Gapor, A.F. Chambers, K.K. Carroll. 1997a. Palm oil tocotrienols and plant flavonoids act synergistically with each other and with Tamoxifen in inhibiting proliferation and growth of estrogen receptor-negative MDA-MB-435 and -positive MCF-7 human breast cancer cells in culture. *Asia Pac. J. Clin. Nutr.*, *6*, 41–45.

Guthrie, N., A. Gapor, A.F. Chambers, K.K. Carroll. 1997b. Inhibition of proliferation of estrogen receptor-negative MDA-MB-435 and -positive MCF–7 human breast cancer cells by palm oil tocotrienols and tamoxifen, alone and in combination. *J. Nutr.*, *127*, 544S–548S.

Guttridge, D.C., C. Albanese, J.Y. Reuther, R.G. Pestell, A.S. Baldwin Jr. 1999. NF-kappaB controls cell growth and differentiation through transcriptional regulation of cyclin D1. *Mol. Cell. Biol.*, *19*, 5785–5799.

Hannah, V.C., J. Ou, A. Luong, J.L. Goldstein, M.S. Brown. 2001. Unsaturated fatty acids down-regulate SREBP isoforms aa and 1c by two mechanisms in HEK-293 cells. *J. Biol. Chem.*, *276*, 4365–4372.

Har, C.H., C.K. Keong. 2005. Effects of tocotrienols on cell viability and apoptosis in normal murine liver cells (BNL CL.2) and liver cancer cells (BNL 1ME A.7R.1) *in vitro*. *Asia Pac. J. Clin. Nutr.*, *14*, 374–380.

Hayden, M.S., A.P. West, S. Ghosh. 2006. SnapShot: NF-kB signaling pathways. *Cell*, *127*, 1286.

Hayes, K.C., A. Pronczuk, J.S. Liang. 1993. Differences in the plasma transport and tissue concentrations of tocopherols and tocotrienols: Observations in humans and hamsters. *Proc. Soc. Exp. Biol. Med.*, *202*, 353–359.

He, L., H. Mo, S. Hadisusilo, A.A. Qureshi, C.E. Elson. 1997. Isoprenoids suppress the growth of murine B16 melanomas *in vitro* and *in vivo*. *J. Nutr.*, *127*, 668–674.

Hentosh, P., S.H. Yuh, C.E. Elson, D.M. Peffley. 2001. Sterol-independent regulation of 3-hydroxy-3-methylglutaryl coenzyme A reductase in tumor cells. *Mol. Carcinog.*, *32*, 154–166.

Herbst, R.S. 2006. Therapeutic options to target angiogenesis in human malignancies. *Expert Opin. Emerg. Drugs*, *11*, 635–650.

Herr, I., K.M. Debatin. 2001. Cellular stress response and apoptosis in cancer therapy. *Blood*, *98*, 2603–2614.

Hinz, M., D. Krappmann, A. Eichten, A. Heder, C. Scheidereit, M. Strauss. 1999. NF-kappaB function in growth control: Regulation of cyclin D1 expression and G0/G1-to-S-phase transition. *Mol. Cell. Biol.*, *19*, 2690–2698.

Horiguchi, A., M. Sumitomo, J. Asakuma, T. Asano, M. Hayakawa. 2004. 3-hydroxy-3-methylglutaryl-coenzymel a reductase inhibitor, fluvastatin, as a novel agent for prophylaxis of renal cancer metastasis. *Clin. Cancer Res.*, *10*, 8648–8655.

Horton, J.D., J.L. Goldstein, M.S. Brown. 2002. SREBPs: Activators of the complete program of cholesterol and fatty acid synthesis in the liver. *J. Clin. Invest.*, *109*, 1125–1131.

Hua, X., A. Nohturfft, J.L. Goldstein, M.S. Brown. 1996. Sterol resistance in CHO cells traced to point mutation in SREBP cleavage-activating protein. *Cell*, *87*, 415–426.

Ikeda, S., T. Niwa, K. Yamashita. 2000. Selective uptake of dietary tocotrienols into rat skin. *J. Nutr. Sci. Vitaminol. (Tokyo)*, *46*, 141–143.

Inokuchi, H., H. Hirokane, T. Tsuzuki, K. Nakagawa, M. Igarashi, T. Miyazawa. 2003. Anti-angiogenic activity of tocotrienol. *Biosci. Biotechnol. Biochem.*, *67*, 1623–1627.

Iqbal, J., M. Minhajuddin, Z.H. Beg. 2003. Suppression of 7,12-dimethylbenz α anthracene-induced carcinogenesis and hypercholesterolaemia in rats by tocotrienol-rich fraction isolated from rice bran oil. *Eur. J. Cancer Prev.*, *12*, 447–453.

Issat, T., D. Nowis, M. Jakobisiak, J. Golab. 2004. Lovastatin potentiates antitumor effects of saquinavir against human lymphoma cells. *Oncol. Rep.*, *12*, 1371–1375.

Jakobisiak, M., S. Bruno, J.S. Skierski, Z. Darzynkiewicz. 1991. Cell cycle-specific effects of lovastatin. *Proc. Natl. Acad. Sci. USA*, *88*, 3628–3632.

Jakobisiak, M., J. Golab. 2003. Potential antitumor effects of statins (Review). *Int. J. Oncol.*, *23*, 1055–1069.

Jakowlew, S.B. 2006. Transforming growth factor-β in cancer and metastasis. *Cancer Metastasis Rev.*, *25*, 435–457.

Jiang, Q., J. Wong, H. Fyrst, J.D. Saba, B.N. Ames. 2004. Gamma-tocopherol or combinations of vitamin E forms induce cell death in human prostate cancer cells by interrupting sphingolipid synthesis. *Proc. Natl. Acad. Sci. USA*, *101*, 17825–17830.

Jones, K.D., W.T. Couldwell, D.R. Hinton, Y. Su, S. He, L. Anker, R.E. Law. 1994. Lovastatin induces growth inhibition and apoptosis in human malignant glioma cells. *Biochem. Biophys. Res. Commun.*, *205*, 1681–1687.

Keyomarsi, K., L. Sandoval, V. Band, A.B. Pardee. 1991. Synchronization of tumor and normal cells from G1 to multiple cell cycles by lovastatin. *Cancer Res.*, *51*, 3602–3609.

Khor, H.T., D.Y. Chieng, K.K. Ong. 1995. Tocotrienols inhibit HMG CoA reductase activity in the guinea pig. *Nutr. Res.*, *15*, 537–544.

Khor, H.T., T.T. Ng. 2000. Effects of administration of α-tocopherol and tocotrienols on serum lipids and liver HMG CoA reductase activity. *Int. J. Food Sci. Nutr.*, *51*, S3–11.

Khosla, P., V. Patel, J.M. Whinter, S. Khanna, M. Rakhkovskaya, S. Riy, C.K. Sen. 2006. Postprandial levels of the natural vitamin E tocotrienol in human circulation. *Antioxid. Redox Signal.*, *8*, 1059–1068.

Kim, W.S., M.M. Kim, H.J. Choi, S.S. Yoon, M.H. Lee, K. Park, C.H. Park, W.K. Kang. 2001. Phase II study of high-dose lovastatin in patients with advanced gastric adenocarcinoma. *Invest. New Drugs*, *19*, 81–83.

Komiyama, K., K. Iizuka, M. Yamaoka, H. Watanabe, N. Tsuchiya, I. Umezawa. 1989. Studies on the biological activity of tocotrienols. *Chem. Pharm. Bull. (Tokyo)*, *37*, 1369–1371.

Kumar, K.S., M. Raghavan, K. Hieber, C. Ege, S. Mog, N. Parra, A. Hildabrand, V. Singh, V. Srinivasan, R. Toles, P. Karikari, G. Petrovics, T. Seed, S. Srivastava, A. Papas. 2006. Preferential radiation sensitization of prostate cancer in nude mice by nutraceutical antioxidant gamma-tocotrienol. *Life Sci.*, *78*, 2099–2104.

Lamkanfi, M., N. Festjens, W. Declercq, T. Vanden Berghe, P. Vandenabeele. 2007. Caspases in cell survival, proliferation and differentiation. *Cell Death Differ.*, *14*, 44–55.

Lee, J.T. Jr., J.A. McCubrey. 2002. The Raf/MEK/ERK signal transduction cascade as a target for chemotherapeutic intervention in leukemia. *Leukemia*, *16*, 486–507.

Lee, S.J., M.J. Ha, J. Lee, P. Nguyen, Y.H. Choi, F. Pirnia, W.K. Kang, X.F. Wang, S.J. Kim, J.B. Trepel. 1998. Inhibition of the 3-hydroxy-3-methylglutaryl-coenzymel A reductase pathway induces p53-independent transcriptional regulation of p21(WAF1/CIP1) in human prostate carcinoma cells. *J. Biol. Chem.*, *273*, 10618–10623.

Lehoux, J.G., N. Kandalaft, S. Belisle, D. Bellabarba, B. Benard, A. Lefebvre. 1984. Increased 3-hydroxy-3-methyl-glutaryl coenzyme A reductase activity in a virilizing adrenal carcinoma. *J. Steroid Biochem.*, *21*, 329–342.

Li, X., L. Liu, J.C. Tupper, D.D. Bannerman, R.K. Winn, S.M. Sebti, A.D. Hamilton, J.M. Harlan. 2002. Inhibition of protein geranylgeranylation and RhoA/RhoA kinase pathway induces apoptosis in human endothelial cells. *J. Biol. Chem.*, *277*, 15309–15316.

Macaulay, R.J., W. Wang, J. Dimitroulakos, L.E. Becker, H. Yeger. 1999. Lovastatin-induced apoptosis of human medulloblastoma cell lines *in vitro*. *J. Neurooncol.*, *42*, 1–11.

Makpol, S., N.A. Shamaan, Z. Jarien, A.G. Top, B.A. Khalid, W.Z. Wan Ngah. 1997. Different starting times of α-tocopherol and gamma-tocotrienol supplementation and tumor marker enzyme activities in the rat chemically induced with cancer. *Gen. Pharmacol.*, *28*, 589–592.

Marcelli, M., G.R. Cunningham, S.J. Haidacher, S.J. Padayatty, L. Sturgis, C. Kagan, L. Denner. 1998. Caspase-7 is activated during lovastatin-induced apoptosis of the prostate cancer cell line LNCaP. *Cancer Res.*, *58*, 76–83.

McAnally, J.A., J. Gupta, S. Sodhani, L. Bravo, H. Mo. 2007. Tocotrienols potentiate lovastatin-mediated growth suppression *in vitro* and *in vivo*. *Exp. Biol. Med. (Maywood)*, *232*, 523–531.

McGuire, T.F., X.Q. Xu, S.J. Corey, G.G. Romero, S.M. Sebti. 1994. Lovastatin disrupts early events in insulin signaling: A potential mechanism of lovastatin's anti-mitogenic activity. *Biochem. Biophys. Res. Commun.*, *204*, 399–406.

McIntyre, B.S., K.P. Briski, A. Gapor, P.W. Sylvester. 2000a. Antiproliferative and apoptotic effects of tocopherols and tocotrienols on preneoplastic and neoplastic mouse mammary epithelial cells. *Proc. Soc. Exp. Biol. Med.*, *224*, 292–301.

McIntyre, B.S., K.P. Briski, M.A. Tirmenstein, M.W. Fariss, A. Gapor, P.W. Sylvester. 2000b. Antiproliferative and apoptotic effects of tocopherols and tocotrienols on normal mouse mammary epithelial cells. *Lipids*, *35*, 171–180.

Mehta, N., J. Hordines, D. Sykes, R.J. Doerr, S.A. Cohen. 1998. Low density lipoproteins and Lovastatin modulate the organ-specific transendothelial migration of primary and metastatic human colon adenocarcinoma cell lines *in vitro*. *Clin. Exp. Metastasis*, *16*, 587–594.

Meric-Bernstam, F., M.C. Hung. 2006. Advances in targeting human epidermal growth factor receptor-2 signaling for cancer therapy. *Clin. Cancer Res.*, *12*, 6326–6330.

Miquel, K., A. Pradines, G. Favre. 1996. Farnesol and geranylgeraniol induce actin cytoskeleton disorganization and apoptosis in A549 lung adenocarcinoma cells. *Biochem. Biophys. Res. Commun.*, *225*, 869–876.

Mitchell, A.D., T.D. Pugh, S. Goldfarb. 1978. Partial "feedback control" of β-hydroxy-β-methylglutaryl coenzyme A reductase activity in primary hepatocellular carcinomas. *Cancer Res.*, *38*, 4474–4477.

Miyazawa, T., H. Inokuchi, H. Hirokane, T. Tsuzuki, K. Nakagawa, M. Igarashi. 2004. Anti-angiogenic potential of tocotrienol *in vitro*. *Biochem. (Moscow)*, *69*, 85–88.

Mizushina, Y., K. Nakagawa, A. Shibata, Y. Awata, I. Kuriyama, N. Shimazaki, O. Koiwai, Y. Uchiyama, K. Sakaguchi, T. Miyazawa, H. Yoshida. 2006. Inhibitory effect of tocotrienol on eukaryotic DNA polymerase lambda and angiogenesis. *Biochem. Biophys. Res. Commun.*, *339*, 949–955.

Mo, H., C.E. Elson. 1999. Apoptosis and cell-cycle arrest in human and murine tumor cells are initiated by isoprenoids. *J. Nutr.*, *129*, 804–813.

Mo, H., C.E. Elson. 2004. Studies of the isoprenoid-mediated inhibition of mevalonate synthesis applied to cancer chemotherapy and chemoprevention. *Exp. Biol. Med. (Maywood)*, *229*, 567–585.

Mo, H., J. Gupta, S. Sodhani, S. Jones. 2005. A blend of δ-tocotrienol and low-dose lovastatin suppresses the growth of murine B16 melanomas. *FASEB J.*, *19*, A79.

Montaner, S., R. Perona, L. Saniger, J.C. Lacal. 1998. Multiple signalling pathways lead to the activation of the nuclear factor kappaB by the Rho family of GTPases. *J. Biol. Chem.*, *273*, 12779–12785.

Morris, T.J., S.L. Palm, L.L. Furcht, H. Buchwald. 1995. Effect of lovastatin alone and as an adjuvant chemotherapeutic agent on hepatoma tissue culture-4 cell growth. *Ann. Surg. Oncol.*, *2*, 266–274.

Muller, C., A.G. Bockhorn, S. Klusmeier, M. Kiehl, C. Roeder, H. Kalthoff, O.M. Koch. 1998. Lovastatin inhibits proliferation of pancreatic cancer cell lines with mutant as well as with wild-type K-ras oncogene but has different effects on protein phosphorylation and induction of apoptosis. *Int. J. Oncol.*, *12*, 717–723.

Nakagawa, K., T. Eitsuka, H. Inokuchi, T. Miyazawa. 2004. DNA chip analysis of comprehensive food function: Inhibition of angiogenesis and telomerase activity with unsaturated vitamin E, tocotrienol. *Biofactors*, *21*, 5–10.

Nakanishi, M., J.L. Goldstein, M.S. Brown. 1988. Multivalent control of 3-hydroxy-3-methylglutaryl coenzyme A reductase. Mevalonate-derived product inhibits translation of mRNA and accelerates degradation of enzyme. *J. Biol. Chem.*, *263*, 8929–8937.

Nesaretnam, K., R. Ambra, K.R. Selvaduray, A. Radhakrishnan, K. Reimann, G. Razak, F. Virgili. 2004. Tocotrienol-rich fraction from palm oil affects gene expression in tumors resulting from MCF-7 cell inoculation in athymic mice. *Lipids*, *39*, 459–467.

Nesaretnam, K., S. Dorasamy, P.D. Darbre. 2000. Tocotrienols inhibit growth of ZR-75-1 breast cancer cells. *Int. J. Food Sci. Nutr.*, *51*, S95–103.

Nesaretnam, K., N. Guthrie, A.F. Chambers, K.K. Carroll. 1995. Effect of tocotrienols on the growth of a human breast cancer cell line in culture. *Lipids*, *30*, 1139–1143.

Nesaretnam, K., H.T. Khor, J. Ganeson, et al. 1992. The effect of vitamin E tocotrienols from palm oil on chemically induced mammary carcinogenesis in female rats. *Nutr. Res.*, *12*, 879–892.

Nesaretnam, K., R. Stephen, R. Dils, P. Darbre. 1998. Tocotrienols inhibit the growth of human breast cancer cells irrespective of estrogen receptor status. *Lipids*, *33*, 461–469.

Neuzil, J., M. Tomasetti, Y. Zhao, L.F. Dong, M. Birringer, X.F. Wang, P. Low, K. Wu, B.A. Salvatore, S.J. Ralph. 2007. Vitamin e analogs, a novel group of "mitocans," as anticancer agents: the importance of being redox–silent. *Mol. Pharmacol.* , *71*, 1185-1199.

Newman, A., R.D. Clutterbuck, R.L. Powles, D. Catovsky, J.L. Millar. 1997. A comparison of the effect of the 3-hydroxy-3-methylglutaryl coenzyme A (HMG-CoA) reductase inhibitors simvastatin, lovastatin and pravastatin on leukaemic and normal bone marrow progenitors. *Leuk. Lymphoma, 24*, 533–537.

Newman, A., R.D. Clutterbuck, R.L. Powles, J.L. Millar. 1994. Selective inhibition of primary acute myeloid leukaemia cell growth by lovastatin. *Leukemia, 8*, 274–280.

Ngah, W.Z., Z. Jarien, M.M. San, A. Marzuki, G.M. Top, N.A. Shamaan, K.A. Kadir. 1991. Effect of tocotrienols on hepatocarcinogenesis induced by 2-acetylaminofluorene in rats. *Am. J. Clin. Nutr., 53*, 1076S–1081S.

Nishida, S., H. Matsuoka, M. Tsubaki, Y. Tanimori, M. Yanae, Y. Fujii, M. Iwaki. 2005. Mevastatin induces apoptosis in HL60 cells dependently on decrease in phosphorylated ERK. *Mol. Cell. Biochem., 269*, 109–114.

Notarnicola, M., C. Messa, M. Pricci, V. Guerra, D.F. Altomare, S. Montemurro, M.G. Caruso. 2004. Up-regulation of 3-hydroxy-3-methylglutaryl coenzyme A reductase activity in left-sided human colon cancer. *Anticancer Res., 24*, 3837–3842.

Odysseos, A.D., P. Vraka, S. Bouralexis, D.M. Frindlay, A. Papas, A. Evdokiou. 2002. Gamma-tocotrienol triggers caspase-mediated induction of apoptosis in androgen-responsive, but not androgen unresponsive prostate cancer cells *in vitro. Free Radical Res., 36*, 116–117.

Okabe, M., M. Oji, I. Ikeda, H. Tachibana, K. Yamada. 2002. Tocotrienol levels in various tissues of Sprague-Dawley rats after intragastric administration of tocotrienols. *Biosci. Biotechnol. Biochem., 66*, 1768–1771.

Osborne, T.F. 2000. Sterol regulatory element-binding proteins (SREBPs): Key regulators of nutritional homeostasis and insulin action. *J. Biol. Chem., 275*, 32379–32382.

Padayatty, S.J., M. Marcelli, T.C. Shao, G.R. Cunningham. 1997. Lovastatin-induced apoptosis in prostate stromal cells. *J. Clin. Endocrinol. Metab., 82*, 1434–1439.

Park, C., I. Lee, W.K. Kang. 2001. Lovastatin-induced E2F-1 modulation and its effect on prostate cancer cell death. *Carcinogenesis, 22*, 1727–1731.

Park, W.H., Y.Y. Lee, E.S. Kim, J.G. Seol, C.W. Jung, C.C. Lee, B.K. Kim. 1999. Lovastatin-induced inhibition of HL-60 cell proliferation via cell cycle arrest and apoptosis. *Anticancer Res., 19*, 3133–3140.

Parker, R.A., B.C. Pearce, R.W. Clark, D.A. Gordon, J.J. Wright. 1993. Tocotrienols regulate cholesterol production in mammalian cells by post-transcriptional suppression of 3-hydroxy-3-methylglutaryl-coenzymel A reductase. *J. Biol. Chem., 268*, 11230–11238.

Peffley, D.M. 1992. Regulation of 3-hydroxy-3-methylglutaryl coenzyme A reductase synthesis in Syrian hamster C100 cells by mevinolin, 25-hydroxycholesterol and mevalonate: The role of posttranscriptional control. *Somat. Cell Mol. Genet., 18*, 19–32.

Peffley, D.M., A.K. Gayen. 1997. Inhibition of squalene synthase but not squalene cyclase prevents mevalonate-mediated suppression of 3-hydroxy-3-methylglutaryl coenzyme A reductase synthesis at a posttranscriptional level. *Arch. Biochem. Biophys., 337*, 251–260.

Peffley, D.M., A.K. Gayen, O.H. Morand. 1998. Down-regulation of 3-hydroxy-3-methylglutaryl coenzyme A reductase mRNA levels and synthesis in Syrian hamster C100 cells by the oxidosqualene cyclase inhibitor 4'-(6-allyl-ethyl-amino-hexyloxy)-2'-fluoro-phenyl -(4-bromophenyl) me thanone (Ro 48-8071): Comparison to simvastatin. *Biochem. Pharmacol., 56*, 439–449.

Peffley, D., M. Sinensky. 1985. Regulation of 3-hydroxy-3-methylglutaryl coenzyme A reductase synthesis by a non-sterol mevalonate-derived product in Mev-1 cells. Apparent translational control. *J. Biol. Chem., 260*, 9949–9952.

Perez-Sala, D., D. Collado-Escobar, F. Mollinedo. 1995. Intracellular alkalinization suppresses lovastatin-induced apoptosis in HL-60 cells through the inactivation of a pH-dependent endonuclease. *J. Biol. Chem., 270*, 6235–6242.

Perez-Sala, D., F. Mollinedo. 1994. Inhibition of isoprenoid biosynthesis induces apoptosis in human promyelocytic HL-60 cells. *Biochem. Biophys. Res. Commun., 199*, 1209–1215.

Perona, R., S. Montaner, L. Saniger, I. Sanchez-Perez, R. Bravo, J.C. Lacal. 1997. Activation of the nuclear factor-kappaB by Rho, CDC42 and Rac-1 proteins. *Genes Dev., 11*, 463–475.

Philippot, J.R., A.G. Cooper, D.F. Wallach. 1977. Regulation of cholesterol biosynthesis by normal and leukemic (L2C) guinea pig lymphocytes. 1996. *Proc. Natl. Acad. Sci. USA, 74*, 956–960.

Podda, M., C. Weber, M.G. Traber, L. Packer. 1996. Simultaneous determination of tissue tocopherols, tocotrienols, ubiquinols and ubiquinones. *J. Lipid Res., 37*, 893–901.

Potter, V.R. 1958. The biochemical approach to the cancer problem. *Fed. Proc., 17*, 691–697.

Prasanna, P., A. Thibault, L. Liu, D. Samid. 1996. Lipid metabolism as a target for brain cancer therapy: Synergistic activity of lovastatin and sodium phenylacetate against human glioma cells. *J. Neurochem.*, *66*, 710–716.

Qureshi, A.A., W.C. Burger, D.A. Peterson, C.E. Elson. 1986. The structure of an inhibitor of cholesterol biosynthesis isolated from barley. *J. Biol. Chem.*, *261*, 10544–10550.

Qureshi, A.A., B.C. Pearce, R.M. Nor, A. Gapor, D.M. Peterson, C.E. Elson. 1996. Dietary α-tocopherol attenuates the impact of gamma-tocotrienol on hepatic 3-hydroxy-3-methylglutaryl coenzyme A reductase activity in chickens. *J. Nutr.*, *126*, 389–394.

Qureshi, A.A., N. Qureshi, J.J. Wright, Z. Shen, G. Kramer, A. Gapor, Y.H. Chong, G. DeWitt, A. Ong, D.M. Peterson, B.A. Bradlow. 1991. Lowering of serum cholesterol in hypercholesterolemic humans by tocotrienols (palmvitee). *Am. J. Clin. Nutr.*, *53*, 1021S–1026S.

Raederstorff, D., V. Elste, C. Aebischer, P. Weber. 2002. Effect of either gamma-tocotrienol or a tocotrienol mixture on the plasma lipid profile in hamsters. *Ann. Nutr. Metab.*, *46*, 17–23.

Rahmat, A., W.Z.W. Ngah, A. Marzuki, Z. Jarien, R. Ismail, K.A. Kadir, N.A. Shamaan. 1993a. Effect of gamma-tocotrienol and α-tocopherol on blood glutathione and tumor marker enzymes during chemical hepatocarcinogenesis in the rat. *J. Clin. Biochem. Nutr.*, 15, 195–202.

Rahmat, A., W.Z. Ngah, N.A. Shamaan, A. Gapor, K. Abdul Kadir. 1993b. Long-term administration of tocotrienols and tumor-marker enzyme activities during hepatocarcinogenesis in rats. *Nutrition, 9*, 229–232.

Rao, S., M. Lowe, T.W. Herliczek, T.W., K. Keyomarsi. 1998. Lovastatin mediated G1 arrest in normal and tumor breast cells is through inhibition of CDK2 activity and redistribution of p21 and p27, independent of p53. *Oncogene*, *17*, 2393–2402.

Roos, W.P., B. Kaina. 2006. DNA damage-induced cell death by apoptosis. *Trends Mol. Med.*, *12*, 440–450.

Rossiello, M.R., P. Rao, S. Rajalakshmi, D.A.R. Sarma. 1994. Similar patterns of hypomethylation in the β-hydroxy-β-methylglutaryl cenzyme A reductase gene in hepatic nodules induced by different carcinogens. *Mol. Carcinogenesis, 10*, 237–245.

Rozados, V.R., L.I. Hinrichsen, J. McDonnell, O.G. Scharovsky. 2005. Lovastatin enhances *in vitro* radiation-induced apoptosis of rat B–cell lymphoma cells. *J. Exp. Clin. Cancer Res.* , *24*, 55–61.

Rubins, J.B., T. Greatens, R.A. Kratzke, A.T. Tan, V.A. Polunovsky, P. Bitterman. Lovastatin induces apoptosis in malignant mesothelioma cells. *Am. J. Respir. Crit. Care Med.* 1998, *157*, 1616–1622.

Sakai, M.M., H. Hachibana, K. Yamada. 2006. Apoptosis induction by gamma-tocotrienol in human hepatoma Hep3B cells. *J. Nutr. Biochem.*, *17*, 672–676.

Sakai, M., M. Okabe, M.Yamasaki, H. Tachibana, K. Yamada. 2004. Induction of apoptosis by tocotrienol in rat hepatoma dRLh-84 cells. *Anticancer Res., 24*, 1683–1688.

Samant, G.V., P.W. Sylvester. 2006. Gamma-tocotrienol inhibits ErbB3-dependent PI3K/Akt mitogenic signalling in neoplastic mammary epithelial cells. *Cell Prolif.*, *39*, 563–574.

Satoh, T., H. Isobe, K. Ayukawa, H. Sakai, H. Nawata. 1996. The effects of pravastatin, an HMG-CoA reductase inhibitor, on cell viability and DNA production of rat hepatocytes. *Life Sci., 59*, 1103–1108.

Schumm, K., S. Rocha, J. Caamano, N.D. Perkins. 2006. Regulation of p53 tumour suppressor target gene expression by the p52 NF-kappaB subunit. *EMBO J.*, *25*, 4820–4832.

Sears, R.C., J.R. Nevins. 2002. Signaling networks that link cell proliferation and cell fate. *J. Biol. Chem.*, *277*, 11617–11620.

Sen, C.K., S. Khanna, S. Roy, L. Packer. 2000. Molecular basis of vitamin E action. Tocotrienol potently inhibits glutamate-induced pp60(c-Src) kinase activation and death of HT4 neuronal cells. *J. Biol. Chem., 275*, 13049–13055.

Sever, N., B.L. Song, D. Yabe, J.L. Goldstein, M.S. Brown, R.A. DeBose-Boyd. 2003a. Insig-dependent ubiquitination and degradation of mammalian 3-hydroxy-3-methylglutaryl-CoA reductase stimulated by sterols and geranylgeraniol. *J. Biol. Chem.*, *278*, 52479–52490.

Sever, N., T. Yang, M.S. Brown, J.L. Goldstein, R.A. DeBose-Boyd. 2003b. Accelerated degradation of HMG CoA reductase mediated by binding of insig-1 to its sterol-sensing domain. *Mol. Cell, 11*, 25–33.

Shah, S., A. Gapor, P.W. Sylvester. 2003. Role of caspase-8 activation in mediating vitamin E-induced apoptosis in murine mammary cancer cells. *Nutr. Cancer, 45*, 236–246.

Shah, S., P.W. Sylvester. 2004. Tocotrienol-induced caspase-8 activation is unrelated to death receptor apoptotic signaling in neoplastic mammary epithelial cells. *Exp. Biol. Med. (Maywood)*, *229*, 745–755.

Shah, S.J., P.W. Sylvester. 2005a. Gamma-tocotrienol inhibits neoplastic mammary epithelial cell proliferation by decreasing Akt and nuclear factor kappaB activity. *Exp. Biol. Med. (Maywood)*, *230*, 235–241.

Shah, S.J., P.W. Sylvester. 2005b. Tocotrienol-induced cytotoxicity is unrelated to mitochondrial stress apoptotic signaling in neoplastic mammary epithelial cells. *Biochem. Cell Biol., 83,* 86–95.

Shamaan, N.A., W.Z. Wan Ngah, R. Ibrahim, Z. Jarien, A.G. Top, K. Abdul Kadir. 1993. Effect of tocotrienol on the activities of cytosolic glutathione-dependent enzymes in rats treated with 2-acetylaminofluorene. *Biochem. Pharmacol., 45,* 1517–1519.

Shellman, Y.G., D. Ribble, L. Miller, J. Gendall, K. Vanbuskirk, D. Kelly, D.A. Norris, R.P. Dellavalle. 2005. Lovastatin-induced apoptosis in human melanoma cell lines. *Melanoma Res., 15,* 83–89.

Sherr, C.J. 2004. Principles of tumor suppression. *Cell, 116,* 235–246.

Shibata, M.A., Y. Ito, J. Morimoto, Y. Otsuki. 2004. Lovastatin inhibits tumor growth and lung metastasis in mouse mammary carcinoma model: A p53-independent mitochondrial-mediated apoptotic mechanism. *Carcinogenesis, 25,* 1887–1898.

Shibata, M.A., C. Kavanaugh, E. Shibata, H. Abe, P. Nguyen, Y. Otsuki, J.B. Trepel, J.E. Green. 2003. Comparative effects of lovastatin on mammary and prostate oncogenesis in transgénic mouse models. *Carcinogenesis, 24,* 453–459.

Shimano, H., J.D. Horton, R.E. Hammer, I. Shimomura, M.S. Brown, J.L. Goldstein. 1996. Overproduction of cholesterol and fatty acids causes massive liver enlargement in transgenic mice expressing truncated SREBP-1a. *J. Clin. Invest., 98,* 1575–1584.

Shimano, H., J.D. Horton, I. Shimomura, R.E. Hammer, M.S. Brown, J.L. Goldstein. 1997. Isoform 1c of sterol regulatory element binding protein is less active than isoform 1a in livers of transgenic mice and in cultured cells. *J. Clin. Invest., 99,* 846–854.

Shimomura, I., H. Shimano, J.D. Horton, J.L. Goldstein, M.S. Brown. 1997. Differential expression of exons 1a and 1c in mRNAs for sterol regulatory element binding protein-1 in human and mouse organs and cultured cells. *J. Clin. Invest., 99,* 838–845.

Shun, M.C., W. Yu, A. Gapor, R. Parsons, J. Atkinson, B.G. Sanders, K. Kline. 2004. Pro-apoptotic mechanisms of action of a novel vitamin E analog (α-TEA) and a naturally occurring form of vitamin E (δ-tocotrienol) in MDA-MB-435 human breast cancer cells. *Nutr. Cancer, 48,* 95–105.

Singh, R.P., R. Kumar, N. Kapur. 2003. Molecular regulation of cholesterol biosynthesis: Implications in carcinogenesis. *J. Environ. Pathol. Toxicol. Oncol., 22,* 75–92.

Siperstein, M.D., V.M. Fagan. 1964. Deletion of the cholesterol-negative feedback system in liver tumors. *Cancer Res., 24,* 1108–1115.

Siperstein, M.D., A. M. Gyde, H.P. Morris. 1971. Loss of feedback control of hydroxymethyl glutaryl coenzyme A reductase in hepatomas. *Proc. Natl. Acad. Sci. USA, 68,* 315–317.

Sivaprasad, U., T. Abbas, A. Dutta. 2006. Differential efficacy of 3-hydroxy-3-methylglutaryl CoA reductase inhibitors on the cell cycle of prostate cancer cells. *Mol. Cancer Ther., 5,* 2310–2316.

Soma, M.R., R. Baetta, S. Bergamaschi, M.R. De Renzis, C. Davegna, F. Battaini, R. Fumagalli, S. Govoni. 1994. PKC activity in rat C6 glioma cells: Changes associated with cell cycle and simvastatin treatment. *Biochem. Biophys. Res. Commun., 200,* 1143–1149.

Soma, M.R., R. Baetta, M.R. De Renzis, G. Mazzini, C. Davegna, L. Magrassi, G. Butti, S. Pezzotta, R. Paoletti, R. Fumagalli. 1995. *In vivo* enhanced antitumor activity of carmustine N,N'-bis(2-chloroethyl)-N-nitrosourea by simvastatin. *Cancer Res., 55,* 597–602.

Song, B.L., R.A. DeBose-Boyd. 2006. Insig-dependent ubiquination and degradation of 3-hydroxy-3-methylglutaryl coenzyme A reductase stimulated by δ- and gamma-tocotrienols. *J. Biol. Chem., 281,* 25054–25061.

Song, B.L., N.B. Javitt, R.A. DeBose-Boyd. 2005a. Insig-mediated degradation of HMG CoA reductase stimulated by lanosterol, an intermediate in the synthesis of cholesterol. *Cell metab., 1,* 179–189.

Song, B.L, N. Sever, R.A. DeBose-Boyd. 2005b. Gp78, a membrane-anchored ubiquitin ligase, associates with Insig-1 and couples sterol-regulated ubiquitination to degradation of HMG CoA reductase. *Mol. Cell, 19,* 829–840.

Sora, M.K., A.A. Kruszewski, T. Stoklosa, J. Czyzyk, W. Lasek, J. Malejczyk, M. Jakobisiak. 1994. Synergistic antiproliferative activity of tumor necrosis factor α (TNF-α) and lovastatin. *Arch. Immunol. Ther. Exp., 42,* 269–274.

Srivastava, J.K., S. Gupta. 2006. Tocotrienol-rich fraction of palm oil induces cell cycle arrest and apoptosis selectively in human prostate cancer cells. *Biochem. Biophys. Res. Commun., 346,* 447–453.

Stewart, S.A., R.A. Weinberg. 2006. Telomeres: Cancer to human aging. *Ann. Rev. Cell Dev. Biol., 22,* 531–557.

Straka, M.S., S.R. Panini. 1995. Post-transcriptional regulation of 3-hydroxy-3-methylglutaryl coenzyme A reductase by mevalonate. *Arch. Biochem. Biophys., 317,* 235–243.

Sun, L.P., L. Li, J.L. Goldstein, M.S. Brown. 2005. Insig required for sterol-mediated inhibition of Scap/SREBP binding to COPII proteins *in vitro*. *J. Biol. Chem., 280,* 26483–26490.

Sutherland, R.L., E.A. Musgrove. 2004. Cyclins and breast cancer. *J. Mammary Gland Biol. Neoplasia, 9,* 95–104.

Sylvester, P.W., B. S. McIntyre, A. Gapor, K.P. Briski. 2001. Vitamin E inhibition of normal mammary epithelial cell growth is associated with a reduction in protein kinase C (α) activation. *Cell Prolif., 34,* 347–357.

Sylvester, P.W., A. Nachnani, S. Shah, K.P. Briski. 2002. Role of GTP-binding proteins in reversing the antiproliferative effects of tocotrienols in preneoplastic mammary epithelial cells. *Asia Pac. J. Clin. Nutr., 11,* S452–459.

Sylvester, P.W., S.J. Shah. 2005a. Intracellular mechanisms mediating tocotrienol-induced apoptosis in neoplastic mammary epithelial cells. *Asia Pac. J. Clin. Nutr., 14,* 366–373.

Sylvester, P.W., S.J. Shah. 2005b. Mechanisms mediating the antiproliferative and apoptotic effects of vitamin E in mammary cancer cells. *Front Biosci., 10,* 699–709.

Sylvester, P.W., S.J. Shah, G.V. Samant. 2005. Intracellular signaling mechanisms mediating the antiproliferative and apoptotic effects of gamma-tocotrienol in neoplastic mammary epithelial cells. *J. Plant Physiol., 162,* 803–810.

Tabacik, C., S. Aliau, J. Sainte-Marie. 1987. Regulation of cholesterol biosynthesis at a stage after the 3-hydroxy-3-methylglutaryl-CoA reductase step, in normal and leukemic (L2C) guinea pig lymphocytes. *Biochim. Biophys. Acta., 921,* 405–410.

Takada, Y., F.R. Khuri, B.B. Aggarwal. 2004. Protein farnesyltransferase inhibitor (SCH 66336) abolishes NF-kappaB activation induced by various carcinogens and inflammatory stimuli leading to suppression of NF-kappaB-regulated gene expression and up-regulation of apoptosis. *J. Biol. Chem., 279,* 26287–26299.

Takada, Y., A. Murakami, B.B. Aggarwal. 2005. Zerumbone abolishes NF–kappaB and IkappaBα kinase activation leading to suppression of antiapoptotic and metastatic gene expression, upregulation of apoptosis and downregulation of invasion. *Oncogene, 24,* 6957–6969.

Takahashi, K., G. Loo. 2004. Disruption of mitochondria during tocotrienol-induced apoptosis in MDA-MB-231 human breast cancer cells. *Biochem. Pharmacol., 67,* 315–324.

Takebayashi, T., H. Higashi, H. Sudo, H. Ozawa, E. Suzuki, O. Shirado, H. Katoh, M. Hatakeyama. 2003. NF-κ B-dependent induction of cyclin D1 by retinoblastoma protein (pRB) family proteins and tumor-derived pRB mutants. *J. Biol. Chem. , 278,* 14897–14905.

Taras, D., J.F. Blanc, A. Rullier, N. Dugot-Senant, I. Laurendeau, M. Vidaud, J. Rosenbaum. 2007. Pravastatin reduces lung metastasis of rat hepatocellular carcinoma via a coordinated decrease of MMP expression and activity. *J. Hepatol., 46,* 69–76.

Teicher, B.A. 2006. Protein kinase C as a therapeutic target. *Clin. Cancer Res., 12,* 5336–5345.

Theriault, A., Q. Wang, A. Gapor, K. Adeli. 1999. Effects of gamma-tocotrienol on ApoB synthesis, degradation and secretion in HepG2 cells. *Arterioscler. Thromb. Vasc. Biol., 19,* 704–712.

Thibault, A., D. Samid, A.C. Tompkins, W.D. Figg, M.R. Cooper , R.J. Hohl, J. Trepel, B. Liang, N. Patronas, D.J. Venzon, E. Reed, C.E. Myers. 1996. Phase I study of lovastatin, an inhibitor of the mevalonate pathway, in patients with cancer. *Clin. Cancer Res., 2,* 483–491.

Traber, M.G., M. Rallis, M. Podda, C. Weber, H.I. Maibach, L. Packer. 1998. Penetration and distribution of α-tocopherol, α- or gamma-tocotrienols applied individually onto murine skin. *Lipids, 33,* 87–91.

Ukomadu, C., A. Dutta. 2003a. p21-dependent inhibition of colon cancer cell growth by mevastatin is independent of inhibition of G1 cyclin-dependent kinases. *J. Biol. Chem., 278,* 43586–43594.

Ukomadu, C., A. Dutta. 2003b. Inhibition of cdk2 activating phosphorylation by mevastatin. *J. Biol. Chem., 278,* 4840–4846.

van de Donk, N.W., D. Schotte, M.M. Kamphuis, A.M. van Marion, B. van Kessel, A.C. Bloem, H.M. Lokhorst. 2003. Protein geranylgeranylation is critical for the regulation of survival and proliferation of lymphoma tumor cells. *Clin. Cancer Res., 9,* 5735–5748.

Viallard, J.F., F. Lacombe, F. Belloc, J.L. Pellegrin, J. Reiffers. 2001. Molecular mechanisms controlling the cell cycle: Fundamental aspects and implications for oncology. *Cancer Radiother., 5,* 109–129.

Vitols, S., S. Norgren, G. Juliusson, L. Tatidis, H. Luthman. 1994. Multilevel regulation of low-density lipoprotein receptor and 3-hydroxy-3-methylglutaryl coenzyme A reductase gene expression in normal and leukemic cells. *Blood, 84,* 2689–2698.

Wachtershauser, A., B. Akoglu, J. Stein. 2001. HMG-CoA reductase inhibitor mevastatin enhances the growth inhibitory effect of butyrate in the colorectal carcinoma cell line Caco-2. *Carcinogenesis*, *22*, 1061–1067.

Wada, S., Y. Satomi, M. Murakoshi, N. Noguchi, T. Yoshikawa, H. Nishino. 2005. Tumor suppressive effects of tocotrienol *in vivo* and *in vitro*. *Cancer Lett.*, *229*, 181–191.

Wali, V., P. Sylvester. 2006. Antiproliferative effects of HMG-CoA reductase inhibitors (statins) are significantly enhanced when used in combination with gamma-tocotrienol in neoplastic mammary epithelial cells in culture. *Am. Assoc. Cancer Res.*, *47*, A1347.

Wejde, J., H. Blegen, O. Larsson. 1992. Requirement for mevalonate in the control of proliferation of human breast cancer cells. *Anticancer Res.*, *12*, 317–324.

Wong, W.W.L., J. Dimitroulakos, M.D. Minden, L.Z. Penn. 2002. HMG-CoA reductase inhibitors and the malignant cell: The statin family of drugs as triggers of tumor-specific apoptosis. *Leukemia*, *16*, 508–519.

Wong, W.W., M.M. Tan, Z. Xia, J. Dimitroulakos, M.D. Minden, L.Z. Penn. 2001. Cerivastatin triggers tumor–specific apoptosis with higher efficacy than lovastatin. *Clin. Cancer Res.*, *7*, 2067–2075.

Wu, J., W.W.L. Wong, F. Khosravi, M.D. Minden, L.Z. Penn. 2004. Blocking the Raf-MEK-ERK pathway sensitizes acute myelogenous leukemia cells to lovastatin-induced apoptosis. *Cancer Res.*, *64*, 6461–6468.

Yachnin, S., D.B. Toub, V. Mannickarottu. 1984. Divergence in cholesterol biosynthetic rates and 3-hydroxy-3-methylglutaryl-CoA reductase activity as a consequence of granulocyte versus monocyte-macrophage differentiation in HL-60 cells. *Proc. Natl. Acad. Sci. USA*, *81*, 894–897.

Yang, T., P.J. Espenshade, M.E. Wright, D. Yabe, Y. Gong, R. Aebersold, J.L. Goldstein, M.S. Brown. 2002. Crucial step in cholesterol homeostasis: Sterols promote binding of SCAP to INSIG-1, a membrane protein that facilitates retention of SREBPs in ER. *Cell*, *110*, 489–500.

Yano, Y., H. Satoh, K. Fukumoto, I. Kumadaki, T. Ichikawa, K. Yamada, K. Hagiwara, T. Yano. 2005. Induction of cytotoxicity in human lung adenocarcinoma cells by 6-O-carboxypropyl-α-tocotrienol, a redox-silent derivative of α-tocotrienol. *Int. J. Cancer*, *115*, 839–846.

Yap, S.P., K.H. Yuen, J.W. Wong. 2001. Pharmacokinetics and bioavailability of α-, gamma- and δ-tocotrienols under different food status. *J. Pharm. Pharmacol.*, *53*, 67–71.

Yin, L., A.K. Hubbard, C. Giardina. 2000. NF-κ B regulates transcription of the mouse telomerase catalytic subunit. *J. Biol. Chem.*, *275*, 36671–36675.

Yin, X.M. 2006. Bid, a BH3-only multi-functional molecule, is at the cross road of life and death. *Gene*, *369*, 7–19.

Yu, W., M. Simmons-Menchaca, A. Gapor, B.G. Sanders, K. Kline. 1999. Induction of apoptosis in human breast cancer cells by tocopherols and tocotrienols. *Nutr. Cancer*, *33*, 26–32.

Zelvyte, I., R. Dominaitiene, M. Crisby, S. Janciauskiene. 2002. Modulation of inflammatory mediators and PPARgamma and NFkappaB expression by pravastatin in response to lipoproteins in human monocytes *in vitro*. *Pharmacol. Res.*, *45*, 147–154.

Zhong, W.B., C.Y. Wang, T.C. Chang, W.S. Lee. 2003. Lovastatin induces apoptosis of anaplastic thyroid cancer cells via inhibition of protein geranylgeranylation and *de novo* protein synthesis. *Endocrinology*, *144*, 3852–3859.

16 Telomerase Inhibition

Takahiro Eitsuka, Kiyotaka Nakagawa and Teruo Miyazawa

CONTENTS

16.1 INTRODUCTION

The ends of linear eukaryotic chromosomes contain specialized structures called telomeres that are essential for preserving the stability of the genome and maintaining cell viability by preventing aberrant recombination and degradation (McEachern et al., 2000). Human telomeres consist of tandem arrays of the hexameric sequence TTAGGG. Due to an "end-replication problem," DNA polymerase is not able to completely copy the end of the chromosome in lagging strand synthesis, resulting in a loss of telomeric repeats during each round of replication. Eventually, telomeres reach a critical length, and cell senescence occurs.

Human telomerase is a ribonucleoprotein that adds the tandem arrays of TTAGGG repeats to telomere ends (Morin, 1989). In human cells, the enzyme comprises three main components, hTR (human telomerase RNA component) (Feng et al., 1995), TP1 (telomerase-associated protein 1) (Harrington et al., 1997), and hTERT (human telomerase reverse transcriptase) (Meyerson et al., 1997; Nakamura et al., 1997), the last of which plays a key role in telomerase activation. Telomerase activity is not detectable in normal cells, with the exception of germ cells and renewal tissues, but is present in immortalized cell lines and in 80–90% of human cancer specimens (Kim et al., 1994). This indicates that telomere maintenance is essential for the proliferation of tumor cells, and that human telomerase is a novel and potentially highly selective target for cancer therapy.

The expression of hTERT mRNA parallels the enzymatic activity of telomerase in cancer cells, while it is repressed in most normal human somatic cells (Takakura et al., 1998). However, hTR and TP1 are generally expressed in normal tissues (Feng et al., 1995; Harrington et al., 1997), and overexpression of hTERT in telomerase negative cells is sufficient for the enzyme activity (Weinrich et al., 1997), indicating that transcriptional activation of the hTERT gene is the rate-limiting step in telomerase activity. Recently, the promoter region of hTERT has been cloned and sequenced (Cong et al., 1999; Horikawa et al., 1999; Takakura et al., 1999). Its region contains recognition sequences for several transcription factors including SP1, AP2 and c-Myc. In fact, c-Myc activates hTERT transcription by directly interacting with its promoter, leading to increased promoter activity (Wu et al., 1999). Moreover, protein kinase C (PKC) is known to up-regulate telomerase activity. PKC is involved with the posttranscriptional control of telomerase activity (Li et al., 1998) and the modulation of hTERT expression (Sheng et al., 2003). Other cellular factors such as human papillomavirus type-16 E6 protein, Mad1, p53 and retinoblastoma protein are also implicated in the modulation of telomerase (Liu, 1999).

We and other researchers reported that tocotrienol has potential anticancer properties *in vitro* and *in vivo* (Inokuchi et al., 2003; Miyazawa et al., 2004a; Miyazawa et al., 2004b; Nakagawa et al., 2004; Eitsuka et al., 2006; Mizushina et al., 2006; Sen et al., 2006). The proposed mechanism for this anti-tumor action is thought to be growth inhibition, apoptosis induction, antiangiogenesis or telomerase inhibition. In this chapter, we take a closer look at the anticancer effect of tocotrienol, with particular emphasis on telomerase inhibition, and discuss the molecular mechanism for telomerase regulation by tocotorienol.

16.2 INHIBITORY EFFECT OF TOCOTRIENOL ON CELLULAR TELOMERASE ACTIVITY

Telomerase activity was examined using a semi-quantitative telomerase assay (stretch PCR) (Tatematsu et al., 1996). In this assay, DNA amplified from telomerase products by the stretch PCR reaction was separated by electrophoresis and detected on the gel as a ladder consisting of bands spaced six base pairs apart (refer to the ladder presented for control in Figure 16.1A). After culturing DLD-1 (human colorectal adenocarcinoma) cells with tocotrienols for 24 h, a decrease in intensity of the six-base ladders was documented (Figure 16.1a), indicating that these tocotrienols can modulate telomerase activity. Figure 16.1b shows that treatment of DLD-1 cells with 5-30 μM β-, γ- and δ-tocotrienols for 24 h resulted in a dose-dependent decrease in telomerase activity. The inhibitory potency of each tocotrienol isomer varied as the following order; δ- > β- > γ- > α-tocotrienol. To examine the time-dependent telomerase inhibition, DLD-1 cells were cultured with β- and δ-tocotrienols (each 20 μM) for 6–72 h. Telomerase activity was time-dependently decreased, and δ-tocotrienol efficiently inhibited the enzyme activity compared with β-isomer (Figure 16.1c). Interestingly, in contrast to tocotrienols, tocopherols (α-, β-, γ- and δ-isomers) exhibited very weak telomerase inhibition (data not shown). It is therefore likely that the telomerase-inhibitory potency of tocotrienol is much higher than that of tocopherol.

Tocotrienol isomers were shown to possess different anti-telomerase activity, and the ranked order of this inhibitory effect was δ- > β- > γ- > α-tocotrienol (Figure 16.1). The finding indicated that the number and position of methyl substitution on the chromanol ring would be a principal factor influencing telomerase activity, and suggested that the inhibitory potency was elevated with a decrease in the number of methyl substitutions. In β- and γ-tocotrienols with an equal number of methyl substitutions, anti-telomerase activity of β-tocotrienol was superior to that of γ-isomer. Thus, tocotrienol without the 7-methyl group would play a key role in exhibiting a potent telomerase-inhibitory effect. Structurally, tocopherol and tocotrienol are distinguished by their side chains. It has been demonstrated that the unsaturated side chain of tocotrienol allows it to pass through cell membranes more efficiently and at a faster rate than the saturated side chain of tocopherol (Traber and Packer, 1995). Therefore, it is possible that the greater telomerase-inhibitory effect of tocotrienols would be due, in part, to their effective incorporation into DLD-1 cells.

16.3 MOLECULAR MECHANISM FOR TELOMERASE INHIBITION BY TOCOTRIENOL

hTERT, the catalytic subunit of telomerase, plays an important role in telomerase activation (Takakura et al., 1998). Therefore, to evaluate the mechanism for telomerase inhibition by tocotrienol, we investigated the effect of tocotrienol on hTERT expression in DLD-1 cells using a real-time RT-PCR. As shown in Figure 16.2a, tocotrienol effectively inhibited the expression of hTERT mRNA in a dose-dependent manner, indicating that telomerase activity is controlled at the transcriptional level. Since oncogene c-myc is a well-known regulator of hTERT expression (Wu et al., 1999), we then examined and found that tocotrienol caused a significant decrease in c-myc mRNA expression (Figure 16.2b). Finally, because PKC participates in the up-regulation of c-myc mRNA

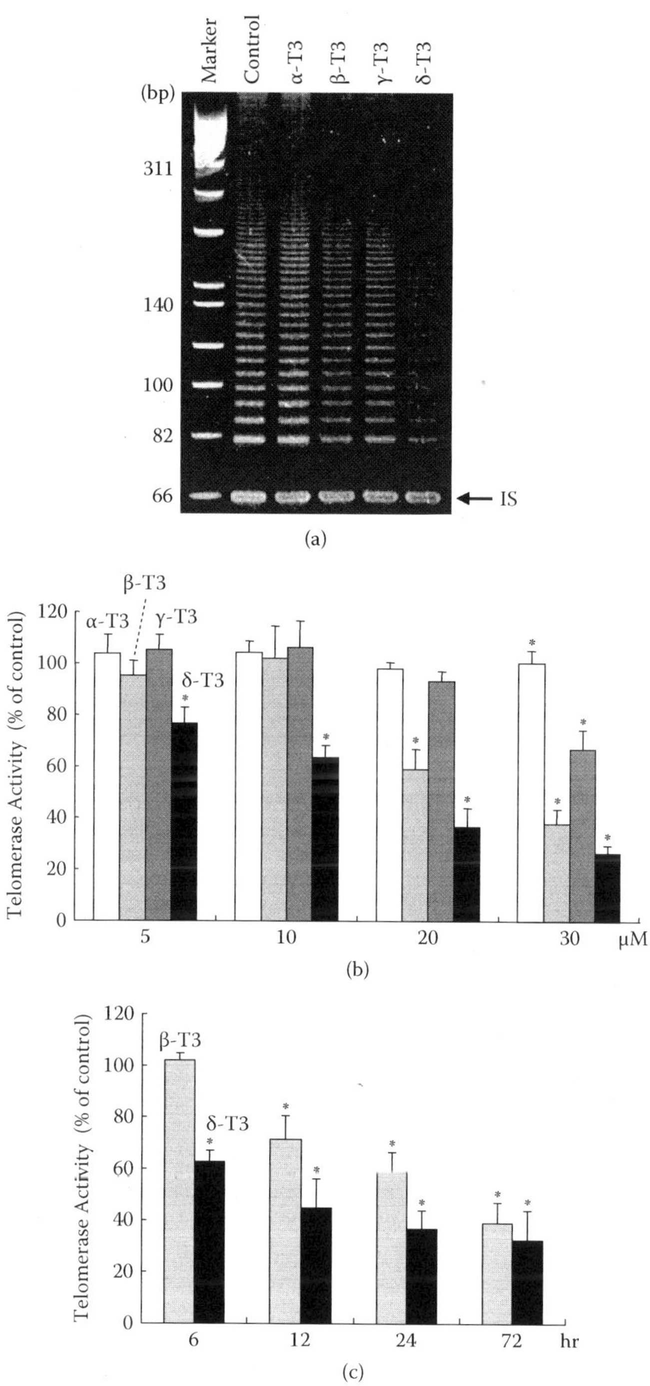

FIGURE 16.1 Cellular telomerase activity is decreased by treatment with tocotrienol. (a) DLD-1 cells were cultured with or without 20 μM tocotrienol for 24 h. Subsequently, telomerase activity in the cell extracts was measured by the stretch PCR assay. The PCR product was separated by 10% non-denaturing polyacrylamide gel electrophoresis and visualized with SYBR Green I. IS, internal standard. (b) The dose-dependent inhibition of telomerase activity was evaluated by treating DLD-1 cells with 5-30 μM tocotrienol or without sample (control) for 24 h. (c) The time-dependent inhibition of telomerase activity was investigated by treating DLD-1 cells in the presence or absence of 20 μM tocotrienol for 6–72 h. Telomerase activity is expressed as a percentage of the control. Values are means ± S.D. from three independent experiments; $^*P < 0.05$ compared with control.

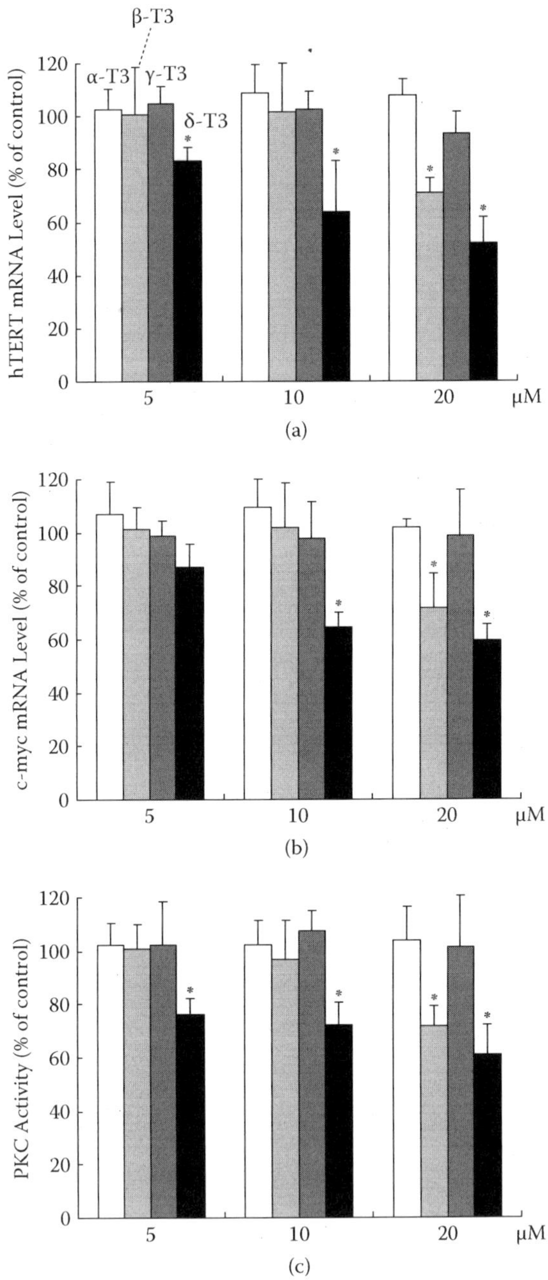

FIGURE 16.2 Inhibitory effect of tocotrienol on mRNA expression of hTERT and c-myc and on cellular PKC activity. DLD-1 cells were cultured with 5-20 μM tocotrienol or without sample (control) for 24 h. The mRNA expression levels of hTERT (a) and c-myc (b) were then measured by real-time RT-PCR and are expressed as percentages of the control. The mRNA level of β-actin was used as an internal control. (c) PKC activity in DLD-1 cells cultured in the presence or absence of 5–20 μM tocotrienol for 24 h was examined and is expressed as a percentage of the control. Values are means ± S.D. from three independent experiments; $*P < 0.05$ compared with control.

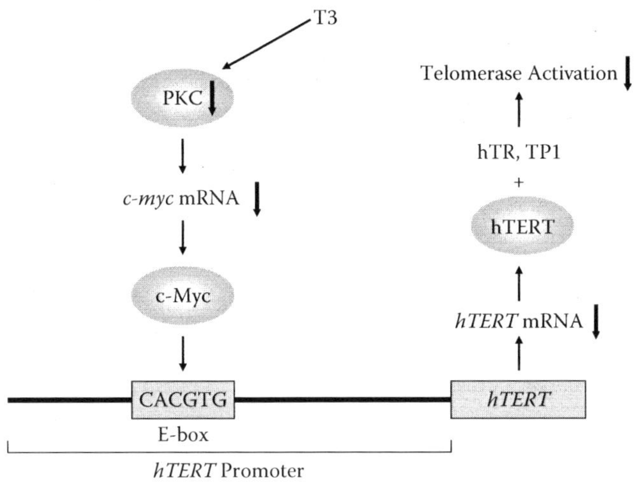

FIGURE 16.3 Molecular mechanism for telomerase inhibition by tocotrienol.

expression (Coughlin et al., 1985), we investigated and confirmed that tocotrienol inhibited cellular PKC activity (Figure 16.2c). These observations suggested that tocotrienol reduced telomerase activity by down-regulating hTERT and c-myc expression through inhibition of PKC activity.

PKC is known to participate in both the posttranscriptional control of telomerase activity (Li et al., 1998) and the modulation of hTERT expression (Sheng et al., 2003). As shown in Figures 16.1 and 16.2, there were proportional correlations among telomerase activity, hTERT expression and PKC activity. Therefore, telomerase inhibition via suppression of PKC activity by tocotrienol could be assigned to the transcriptional inhibition of hTERT expression. This result is in an agreement with recent studies showing that ceramide and curcumin, as inhibitors of PKC, can repress telomerase activity through down-regulation of hTERT (Ogretmen et al., 2001; Ramachandran et al., 2002). Moreover, both direct activators of PKC and hormones which induce PKC via receptor-mediated phosphoinositide turnover elicit a rapid increase in c-myc mRNA expression, suggesting that c-myc expression is controlled through a PKC signaling pathway (Coughlin et al., 1985). Thus, we deduced that down-regulation of c-myc (Figure 16.2b) would be due to the inhibition of PKC activity by tocotrienol (Figure 16.2c). Considering these findings, the following mechanism is conceivable for telomerase inhibition by tocotrienol: tocotrienol inhibits PKC activity, leading to down-regulation of c-myc mRNA, resulting in repression of hTERT expression, thereby reducing telomerase activity (Figure 16.3).

It is reported that PKCα and ζ modulate telomerase activity in breast and nasopharyngeal cancer cells, respectively (Li et al., 1998; Yu et al., 2001). The findings indicate that different PKC isoforms are involved in the regulation of telomerase activity in different cancer cell types. In colorectal cancer cells (such as DLD-1), it is not clear which PKC subtypes participate in the control of telomerase activity. However, Murray et al. demonstrated that elevated expression of PKCβII is implicated in colon carcinogenesis (Murray et al., 1999). It is therefore plausible that PKCβII might regulate telomerase in DLD-1 cells and that PKCβII inhibition with tocotrienol may cause reduction of telomerase activity. Further studies are needed to clarify the inhibitory mechanism for the PKC isoform by tocotrienol.

Tocotrienol has been shown to posttranscriptionally attenuate 3-hydroxy-3-methylglutaryl-coenzyme A (HMG-CoA) reductase activity (Parker et al., 1993). Recent studies have revealed that the HMG-CoA reductase inhibitors such as lovastatin can induce cell cycle arrest and therefore have potential as novel chemotherapeutic agents (Mo and Elson, 2004). Thus, it is likely that the anti-proliferative property of tocotrienol may partly participate in the inhibition of HMG-CoA reductase. Interestingly, lovastatin represses the E2F-1-regulated expression of several cell cycle genes including c-myc (Park et al., 2001). These findings raise the possibility that tocotrienol may inhibit telomerase through not only the reduction of PKC activity but also the suppression of HMG-CoA reductase. Further investigation of telomerase inhibition by tocotrienol will help to develop mechanism-based strategies for cancer prevention.

16.4 CONCLUSION

Telomerase is not detectable in most somatic tissues, whereas it is activated in the majority of cancer cells and malignant tumors (Kim et al., 1994), implying that telomerase is essential for cell immortalization and tumorigenesis. Therefore, telomerase is a novel and potentially highly selective target for cancer therapy. In such a context, there is considerable work being undertaken to screen potential telomerase inhibitors. The dietary constituents (i.e., flavonoids [Naasani et al., 1998], ceramide [Ogretmen et al., 2001] and curcumin [Ramachandran et al., 2002]) have been shown to inhibit telomerase activity *in vitro*. In our recent studies, some lipids (i.e., sulfoquinvosyldiacylglycerol [Eitsuka et al., 2004a], polyunsaturated fatty acids [Eitsuka et al., 2004b; Eitsuka et al., 2005] and tocotrienol [Eitsuka et al., 2006]) appeared to act as powerful telomerase inhibitors. Hence, these dietary compounds have potential use as therapeutic supplements for telomerase inhibition.

In cancer chemotherapy, telomerase inhibitors might act in a synergistic fashion with existing therapeutic modalities and amplify their effectiveness. A telomerase inhibitor will progressively reduce telomere length, although there is an expected time delay until cell death. An angiogenesis inhibitor will maintain a reduced tumor burden, but will not eradicate the tumor or affect telomere length. Thus, combinations of angiogenesis inhibitors with telomerase inhibitors would be predicted to maintain a reduced tumor burden while producing progressively shortened telomeres, potentially leading to preventing or delaying tumor recurrences (Shay and Wright, 2002). Interestingly, tocotrienol has been shown to possess both anti-angiogenic and anti-telomerase properties, which may effectively contribute to cancer prevention.

In conclusion, tocotrienol exhibited the inhibitory effect on cellular telomerase activity and the inhibitory potency of tocotrienol is much superior to that of tocopherol. Tocotrienol modulated telomerase by repressing hTERT and c-myc expression via inhibition of PKC activity. These results support the anti-proliferative function of tocotrienol, and indicate that tocotrienol is a potent candidate regulator of telomerase.

ACKNOWLEDGMENTS

This study was supported in part by a Grant-in-Aid from the Bio-oriented Technology Research Advancement Center of the National Agricultural and Biological Research Organization, Japan.

REFERENCES

Cong, Y.S., J. Wen, S. Bacchetti. 1999. The human telomerase catalytic subunit hTERT: Organization of the gene and characterization of the promoter. *Hum. Mol. Genet.*, *8*, 137–142.

Coughlin, S.R., W.M.F. Lee, P.W. Williams, G.M. Giels, L.T. Williams. 1985. c-myc gene expression is stimulated by agents that activate protein kinase C and does not account for the mitogenic effect of PDGF. *Cell*, *43*, 243–251.

Eitsuka, T., K. Nakagawa, M. Igarashi, T. Miyazawa. 2004a. Telomerase inhibition by sulfoquinovosyldiacylglycerol from edible purple laver (*Porphyra yezoensis*). *Cancer Lett.*, *212*, 15–20.

Eitsuka, T., K. Nakagawa, T. Miyazawa. 2004b. Dual mechanisms for telomerase inhibition in DLD-1 human colorectal adenocarcinoma cells by polyunsaturated fatty acids. *Biofactors*, *21*, 19–21.

Eitsuka, T., K. Nakagawa, T. Suzuki, T. Miyazawa. 2005. Polyunsaturated fatty acids inhibit telomerase activity in DLD-1 human colorectal adenocarcinoma cells: A dual mechanism approach. *Biochim. Biophys. Acta*, *1737*, 1–10.

Eitsuka, T., K. Nakagawa, T. Miyazawa. 2006. Down-regulation of telomerase activity in DLD-1 human colorectal adenocarcinoma cells by tocotrienol. *Biochem. Biophys. Res. Commun.*, *348*, 170–175.

Feng, J., W.D. Funk, S.S. Wang, S.L. Weinrich, A.A. Avilion, C.P. Chiu, R.R. Adams, E. Chang, R.C. Allsopp, J. Yu, S. Le, M.D. West, C.B. Harley, W.H. Andrews, C.W. Greider, B. Villeponteau. 1995. The RNA component of human telomerase. *Science*, *269*, 1236–1241.

Harrington, L., T. McPhail, V. Mar, W. Zhou, R. Oulton, M.B. Bass, I. Arruda, M.O. Robinson. 1997. A mammalian telomerase-associated protein. *Science*, *275*, 973–977.

Horikawa, I., P.L. Cable, C. Afshari, J.C. Barrett. 1999. Cloning and characterization of the promoter region of human telomerase reverse transcriptase gene. *Cancer Res.*, *59*, 826–830.

Inokuchi, H., H. Hirokane, T. Tsuzuki, K. Nakagawa, M. Igarashi, T. Miyazawa. 2003. Anti-angiogenic activity of tocotrienol. *Biosci. Biotechnol. Biochem.*, *67*, 1623–1627.

Kim, N.W., M.A. Piatyszek, K.R. Prowse, C.B. Harley, M.D. West, P.L.C. Ho, G.M. Coviello, W.E. Wright, S.L. Weinrich, J.W. Shay. 1994. Specific association of human telomerase activity with immortal cells and cancers. *Science*, *266*, 2011–2015.

Li, H., L. Zhao, Z. Yang, J.W. Funder, J.P. Liu. 1998. Telomerase is controlled by protein kinase Cα in human breast cancer cells. *J. Biol. Chem.*, *273*, 33436–33442.

Liu, J.P. 1999. Studies of the molecular mechanisms in the regulation of telomerase activity. *FASEB J.*, *13*, 2091–2104.

McEachern, M.J., A. Krauskopf, E.H. Blackburn. 2000. Telomeres and their control. *Annu. Rev. Genet.*, *34*, 331–358.

Meyerson, M., C.M. Counter, E.N. Eaton, L.W. Ellisen, P. Steiner, S.D. Caddle, L. Ziaugra, R.L. Beijersbergen, M.J. Davidoff, Q. Liu, S. Bacchetti, D.A. Haber, R.A. Weinberg. 1997. hEST2, the putative human telomerase catalytic subunit gene, is up-regulated in tumor cells and during immortalization. *Cell*, *90*, 785–795.

Miyazawa, T., H. Inokuchi, H. Hirokane, T. Tsuzuki, K. Nakagawa, M. Igarashi. 2004a. Anti-angiogenic potential of tocotrienol *in vitro*. *Biochemistry (Mosc)*, *69*, 67–69.

Miyazawa, T., T. Tsuzuki, K. Nakagawa, M. Igarashi. 2004b. Antiangiogenic potency of vitamin E. *Ann. N.Y. Acad. Sci.*, *1031*, 401–404.

Mizushina, Y., K. Nakagawa, A. Shibata, Y. Awata, I. Kuriyama, N. Shimazaki, O. Koiwai, Y. Uchiyama, K. Sakaguchi, T. Miyazawa, H. Yoshida. 2006. Inhibitory effect of tocotrienol on eukaryotic DNA polymerase lambda and angiogenesis. *Biochem. Biophys. Res. Commun.*, *339*, 949–955.

Mo, H., C.E. Elson. 2004. Studies of the isoprenoid-mediated inhibition of mevalonate synthesis applied to cancer chemotherapy and chemoprevention. *Exp. Biol. Med.*, *229*, 567–585.

Morin, G.B. 1989. The human telomere terminal transferase enzyme is a ribonucleoprotein that synthesizes TTAGGG repeats. *Cell*, *59*, 521–529.

Murray, N.R., L.A. Davidson, R.S. Chapkin, W.C. Gustafson, D.G. Schattenberg, A.P. Fields. 1999. Overexpression of protein kinase C βII induces colonic hyperproliferation and induces sensitivity to colon carcinogenesis. *J. Cell Biol.*, 145, 699–711.

Naasani, I., H. Seimiya, T. Tsuruo. 1998. Telomerase inhibition, telomere shortening, and senescence of cancer cells by tea catechins. *Biochem. Biophys. Res. Commun.*, *249*, 391–396.

Nakagawa, K., T. Eitsuka, H. Inokuchi, T. Miyazawa. 2004. DNA chip analysis of comprehensive food function: Inhibition of angiogenesis and telomerase activity with unsaturated vitamin E, tocotrienol. *Biofactors*, *21*, 5–10.

Nakamura, T.M., G.B. Morin, K.B. Chapman, S.L. Weinrich, W.H. Andrews, J. Lingner, C.B. Harley, T.R. Cech. 1997. Telomerase catalytic subunit homologs from fission yeast and human. *Science*, *277*, 955–959.

Ogretmen, B., J.M. Kraveka, D. Schady, J. Usta, Y.A. Hannun, L.M. Obeid. 2001. Molecular mechanisms of ceramide-mediated telomerase inhibition in the A549 human lung adenocarcinoma cell line. *J. Biol. Chem.*, *276*, 32506–32514.

Park, C., I. Lee, W.K. Kang. 2001. Lovastatin-induced E2F-1 modulation and its effect on prostate cancer cell death. *Carcinogenesis*, *22*, 1727–1731.

Parker, R.A., B.C. Pearce, R.W. Clark, D.A. Gordon, J.J.K. Wright. 1993. Tocotrienols regulate cholesterol production in mammalian cells by post-transcriptional suppression of 3-hydroxy-3-methylglutaryl-coenzyme A reductase. *J. Biol. Chem.*, *268*, 11230–11238.

Ramachandran, C., H.B. Fonseca, P. Jhabvala, E.A. Escalon, S.J. Melnick. 2002. Curcumin inhibits telomerase activity through human telomerase reverse transcriptase in MCF-7 breast cancer cell line. *Cancer Lett.*, *184*, 1–6.

Sen, C.K., S. Khanna, S. Roy. 2006. Tocotrienols: Vitamin E beyond tocopherols. *Life Sci.*, *78*, 2088–2098.

Shay, J.W., W.E. Wright. 2002. Telomerase: A target for cancer therapeutics. *Cancer Cell*, *2*, 257–265.

Sheng, W.Y., Y.L. Chien, T.C.V. Wang. 2003. The dual role of protein kinase C in the regulation of telomerase activity in human lymphocytes. *FEBS Lett.*, *540*, 91–95.

Takakura, M., S. Kyo, T. Kanaya, M. Tanaka, M. Inoue. 1998. Expression of human telomerase subunits and correlation with telomerase activity in cervical cancer. *Cancer Res.*, *58*, 1558–1561.

Takakura, M., S. Kyo, T. Kanaya, H. Hirano, J. Takeda, M. Yutsudo, M. Inoue. 1999. Cloning of human telomerase catalytic subunit (hTERT) gene promoter and identification of proximal promoter sequences essential for transcriptional activation in immortalized and cancer cells. *Cancer Res.*, *59*, 551–557.

Tatematsu, K., J. Nakayama, M. Danbara, S. Shionoya, H. Sato, M. Omine, F. Ishikawa. 1996. A novel quantitative "stretch PCR assay," that detects a dramatic increase in telomerase activity during the progression of myeloid leukemias. *Oncogene*, *13*, 2265–2274.

Traber, M.G., L. Packer. 1995. Vitamin E: Beyond antioxidant function. *Am. J. Clin. Nutr.*, *62*, 1501S–1509S.

Weinrich, S.L., R. Pruzan, L. Ma, M. Ouellette, V.M. Tesmer, S.E. Holt, A.G. Bodnar, S. Lichsterner, N.W. Kim, J.B. Trager, R.D. Taylor, R. Carlos, W.H. Andrews, W.E. Wright, J.W. Shay, C.B. Harley, G.B. Morin. 1997. Reconstitution of human telomerase with template RNA component hTERC and the catalytic protein subunit hTERT. *Nat. Genet.*, *17*, 498–502.

Wu, K.J., C. Grandori, M. Amacker, N. Simon-Vermot, A. Polack, J. Lingner, R. Dalla-Favera. 1999. Direct activation of TERT transcription by c-MYC. *Nat. Genet.*, *21*, 220–224.

Yu, C.C., S.C. Lo, T.C.V. Wang. 2001. Telomerase is regulated by protein kinase C-ζ in human nasopharyngeal cancer cells. *Biochem. J.*, *355*, 459–464.

Part F

Heart Disease

17 Tocopherol and Tocotrienols: Role in Heart Disease Care and Prevention

Vijaya Juturu

CONTENTS

17.1 PREVALENCE OF HEART DISEASE

Cardiovascular disease (CVD) was the leading cause of deaths in 2004, or, in the same year, one of every five deaths in the United States (Minino et al. 2006). Nearly 2,400 Americans die of CVD each day, an average of one death every 36 seconds. The CVD death rates in 2004 were 341.8 for males and 246.3 for females. Overall death rate from diabetes was 24.4. At least 65 percent of people with diabetes mellitus die of some form of heart disease or stroke (Rosamond et al., 2006). Diabetes increases the risk of stroke, with the relative risk ranging from 1.8 to almost 6.0. (Goldstein et al. 2001). The estimated direct and indirect cost of CVD in the United States for 2007 is $431.8 billion and $151.6 billion, respectively.

Atherosclerosis manifests as advanced fatty deposits (also called atheromas or plaques) on the interior artery lining. The fatty deposits central to atherosclerosis comprise lipids, complex carbohydrates, proteins, fibrous tissue and calcium. The formation of plaques begins as a process called atherogenesis, during which fatty streaks deposit lipids in the subendothelium between the intima lining and muscular portion of the artery wall. The modifiable risk factors of CVD are blood pressure, obesity, blood sugar, lipids and lipoproteins, smoking, improving physical activity, stress and dietary factors including trans fats and saturated fatty acids. The nonmodifiable risk factors are age, sex, heredity, race and ethnicity. The other contributing risk factors are pro-inflammatory markers, pro-coagulation factors, endothelial dysfunction and oxidation of lipids (Figure 17.1).

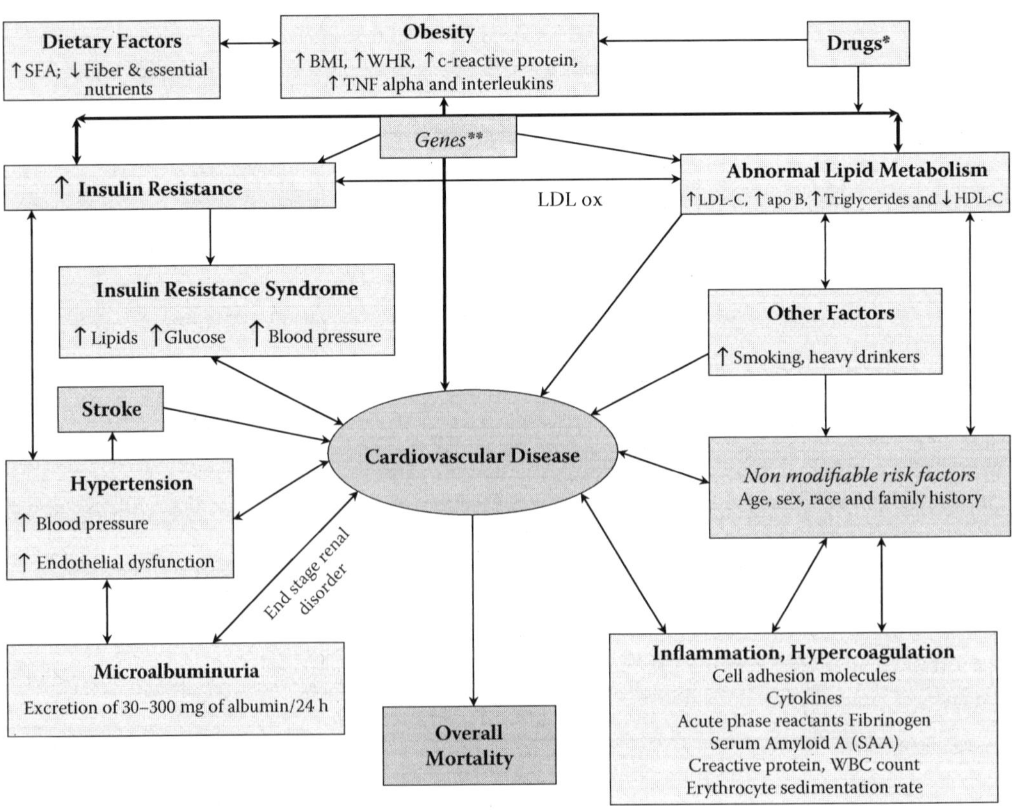

FIGURE 17.1 Contributing risk factors for cardiovascular disease.

17.2 OXIDATION IN ATHEROSCLEROSIS

17.2.1 LDL Oxidation and CVD

Oxidation of low-density lipoprotein (LDL) is an early event of atherogenesis. Cardiovascular disease risk is directly related to elevated oxidized LDL (Tsimikas, 2006). Endothelial injury, associated with increased production of free radicals during oxidative stress, is associated with increased prostaglandin synthesis and platelet adhesion/activation. These processes are associated with the release of aldehydes, which induce the oxidative modification of LDL. The increase of circulating oxidized LDL is most probably independent of plaque instability.

17.3 ANTIOXIDANTS AND CARDIOVASCULAR DISEASE

Over the past decade, the medicinal use of alternative medicines has increased dramatically. In the NHANES survey (1999–2000), 52% of adults reported taking a dietary supplement; 35% took a multivitamin/multimineral and 12% to 13% of them are using vitamin E supplements (Radimer et al., 2004). The supplements are used as an alternative medical nutritional therapy to maintain health status or disease conditions. The purpose of this chapter is to evaluate the available evidence for the role of tocopherol and tocotrienols in prevention and treatment of CVD.

17.4 TOCOPHEROL AND TOCOTRIENOLS

17.4.1 Structure

The four tocopherols and the four tocotrienols have an alpha, beta, gamma and delta form—named on the basis of the number and position of the methyl groups on the chromanol ring. The alpha form has three methyl groups, the beta and gamma forms have two and the delta has only one.

Vitamin E (also known as the tocopherols) occurs naturally in foods such as nuts and seeds, whole grains, cold-pressed vegetable oils and dark green leafy vegetables. D-alpha tocopherol accounts for 80% of the activity of the vitamin; d,l-alpha tocopherol is the name given to synthetic derivatives composed of equal amounts of all the stereoisomers. In the presence of fat, a mixture of tocopherols and tocotrienols are better absorbed and may provide optimal health benefits of vitamin E.

Table 17.1 shows the biological functions of tocopherols and tocotrienols. Vitamin E has shown several beneficial effects *in vitro* and *in vivo* (Azzi et al., 2000).

17.5 DIETARY TOCOPHEROL INTAKE AND CVD

17.5.1 The Rotterdam Study

In the Rotterdam study (Klipstein-Grobusch et al., 2001), the relationship of vitamin E with disease of the arteries was reported in 4,367 Netherland subjects aged 55–94 years who had no previous cardiovascular disease at baseline. In men, vitamin E intake was associated with lower arterial disease. Vitamin E intake was inversely associated with peripheral arterial disease. In the SECURE trial (Study to Evaluate Carotid Ultrasound changes in patients treated with Ramipril and vitamin E), a total of 732 patients >/=55 years of age who had vascular disease or diabetes and at least one other risk factor and who did not have heart failure or a low left ventricular ejection fraction randomly received ramipril 2.5 mg/d or 10 mg/d and vitamin E (RRR-alpha-tocopheryl acetate) 400 IU/d or their matching placebos (Lonn et al., 2001). There were no differences in atherosclerosis progression rates between the treatments after 4 years of follow up.

TABLE 17.1
Biological Function of Tocopherol and Tocotrienols

Tocopherol	Tocotrienol
Antioxidant activity	Suppressing inducible Pp60 C-Src kinase activation
Inhibition of protein kinase c (PKC) activity	Suppressing inducible 12-lipoxygenase activation
Modulation of gene expression	Inducing Ikbkap expression
Inhibition of vascular smooth muscle cell proliferation inhibits platelet aggregation	Potent neuroprotection
Delay intra-arterial thrombus formation	Inhibiting cholesterogenesis by suppressing hmg-coa reductase
Attenuation of P47(Phox) phosphorylation	Stimulating Apob degradation
Membrane translocation	Preventing increased blood pressure
Inhibition of monocyte adhesion	Decreasing platelet aggregation
Inhibition of α-tropomyosin expression	Reducing lipid peroxides in plasma & blood vessels
Inhibition of liver collagen α1 (I) expression	Enhancing total antioxidant status
Inhibition of scavenger receptors Cd36	Protecting against free radical-induced impairment of erythrocyte deformability
Inhibition of ICAM-1 And VCAM-1 expression	Reducing the accumulation of protein carbonyl
Preservation of endothelial function	Reducing LDL oxidation
Inhibition of the oxygen burst in neutrophils	Inhibiting monocyte-endothelial cell
Enhancement of immune responses, interference with sex-steroid signaling	Endothelial cell proliferation
Suppression of tumor angiogenesis	Inhibiting proliferation of estrogen receptor-negative Mda-Mb-435 and -positive Mcf-7 breast cancer cells
	Inhibiting growth of Zr-75-1 breast cancer cells
	Modulating normal mammary gland growth, function and remodeling
	Antiproliferative and apoptotic effects
	Inhibiting angiogenesis and telomerase activity
	Inhibiting of adhesion molecule (e.g., Icam-1 and Vcam-1)
	Expression and monocyte cell adherence

17.5.2 Continuing Survey of Food Intakes by Individuals (1994–1996)

CSFII study intake data from the 1994 to 1996 (Continuing Survey of Food Intakes by Individuals), involving 5,056 men and 4,703 women aged 20 years and older, indicated that vitamin E intakes were low for a large percentage of adolescent girls and an overt deficiency of vitamin E (Marras et al., 2004).

17.5.3 National Health and Nutrition Examination Survey (NHANES)

The Second National Health and Nutrition Examination Survey (NHANES II) reported mean intakes of vitamin E at 9.6 and 7.0 mg/d of alpha-tocopherol equivalents for men and women, respectively (Murphy et al., 1990). In the National Health and Nutrition Examination Survey (NHANES 1999–2000, Ahuja et al., 2004) data reported the dietary intakes of alpha-tocopherol in men and women, aged 19 and older, were 7.8 and 6.3 mg/d, respectively, and that only 10% of men and 4% of women met the new EAR for vitamin E.

17.5.4 The NHLBI Growth and Health Study

In a longitudinal analysis, regardless of race (White or African American girls, 81% to 99.0%), the intake of vitamin E is less than the estimated average requirement (Affenito et al., 2007).

17.6 TOCOPHEROL AND CARDIOVASCULAR DISEASE

17.6.1 Interventional Studies

17.6.1.1 Primary Prevention Studies

Table 17.2 provides the summary findings of the effects of tocopherol on the primary and secondary prevention of CVD.

The primary prevention studies (Rapola et al., 1997; Takamatsu et al., 1995; The ATBC Study Group, 1994; Tornwall et al., 2004; Virtamo et al., 1998), suggest that there is insufficient evidence to support a relationship between vitamin E and the reduction of risk of CVD.

The vitamin E-supplemented group had lower mortality of ischemic heart disease (602/637) and ischemic stroke death rates (56/67) than the non-supplemented group (The ATBC Study Group, 1994). In the secondary analyses, (Rapola et al., 1997) a statistically significant beneficial effect for vitamin E on the incidence of angina pectoris was observed, but no beneficial effects for the incidence of major coronary events (Virtamo et al., 1998) or intermittent claudication (Tornwall et al., 2004). Takamatsu et al. (1995) observed that the frequency of coronary disorders was higher in the control group compared with the group receiving vitamin E. Some of these studies were not designed to measure the association between vitamin E and reduced risk of CVD. Seven studies were reported in Table 17.2 (N=64,768); the two large studies have other severe chronic conditions such as cancer and other risk factors. Two studies observed significant effects of tocopherol on reducing LDL oxidation. In two studies, patients with hyperlipidemia had shown a slight reduction in the progression of disease (Table 17.2). Further studies are required to focus on the effect of tocopherol and CVD mortality risk and the progression or regression of heart disease only (with no other chronic conditions) in long-term trials.

17.6.1.2 Secondary Prevention Studies

Since the 1990s, 19 secondary prevention studies have been reported (Table 17.2, N = 171586). GISSI Investigators (1999) found no benefit from 330 IU/day of vitamin E supplementation. De Maio et al. (1992) reported no association between vitamin E (1200 IU/day) and recurrent stenosis. The Heart Outcomes Prevention Evaluation (HOPE) study showed a neutral impact for vitamin E (400 IU/day with 5 years of follow-up) on a range of CVD outcomes (Lonn et al., 2002). Williams et al. (1971) showed benefits of vitamin E for intermittent claudication. In another small double blind crossover study no relationship between 1600 IU/day of vitamin E and symptoms of angina were observed (Gillilan et al., 1977). Overall, the evidence of tocopherol on secondary prevention is inconclusive.

17.6.1.3 Observational Studies

Relationship of vitamin E intake and change in tissue levels were associated with decreased risk of CVD in case-control and prospective cohort studies. Overall, the studies support that vitamin E intake from food or supplements may reduce cardiac events. (Kushi et al., 1996; Rimm et al., 1993; Stampfer et al., 1993; Knekt et al., 1994; Bolton-Smith et al., 1991; Keli et al., 1996; Losonczy et al., 1996; Meyer et al., 1996; Sahyoun et al., 1996; Ascherio et al., 1999; Donnan et al., 1993; Klipstein-Grobusch et al., 1999; Kritchevsky et al., 1995). In two studies, no benefit from vitamin E supplementation on stroke (Keli et al., 1996) or myocardial infarction (MI) (Klipstein-Grobusch et al., 1999) was observed. Low levels of alpha-tocopherol have been associated with increased risk for coronary artery disease. Higher serum concentrations of alpha-tocopherol (up to 13–14 mg/L, which is within the normal range) are associated with moderately lower total and cause-specific mortality in older male smokers (Wright et al., 2006).

TABLE 17.2
Effect of Tocopherol on Heart Disease and Risk Factors

Author, year	Study	N	Subject population	Dose	Study Duration	Results
Salonen et al., 2000	ASAP	520	Hyperlipidemia smoking and nonsmoking men and postmenopausal women	136 IU twice a day+ 250 mg of slow-release vitamin C	3	The proportion of men with progression was reduced by 74% (95% CI 36-89%, P = 0.003) by supplementation.
Salonen et al., 2003	ASAP follow up	520	Hyperlipidemia smoking and nonsmoking men and postmenopausal women	136 IU twice a day+ 250 mg of slow-release vitamin C	6	Combination of vitamin E and slow-release vitamin C slows down atherosclerotic progression in hypercholesterolemic persons.
Tornwall et al., 2004	ATBC	29,133	Male smokers from Finland	50 IU/d	5–8	AT therapy had no significant effect on the first major coronary event (fatal and nonfatal).
Blot et al., 1993	Linxian	30,000	Subjects at risk for stomach cancer in southwestern China and had a very high incidence of carcinoma of the esophagus and stomach	30 mg	5.25	Little or no reduction in mortality from cardiovascular disease among subjects receiving the supplement combination that included vitamin E (no data provided), and a 10% reduction in mortality from cerebrovascular disease.
Porkkala-Sarataho et al., 1998	MASI	60	Healthy smokers	200 mg	2 mo	200 mg oral RRR-alpha-tocopheryl acetate/d had a clear effect on the in vitro oxidation of VLDL+LDL in smoking men.
Fang et al., 2002	Transplant Associated Arteriosclerosis Study	40	Transplant Associated Arteriolosclerosis in patients (0-2 years after cardiac transplantation)	800 IU/d RRR-AT and 1 g/d vitamin C	1 yr	There was a significant reduction compared with placebo in maximum intimal thickness and plaque area and a significant increase in AT and ascorbate levels in the antioxidant group.
Collaborative Group of the Primary Prevention Project, 2001	PPP	4,495	Patients with risk factors for cardiovascular disease	500 mg	3.6	46% reduction in the incidence of peripheral artery disease among patients taking vitamin E (P = 0.043); it decreased LDL oxidation.

GISSI-Prevenzione Investigators, 1999	GISSI	11,324	Post-MI adults	300 mg (synthetic)	3.5	No effect on MI + CVD death + stroke
Lonn et al., 2002	HOPE	9,541	High CVD risk	400 IU (natural)	4.5	No effect on MI + CVD death + stroke
Palumbo et al., 2000	PPP	4,495	At risk of CVD	300 mg (synthetic)	3.6	No effect on MI + CVD death + stroke
Lonn et al., 2002	MICRO-HOPE	3,654	Diabetes	400 IU (natural)	4.5	No effect on MI + CVD death + stroke
Hodis et al., 2002	VEAPS	353	Elevated LDL-C	400 IU dl-α-tocopherol	3	No effect on intima-media thickness + clinical events
Stephens et al., 1996	CHAOS	2,002	Coronary disease	800 or 400 IU	1.4	Decreased nonfatal acute MI
Heart Protection Study Collaborative Group, 2002	MRC/BHFHeart Protection Study	20,536	Preexisting coronary artery disease, peripheral vascular disease, or diabetes	600 mg	5	Antioxidant vitamin therapy significantly increased plasma antioxidant levels. There was also a significant increase in plasma cholesterol and triglycerides. They did not appear to show any significant effect on HDL cholesterol levels.
Tardif et al., 1997	MVP	317	Patients scheduled for percutaneous angioplasty and having preexisting coronary artery disease	700 IU; probucol (500 mg)	Patients were treated for 4 weeks before and 6 months after angioplasty	Restenosis rates per segment were 20.7% in the probucol group, 28.9% in the combined-treatment group, 40.3% in the multivitamin group, and 38.9% in the placebo group (P = 0.003 for probucol vs. no probucol). The rates of repeat angioplasty were 11.25% 16.2%, 24.4%, and 26.6%, respectively (P = 0.009 for probucol vs. no probucol).
Kelemen et al., 2005	Women's Angiographic Vitamin and Estrogen Trial	423	Postmenopausal women with at least one 15–75% coronary stenosis at baseline	800 IU/d of all-rac-AT and 1 g/d vitamin C	6 mo	Antioxidants had no effect on blood lipids, but significantly increased plasma AT levels and ascorbate. Vitamin treatment was associated with a nonsignificant change in minimum luminal diameter.

Continued

TABLE 17.2 (Continued)
Effect of Tocopherol on Heart Disease and Risk Factors

Author, year	Study	N	Subject population	Dose	Study Duration	Results
Brown et al., 2001	HATS	160	CAD and a low HDL cholesterol	800 IU/d of RRR-AT, 1000 mg/d of vitamin C, 25 mg/d of ß-carotene, and 100 μg/d of selenium	3	The antioxidant cocktail significantly prolonged (35%) the lag phase of LDL oxidation; the antioxidant cocktail resulted in 50% reduction in the percentage of stenosis.
Virtamo et al., 1998	ATBC	1,862	Smokers who had an MI	50 IU vitamin E	5.3	38% reduction in nonfatal MIFatal coronary end points not reduced.
Boaz et al., 2000	SPACE	196	Hemodialysis patients	800 IU	2	Decreases acute MI + stroke + peripheral vascular disease + unstable angina.
Kang et al., 2006	Womens health study	87,245	Female nurses free of diagnosed cardiovascular disease and cancer	600 IU	>2	41% reduction in risk of heart disease among nurses who had taken vitamin E for more than 2 years.
Rimm et al., 1993	HPPS	40,000 men	U.S. male health professionals	400 IU	>2	Had a 37% lower risk of heart disease than men who had not taken supplements of vitamin E.
Engelen et al., 2000	DM trial	44	Type 1 DM	750 IU	1	There was a decrease in lipoprotein peroxidizability. Within 3 months after stopping supplementation, serum vitamin E levels returned to baseline.
Beckman et al., 2003	Diabetes	26/23/15	Type 1 /Type 2 DM/Healthy matched Controls	800 IU	1	Oral antioxidant therapy improves EDV in T1 but not T2 diabetes.
Leichtle et al., 2006	CHD	12/12	patients with coronary heart disease and healthy subjects	RRR-α.-tocopherol at 100, 200 and 400 mg/day	3 wks /dose	Supplementation (200 mg/day) caused a significant decrease of the acute phase plasma proteins C-reactive protein (CRP) (–65%) and fibrinogen (–24%).

Note: MI indicates myocardial infarction; CHAOS, Cambridge Heart AntiOxidant Study; SPACE, Secondary Prevention with Antioxidants of Cardiovascular disease in End-stage renal disease; ATBC, Alpha-Tocopherol-Beta-Carotene Cancer Prevention study; ASAP, Antioxidant Supplementation in Atherosclerosis Prevention study; and IVUS, Intravascular Ultrasonography Study; HDL-Atherosclerosis Treatment Study (HATS). ASAP: The Antioxidant Supplementation in Atherosclerosis Prevention Study; ATBC :the Alpha Tocopherol Beta Carotene trial; Linxian: The Linxian Nutrition Intervention trial; The Primary Prevention trial (PPP).

17.6.1.4 Hypercoagulabilty/Atherosclerosis

A higher dietary intake of vitamin E as tocopherol was associated with less development of preclinical carotid atherosclerosis in women (Iannuzzi et al., 2002) and reduced lipid peroxidation in non-smoking adults (Huang et al., 2002).

17.6.1.5 Intermittent Claudication

Vitamin E supplementation (tocopherol) may lead to intermittent claudication (Kleijnen and Mackerras, 2007), which is is a cramping pain caused by an inadequate blood flow to the calf and leg muscles. It is a symptom of atherosclerosis, a disease where fatty deposits build up in the arteries, blocking blood flow.

17.6.1.6 Vasculitis

Vitamin E (tocopherol) may protect the lysosomal membranes from rupturing and destroying the cells and is beneficial at minimum doses in the treatment of several acute and chronic pulmonary injuries by inhibiting the vasoconstrictive and mitogenic activity of angiotensin II (Molteni et al., 2004).

17.6.1.7 Aneurysmal Disease

Vitamin E (tocopherol) concentrations were highest in peripheral occlusive diseased tissue and as much as three times greater in organ donors than in patients with aortic occlusive disease and aneurysmal disease. Signs of lipid peroxidation were markedly elevated in all diseased arterial tissue compared with controls. These data supply evidence of altered vitamin E metabolism and free radical processes in the tissues of patients with various manifestations of atherosclerosis (Killion et al., 1996).

17.6.1.8 Oxidative Stress and CVD

Pharmacological doses of vitamin E supplementation (tocopherol: 300, 600, and 1200 mg/day) for 3 consecutive weeks had no detectable effects on lipid peroxidation and thromboxane biosynthesis in 46 healthy moderate cigarette smokers (Cipollone et al., 2000). Similar observations were observed in randomized supplementation trials. Vitamin E decreases systemic oxidative stress and 8-isoprostane concentrations in overweight/obese individuals. A decrease in plasma 8-isoprostane has the potential to reduce risk of cardiovascular disease in obesity (Wayne et al., 2007).

17.6.1.9 LDL Oxidation

Vitamin E may inhibit the development and proliferation of LDL oxidation but no reduction in atheroma size (Kaikkonen et al., 2000). In the Antioxidant Supplementation in Atherosclerosis Prevention (ASAP) study, a combined supplementation with reasonable doses of both vitamin E and slow-release vitamin C can retard the progression of common carotid atherosclerosis in men (Salonen et al., 2000; 2003). Vitamin E supplementation improves the imbalance of oxidative stress and antioxidant status in plasma but not in plaques (Micheletta et al., 2004).

17.6.1.10 Stroke

In stroke, the third leading cause of death in the United States, vitamin E supplementation may prevent ischemic stroke in high-risk hypertensive patients (Leppala et al., 2000). Further studies are required to see the effects of different doses on high-risk patients and incidence of strokes.

17.6.1.11 Type II Diabetes

Diabetes appears to increase oxidative stress. Antioxidants such as vitamin E may reduce oxidative stress in type I diabetes (Jain et al., 1996). Another study showed that vitamin E (680 IU) along with

TABLE 17.3
Evidence-Based Category for Vitamin E and Cardiovascular Disease

Grade A	Grade B	Grade C	Grade D
Vitamin E deficiency	—	Angina	Heart disease prevention
		Antioxidant	Stroke
		Atherosclerosis	
		Cardiovascular disease in dialysis patients	
		Diabetes mellitus	
		Glomerulosclerosis (kidney disease)	
		High cholesterol	
		Immune system function	
		Intermittent claudication	

Note: A–Strong scientific evidence for this use; B–Good scientific evidence for this use; C–Unclear scientific evidence for this use; D–Fair scientific evidence against this use (it may not work).

Source: http://www.mayoclinic.com/health/vitamin-e/NS_patient-vitamin-e; Nov 1, 2005 (accessed on May 3, 2007).

vitamin C (1200mg) will reduce the albumin excretion rate in urine which reduces the risk of end stage renal disease associated with diabetes (Gaede et al., 2001) and other studies using 900 to 1,600 IU of synthetic alpha-tocopherol daily found either minimal or no improvement, respectively (Paolisso et al., 1993; Reaven et al., 1995). Giannini et al. (2007) demonstrated that the high dose of vitamin E (1200 mg/d) supplementation reduces markers of oxidative stress and improves antioxidant defense in young patients with T1DM. It does not reduce albumin excretion rate in patients with T1DM and persistent microalbuminuria. In another study, alpha tocopherol and mixed tocopherol supplementation resulted in reduced plasma F(2)-isoprostanes but did not affect 24-h urinary F(2)-isoprostanes or erythrocyte antioxidant enzyme activities (Wu et al., 2007). Based on the evidence analysis, vitamin E had no significant evidence of reducing the risk of cardiovascular disease events (Table 17.3).

17.6.1.12 Chronic Kidney Disease

Cardiovascular disease patients are more prone to chronic kidney disease (CKD). Nanayakkara et al. (2007) reported that in a randomized double blind trial vitamin E supplementation (300 mg/d)was added to the pravastatin (40mg/d) treatment regimen 6 months later. In patients with mild to moderate nondiabetic CKD who had no manifest arterial occlusive disease and well controlled blood pressure, 18 months of treatment with an oxidative stress-lowering strategy resulted in a statistically significant reduction in common carotid intima-media thickness (CC-IMT, $p<0.001$) and a statistically significant improvement in brachial artery-flow mediated dilatation (BA-FMD, $p=0.001$) and no significant effect on GFR ($p=0.89$).

17.6.1.13 Qualified Health Claim for Vitamin E Is Declined

The FDA has concluded that there is no significant scientific agreement for a relationship between vitamin E supplements and CVD risk, and that the scientific evidence for a relationship is outweighed by the scientific evidence against the relationship (Trumbo, 2005).

17.7 TOCOTRIENOL AND CARDIOVASCULAR DISEASE

Tocotrienols (found in high concentrations in palm oil) are many times more potent as antioxidants and they are poorly assimilated by digestion, are poorly distributed to tissues in blood and are rapidly metabolized and eliminated from the body. They are well-absorbed by the skin and well suited for use as a vitamin E cream. *In vitro* and *in vivo* studies suggest cardioprotective effects of tocotrienols in different models.

17.7.1 Dietary Intakes of Tocotrienols Intake and CVD

17.7.1.1 Tocotrienol Supplementation and CVD Risk

Tocotrienols in general and gamma-tocotrienol in particular decreased total and LDL cholesterol in animals (Minhajuddin et al., 2005; Poveda et al., 2005; Nafeeza et al., 2001). There are no primary and secondary prevention trials reported for tocotrienols. Further studies are needed to explore their role in the regression of atherosclerosis and cardiac events.

17.7.1.2 Stroke-Induced Injuries

Oral supplementation of the palm tocotrienol complex acts on key molecular checkpoints (c-Src and 12-Lipoxygenase) to protect against glutamate- and stroke-induced neurodegeneration and ultimately may protect against stroke *in vivo* (Khanna et al., 2005).

17.7.1.3 Reversal of Arterial Blockage in Carotid Stenosis Patients

Palm tocotrienol complex has the ability to reverse arterial blockage of the carotid artery in carotid stenosis patients.

17.7.1.4 Lipid Metabolism

Cardiovascular risk factors such as total cholesterol, LDL cholesterol, apo lipoprotein A and thromboxane and platelet factor 4 were reduced with tocotrienols (Tomeo et al., 1995; Qureshi et al., 1991, 1995; Ajuluchukwu et al., 2007). In animal studies, tocotrienols were shown to reduce total cholesterol by 30% and LDL by 67% compared with controls in rats with induced hypercholesterolemia. Tocotrienols were also shown to significantly reduce HMG-CoA activity. (Iqbal et al., 2003; Hasselwander et al., 2002) . Tocotrienol-rich fraction (TRF) mediated decrease on elevated blood glucose and glycated hemoglobin A(1C) (HbA(1C)) in diabetic rats. Tocotrienols, especially delta- and gamma-tocotrienols, were shown to be effective nutritional agents to treat high cholesterol in recent research programs. In particular, gamma-tocotrienol appears to act on a specific enzyme called 3-hydroxy-3-methylglutaryl-coenzyme and suppresses the production of this enzyme, which results in less cholesterol being manufactured by liver cells.

17.7.1.5 Carbohydrate Metabolism

Intakes of alpha-tocopherol, gamma-tocopherol, delta-tocopherol, and beta-tocotrienol were inversely related to a risk of type II diabetes. Thus the development of type II diabetes may be reduced by the intake of antioxidants in the diet (Montonen et al., 2004). In type II diabetic subjects with hyperlipidemia, TRF showed an average decline of 23, 30, and 42% in serum total lipids, TC and LDL-C, respectively, and a reduction of LDL-C from an average of 179 mg/dl to 104 mg/dl (Baliarsingh et al., 2005).

17.7.1.6 Antioxidant Activity

The cardioprotective properties of TRF appear to be due to inhibition of c-Src activation and proteasome stabilization in isolated heart rats perfused for 15 minutes (Das et al., 2005, 2007; Ajuluchukwu et al., 2007), as evidenced by their ability to improve post-ischemic ventricular function and reduce myocardial infarct size.

17.7.1.7 Hypertension

Gamma-tocotrienol could cause natriuresis and diuresis in rats, stimulating sodium excretion *in vivo*, suggesting that it has a hormone-like natriuretic function (Saito et al., 2003). Gamma-tocotrienol may prevent development of increased blood pressure, reduce lipid peroxides in plasma and blood vessels and enhance total antioxidant status including SOD activity (Newaz and Nawal, 1999).

17.8 SUMMARY

The results from primary and secondary prevention studies suggest that the use of vitamin E for cardiovascular disease is inconclusive. The study designs have limitations and are reported in subjects who have other chronic diseases. Overall, from these studies, it was suggested that less than 400 mcg tocopherol is safe and adverse events were observed at higher doses. There are no studies supporting the evidence of tocopherol and tocotrienols in reducing the risk of cardiac disease and cardiac events. Well-controlled studies are required to see the evidence of beneficial effects of tocopherol and tocotrienols in the regression of atherosclerosis and cardiac events in males and females. *In vitro* and *in vivo* studies are suggesting its functional importance in reducing cardiovascular disease. Observational studies also show the association of dietary vitamin E intake and reduction in cardiovascular disease relative to risk. However, some of the limitations restrict the recommendation of vitamin E for cardiovascular disease. The discrepancies in the trials may be due to the type and form, whether the nutrient is administered alone or in combinations, single dose vs. multiple doses, study designs, outcome measures, duration of the study, populations and whether the subjects have CVD alone or a combination with other chronic conditions. It is very clear that in chronic conditions like CVD, diabetes and hypertension, additional requirement of vitamins and minerals may help to improve the immune status and health. Data is required to suggest that consuming tocopherols and tocotrienols from foods or supplements, and at what levels, will support additional benefit with regard to CVD risk reduction.

REFERENCES

Affenito, S. G., D. R. Thompson, D. L. Franko, R. H. Striegel-Moore, S. R. Daniels, B. A. Barton, G. B. Schreiber, M. Schmidt, P. B. Crawford. 2007. Longitudinal assessment of micronutrient intake among African-American and White girls: The National Heart, Lung, and Blood Institute Growth and Health Study. *J Am Diet Assoc*, 107(7), 1113–23.

Ahuja, J. K., J. D. Goldman, A. J. Moshfegh. 2004. Current status of vitamin E nutriture. *Ann N Y Acad Sci*, 1031, 387–90.

Ajuluchukwu, J. N., N. U. Okubadejo, M. Mabayoje, F. I. Ojini, R. N. Okwudiafor, A. C. Mbakwem, O. A. Fasanmade, D. A. Oke. 2007. Comparative study of the effect of tocotrienols and tocopherol on fasting serum lipid profiles in patients with mild hypercholesterolaemia: A preliminary report. *Nig Postgrad Med J, 14(1)*, 30–3.

Alpha-Tocopherol, Beta-Carotene Cancer Prevention Study Group. 1994. The effect of vitamin E and beta-carotene on the incidence of lung cancer and other cancers in male smokers. *N Engl J Med, 330*, 1029–1035.

Ascherio, A., E. B. Rimm, M. A. Hernan, E. Giovannucci, I. Kawachi, M. J. Stampfer, W. C. Willett. 1999. Relation of consumption of vitamin E, vitamin C, and carotenoids to risk for stroke among men in the United States. *Ann Intern Med, 130*, 963–970.

Azzi, A., I. Breyer, M. Feher, M. Pastori, R. Ricciarelli, S. Spycher, M. Staffieri, A. Stocker, S. Zimmer, J. M. Zingg. 2000. Specific cellular responses to alpha-tocopherol. *J Nutr, 130*, 1649–52.

Baliarsingh, S., Z. H. Beg, J. Ahmad. 2005. The therapeutic impacts of tocotrienols in type 2 diabetic patients with hyperlipidemia. *Atherosclerosis, 182(2)*, 367–74.

Beckman, J. A., A. B. Goldfine, M. B. Gordon, L. A. Garrett, J. F. Keaney Jr, M. A. Creager. 2003. Oral antioxidant therapy improves endothelial function in Type 1 but not Type 2 diabetes mellitus. *Am J Physiol Heart Circ Physiol, 285(6)*, H2392–8.

Blot, W. J., J. Y. Li, P. R. Taylor, W. Guo, D. Sawsey, W. G. Qang, C. S. Yang, S. F. Zheng, M. Gail, G. Y. Li. 1993. Nutrition intervention trials in Linxian China: Supplementation with specific vitamin/mineral combinations, cancer incidence, and disease-specific mortality in the general population. *J Natl Cancer Inst*, *85*, 1483–92.

Boaz, M., S. Smetana, T. Weinstein, Z. Matas, U. Gafter, A. Iaina, A. Knecht, Y. Weissgarten, D. Brunner, M. Fainaru, M. S. Green. 2000. Secondary prevention with antioxidants of cardiovascular disease in end-stage renal disease (SPACE): Randomized placebo controlled trial. *Lancet*, *356*, 1213–1218.

Bolton-Smith, C., C. E. Casey, K. F. Gey, W. C. Smith, H. Tunstall-Pedoe. 1991. Antioxidant vitamin intakes assessed using a food-frequency questionnaire: Correlation with biochemical status in smokers and non-smokers. *Br J Nutr.*, *65(3)*, 337–46.

Brown, B. G., X. Q. Zhao, A. Chait, L. D. Fisher, M. C. Cheung, J. S. Morse, A. A. Dowdy, E. K. Marino, E. L. Bolson, P. Alaupovic, J. Frohlich, J. J. Albers. 2001. Simvastatin and niacin, antioxidant vitamins, or the combination for the prevention of coronary disease. *N Engl J Med*, *345(22)*, 1583–92

Bruunsgaard, H., H. E. Poulsen, B. K. Pedersen, K. Nyyssonen, J. Kaikkonen, J. T. Salonen. 2003. Long-term combined supplementations with alpha-tocopherol and vitamin C have no detectable anti-inflammatory effects in healthy men. *J Nutr*, *133(4)*, 1170–3.

Cipollone, F., G. Ciabattoni, P. Patrignani, M. Pasquale, D. Di Gregorio, T. Bucciarelli, G. Davi, F. Cuccurullo, C. Patrono. 2000. Oxidant stress and aspirin-insensitive thromboxane biosynthesis in severe unstable angina. *Circulation*, *102(9)*, 1007–13.

Collaborative Group of the Primary Prevention Project (PPP). 2001. Low-dose aspirin and vitamin E in people at cardiovascular risk: A randomized trial in general practice. *Lancet*, *357(9250)*, 89–95.

Das S., K. Nesaretnam, D. K. Das. 2007. Tocotrienols in cardioprotection. *Vitam Horm*, *75*, 285–99

Das, S., S. R. Powell, P. Wang, A. Divald, K. Nesaretnam, A. Tosaki, G. A. Cordis, N. Maulik;D. K. Das. 2005. Cardioprotection with palm tocotrienol: Antioxidant activity of tocotrienol is linked with its ability to stabilize proteasomes. *Am J Physiol Heart Circ Physiol*, *289(1)*, H361–7.

DeMaio, S. J., S. B. King, 3rd, N. J. Lembo, G. S. Roubin, J. A. Hearn, H. N. Bhagavan, D. S. Sgoutas. 1992. Vitamin E supplementaiton, plasma lipids and incidence of restenosis after percutaneous transluminal coronary angioplasty (PTCA). *J Am Coll Nutr*, *11*, 68–73.

Donnan, P. T., M. Thomson, F. G. Fowkes, R. J. Prescott, E. Housley. 1993. Diet as a risk factor for peripheral arterial disease in the general population: The Edinburgh Artery Study. *Am J Clin Nutr*, *57(6)*, 917–21.

Engelen, W., B. M. Keenoy, J. Vertommen, I. De Leeuw. 2000. Effects of long-term supplementation with moderate pharmacologic doses of vitamin E are saturable and reversible in patients with type 1 diabetes. *Am J Clin Nutr*, *72(5)*, 1142–9.

Fang J. C., S. Kinlay, J. Beltrame, H. Hikiti, M. Wainstein, D. Behrendt, J. Suh, B. Frei, G. H. Mudge, A. P. Selwyn, P. Ganz. 2002. Effect of vitamins C and E on progression of transplant-associated arteriosclerosis: A randomized trial. *Lancet*, *359(9312)*, 1108–13.

Gaede, P., H. E. Poulsen, H. H. Parving, O. Pedersen. 2001. Double-blind, randomised study of the effect of combined treatment with vitamin C and E on albuminuria in Type 2 diabetic patients. *Diabet Med*, *18*, 756–760.

Giannini, C., F. Lombardo, F. Curro, M. Pomilio, T. Bucciarelli, F. Chiarelli, A. Mohn. 2007. Effects of high-dose vitamin E supplementation on oxidative stress and microalbuminuria in young adult patients with childhood onset type 1 diabetes mellitus. *Diabetes Metab Res Rev* Feb 1, [Epub ahead of print].

Gillilan, R. E., B. Mondell, J. R. Warbasse. 1977. Quantitative evaluation of vitamin E in the treatment of angina pectoris. *Am Heart J*, *93(4)*, 444–9.

GISSI-Prevenzione Investigators. 1999. Dietary supplementation with n-3 polyunsaturated fatty acids and vitamin E after myocardial infarction: Results of the GISSI-Prevenzione Trial. *Lancet*, *354*, 447–455.

Goldstein, L. B., R. Adams, K. Becker, C. D. Furberg, P. B. Gorelick, G. Hademenos, M. Hill, G. Howard, V. J. Howard, B. Jacobs, S. R. Levine, L. Mosca, R. L. Sacco, D. G. Sherman, P. A. Wolf, G. J. del Zoppo. 2001. Primary prevention of ischemic stroke: A statement for healthcare professionals from the Stroke Council of the American Heart Association. *Stroke*, *32*, 280–299.

Hasselwander, O., K. Kramer, P. P. Hoppe. 2002. Effects of feeding various tocotrienol sources on plasma lipids and aortic atherosclerotic lesions in cholesterol-fed rabbits. Food *Res Intern*, *35 (2–3)*, 245–251.

Heart Protection Study Collaborative Group. 2002. MRC/BHF Heart Protection Study of antioxidant vitamin supplementation in 20,536 high-risk individuals: A randomised placebo-controlled trial. *Lancet*, *360*, 23–33.

Hodis, H. N., W. J. Mack, L. LaBree, P. R. Mahrer, A. Sevanian, C. R. Liu, C. H. Liu, J. Hwang, R. H. Selzer, S. P. Azen. VEAPS Research Group. 2002. Alpha-tocopherol supplementation in healthy individuals reduces low-density lipoprotein oxidation but not atherosclerosis: The Vitamin E Atherosclerosis Prevention Study (VEAPS). *Circulation*, *106*, 1453–1459.

Huang, H. Y., L. J. Appel, K. D. Croft, E. R. Miller 3rd, T. A. Mori, I. B. Puddey. 2002. Effects of vitamin C and vitamin E on *in vivo* lipid peroxidation: Results of a randomized controlled trial. *Am J Clin Nutr, 76(3),* 549–55.

Iannuzzi, A., E. Celentano, S. Panico, R. Galasso, G. Covetti, L. Sacchetti, F. Zarrilli, M. De Michele, P. Rubba. 2002. Dietary and circulating antioxidant vitamins in relation to carotid plaques in middle-aged women. *Am J Clin Nutr, 76(3),* 582–7.

Iqbal, J., M. Minhajuddin, Z. H. Beg. 2003. Suppression of 7, 12-dimethylbenz[alpha]anthracene-induced carcinogenesis and hypercholesterolaemia in rats by tocotrienol-rich fraction isolated from rice bran oil. *Eur J Cancer Prev, 12(6),* 447–53.

Jain, S. K., R. McVie, J. J. Jaramillo, M. Palmer, T. Smith. 1996. Effect of modest vitamin E supplementation on blood glycated hemoglobin and triglyceride levels and red cell indices in type I diabetic patients. J *Am Coll Nutr, 15(5),* 458–461.

Kaikkonen, J., K. Nyyssonen, A. Tomasi, A. Iannone, T. P. Tuomainen, E. Porkkala-Sarataho, J. T. Salonen. 2000. Antioxidative efficacy of parallel and combined supplementation with coenzyme Q10 and d–alpha-tocopherol in mildly hypercholesterolemic subjects: A randomized placebo-controlled clinical study. *Free Radic Res, 33(3),* 329–40.

Kang J. H., N. Cook, J. Manson, J. E. Buring, F. Grodstein. 2006. A randomized trial of vitamin E supplementation and cognitive function in women. *Arch Intern Med, 166,* 2462–2468.

Kelemen, M., D. Vaidya, D. D. Waters, B. V. Howard, F. Cobb, N. Younes, M. Tripputti, P. Ouyang. 2005. Hormone therapy and antioxidant vitamins do not improve endothelial vasodilator function in postmenopausal women with established coronary artery disease: A sub study of the Women's Angiographic Vitamin and Estrogen (WAVE) trial. *Atherosclerosis, 179(1),* 193–200.

Keli, S. O., M. G. Hertog, E. J. Feskens, D. Kromhout. 1996. Dietary flavonoids, antioxidant vitamins, and incidence of stroke: The Zutphen study. *Arch Intern Med, 156,* 637–642.

Khanna, S., S . Roy, A. Slivka, T. K. Craft, S. Chaki, C. Rink, M. A. Notestine, A. C. DeVries, N. L. Parinandi, C. K. Sen. 2005. Neuroprotective properties of the natural vitamin E alpha-tocotrienol, *Stroke, 36(10),* 2258–64.

Killion, S. L., G. C. Hunter, C. D. Eskelson, M. A. Dubick, C. W. Putnam, K. A. Hall, C. A. Luedke, R. L. Misiorowski, J. D. Schilling, K. E. McIntyre. 1996. Vitamin E levels in human atherosclerotic plaque: The influence of risk factors. *Atherosclerosis, 126(2),* 289–97.

Kleijnen, J., D Mackerras. 2007. Vitamin E for intermittent claudication. Cochrane Database of Systematic Reviews Issue 2.

Klipstein-Grobusch, K. J., M. Geleijnse, J. H. den Breeijen, H. Boeing, A. Hofman, D. E. Grobbee, J. C. Witteman. 1999. Dietary antioxidants and risk of myocardial infarction in the elderly: The Rotterdam Study. *Am J Clin Nutr, 69,* 261–266.

Klipstein-Grobusch, K., J. H. den Breeijen, D. E. Grobbee, H. Boeing, A. Hofman, J. C. Witteman. 2001. Dietary antioxidants and peripheral arterial disease: The Rotterdam Study. *Am J Epidemiol, 154(2),* 145–9.

Knekt, P., A. Reunanen, R. Jarvinen, R. Seppanen, M. Heliovaara, A. Aromaa. 1994. Antioxidant vitamin intake and coronary mortality in a longitudinal population study. *Am J Epidemiol, 139,* 1180–1189.

Kritchevsky, S. B., T. Shimakawa, G. S. Tell, B. Dennis, M. Carpenter, J. H. Eckfeldt, H. Peacher-Ryan, G. Heiss. 1995. Dietary antioxidants and carotid artery wall thickness. The ARIC Study. Atherosclerosis Risk in Communities Study. *Circulation, 92(8),* 2142–50.

Kushi, L. H., A. R. Folsom, R. J. Prineas, P. J. Mink, Y. Wu, R. M. Bostick. 1996. Dietary antioxidant vitamins and death from coronary heart disease in postmenopausal women. *N Engl J Med, 334,* 1156–1162.

Lee, I. M., N. R. Cook, J. M. Gaziano, D. Gordon, P. M. Ridker, J. E. Manson, C. H. Hennekens, J. E. Buring, 2005. Vitamin E in the primary prevention of cardiovascular disease and cancer: The Women's Health Study: A randomized controlled trial. *JAMA, 294(1),* 56–65.

Leichtle, A., D. Teupser, J. Thiery. 2006. Alpha-tocopherol distribution in lipoproteins and anti-inflammatory effects differ between CHD-patients and healthy subjects. *J Am Coll Nutr, 25(5),* 420–8.

Leppälä, J. M., J. Virtamo, R. Fogelholm, J. K. Huttunen, D. Albanes, P. R. Taylor, O. P. Heinonen. 2000. Controlled trial of alpha-tocopherol and beta-carotene supplements on stroke incidence and mortality in male smokers. *Arterioscler Thromb Vasc Biol, 20,* 230–235.

Lonn, E., S. Yusuf, V. Dzavik, C. Doris, Q. Yi, S. Smith, A. Moore-Cox, J. Bosch, W. Riley, K. Teo. 2001. SECURE Investigators. Effects of ramipril and vitamin E on atherosclerosis: The study to evaluate carotid ultrasound changes in patients treated with ramipril and vitamin E (SECURE). *Circulation, 103(7),* 919–25.

Lonn, E., S. Yusuf, B. Hoogwerf, J. Pogue, Q. Yi, B. Zinman, J. Bosch, G. Dagenais, J. F. Mann, H. C. Gerstein. 2002. HOPE Study/ MICRO-HOPE Study. Effects of vitamin E on cardiovascular and microvascular outcomes in high-risk patients with diabetes: Results of the HOPE study and MICRO-HOPE substudy. *Diabetes Care, 25,* 1919–1927.

Losonczy, K. G., T. B. Harris, R. J. Havlik. 1996. Vitamin E and vitamin C supplement use and risk of all-cause and coronary heart disease mortality in older persons: The Established Populations for Epidemiologic Studies of the Elderly. *Am J Clin Nutr, 64(2),* 190–6.

Maras, J. E., O. I. Bermudez, N. Qiao, P. J. Bakun, E. L. Boody-Alter, K. L Tucker. 2004. Intake of alpha-tocopherol is limited among US adults. *J Am Diet Assoc, 104(4),* 567–75.

Meyer, F., I Bairati, GR Dagenais. 1996. Lower ischemic heart disease incidence and mortality among vitamin supplement users. *Can J Cardiol, 12(10),* 930–4.

Micheletta, F., S. Natoli, M. Misuraca, E. Sbarigia, U. Diczfalusy, L. Iuliano. 2004. Vitamin E supplementation in patients with carotid atherosclerosis: Reversal of altered oxidative stress status in plasma but not in plaque *Arterioscler. Thromb. Vasc. Biol, 24(1),* 136–140.

Minhajuddin, M., Z. H. Beg, J. Iqbal. 2005. Hypolipidemic and antioxidant properties of tocotrienol rich fraction isolated from rice bran oil in experimentally induced hyperlipidemic rats. *Food Chem Toxicol,* 43(5), 747–53.

Minino, A. M., M. P. Heron, B. L. Smith. 2006. Preliminary Data for 2004 National Vital Statistics Reports, Hyattsville, MD: National Center for Health Statistics, 54 (16).

Molteni, A., B. L. Herndon, A. Kamal, W. J. Castellani, S. Reppert, Y. Xue, J. Humbehr, R. C. Baybutt. 2004. Effect of the antioxidant α–tocopherol in an experimental model of pulmonary hypertension and fibrosis: Administration of monocrotaline. *Nutr Res, 24(9),* 707–720.

Montonen, J, P. Knekt, R. Jarvinen, A. Reunanen. 2004. Dietary antioxidant intake and risk of type 2 diabetes. *Diabetes Care, 27(2),* 362–6.

Murphy, S. P., A. F. Subar, G. Block. 1990. Vitamin E intakes and sources in the United States. *Am J Clin Nutr,* 52, 361–7.

Nafeeza, M. I., A. G. Norzana, H. L. Jalaluddin, M. T. Gapor. 2001. The effects of a tocotrienol-rich fraction on experimentally induced atherosclerosis in the aorta of rabbits. *Malay J Pathol, 23(1),* 17–25.

Nanayakkara, P. et al. 2007. Results from the Anti-Oxidant Therapy in Chronic Renal Insufficiency (ATIC) Study. *Arch Intern Med, 167(12),* 1262–1270.

Newaz, M. A., Nawal, N. N. 1999. Effect of gamma-tocotrienol on blood pressure, lipid peroxidation and total antioxidant status in spontaneously hypertensive rats (SHR). *Clin Exp Hypertens,* 21*(8),* 1297–313.

Palumbo, G., F. Avanzini, C. Alli, M. C. Roncaglioni, E. Ronchi, M. Cristofari, A. Capra, S. Rossi, L. Nosotti, C. Costantini, C. Cavalera. 2000. Effects of vitamin E on clinic and ambulatory blood pressure in treated hypertensive patients. Collaborative Group of the Primary Prevention Project (PPP)-Hypertension study. *Am J Hypertens, 13(5 Pt 1),* 564–7.

Paolisso, G, A. D'Amore, D. Galzerano. 1993. Daily vitamin E supplements improve metabolic control but not insulin secretion in elderly type II diabetic patients. *Diabetes Care, 16(11),* 1433–1437.

Porkkala-Sarataho, E. K., M. K. Nyyssonen, J. E. Kaikkonen et al. 1998. A randomized, single-blind, placebo-controlled trial of the effects of 200 mg alpha-tocopherol on the oxidation resistance of atherogenic lipoproteins. *Am J Clin Nutr,* 1034–41.

Poveda, E., P. Ayala, R. Milena, E. Ordonez, C. Baracaldo, W. Delgado, M. Guerra. 2005. Effects of vegetable oil supplementation on the lipid profile of Wistar rats. *Biomedica, 25(1),* 101–9.

Prieme, H., S. Loft, K. Nyyssonen, J. T. Salonen, H. E Poulsen. 1997. No effect of supplementation with vitamin E, ascorbic acid, or coenzyme Q10 on oxidative DNA damage estimated by 8-oxo-7, 8-dihydro-29-deoxyguanosine excretion in smokers. *Am J Clin Nutr,* 65, 503–507.

Qureshi, A, A,, B. A. Bradlow, L. Brace, M. Janganello, D. M. Peterson, B. C. Pearce, J. J. Wright, A, Gapor, C. E. Elson. 1995. Response of hypercholesterolemic subjects to administration of tocotrienols. *Lipids, 30(12),* 1171–7.

Qureshi, A. A., N. Qureshi, J. J. Wright, Z. Shen, G. Kramer, A. Gapor, Y. H. Chong, G. DeWitt, A. Ong, D. M. Peterson. 1991. Lowering of serum cholesterol in hypercholesterolemic humans by tocotrienols (palmvitee). *Am J Clin Nutr, 53(4 Suppl),* 1021S–1026S.

Radimer, K., B. Bindewald, J. Hughes, B. Ervin, C. Swanson, M. F. Picciano. 2004. Dietary supplement use by US adults: Data from the National Health and Nutrition Examination Survey, 1999–2000. *Am J Epidemiol, 160(4),* 339–349

Rapola, J. M, V. Jirtamo, R. Sipatti, J. K. Huttunen, D. Albanes, P. R. Taylor, O. P. Heinonen. 1997. Randomized trial of alpha-tocopherol and beta-carotene supplements on incidence of major coronary events in men with previous myocardial infarction. *Lancet, 349*, 1715–1720.

Reaven, P. D., D. A. Herold, J. Barnett, S. Edelman. 1995. Effects of Vitamin E on susceptibility of low-density lipoprotein and low-density lipoprotein subfractions to oxidation and on protein glycation in NIDDM. *Diabetes Care, 18(6),* 807–816

Rimm, E. B., M. J. Stampfer, A. A. scherio, E. Giovannucci, G. A. Colditz, W. C. Willett. 1993. Vitamin E consumption and the risk of coronary heart disease in men. *N Engl J Med, 328*, 1450–1456.

Rodes, J., G. Cote, J. Lesperance, M. G. Bourassa, S. Douc, L. Bilodeau, O. F. Bertrand, F. Harel, R. Gallo, J. C. Tardif. 1998. Prevention of restenosis after angioplasty in small coronary arteries with probucol. *Circulation, 97(5),* 429–36.

Rosamond, W., K. Flegal, G. Friday, K. Furie, A. Go, K. Greenlund, N. Haase, M. Ho, V. Howard, B. Kissela, S. Kittner, D. Lloyd-Jones, M. McDermott, J. Meigs, C. Moy, G. Nichol, C. J. O'Donnell, V. Roger, J. Rumsfeld, P. Sorlie, J. Steinberger, T. Thom, S. Wasserthiel-Smoller, Y. Hong. American Heart Association Statistics Committee and Stroke Statistics Subcommittee. 2006. Heart disease and stroke statistics–2007 update: A report from the American Heart Association Statistics Committee and Stroke Statistics Subcommittee. *Circulation, 113.* e69–171.

Sahyoun, N. R., P. F. Jacques, R. M. Russell. 1996. Carotenoids, vitamins C and E, and mortality in an elderly population. *Am J Epidemiol, 144(5)*, 501–11.

Saito, H., C. Kiyose, H. Yoshimura, T. Ueda, K. Kondo, O. Igarashi. 2003. γ–Tocotrienol, a vitamin E homolog, is a natriuretic hormone precursor . *J Lipid Res, 44*, 1530–1535.

Salonen, J. T., K. Nyyssonen, R. Salonen, H. M. Lakka, J. Kaikkonen, E. Porkkala-Sarataho, S. Voutilainen, T. A. Lakka, T. Rissanen, L. Leskinen, T. P. Tuomainen, V. P. Valkonen, U. Ristonmaa, H. E. Poulsen. 2000. Antioxidant Supplementation in Atherosclerosis Prevention (ASAP) study: A randomized trial of the effect of vitamins E and C on 3-year progression of carotid atherosclerosis. *J Intern Med, 248,* 377–386

Salonen, R. M., K. Nyyssonen, J. Kaikkonen, E. Porkkala-Sarataho, S. Voutilainen, T. H. Rissanen, T. P. Tuomainen, V. P. Valkonen, U. Ristonmaa, H. M. Lakka, M. Vanharanta, J. T. Salonen, H. E. Poulsen. 2003. Antioxidant Supplementation in Atherosclerosis Prevention Study. Six-year effect of combined vitamin C and E supplementation on atherosclerotic progression: The Antioxidant Supplementation in Atherosclerosis Prevention (ASAP) Study. *Circulation, 107(7),* 947–53.

Stampfer, M. J., C. H. Hennekens, J. E. Manson, G. A. Colditz, B. Rosner, W. C. Willett. 1993. Vitamin E consumption and the risk of coronary disease in women. *N Engl J Med, 328*, 1444–1449.

Stephens, N. G., P. M. Parsons, P. M. Schofield, M. J. Brown. 1996. Randomized Controlled trial of vitamin E in patients with coronary heart disease: Cambridge Heart Antioxidant Study (CHAOS). *Lancet, 349,* 781–786.

Takamatsu, S., M. Takamatsu, S. Katoh, T. Imaizumi, H. Yoshida, M. Hiramoto, M. Koyama, Y. Ohgushi, S. Mizuno. 1995. Effects on health of dietary supplementation with 100 mg d-alpha-tocopheryl acetate, daily for 6 years. *J Int Med Res, 23(5),* 342–57.

Tardif, J. C., G. Cote, J. Lesperance. 1997. Probucol and multivitamins in the prevention of restenosis after coronary angioplasty. Multivitamins and Probucol Study Group. *N Engl J Med, 337(6)*, 365–72.

The Heart Outcomes Prevention Evaluation Study Investigators. 2000. Vitamin E supplementation and cardiovascular events in high-risk patients. *N Engl J Med, 342,* 154–160.

Tomeo, A. C., M. Geller, T. R. Watkins, A. Gapor, M. L. Bierenbaum. 1995. Antioxidant effects of tocotrienols in patients with hyperlipidemia and carotid stenosis. *Lipids, 30(12),* 1179–83.

Tornwall, M. E., J. Virtamo, J. K. Haukka, D. Albanes, J. K. Huttunen. 2001. Alpha-tocopherol (vitamin E) and beta-carotene supplementation does not affect the risk for large abdominal aortic aneurysm in a controlled trial. *Atherosclerosis, 157(1),* 167–73.

Tornwall, M. E., J. Virtamo, P. A. Korhonen, M. J. Virtanen, P. R. Taylor, D. Albanes, J. K. Huttunen. 2004. Effect of alpha-tocopherol and beta-carotene supplementation on coronary heart disease during the 6-year post-trial follow-up in the ATBC study. *Eur Heart J, 25(13)*, 1171–8.

Trumbo, P. R. 2005. The level of evidence for permitting a qualified health claim: FDA's review of the evidence for selenium and cancer and vitamin E and heart disease. *J. Nutr, 135*, 354–356.

Tsimikas, S. 2006. Oxidative biomarkers in the diagnosis and prognosis of cardiovascular disease. *Am J Cardiol, 98(11A),* 9P–17P.

Virtamo, J., J. M. Rapola, S. Ripatti, O. P. Heinonen, P. R. Taylor, D. Albanes, J. K. Huttunen. 1998. Effect of vitamin E and beta carotene on the incidence of primary nonfatal myocardial infarction and fatal coronary heart disease. *Arch Intern Med, 158(6),* 668–75.

Wayne, H., F. Sutherland, P. J. Manning, R. J. Walker, S A. de Jong, A. R. Ryalls, E. A. Berry. 2007. Vitamin E supplementation and plasma 8–isoprostane and adiponectin in overweight subjects. Obesity, *15*, 386–391.

Williams, H. T. G., D. Fenna, R. A. Macbeth. 1971. Alpha tocopherol in the treatment of intermittent claudication. *Surg Gynecol Obstet, 132,* 662–666.

Wright M. E., K. A. Lawson, S. J. Weinstein, P. Pietinen, P. R. Taylor, J. Virtamo, D. Albanes. 2006. Higher baseline serum concentrations of vitamin E are associated with lower total and cause-specific mortality in the Alpha-Tocopherol, Beta-Carotene Cancer Prevention Study. *Am J Clin Nutr, 84(5),* 1200–7.

Wu, J. H., N. C. Ward, A. P. Indrawan, C. A. Almeida, J. M. Hodgson, J. M. Proudfoot, I. B. Puddey, K. D. Croft. 2007. Effects of alpha-tocopherol and mixed tocopherol supplementation on markers of oxidative stress and inflammation in type 2 diabetes. *Clin Chem, 53(3),* 511–9.

18 Tocotrienols and the Regulation of Cholesterol Biosynthesis

Jian Cao, Wei Qi and Bao-Liang Song

CONTENTS

18.1 CHOLESTEROL AND THE REGULATION OF CHOLESTEROL BIOSYNTHESIS

Cholesterol has multiple functions in humans and animals. It is a component of the phospholipid bilayer that is essential to provide greater stability and modulate fluidity of the cell membrane. Cholesterol is also used as the substrate for bile acids (Russell, 2003) and hormones biosynthesis (Payne and Hales, 2004), and can be converted to oxysterols to regulate orphan nuclear receptors including LXRα (Janowski et al., 1996). Meanwhile, Sonic hedgehog (Shh) is covalently linked to cholesterol during its maturation. The cholesterol modification is necessary for normal Shh signaling (Porter et al., 1996).

18.1.1 Hypercholesterolemia and Diseases

Although cholesterol is so important, high blood cholesterol or hypercholesterolemia, a metabolic derangement derived from genetic disorder or high cholesterol dietary, is a key factor for the development of a series of severe diseases including atherosclerosis, Alzheimer's disease and gallbladder stones (Maxfield and Tabas, 2005).

Atherosclerosis is the primary cause of heart disease and stroke. In developed countries, it is the underlying cause of about 50% of all deaths (Lusis, 2000). The initiation of atherosclerosis is the accumulation of modified low density lipoprotein (LDL) under endothelium. LDL, the major carrier of serum cholesterol in humans, poses a risk for atherosclerosis when it invades the endothelium and becomes the oxidized form. A series of biochemical reactions regulate the formation of oxidized LDL (ox-LDL), mainly stimulated by the presence of free radicals in the endothelium or blood vessel lining. Then, the ox-LDL accumulated in the endothelium induces an inflammation response. Monocytes, a type of leukocyte, are recruited and cross the artery wall from the bloodstream. The monocytes ingest ox-LDL, cumulate cholesterol ester and differentiate into foam cells. Foam cells eventually die and further propagate the inflammatory process, thereby forming atherosclerosis plaque on the endothelium of vasculature. Advanced atherosclerotic lesions lead to progressive narrowing of the vessel lumen and ischemic symptoms. Once the plaque ruptures, plaque lipids and tissue factors will be exposed to blood, leading to acute cardiovascular events such as thrombosis, myocardial infarction and stroke (Glass and Witztum, 2001; Lusis, 2000).

Although several other important environmental and genetic risk factors associated with atherosclerosis have been revealed by epidemiological studies, elevated serum cholesterol alone is sufficient to drive the development of atherosclerosis in humans and experimental animals, even in the absence of other known risk factors (Glass and Witztum, 2001). Therefore, it is very important to control serum cholesterol level in order to reduce the onset of atherosclerosis.

18.1.2 Cholesterol Biosynthesis

Cholesterol required in humans and animals is supplied by the diet and endogenous synthesis. Figure 18.1 briefly illustrates the cholesterol biosynthesis pathway.

Cholesterol is synthesized from acetate precursors, and all of the 27 carbons of cholesterol come from acetyl-CoA proved by ^{14}C incorporation experiment. The acetyl-CoA is first converted to 3-hydroxy-3-methylglutaryl CoA (HMG-CoA) by two steps of condensation reactions successively. Then HMG-CoA is reduced to mevalonate by HMG-CoA reductase. The reduction of HMG-CoA to mevalonate is the rate-limiting step of *de novo* cholesterol biosynthesis, and HMG-CoA reductase is subject to complex regulatory controls on several levels including transcription, mRNA stability, protein degradation and phosphorylation. The regulation of HMG-CoA reductase will be discussed in detail in the following sections.

After the reduction of HMG-CoA, mevalonate is converted to isopentenyl pyrophosphate (IPP) by phosphorylation and decarboxylation. Then isomerization is performed to convert isopentenyl pyrophosphate to dimethylallyl pyrophosphate (DPP), and these two 5-carbon molecules (isopentenyl pyrophosphate and dimethylallyl pyrophosphate) condense to form the 10-carbon geranyl pyrophosphate. After that, one more molecule of isopentenyl pyrophosphate attaches to geranyl pyrophosphate to form 15-carbon farnesyl pyrophosphate.

In the subsequent step, two molecules of farnesyl pyrophosphate condense in a head-to-head manner to form the 30-carbon isoprenoids squalene. Then squalene undergoes cyclinzation to yield lanosterol. Lanosterol, the first sterol intermediate in cholesterol biosynthesis, was identified to be an endogenous regulator for the stability of HMG-CoA reductase protein (Song et al., 2005a). The last stage of cholesterol biosynthesis is to convert lanosterol to cholesterol. Nineteen additional steps of reactions operated by nine membrane-bound enzymes remove three methyl groups and modify

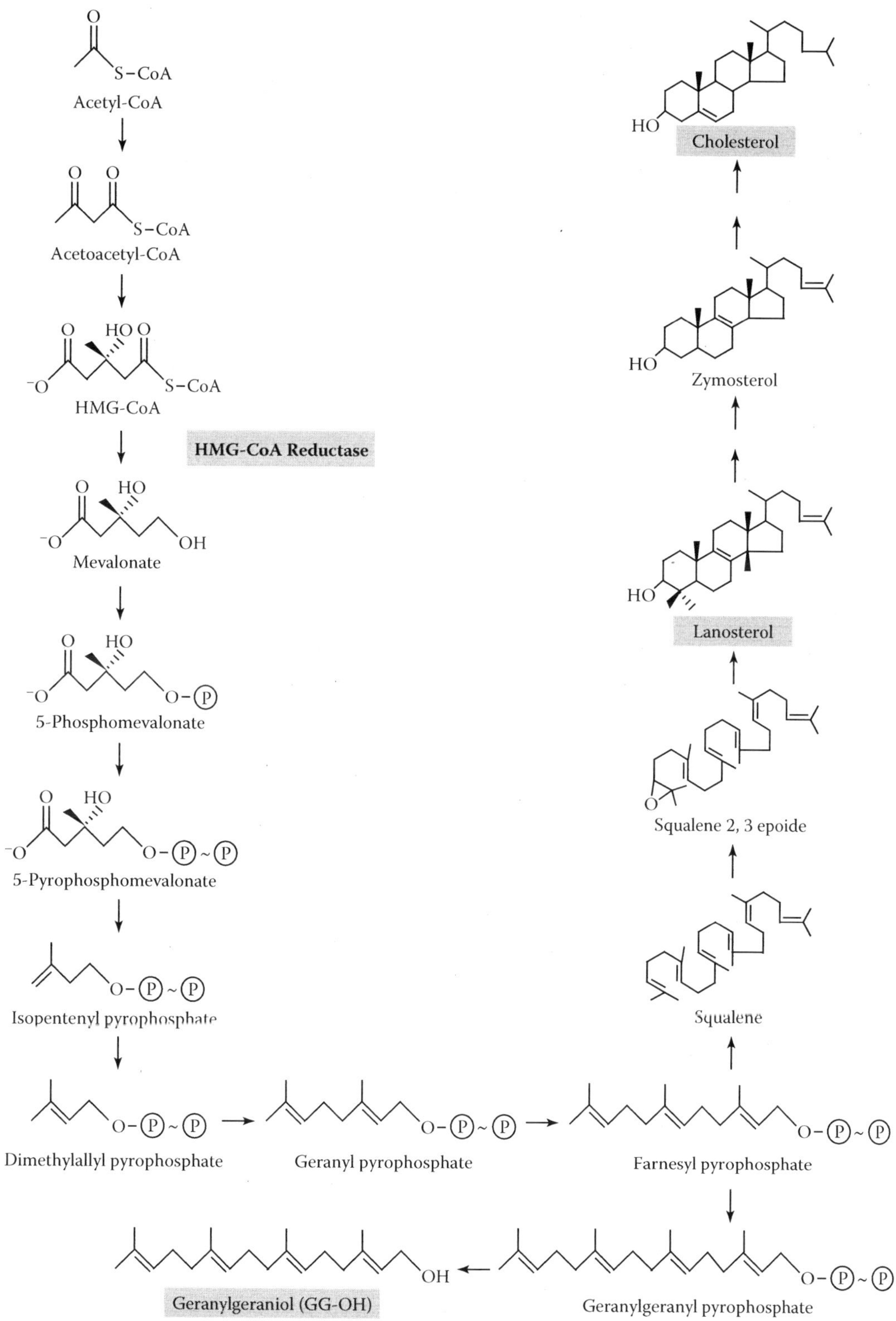

FIGURE 18.1 Schematic representation of the cholesterol biosynthetic pathway in mammalian cells. Acetyl-CoA is converted to cholesterol by about 30 steps. HMG-CoA reductase and three key molecules (geranylgeraniol, lanosterol and cholesterol) are highlighted in gray boxes.

the number and position of double bonds, which finally leads to the 27-carbon product cholesterol (Espenshade and Hughes, 2007; Gaylor, 2002).

Besides the final product, the intermediates of cholesterol synthetic pathway can be diverted to other products, such as Vitamin D, farnesyl and geranylgeranyl ligands that prenylate some of the key cellular proteins and anchor them to cell membranes (Zhang and Casey, 1996), coenzyme Q of the oxidative phosphorylation pathway, side chain of heme A, isopentyl tRNAs for protein synthesis and so on (Grunler et al., 1994).

18.1.3 Regulation of Cholesterol Biosynthesis

To maintain the level of membrane cholesterol, cells have developed several feedback strategies to regulate the endogenous cholesterol biosynthesis. Two of the well-studied are: (1) the sterol regulatory element binding proteins (SREBP) pathway and (2) the regulated degradation of HMG-CoA reductase.

18.1.3.1 SREBP Pathway

SREBP are a family of basic-helix-loop-helix-leucine zipper (bHLH-LZ) transcription factors (Wang et al., 1994). They regulate a multitude of enzymes that are required for the endogenous cholesterol and fatty acid synthesis (Eberle et al., 2004). There are three different forms of SREBP in mammals, named SREBP-1a, SREBP-1c and SREBP-2 (Brown and Goldstein, 1997). SREBP-1a and SREBP-1c are produced from one gene through different transcription initiation sites usage and mRNA alternative splicing. SREBP-2 is encoded by a separated gene (Osborne, 2000). The target genes of SREBP-1 are mainly involved in fatty acid synthesis. And SREBP-2 preferably regulates the genes in cholesterol biosynthesis and uptake (Eberle et al., 2004).

The SREBP protein is first synthesized as a membrane-bound inactive precursor and localized in the endoplasmic reticulum (ER). The precursor of SREBP can be divided into three domains: (1) an amino-terminal region that contains the activation domain for dimerization and DNA binding; (2) two hydrophobic transmembrane spanning helices and a short loop that projects into the ER lumen; and (3) a carboxyl-terminal regulatory domain. Both the amino- and carboxyl-terminus are oriented into cytosol (Goldstein et al., 2006).

Through the regulatory domain, SREBP constitutively binds to another ER membrane protein: SREBP cleavage activating protein (SCAP) (Nohturfft et al., 1998). SCAP protein possesses eight membrane-spanning regions in the amino-terminal and the second to sixth transmembrane regions constitute a sterol sensing domain (SSD) (Goldstein et al., 2002; Radhakrishnan et al., 2004). The carboxyl-terminal cytosolic domain of SCAP interacts with the regulatory domain of SREBP. In sterol-depleted cells, the complex of SCAP and SREBP precursor traffics from ER to Golgi apparatus through secretary machinery (Goldstein et al., 2006). In Golgi, two proteases (called Site-1 protease and Site-2 protease) sequentially cleave SREBP to release the amino-terminal activation domain which is also called nuclear form of SREBP (nSREBP) (Rawson et al., 1998; Duncan et al., 1998). Then this truncated, transcriptional active form of SREBP enters the nucleus and binds to a class of *cis*-elements named sterol regulatory element (SRE) on the promoters of SREBP target genes to upregulate their expression (Figure 18.2, left panel) (Goldstein et al., 2006).

High concentration of cholesterol is able to preserve SCAP-SREBP complex in ER, thereby reducing the expression of SREBP target genes (Espenshade et al., 2002). The mechanism of how cholesterol prevents SCAP-SREBP from exiting ER has been resolved by the Brown-Goldstein lab at the University of Texas Southwestern Medical Center recently. Their research revealed a new player, Insig, and found out that the sterol-regulated binding between SCAP and Insig plays a key role in this process (Yang et al., 2002). There are two homologs for Insig in mammals: Insig-1 and Insig-2. The full name of Insig-1 is insulin-induced gene 1 (Peng et al., 1997; Yabe et al., 2002). However, the stimulation of Insig-1 expression by insulin is not a direct effect. Insig-2 and Insig-1 are very similar both in amino acid sequence and topology pattern (Goldstein et al., 2006; Yabe et

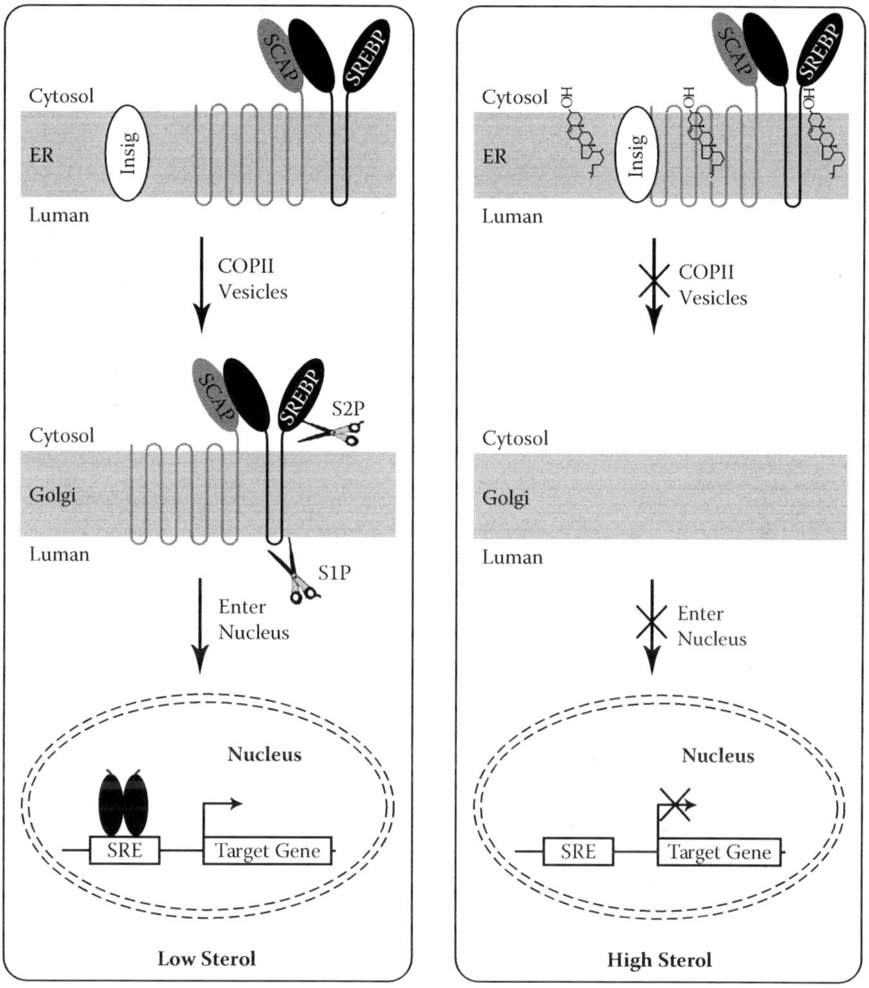

FIGURE 18.2 Sterol-regulated proteolysis of SREBP. (Left) In the absence of sterols, the SCAP-SREBP complex moves to Golgi through COPII vesicles. At Golgi, SREBP is cleaved sequentially by two proteases: Site-1 protease (S1P) and Site-2 protease (S2P), to release the transcription factor domain of SREBP. The transcriptional active form of SREBP enters nucleus, binds to sterol regulatory elements in gene promoters and activates target genes involved in fatty acid synthesis, cholesterol synthesis and uptake. (Right) High level of sterol promotes the binding of SCAP to Insig. Insig blocks SCAP-SREBP transport from ER to Golgi, eventually down regulating the expression of SREBP target genes.

al., 2002). When cholesterol is overloaded, it promotes the binding between SCAP and Insig in the ER membrane (Figure 18.2, right panel) (Adams et al., 2003; Yabe et al., 2002). Their interaction prevents the transportation of SCAP-SREBP complex from exiting the ER via COPII vesicles (Sun et al., 2005). Eventually, cholesterol renders the ER-retention of SREBP, reduces the maturation of SREBP and down-regulates the gene expressions.

18.1.3.2 Regulated Degradation of HMG-CoA Reductase

Sterol-regulated degradation of HMG-CoA reductase is another major feedback regulatory pathway for cholesterol biosynthesis. HMG-CoA reductase converts HMG-CoA to movalonate. This reduction is the rate-limiting reaction in the synthesis of cholesterol and nonsterol isoprenoids (Goldstein and Brown, 1990).

Similar to SCAP, HMG-CoA reductase locates to the ER with eight membrane-spanning regions (Roitelman et al., 1992). HMG-CoA reductase can be divided into two distinguishable parts by structure and function: carboxyl-terminal cytosolic domain and amino-terminal transmembrane domain (Goldstein et al., 2006). The transmembrane domain of reductase contains a sterol sensing domain (SSD) and bears significant similarity with the corresponding region of SCAP in amino acid sequence and the secondary structure (Sever et al., 2003b). The carboxyl-terminal domain of reductase alone exerts all of the catalytic activity of the enzyme; meanwhile, a truncated reductase containing only the amino-terminal domain undergoes sterol-induced degradation as the full-length protein does (Liscum et al., 1985; Gil et al., 1985).

The sterol-regulated degradation of reductase is mediated by the ubiquitin-proteasome pathway (Sever et al., 2003a). Ubiquitination is carried out through the sequential actions of three kinds of enzymes: the ubiquitin-activating enzyme (E1), ubiquitin-conjugating enzymes (E2s), and ubiquitin ligases (E3s). Ubiquitin is first covalently conjugated to a reactive cysteine residue of E1 (E1-Ub), then transferred to a catalytic cysteine of E2 (E2-Ub). Finally, E3 facilitates the transfer of ubiquitin from E2-Ub to a lysine residue on the substrate (or ubiquitin) (Hershko et al., 2000; Pickart, 2001). This reaction can be repeated several times to form polyubiquitin chains. Another model was proposed in which a ubiquitin chain is first preassembled on E2 by ubiquitin ligase. Then the same ubiquitin ligase transfers this ubiquitin chain to its substrate (Li et al., 2007). Finally, polyubiquitin modified protein is moved to 26S proteasome for degradation.

At the situation of HMG-CoA reductase degradation, binding of reductase to Insig-1 or Insig-2 is promoted by sterols and is a prerequisite for ubiquitination and degradation of reductase (Sever et al., 2003a). Four lines of evidence support this notion. First, when reductase is overexpressed in Chinese hamster ovary (CHO) cells by transfection, the enzyme is no longer subjected to sterol accelerated degradation. Overexpression of Insig-1 or -2 restores the regulated degradation of transfected reductase (Sever et al., 2003a; Sever et al., 2003b). Second, the combined knockdown of Insig-1 and -2 through RNA interference (RNAi) abolishes sterol-induced degradation of endogenous reductase (Sever et al., 2003a). Third, in mutant cells lacking Insigs, sterols fail to stimulate the degradation of reductase (Sever et al., 2003a; Lee et al., 2005). Fourth, in the livers of Insig-1 and -2 knockout mice, reductase protein level is increased by hundred folds compared with a 2- to 3-fold increase of its mRNA (Engelking et al., 2005).

Recently, the mechanism of the sterol-regulated degradation of HMG-CoA reductase started to emerge. Using co-immunoprecipitation coupled with mass spectrometry, Song et al. identified that gp78, a membrane anchored ubiquitin ligase, as an Insig-interacting protein (Song et al., 2005b). gp78 contains more than five transmembrane helices that constitutively bind to Insig in the membrane. High concentration of sterol promotes the interaction between HMG-CoA reductase and Insig, through which reductase is recruited to the complex and ubiquitinated at two specific lysine residues by gp78 (Song et al., 2005b).

Along the same vein, our research further revealed that the cytosolic domain of gp78 bound to Ufd1 and VCP. On one hand, Ufd1 functions as a cofactor that enhances the E3 activity of gp78, and accelerates the ubquitin chain assembled in E2. On the other hand, Ufd1 and VCP recognize the polyubiquitin chains, extract ubiquitinated reductase from the ER membrane and present them to 26S proteasome for degradation (Cao et al., 2007).

As a conclusion, sterols induce the binding of HMG-CoA reductase to Insig, thereby forming a complex of gp78, Ubc7 (E2), VCP, Ufd1, Insig and HMG-CoA reductase. gp78 catalyzes the ubiquitin chain assembled on Ubc7, and the reaction is enhanced by Ufd1. Then preassembled ubquitin chain is transferred to HMG-CoA reductase by gp78. Ubiquitinated HMG-CoA reductase is moved to proteasome for degradation. The postubiquitination step of HMG-CoA reductase is stimulated by geranylgeraniol. VCP and Ufd1 are involved in this step. Figure 18.3 illustrates the pathway of sterol stimulated HMG-CoA reductase degradation.

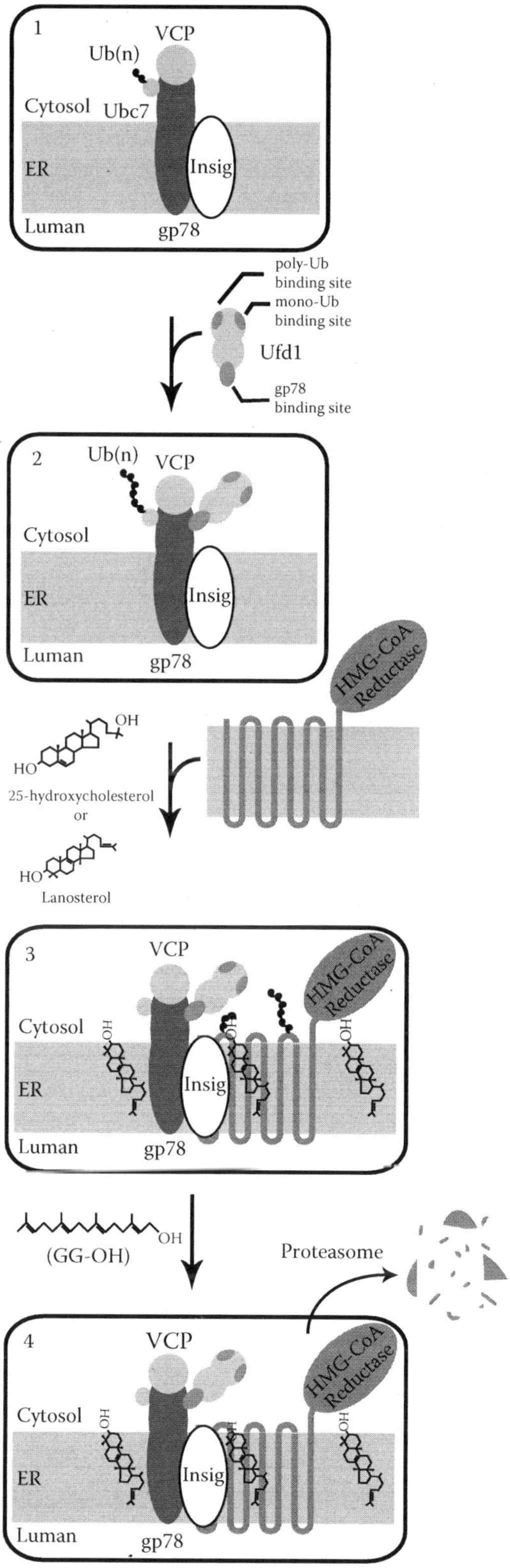

FIGURE 18.3 Sterol-regulated ubiquitination and degradation of HMG-CoA reductase. (1) gp78, a membrane anchored ubiquitin ligase, constitutively binds to Insig, VCP and Ubc7 (E2). (2) Ufd1 interacts with gp78 directly, enhances the E3 activity of gp78 through its monoubiquitin binding site, and elongates the preassembled ubiquitin chain on Ubc7. (3) Lanosterol or 25-hydroxycholesterol triggers the binding between HMG-CoA reductase and Insig. gp78 catalyzes the transformation of ubiquitin chain from Ubc7 to HMG-CoA reductase. (4) Ubiquitinated HMG-CoA reductase is removed to proteasome for degradation, stimulated by geranylgeraniol (GG-OH). VCP and the polyubiquitin binding site of Ufd1 are involved in this post-ubiquitination step.

18.1.3.3 Endogenous Molecules That Regulate the Cholesterol Biosynthesis

Thirty years ago, scientists knew that the cholesterol regulatory system is modified not only by the end product, cholesterol, but also some other small molecules and that they regulate these processes even more efficiently. For example, 25-hydroxycholesterol (25-HC), one form of oxysterols, blocks SREBPs cleavage and accelerates HMG-CoA reductase degradation (Adams et al., 2004; Sever et al., 2003b). It is usually used in laboratory experiments to investigate the mechanism of sterol feedback controls. Recently, studies from Brown-Goldstein lab revealed that cholesterol specifically binds to SCAP and causes the conformational changes of SCAP that can be detected by trypsin digestion assay (Brown et al., 2002; Radhakrishnan et al., 2004; Feramisco et al., 2005). Then SCAP binds to Insig to preserve SCAP-SREBP complex in ER (Yang et al., 2002). However, cholesterol cannot bind to HMG-CoA reductase or promote the ubiquitination of HMG-CoA reductase in permeablized cells or *in vitro* (Song and DeBose-Boyd, 2004; Radhakrishnan et al., 2004). These results suggest that cholesterol is the endogenous ligand of SCAP that specifically regulates SREBP pathway (Radhakrishnan et al., 2004;). 25-HC works differently from cholesterol. 25-HC binds to Insig directly to enhance the Insig-SCAP interaction (Radhakrishnan et al., 2007). It is also possible that 25-HC regulates the degradation of HMG-CoA reductase by the similar mechanism: binding to Insig and promoting the Insig-reductase interaction.

The degradation of HMG-CoA reductase is synergistically stimulated by sterol and nonsterol product. As discussed before, sterol can promote the interaction between reductase and Insig, thereby facilitating the ubiquitination of reductase by gp78 (Song et al., 2005b). The 20-carbon isoprenoid geranylgeraniol (GG-OH), a nonsterol mevalonate derivative, can synergize with sterols in accelerating the degradation of reductase (Sever et al., 2003a). However, GG-OH doesn't promote the ubiquitination of reductase alone, suggesting geranylgeranylated protein may be involved in the post-ubiquitination steps in reductase degradation (Sever et al., 2003a).

Lanosterol, the first sterol produced in the cholesterol biosynthetic pathway, was later identified as an endogenous regulator of reductase ubiquitination and degradation (Song et al., 2005a). Notably, lanosterol doesn't inhibit the cleavage of SREBP, nor binds to SCAP. Song et al. further demonstrated that the 4,4,-dimethyl moiety of lanosterol is the major determinant for reductase regulation (Song et al., 2005a). So, lanosterol is an endogenous small regulatory molecule specific for the degradation of HMG-CoA reductase. We envision this process to be the first in a series of reactions that avoid sterol overaccumulation. When the cholesterol biosynthesis is in excess, more lanosterol would be produced, causing feedback that inhibits the reduction of mevalonate by promoting the degradation of HMG-CoA reductase. Meanwhile, lanosterol doesn't inhibit the maturation of SREBP, which ensures lanosterol to be converted to cholesterol eventually. Whether lanosterol directly binds reductase or Insig remains obscure.

In conclusion, 25-HC inhibits the cleavage of SREBP and promotes the degradation of HMG-CoA reductase. Cholesterol specifically blocks the maturation of SREBP. Lanosterol only stimulates the degradation of reductase. Meanwhile, GG-OH, a nonsterol derivative can potentiate the effect of sterols on the degradation of reductase.

18.2 TOCOTRIENOLS DOWN-REGULATE CHOLESTEROL BIOSYNTHESIS

Hypercholesterolemia is a well recognized risk factor for cardiovascular diseases. Humans with high concentrations of serum cholesterol have correspondingly high mortality rates from cardiovascular diseases (Ross, 1999). Conversely, vegetarians or populations with diets rich in cereal grains and vegetables tend to have a low incidence of cardiovascular diseases (Pearce et al., 1992). After more than 20 years of study, it has been gradually understood that the tocotrienol molecules in grains are the effective ingredient that lowers the cholesterol biosynthesis. Considering the relationship between hypercholesterolemia and cardiovascular diseases, the hypocholesterolemic feature of tocotrienols makes them a group of attractive drug candidates.

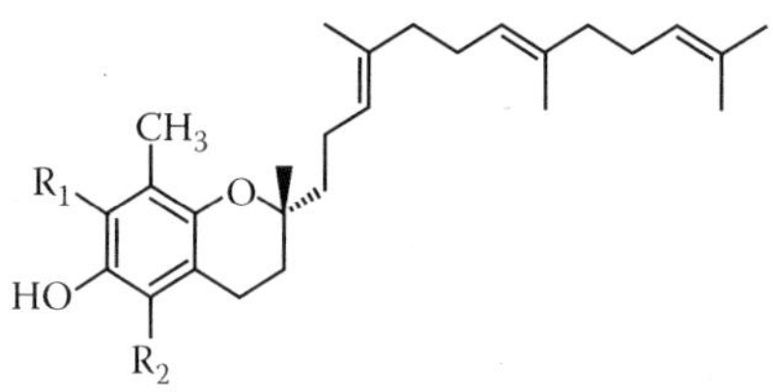

Tocotrienol

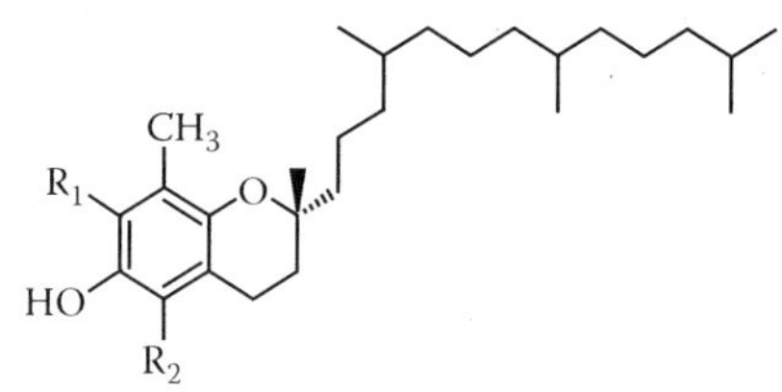

Tocopherol

Compound	R_1	R_2
α–	CH_3	CH_3
β–	H	CH_3
γ–	CH_3	H
δ–	H	H

FIGURE 18.4 Schematic representation of chemical structures of tocotrienols and tocopherols.

18.2.1 Structures of Tocotrienols and Tocopherols

α-tocotrienol was the first identified member of vitamin E, which was discovered in 1922 for its feature of supporting fertility. At present, vitamin E represents a class of compounds containing eight naturally occurring members and can be divided into two subgroups: tocotrienols and tocopherols (Figure 18.4). All of them are synthesized exclusively by plants, and humans absorb them from their daily diets. Tocopherols, the primary form of vitamin E, are found in common vegetable oils such as soybean, canola, wheat germ, and sunflower oils; whereas tocotrienols are mainly present in oat, barley, rye, rice bran and other cereal grains, with the richest source found in palm fruits (Qureshi, Burger et al., 1980).

Tocopherols and tocotrienols both have a polar chromanol ring core and the only difference between these two kinds of vitamin E is the number of their unsaturated bonds (Figure 18.4). Tocotrienol has a fanesyl side chain with three double bonds, while tocopherol has a saturated phytyl side chain. The unsaturated tail of tocotrienol arises from condensation of homogentisate and geranylgeranyl pyrophosphate, and the saturated one of tocopherols is thought to be derived from homogentisate and phytyl pyrophosphate (Sen et al., 2006).

There are four isomers, α, β, γ and δ, found in each subgroup of vitamin E. Different Greek letter prefixes indicate the different numbers and position of methyl substitution on their chromanol ring. Their structural formulas are shown in Figure 18.4.

18.2.2 Supplementing Tocotrienols But Not Tocopherols in Diet Lowers Serum Cholesterol

In some areas of Asia, humans consuming cereal as daily diets have a low incidence of cardiovascular disease. Compared with corn, wheat, oats, and rye, barley is the most effective cereal in lowering blood cholesterol level and liver cholesterol biosynthesis when fed to experimental animals (Qureshi, Burger et al., 1980). Purification has been performed to study the effective ingredient in barley. High-protein barley flour was first identified to be the richest source of the cholesterol-suppressive factors. Then cholesterol-suppressive activity was partially extracted by petroleum ether. Using semipreparative HPLC, investigators further fractionated the petroleum ether-soluble fraction of high-protein barley flour and the cholesterol-suppressive effects of each portion were tested. Finally, two cholesterol inhibitors were identified from the petroleum ether-soluble fraction of high-protein barley flour; one of them is α-tocotrienol (Qureshi, Burger et al., 1986).

The cholesterol-lowering effect of tocotrienols has been studied in many kinds of animal models including chickens (Wang et al., 1993; Qureshi, Pearce et al., 1996; Yu et al., 2006), golden hamsters (Khor and Chieng, 1996), rats (Watkins et al., 1993 ; Iqbal et al., 2003; Minhajuddin et al., 2005), swine (Qureshi, Peterson et al., 2001b), rabbits (Hasselwander et al., 2002), and mice (Qureshi, Salser et al., 2001d; Black et al., 2000). In most of the experiments, supplementation of tocotrienols in the diet for several weeks significantly decreased the serum total cholesterol and LDL cholesterol. Meanwhile, the concentration of HDL cholesterol was increased or showed no significant changes. As a result, the ratio of HDL cholesterol to LDL cholesterol was dramatically raised. The changes in these parameters reflected the improvement of the serum lipid state, which is beneficial in cardiovascular disease.

On the other hand, although tocopherols have been widely used as antioxidants to prevent some chronic diseases, especially those believed to be caused by oxidative damage such as cardiovascular disease, atherosclerosis and cancer, tocopherols do not share the hypocholesterolemic feature of tocotrienols. Animal experiments and clinical studies established that tocopherol supplements in diets produced only a small elevation of HDL cholesterol and showed no significant impact on total cholesterol or LDL cholesterol (Yu et al., 2006). In some cases, tocopherols were used in a double-blind study and showed no significant effect on serum lipid parameters like placebo (Qureshi et al., 1991).

Hyperlipidemia and hypercholesterolemia (HH) swine is a strain of pig bearing spontaneous and genetically hereditary high concentrations of serum triglycerides and cholesterol. The lipid profiles of HH swine are similar to humans with high serum cholesterol. The study on HH swine showed that with dietary supplementation of tocotrienols, serum total cholesterol concentration was decreased by 32% or 34%, and LDL cholesterol concentration was decreased by 35% or 38%, whereas HDL cholesterol levels did not differ among different groups (Qureshi, Peterson et al., 2001b).

Rats treated with 7,12-dimethylbenz [α]anthracene (DMBA) showed induced carcinogenesis as well as hypercholesterolemia. Compared with DMBA treatment alone, combined tocotrienols treatment for 6 months caused a significant decline of 30% in total cholesterol and 67% in LDL cholesterol level. At the same time, tocotrienols also showed anti-carcinogenesis activity, and this effect, just as with statins, may be explained by their mevalonate-suppressive action. (Iqbal et al., 2003)

Apolipoprotein (Apo) E is the major ligand for removing cholesterol-rich chylomicron and VLDL remnants from the blood. Feeding a diet with high triglyceride and cholesterol, heterozygous $ApoE^{+/-}$ mice develop atheromas and are used as a model for hypercholesterolemia and atherosclerosis development. Supplemented with a mixture of vitamin E compounds, the $ApoE^{+/-}$ mice had 60% lower plasma cholesterol than the control group without vitamin E feeding. At the same time, the formation of atherosclerotic lesions of $ApoE^{+/-}$ mice induced by an atherogenic diet was attenuated substantially in the vitamin E-feeding group. Considering the fact that supplementation of α-tocopherol or palm-carotenoids shows no prevention on atherosclerosis, the effect of vitamin E reflects the cholesterol-lowering function of tocotrienols and has nothing to do with their antioxidant properties (Black et al., 2000).

Besides animal experiments, tocotrienol supplements in the daily diet also showed cholesterol-lowering effects in human trials investigated by some clinical studies. Trials were operated with healthy humans (Tan et al., 1991), hypercholesterolemic humans (Qureshi, Quereshi et al., 1991; Qureshi, Bradlow et al., 1995; Qureshi, Bradlow et al., 1997; Qureshi, Sami et al., 2001c; Qureshi, Sami et al., 2002), type 2 diabetic patients (Baliarsingh et al., 2005), or patients with cardiovascular disease (CVD) (Martirosyan et al., 2007). Similar to the results from animal experiments, supplementing tocotrienols for several weeks suppressed serum total cholesterol (Baliarsingh et al., 2005; Tan et al., 1991; Qureshi, Sami et al., 2002; Qureshi, Bradlow et al., 1997; Qureshi, Bradlow et al., 1995; Qureshi, Quereshi et al., 1991; Martirosyan et al., 2007; Qureshi, Sami et al., 2001c) and LDL cholesterol levels (Baliarsingh et al., 2005; Qureshi, Sami et al., 2002; Qureshi, Bradlow et al., 1997; Tan et al., 1991; Qureshi, Quereshi et al., 1991; Martirosyan et al., 2007; Qureshi, Sami et al., 2001c). Other serum lipid parameters also improved when treated with tocotrienols, such as serum total lipids (Baliarsingh et al., 2005), concentration of ApoB (Qureshi, Sami et al., 2002; Qureshi, Bradlow et al., 1995; Qureshi, Quereshi et al., 1991), triglycerides (Qureshi, Sami et al., 2002; Baliarsingh et al., 2005; Martirosyan et al., 2007), plasma thromboxane B2 (Qureshi, Bradlow et al., 1997; Qureshi, Bradlow et al., 1995; Qureshi, Quereshi et al., 1991) and platelet factor 4 (Qureshi, Bradlow et al., 1997; Qureshi, Quereshi et al., 1991).

Among these positive results with animals or humans, a study showed that tocotrienols had little effect on plasma lipids. Hasselwander et al. carried out an experiment of feeding various tocotrienol sources in cholesterol-fed rabbits for 12 weeks (Hasselwander et al., 2002). When all treatments resulted in a significant increase in plasma tocotrienols, a mild 22%–23% decrease in total serum cholesterol and LDL cholesterol was observed following γ-tocotrienol treatment at the intermediate timepoint of 6 weeks. After continued feeding of γ-tocotrienol to 12 weeks, the hypocholesterol effect was smaller, but a 20% reduction in the lesion area was still observed, reflecting its anti-atherogenesis effect. It is unclear whether the weaker response in this specific study was due to a difference in animal models or the tocotrienol isomers. Considering that a 10% decrease in serum cholesterol results in a 20% reduction in mortality from cardiovascular disease and a 17% reduction in the incidence of myocardial infarction (Levine et al., 1995), the potential clinical usage of tocotrienols is still an attractive study field.

18.2.3 Tocotrienols Synergistically Inhibit Cholesterol Biosynthesis with Statins

Statins are a class of drugs widely used to treat hypercholesterolemia. As a competitive inhibitor for HMG-CoA reductase, the statin depletes hepatic cholesterol by lowering cholesterol biosynthesis (Gould et al., 1998; Collins et al., 2002; Pedersen et al., 1994). Then a low concentration of cholesterol in the endoplasmic reticulum triggers the moving of SCAP-SREBP to the Golgi apparatus, where the active forms of SREBP are released to enhance the transcription of their target genes, including LDL receptor and HMG-CoA reductase (Figure 18.2). Increased expression of the LDL receptor promotes LDL clearance from circulation to lower concentration of total and LDL cholesterol in serum (Goldstein and Brown, 1990). On the other hand, increase of HMG-CoA reductase expression compromises the hypocholesterol effect of statins themselves, and the dosage of statin has to be gradually increased to achieve the same effect (Kita et al., 1980). Besides, therapies with large doses of statins encounter several serious side effects. Unlike statins, tocotrienols decrease cholesterol biosynthesis by enhancing HMG-CoA reductase degradation without accumulation of HMG-CoA reductase. Patients on statin drug therapy may achieve further decreases in their blood cholesterol levels and a lower dose of statin can be used when applied together with tocotrienols. Studies have been performed to determine the synergistic effects of statin and different vitamin E members. When applied together, tocotrienols significantly enhanced the hypocholesterolemic effect of lovastatin, a form of statin, in both chickens (Qureshi and Peterson, 2001a) and hypercholesterolemic humans (Qureshi, Sami et al., 2001c). Compared with the control diet or individual supplement groups, combinations of tocotrienols with lovastatin lowered the serum total cholesterol and LDL cholesterol most efficiently (Qureshi and Peterson, 2001a). Meanwhile, hepatic HMG-CoA reductase activity was also greatly decreased in the double treatment group, even more dramatically than with the lovastatin treatment alone. The results of these experiments provided a novel therapeutic direction by combination of tocotrienols and statins.

18.2.4 α-Tocopherol Attenuates Tocotrienols' Hypocholesterolemic Effects

The hypocholesterolemic effects of tocotrienols have been confirmed by a number of investigators. However, some opposite observations are also reported by other scientists (Wahlqvist et al., 1992; Mensink et al., 1999; O'Byrne et al., 2000; Mustad et al., 2002; Rasool et al., 2006). For example, in a study of mildly hypercholsterolemic men, supplement of a vitamin E concentrate rich in tocotrienols showed no improvement in serum lipid parameters compared with placebo plus α-tocopherol

(Mensink et al., 1999). In another study with healthy humans, treatment with a mixture of different isomers of tocotrienols and α-tocopherol significantly increased their concentrations in plasma, but did not dramatically affect serum total or LDL cholesterol (Rasool et al., 2006). One of the potential explanations for these opposite observations is that α-tocopherol attenuates tocotrienols' hypocholesterolemic effects.

Tocotrienols from different sources have been used in previous studies. The most frequently used sources in animal experiments are the tocotrienol-rich fraction of rice bran (Yu et al., 2006; Qureshi, Bradlow et al., 1997;Hasselwander et al., 2002; Baliarsingh et al., 2005; Iqbal et al., 2003; Minhajuddin et al., 2005; Qureshi, Sami et al., 2002; Qureshi, Peterson et al., 2001b; Qureshi, Sami et al., 2001c; Qureshi, Bradlow et al., 1997), tocotrienol-rich fraction of palm oil (Hasselwander et al., 2002; Yu et al., 2006), and purified individual tocotrienols (Hasselwander et al., 2002; O'Byrne et al., 2000). Capsulated palm-oil-vitamin E concentrate (palmvitee) derived from palm oil has also been used in human subject studies (Tan et al., 1991; Qureshi et al., 1991). The different mixtures of vitamin E used in these studies actually contain variant components of tocotrienols and tocopherols. Some of them are rich in α-tocopherol. As studied by Qureshi et al., the presence of large amount of α-tocopherol blocks the hypocholesterolemic effect of tocotrienols by inducing HMG-CoA reductase activity in chicken liver (Qureshi, Pearce et al., 1996). Another study also suggested that α-tocopherol appears to attenuate the tocotrienols' effect *in vivo* but not in isolated liver cells (Pearce et al., 1992). This finding suggests that the transport systems of vitamin E might play a role in this process. Recently, a study in chicken model has compared the purified tocotrienols with tocotrienol-rich fraction of palm or rice bran oil that contains α-tocopherol, and the results demonstrated that the purified tocotrienols are more effective in lowering the serum total and LDL cholesterol levels (Yu et al., 2006). All these evidence indicated that the α-tocopherol diminishes the hypocholesterolemic function of tocotrienols. This information will be useful in the future animal and clinical studies about tocotrienols and the potential drug development.

18.3 THE MECHANISM OF TOCOTRIENOLS' ACTION

Supplementing tocotrienols in the daily diet could lower serum cholesterol concentration and improve serum lipid parameters. Recently, the molecular mechanism for this process was uncovered. It has been revealed that tocotrienols reduce hepatic HMG-CoA reductase protein levels through Insig-dependent ubiquitination and degradation of HMG-CoA reductase to lower cholesterol biosynthesis and eventually decrease serum cholesterol concentration.

18.3.1 Tocotrienols Reduce HMG-CoA Reductase Activity on a Posttranscriptional Process

The inhibition of HMG-CoA reductase activity results in decreasing the speed of cholesterol production, a principle widely used in cholesterol-lowering therapies. From early studies, it was noticed that the hypocholesterolemic capacity of tocotrienols is linked to the reduction of HMG-CoA reductase activity.

In 1980, Qureshi et al. showed that plasma or liver cholesterol was reduced dramatically in chickens after feeding with different barley-based diets. Meanwhile, hepatic HMG-CoA reductase activity also changed in parallel to the cholesterol concentration (Qureshi, Burger et al., 1980). Later, studies revealed that tocotrienol was one of the cholesterol biosynthesis-suppressive factors and inhibited HMG-CoA reductase activity in both rat and chicken hepatocytes in a dose-dependent manner (Qureshi, Burger et al., 1986). Tocotrienol treatment decreased the rate of [^{14}C]-acetate incorporation into cholesterol instead of [^{14}C]-mevalonate incorporation into cholesterol (Parker et al., 1993). These data strongly indicated that tocotrienols influence cholesterol biosynthesis by affecting a step between acetyl-CoA and movalonate, and HMG-CoA reductase is located within these steps. After incubating cells with different concentrations of γ-tocotrienol, cholesterol biosynthesis and microsomal enzyme activity of HMG-CoA reductase were inhibited (Parker et al., 1993). At each concentration point, the rate of cholesterol biosynthesis closely reflected the activity level of reductase, and the parameters of these two curves were linearly correlated, indicating that γ-tocotrienol blocked the cholesterol biosynthesis by down-regulating the activity of HMG-CoA reductase (Parker et al., 1993).

25-hydroxycholesterol and statins also lower the activity of HMG-CoA reductase in intact cells (Adams et al., 2004; Goldstein et al., 2006; Sever et al., 2003a; Gould et al., 1998). But their mechanisms are totally different. 25-hydroxycholesterol reduces HMG-CoA reductase activity by triggering both the retention of SREBP on ER and the degradation of HMG-CoA reductase, thereby the mRNA and protein of HMG-CoA reductase are both decreased (Adams et al., 2004; Goldstein et al., 2006). On the other hand, statins are competitive inhibitors of HMG-CoA reductase and they directly block the activity of HMG-CoA reductase. Through the feedback regulation of cholesterol, treatment with statins induces SREBP cleavage and inhibits the degradation of reductase, resulting in an increase of both mRNA and protein of HMG-CoA reductase (Kita et al., 1980; Goldstein and Brown, 1990).

Along the same vein, Parker et al. performed an experiment of [^{35}S]-methionine incorporation and pulse-chase to study how γ-tocotrienol regulates reductase protein. They showed that γ-tocotrienol treatment decreased the rate of HMG-CoA reductase synthesis to 57% of control, and the half-life of the enzyme was reduced to 1.59 hours compared with 3.73 hours in untreated cells (Parker et al., 1993). Integrating these results, it was concluded that tocotrienols modify cholesterol biosynthesis by decreasing HMG-CoA reductase expression, as 25-hydroxycholesterol does. In fact, treatment with γ-tocotrienol decreased the protein level of HMG-CoA reductase to 26% of control. At the same time, HMG-CoA reductase mRNA was moderately decreased (74% of control), indicating that γ-tocotrienol regulates cholesterol production by suppression of HMG-CoA reductase more on a posttranscriptional process (Parker et al., 1993).

18.3.2 Tocotrienols Stimulate the Degradation of HMG-CoA Reductase

Although tocotrienols were shown to inhibit HMG-CoA reductase at the posttranscriptional level, there are still multiple possibilities: tocotrienols may inhibit translation of HMG-CoA reductase mRNA, or stimulate the degradation of HMG-CoA reductase protein. Song et al. examined the second possibility directly. Chemically synthesized tocotrienols and tocopherols were used in their study and they found that γ- and δ-tocotrienols treatment induces HMG-CoA reductase degradation, whereas tocopherols and α- or β- forms of tocotrienols do not accelerate reductase degradation (Song and DeBose-Boyd, 2006). The degradation of HMG-CoA reductase induced by tocotrienols was blocked in the present of proteasome inhibitors. Meanwhile, tocotrienol-induced polyubiquitin chain assembly on HMG-CoA reductase could be observed in the presence of proteasome inhibitor, indicating that the degradation of HMG-CoA reductase induced by tocotrienols is through the ubiquitin-proteasome pathway (Song and DeBose-Boyd, 2006). Furthermore, the γ- and δ-tocotrienol-induced degradation of HMG-CoA reductase requires Insig-1/2 proteins and Insig–reductase interaction. These results illustrate that γ- and δ-tocotrienols stimulate reductase degradation through the Insig-dependent ubiqutin-proteasome pathway, which is also employed by 25-hydroxysterol and lanosterol in physiological conditions (Song and DeBose-Boyd, 2006).

There are two possible activators responsible for tocotrienol-stimulated ubiquitination and degradation of HMG-CoA reductase: tocotrienols themselves or intermediates of tocotrienols metabolism. An *in vitro* system was used to test whether the γ- and δ-tocotrienols directly promote HMG-CoA reductase degradation. In this system, the cell membrane fraction was isolated and used to provide the membrane proteins, including HMG-CoA reductase, Insigs and gp78. This system has been shown to support the 25-hydroxycholesterol-induced ubiquitination of reductase in the former study (Song and DeBose-Boyd, 2004). Using this system, it was found that γ- or δ-tocotrienols stimulate HMG-CoA reductase ubiquitination directly, as 25-hydroxycholesterol does (Song and

DeBose-Boyd, 2006). Taken together, the results demonstrate that γ- and δ-tocotrienols themselves rather than their metabolic products stimulate the ubiquitination of HMG-CoA reductase.

It has been known for a long time that the mevalonate-derived sterol and non-sterol products can both accelerate the degradation of HMG-CoA reductase. Sterols regulate the HMG-CoA reductase and SREBP pathway at the same time and therefore affect both the mRNA level and protein level of reductase. Nonsterol products, such as 20-carbon isoprenoid geranylgeranoil, can only regulate the degradation of reductase protein but not the mRNA level (Sever et al., 2003a). Early studies found that γ- and δ-tocotrienols affect only the degradation of HMG-CoA reductase, and their corresponding tocopherols have no effect (Sen et al., 2006). The only difference between these two kinds of vitamin E molecules is their side chains: tocotrienols with unsaturated fanesyl side chain and tocopherols with saturated phytyl side chain (Figure 18.4). As a result, it was proposed that tocotrienols accelerate HMG-CoA reductase degradation by its fanesyl side chain, mimicking the action of nonsterol isoprenoids. It is clear now that γ- and δ-tocotrienols mimic sterols, rather than nonsterol products of mevalonate metabolism, to stimulate the ubiquitination and degradation of HMG-CoA reductase. First, mevalonate-derived nonsterol products stimulate HMG-CoA reductase degradation only in the presence of sterols. Mevalonate or GG-OH alone has no effect on the stability of reductase (Sever et al., 2003a). γ- or δ-tocotrienol could stimulate the degradation of reductase by itself. Second, mevalonate can further enhance sterols or tocotrienol-induced reductase degradation (Sever et al., 2003a; Song and DeBose-Boyd, 2006). This finding suggests that tocotrienols and mevalonate are in the different pathways to influence the stability of HMG-CoA reductase. Third, mevalonate-derived isoprenoids accelerate the degradation of reductase on a post-ubiquitination step and do not affect reductase ubiquitination (Sever et al., 2003a). Contrarily, γ- and δ-tocotrienol can dramatically induce the ubiquitination of HMG-CoA reductase (Song and DeBose-Boyd, 2006).

18.3.3 Tocotrienols Have Different Capacities of Lowering Cholesterol Biosynthesis

There are four isomers of tocotrienols, namely α-, β-, δ-, and γ-tocotrienol. Although the only difference between tocotrienol isomers is the number and position of methyl groups on their chromanol ring, tocotrienol isomers have different capacities of lowering cholesterol biosynthesis.

α-tocotrienol was identified as the hypocholesterolemic compound from barley extract. As an enriched source of α-tocotrienol, palm oil extract shows cholesterol suppressive activity. However, synthetic α-tocotrienol is considerably less active than anticipated based on the activity of the palm oil extract, even taking into consideration that synthesized α-tocotrienol is a racemic mixture while natural α-tocotrienol is chiral (Pearce et al., 1992). Later studies identified that the tocotrienol-rich fraction isolated from palm oil consisted of a blend of α-tocotrienol (18%), γ-tocotrienol (27%), and δ-tocotrienol (7%) by chromatographic separation (Pearce et al., 1992). γ- and δ-tocotrienols showed more capacity for lowering cholesterol biosynthesis than the α isomer (Pearce et al., 1992; Yu et al., 2006; Song and DeBose-Boyd, 2006).

In vivo experiments supported that δ- and γ-tocotrienol have stronger hypocholesterolemic activity. Supplement of purified δ- or γ-tocotrienol in chickens' diet yielded a decrease of 32% for serum cholesterol and 66% for LDL cholesterol. That reduction is much greater than the decrease by supplementing α-tocotrinol or a mixture of different tocotrienols (Yu et al., 2006). Through the same effect, γ-tocotrienol treatment in cholesterol-fed rabbits for 6 weeks led to a 20% reduction in the lesion area, whereas α-tocotrienol treatment had no significant effect (Hasselwander et al., 2002).

These results are consistent with the early *in vitro* studies. Both α- and γ-tocotrienol lowered cholesterol biosynthesis in cultured cells (Parker et al., 1993) or isolated hepatocytes (Pearce et al., 1992), measured by the rate of [^{14}C]-acetate incorporation into cholesterol after incubation with tocotrienols. But the efficiency of α-tocotrienol was much lower compared with γ-tocotrienol. The IC_{50} of α-tocotrienol is about 40-fold higher than γ isomer (Parker et al., 1993). The suppression of HMG-CoA reductase activity was correlated with the inhibition of cholesterol biosynthesis between different tocotrienols. α-tocotrienol induced a marginal decrease of HMG-CoA reductase activity, and a lower inhibition of cholesterol biosynthesis, meanwhile γ-tocotrienol inhibited HMG-CoA reductase activity dramatically and blocked most of the cholesterol biosynthesis (Pearce et al., 1992).

Although both γ- and δ-tocotrienol could stimulate the degradation of HMG-CoA reductase, they bear different regulatory activities for SREBP processing. When incubated with cells, δ-tocotrienol works on both sterol regulation pathways; it inhibits SREBP cleavage as well as promotes reductase degradation. γ-tocotrienol affects only HMG-CoA reductase degradation, but does not block SREBP-2 processing (Song and DeBose-Boyd, 2006). Because most of the enzymes involved in cholesterol biosynthesis are SREBP-2 targets (Eberle et al., 2004), blocking SREBP-2 cleavage provides another way for lowering cholesterol biosynthesis.

Apart from the known tocopherols and tocotrienols, two novel tocotrienols, desmethyl tocotrienol and didesmethy tocotrienol, were isolated from rice bran (Qureshi, Mo et al., 2000). The new tocotrienol members showed much more potent hypocholesterolemic capacity than tocotrienols on cell and animal levels (Qureshi, Mo et al., 2000; Qureshi, Sami et al., 2001c; Qureshi, Salser et al., 2001d). The molecular mechanisms of these novel tocotrienols are still unknown and it will be interesting to determine whether these two molecules function through similar pathways.

18.3.4 Structure-Activity Relationships of Tocotrienols

Naturally occurring vitamin E isomers are all chiral molecules possessing the (2R), 3'-trans, 7'-trans configuration and labeled as d-tocopherols or d-tocotrienols. Meanwhile, vitamin E synthesized through chemical reactions are all racemic, labeled as dl-tocopherols or dl-tocotrienols. Although chemically synthesized tocotrienols consist of both normal and their mirror-reflected compounds; no distinct difference was observed in their effect on inhibition of cholesterol biosynthesis compared with natural tocotrienols (Pearce et al., 1992). Therefore, it is likely that the chiral configurations are not the key determinants for their hypocholesterolemic effects.

In contrast with γ- and δ-tocotrienol, none of the four tocopherols stimulates reductase degradation or blocks SREBP cleavage. It is implied that the isoprenoid-like unsaturated farnesyl side chain of tocotrienols is necessary for regulation of both pathways. From another aspect, Pearce et al. compared tocotrienols with the analogues of tocotrienols bearing a short, geranyl-like side chain, and they found the analogues have lower activities in decreasing cholesterol biosynthesis (Pearce et al., 1992). These findings indicate that unsaturated bonds on the farnesyl side chain of tocotrienols are a crucial determinant of their activity on hypocholsterolemia, and the length of the side chain determines the strength of the activity.

All four tocotrienols have unsaturated side chains, but α- and β- tocotrienol contain a methyl substitution in the R2 position of their chromanol ring (Figure 18.4), which abolishes the regulatory activity on reductase degradation and SREBP cleavage. It implies that the methyl substitution in the R2 position blocks the hypocholesterolemic activity of tocotrienols, even though the unsaturated bonds are still present (Song and DeBose-Boyd, 2006).

Both γ- and δ-tocotrienol can lower cholesterol biosynthesis, but the exact mechanisms are not completely the same. γ-tocotrienol stimulates HMG-CoA reductase degradation, but does not efficiently block SREBP-2 processing. On the other hand, δ-tocotrienol regulates both HMG-CoA reductase and SREBP. The difference between these two forms of Vitamin E is the R1 position of their chromanol ring. γ-tocotrienol bears a methyl group substitution in the position and δ-tocotrienol has a hydrogen in the same position. This indicates the substitution in the R1 position of the chromanol ring appears to add an additional level of specificity to the action of tocotrienols. But the mechanism responsible for the specificity of δ- or γ- tocotrienols still needs further study (Song and DeBose-Boyd, 2006).

There are many similarities between two major feedback pathways of cholesterol biosynthesis: the ER retention of SCAP-SREBP and the degradation of HMG-CoA reductase. Insig is involved in both processes and sterols stimulate the binding of Insig to the sterol sensing domain of SCAP or reductase. In fact, SCAP and reductase share a similar topology. Each protein can be divided into two domains: a hydrophobic amino-terminal domain containing eight membrane-spanning helices to anchor the proteins to ER membranes; and a large hydrophilic carboxyl-terminal domain projecting into the cytosol. The carboxyl-terminal domain of reductase exerts the catalytic activity of enzyme, whereas the carboxyl-terminal domain of SCAP mediates association with SREBP. Sterol sensing domains comprise 2–6 transmembrane helices of SCAP or reductase and are responsible for sterol-induced binding to Insig. Mutations within the sterol-sensing domain of SCAP or reductase prevent the interaction with Insig, thereby abolishing sterol-regulated ER retention of SCAP-SREBP and degradation of reductase. Although in both cases sterol stimulates the binding between Insig and sterol sensing domain contained protein, some differences exist in these two pathways. The fates of SSD-containing proteins after binding to Insig are entirely different. Once binding to Insig, SCAP-SREBP is retained in ER, whereas binding to Insig will render HMG-CoA reductase to be ubiquitinated and degraded. Another major difference between SREBP cleavage and HMG-CoA reductase degradation is the regulator specificity for these two pathways. Lanosterol and γ-tocotrienol can stimulate the degradation of HMG-CoA reductase without triggering SREBP cleavage. Cholesterol shows no effect on HMG-CoA reductase stability when inducing SREBP cleavage. 25-hydroxycholesterol and δ-tocotrienol are active in both processes.

Tocotrienols may bind to an accessory protein to bring about the effects on HMG-CoA reductase degradation and SREBP cleavage. Considering the mechanism for the action of 25-hydroxycholsterol on SCAP, tocotrienols may directly bind the sterol-sensing domains of HMG-CoA reductase and SCAP. Conformational changes of these SSD-containing proteins further allow Insig binding, then degradation or ER retention is facilitated. The different effects of γ- and δ-tocotrienol may reflect the difference in binding pockets between these SSDs: binding pockets in reductase may be larger than the corresponding region in SCAP so that the R1 methyl group of γ-tocotrienol can be incorporated only on reductase. The hypothesis is consistent with the situation of cholesterol and lanosterol. With three more methyl groups on its chroman ring than cholesterol, lanosterol has no effect on SREBP cleavage while cholesterol has.

18.4 CONCLUSIONS

Besides antioxidation, tocotrienols have some additional beneficial therapeutic properties over tocopherols. γ- and δ-tocotrienols can induce the ubiquitination and degradation of HMG-CoA reductase, the rate-limited enzyme on cholesterol biosynthesis, and this process is mediated through an Insig-dependent pathway. Tocotrienol-mediated down-regulation of HMG-CoA reductase lowers *de novo* cholesterol biosynthesis. Tocotrienols manifest an intrinsic hypocholesterolemic activity when administered in the diet to animals, including humans. γ- and δ-isomers are more potent than the other two tocotrienol isomers. The relationship between tocotrienols and the regulation of cholesterol biosynthesis may be beneficial for the development of hypocholesterolemic therapies.

REFERENCES

Adams, C. M., J. L. Goldstein and M. S. Brown. 2003. Cholesterol-induced conformational change in SCAP enhanced by Insig proteins and mimicked by cationic amphiphiles. *Proc. Natl. Acad. Sci. USA*, 100, 10647–10652.

Adams, C. M., J. Reitz, J. K. De Brabander, J. D. Feramisco, L. Li, M. S. Brown and J. L. Goldstein. 2004. Cholesterol and 25-hydroxycholesterol inhibit activation of SREBPs by different mechanisms, both involving SCAP and Insigs. *J. Biol. Chem.*, 279, 52772–52780.

Baliarsingh, S., Z. H. Beg and J. Ahmad. 2005. The therapeutic impacts of tocotrienols in type 2 diabetic patients with hyperlipidemia. *Atherosclerosis*, 182, 367–374.

Black, T. M., P. Wang, N. Maeda and R. A. Coleman. 2000. Palm tocotrienols protect ApoE +/– mice from diet-induced atheroma formation. *J. Nutr.*, 130, 2420–2426.

Brown, M. S. and J. L. Goldstein. 1997. The SREBP pathway: Regulation of cholesterol metabolism by proteolysis of a membrane-bound transcription factor. *Cell,* 89, 331–340.

Brown, A. J., L. Sun, J. D. Feramisco, M. S. Brown and J. L. Goldstein. 2002. Cholesterol addition to ER membranes alters conformation of SCAP, the SREBP escort protein that regulates cholesterol metabolism. *Mol. Cell,* 10, 237–245.

Cao, J., J. Wang, W. Qi, H. H. Miao, J. Wang, L. Ge, R. A. DeBose-Boyd, J. J. Tang, B. L. Li and B. L. Song. 2007. Ufd1 is a cofactor of gp78 and plays a key role in cholesterol metabolism by regulating the stability of HMG-CoA reductase. *Cell Metab.,* 6, 115–128.

Chen, C. W. and H. H. Cheng. 2006. A rice bran oil diet increases LDL–receptor and HMG–CoA reductase mRNA expressions and insulin sensitivity in rats with streptozotocin/nicotinamide-induced type 2 diabetes. *J. Nutr.,* 136, 1472–1476.

Collins, R., J. Armitage, S. Parish, P. Sleight and R. Peto. 2002. MRC/BHF Heart Protection Study of cholesterol lowering with simvastatin in 20536 high-risk individuals: A randomised placebo-controlled trial. *Lancet*, 360, 7–22.

Duncan, E. A., U. P. Dave, J. Sakai, J. L. Goldstein and M. S. Brown. 1998. Second-site cleavage in sterol regulatory element-binding protein occurs at transmembrane junction as determined by cysteine panning. *J. Biol. Chem.,* 273, 17801–17809.

Eberle, D., B. Hegarty, P. Bossard, P. Ferre and F. Foufelle. 2004. SREBP transcription factors: Master regulators of lipid homeostasis. *Biochimie*, 86, 839–848.

Engelking, L. J., G. Liang, R. E. Hammer, K. Takaishi, H. Kuriyama, B. M. Evers, W. P. Li, J. D. Horton, J. L. Goldstein, M. S. Brown. 2005. Schoenheimer effect explained–feedback regulation of cholesterol synthesis in mice mediated by Insig proteins. *J. Clin. Invest.*, 115, 2489–2498.

Espenshade, P. J., W. P. Li and D. Yabe. 2002. Sterols block binding of COPII proteins to SCAP, thereby controlling SCAP sorting in ER. *Proc. Natl. Acad. Sci. USA*, 99, 11694–11699.

Espenshade, P. J. and A. L. Hughes. 2007. Regulation of sterol synthesis in eukaryotes. *Annu. Rev. Genet.*, 41, 401–427.

Fairus, S., R. M. Nor, H. M. Cheng and K. Sundram. 2006. Postprandial metabolic fate of tocotrienol-rich vitamin E differs significantly from that of α-tocopherol. *Am. J. Clin. Nutr.*, 84, 835–842.

Feramisco, J. D., A. Radhakrishnan, Y. Ikeda, J. Reitz, M. S. Brown and J. L. Goldstein. 2005. Intramembrane aspartic acid in SCAP protein governs cholesterol-induced conformational change. *Proc. Natl. Acad. Sci. USA*, 102, 3242–3247.

Gaylor, J. L. 2002. Membrane-bound enzymes of cholesterol synthesis from lanosterol. *Biochem. Biophys. Res. Commun.*, 292, 1139–1146.

Gil, G., J. R. Faust, D. J. Chin, J. L. Goldstein and M. S. Brown. 1985. Membrane-bound domain of HMG CoA reductase is required for sterol-enhanced degradation of the enzyme. *Cell*, 41, 249–258.

Glass, C. K. and J. L. Witztum. 2001. Atherosclerosis: The road ahead. *Cell*, 104, 503–516.

Goldstein, J. L. and M. S. Brown. 1990. Regulation of the mevalonate pathway. *Nature*, 343, 425–430.

Goldstein, J. L., R. B. Rawson and M. S. Brown. 2002. Mutant mammalian cells as tools to delineate the sterol regulatory element-binding protein pathway for feedback regulation of lipid synthesis. *Arch. Biochem. Biophys.*, 397, 139–148.

Goldstein, J. L., R. A. DeBose-Boyd and M. S. Brown. 2006. Protein sensors for membrane sterols. *Cell*, 124, 35–46.

Gould, A. L., J. E. Rossouw, N. C. Santanello, J. F. Heyse and C. D. Furberg. 1998. Cholesterol reduction yields clinical benefit: impact of statin trials. *Circulation*, 97, 946–952.

Grunler, J., J. Ericsson and G. Dallner. 1994. Branch-point reactions in the biosynthesis of cholesterol, dolichol, ubiquinone and prenylated proteins. *Biochim. Biophys. Acta*, 1212, 259–277.

Hasselwander, O., K. Kramer, P. P. Hoppe, U. Oberfrank, K. Baldenius, H. Schroder, W. Kaufmann, R. Bahnemann and B. Nowakowsky. 2002. Effects of feeding various tocotrienol sources on plasma lipids and aortic atherosclerotic lesions in cholesterol–fed rabbits. *Food Res. Int.*, 35, 245–251.

Hershko, A., A. Ciechanover and A. Varshavsky. 2000. Basic Medical Research Award. The ubiquitin system. *Nat. Med.*, 6, 1073–1081.

Iqbal, J., M. Minhajuddin and Z. H. Beg. 2003. Suppression of 7,12–dimethylbenz[α]anthracene-induced carcinogenesis and hypercholesterolaemia in rats by tocotrienol–rich fraction isolated from rice bran oil. *Eur. J. Cancer Prev.*, 12, 447–453.

Janowski, B. A., P. J. Willy, T. R. Devi, J. R. Falck and D. J. Mangelsdorf. 1996. An oxysterol signalling pathway mediated by the nuclear receptor LXR α. *Nature*, 383, 728–731.

Khor, H. T. and D. Y. Chieng. 1996. Effect of dietary supplementation of tocotrienols and tocopherols on serum lipids in the hamster. *Nutr. Res.*, 16, 1393–1401.

Kita, T., M. S. Brown and J. L. Goldstein. 1980. Feedback regulation of 3-hydroxy-3-methylglutaryl coenzyme A reductase in livers of mice treated with mevinolin, a competitive inhibitor of the reductase. *J. Clin. Invest.*, 66, 1094–1100.

Lee, P. C., N. Sever and R. A. DeBose-Boyd. 2005. Isolation of sterol-resistant Chinese hamster ovary cells with genetic deficiencies in both Insig-1 and Insig-2. *J. Biol. Chem.*, 280, 25242–25249.

Levine, G. N., J. F. Keaney, Jr. and J. A. Vita. 1995. Cholesterol reduction in cardiovascular disease. Clinical benefits and possible mechanisms. *N. Engl. J. Med.*, 332, 512–521.

Li, W., D. Tu, A. T. Brunger and Y. Ye. 2007. A ubiquitin ligase transfers preformed polyubiquitin chains from a conjugating enzyme to a substrate. *Nature*, 446, 333–337.

Liscum, L., J. Finer–Moore, R. M. Stroud, K. L. Luskey, M. S. Brown and J. L. Goldstein. 1985. Domain structure of 3-hydroxy-3-methylglutaryl coenzyme A reductase, a glycoprotein of the endoplasmic reticulum. *J. Biol. Chem.*, 260, 522–530.

Lusis, A. J. 2000. Atherosclerosis. *Nature*, 407, 233–241.

Martirosyan, D. M., L. A. Miroshnichenko, S. N. Kulakova, A. V. Pogojeva and V. I. Zoloedov. 2007. Amaranth oil application for coronary heart disease and hypertension. *Lipids Health Dis.*, 6, 1–12.

Maxfield, F. R. and I. Tabas. 2005. Role of cholesterol and lipid organization in disease. *Nature*, 438, 612–621.

Mensink, R. P., A. C. van Houwelingen, D. Kromhout and G. Hornstra. 1999. A vitamin E concentrate rich in tocotrienols had no effect on serum lipids, lipoproteins, or platelet function in men with mildly elevated serum lipid concentrations. *Am. J. Clin. Nutr.*, 69, 213–219.

Minhajuddin, M., Z. H. Beg and J. Iqbal. 2005. Hypolipidemic and antioxidant properties of tocotrienol rich fraction isolated from rice bran oil in experimentally induced hyperlipidemic rats. *Food Chem. Toxicol.*, 43, 747–753.

Mustad, V. A., C. A. Smith, P. P. Ruey, N. K. Edens and S. J. DeMichele. 2002. Supplementation with 3 compositionally different tocotrienol supplements does not improve cardiovascular disease risk factors in men and women with hypercholesterolemia. *Am. J. Clin. Nutr.*, 76, 1237–1243.

Nohturfft, A., M. S. Brown and J. L. Goldstein. 1998. Topology of SREBP cleavage-activating protein, a polytopic membrane protein with a sterol-sensing domain. *J. Biol. Chem.*, 273, 17243–17250.

O'Byrne, D., S. Grundy, L. Packer, S. Devaraj, K. Baldenius, P. P. Hoppe, K. Kraemer, I. Jialal and M. G. Traber. 2000. Studies of LDL oxidation following α-, γ-, or δ-tocotrienyl acetate supplementation of hypercholesterolemic humans. *Free Rad. Biol. Med.*, 29, 834–845.

Osborne, T. F. 2000. Sterol regulatory element-binding proteins (SREBPs): Key regulators of nutritional homeostasis and insulin action. *J. Biol. Chem.*, 275, 32379–32382.

Parker, R. A., B. C. Pearce, R. W. Clark, D. A. Gordon and J. J. Wright. 1993. Tocotrienols regulate cholesterol production in mammalian cells by post-transcriptional suppression of 3-hydroxy-3-methylglutaryl-coenzyme A reductase. *J. Biol. Chem.*, 268, 11230–11238.

Payne, A. H. and D. B. Hales. 2004. Overview of steroidogenic enzymes in the pathway from cholesterol to active steroid hormones. *Endocr. Rev.*, 25, 947–970.

Pearce, B. C., R. A. Parker, M. E. Deason, A. A. Qureshi and J. J. Wright. 1992. Hypocholesterolemic activity of synthetic and natural tocotrienols. *J. Med. Chem.*, 35, 3595–3606.

Pedersen, T. R. et al. 1994. Randomized trial of cholesterol-lowering in 4444 patients with coronary-heart-disease—the Scandinavian Simvastatin Survival Study (4S). *Lancet*, 344, 1383–1389.

Peng, Y., E. J. Schwarz, M. A. Lazar, A. Genin, N. B. Spinner and R. Taub. 1997. Cloning, human chromosomal assignment and adipose and hepatic expression of the CL-6/INSIG1 gene. *Genomics*, 43, 278–284.

Pickart, C. M. 2001. Mechanisms underlying ubiquitination. *Annu. Rev. Biochem.*, 70, 503–533.

Porter, J. A., K. E. Young and P. A. Beachy. 1996. Cholesterol modification of hedgehog signaling proteins in animal development. *Science*, 274, 255–259.

Qureshi, A. A., W. C. Burger, N. Prentice, H. R. Bird and M. L. Sunde. 1980. Regulation of lipid metabolism in chicken liver by dietary cereals. *J. Nutr.*, 110, 388–393.

Qureshi, A. A., W. C. Burger, D. M. Peterson and C. E. Elson. 1986. The structure of an inhibitor of cholesterol biosynthesis isolated from barley. *J. Biol. Chem.*, 261, 10544–10550.

Qureshi, A. A., N, Qureshi, J. J. Wright, Z. Shen, G. Kramer, A. Gapor, Y. H. Chong, G. DeWitt, A. Ong and D. M. Peterson. 1991. Lowering of serum cholesterol in hypercholesterolemic humans by tocotrienols (palmvitee). *Am. J. Clin. Nutr.*, 53, 1021S–1026S.

Qureshi, A. A., B. A. Bradlow, L. Brace, J. Manganello, D. M. Peterson, B. C. Pearce, J. J. Wright, A. Gapor and C. E. Elson. 1995. Response of hypercholesterolemic subjects to administration of tocotrienols. *Lipids*, 30, 1171–1177.

Qureshi, A. A., B. C. Pearce, R. M. Nor, A. Gapor, D. M. Peterson and C. E. Elson. 1996. Dietary α-tocopherol attenuates the impact of γ-tocotrienol on hepatic 3-hydroxy-3-methylglutaryl coenzyme A reductase activity in chickens. *J. Nutr.*, 126, 389–394.

Qureshi, A. A., B. A. Bradlow, W. A. Salser and L. D. Brace. 1997. Novel tocotrienols of rice bran modulate cardiovascular disease risk parameters of hypercholesterolemic humans. *J. Nutr. Chem.*, 8, 290–298.

Qureshi, A. A., H. Mo, L. Packer and D. M. Peterson. 2000. Isolation and identification of novel tocotrienols from rice bran with hypocholesterolemic, antioxidant and antitumor properties. *J. Agric. Food Chem.*, 48, 3130–3140.

Qureshi, A. A. and D. M. Peterson. 2001a. The combined effects of novel tocotrienols and lovastatin on lipid metabolism in chickens. *Atherosclerosis*, 156, 39–47.

Qureshi, A. A., D. M. Peterson, J. O. Hasler-Rapacz and J. Rapacz. 2001b. Novel tocotrienols of rice bran suppress cholesterogenesis in hereditary hypercholesterolemic swine. *J. Nutr.*, 131, 223–230.

Qureshi, A. A., S. A. Sami, W. A. Salser and F. A. Khan. 2001c. Synergistic effect of tocotrienol-rich fraction (TRF(25)) of rice bran and lovastatin on lipid parameters in hypercholesterolemic humans. *J. Nutr. Biochem.*, 12, 318–329.

Qureshi, A. A., W. A. Salser, R. Parmar and E. E. Emeson. 2001d. Novel tocotrienols of rice bran inhibit atherosclerotic lesions in C57BL/6 ApoE-deficient mice. *J. Nutr.*, 131, 2606–2618.

Qureshi, A. A., S. A. Sami, W. A. Salser and F. A. Khan. 2002. Dose-dependent suppression of serum cholesterol by tocotrienol-rich fraction (TRF25) of rice bran in hypercholesterolemic humans. *Atherosclerosis*, 161, 199–207.

Radhakrishnan, A., L. P. Sun, H. J. Kwon, M. S. Brown and J. L. Goldstein. 2004. Direct binding of cholesterol to the purified membrane region of SCAP: Mechanism for a sterol-sensing domain. *Mol. Cell*, 15, 259–268.

Radhakrishnan, A., Y. Ikeda, H. J. Kwon, M. S. Brown and J. L. Goldstein. 2007. Sterol-regulated transport of SREBPs from endoplasmic reticulum to Golgi: Oxysterols block transport by binding to Insig. *Proc. Natl. Acad. Sci. USA*, 104, 6511–6518.

Rasool, A. H., K. H. Yuen, K. Yusoff, A. R. Wong and A. R. Rahman. 2006. Dose dependent elevation of plasma tocotrienol levels and its effect on arterial compliance, plasma total antioxidant status and lipid profile in healthy humans supplemented with tocotrienol rich vitamin E. *J. Nutr. Sci. Vitaminol.* (Tokyo), 52, 473–478.

Rawson, R. B., D. Cheng, M. S. Brown and J. L. Goldstein. 1998. Isolation of cholesterol-requiring mutant Chinese hamster ovary cells with defects in cleavage of sterol regulatory element–binding proteins at site 1. *J. Biol. Chem.*, 273, 28261–28269.

Roitelman, J., E. H. Olender, S. Bar-Nun, W. A. Dunn, Jr. and R. D. Simoni. 1992. Immunological evidence for eight spans in the membrane domain of 3-hydroxy-3-methylglutaryl coenzyme A reductase: Implications for enzyme degradation in the endoplasmic reticulum. *J. Cell Biol.*, 117, 959–973.

Ross, R. 1999. Atherosclerosis—an inflammatory disease. N. Engl. J. Med., 340, 115–126.

Russell, D. W. 2003. The enzymes, regulation and genetics of bile acid synthesis. *Annu. Rev. Biochem.*, 72, 137–174.

Sen, C. K., S. Khanna and S. Roy. 2006. Tocotrienols: Vitamin E beyond tocopherols. *Life Sci.*, 78, 2088–2098.

Sever, N., B. L. Song, D. Yabe, J. L. Goldstein, M. S. Brown and R. A. DeBose-Boyd. 2003a. Insig-dependent ubiquitination and degradation of mammalian 3-hydroxy-3-methylglutaryl-coa reductase stimulated by sterols and geranylgeraniol. *J. Biol. Chem.*, 278, 52479–52490.

Sever, N., T. Yang, M. S. Brown, J. L. Goldstein and R. A. DeBose-Boyd. 2003b. Accelerated degradation of HMG CoA reductase mediated by binding of insig-1 to its sterol-sensing domain. *Mol. Cell*, 11, 25–33.

Song, B. L. and R. A. DeBose-Boyd. 2004. Ubiquitination of 3-hydroxy-3-methylglutaryl-CoA reductase in permeabilized cells mediated by cytosolic E1 and a putative membrane-bound ubiquitin ligase. *J. Biol. Chem.*, 279, 28798–28806.

Song, B. L., N. B. Javitt and R. A. DeBose-Boyd. 2005a. Insig-mediated degradation of HMG CoA reductase stimulated by lanosterol, an intermediate in the synthesis of cholesterol. *Cell Metab.*, 1, 179–189.

Song, B. L., N. Sever and R. A. DeBose-Boyd. 2005b. gp78, a membrane-anchored ubiquitin ligase, associates with Insig-1 and couples sterol-regulated ubiquitination to degradation of HMG CoA reductase. *Mol. Cell*, 19, 829–840.

Song, B. L. and R. A. DeBose-Boyd. 2006. Insig-dependent ubiquitination and degradation of 3-hydroxy-3-methylglutaryl coenzyme a reductase stimulated by δ- and γ-tocotrienols. *J. Biol. Chem.*, 281, 25054–25061.

Sontag, T. J. and R. S. Parker. 2002. Cytochrome P450 omega-hydroxylase pathway of tocopherol catabolism. Novel mechanism of regulation of vitamin E status. *J. Biol. Chem.*, 277, 25290–25296.

Sun, L. P., L. Li, J. L. Goldstein and M. S. Brown. 2005. Insig required for sterol-mediated inhibition of Scap/SREBP binding to COPII proteins in vitro. *J. Biol. Chem.*, 280, 26483–26490.

Tan, D. T., H. T. Khor, W. H. Low, A. Ali and A. Gapor. 1991. Effect of a palm-oil–vitamin E concentrate on the serum and lipoprotein lipids in humans. *Am. J. Clin. Nutr.*, 53, 1027S–1030S.

Traber, M. G. and H. Sies. 1996. Vitamin E in humans: Demand and delivery. *Ann. Rev. Nutr.*, 16, 321–347.

Wahlqvist, M. L., Z. Krivokucabogetic, C. S. Lo, B. Hage, R. Smith and W. Lukito. 1992. Differential serum responses of tocopherols and tocotrienols during vitamin supplementation in hypercholesterolemic individuals without change in coronary risk-factors. *Nutr. Res.*, 12, S181–S201.

Wang, L., R. K. Newman, C. W. Newman, L. L. Jackson and P. J. Hofer. 1993. Tocotrienol and fatty acid composition of barley oil and their effects on lipid metabolism. *Plant Foods Hum. Nutr.*, 9–17.

Wang, X., R. Sato, M. S. Brown, X. Hua and J. L. Goldstein. 1994. SREBP-1, a membrane-bound transcription factor released by sterol-regulated proteolysis. *Cell*, 77, 53–62.

Watkins, T., P. Lenz, A. Gapor, M. Struck, A. Tomeo and M. Bierenbaum. 1993. γ-tocotrienol as a hypocholesterolemic and antioxidant agent in rats fed atherogenic diets. *Lipids*, 28, 1113–1118.

Yabe, D., M. S. Brown and J. L. Goldstein. 2002. Insig-2, a second endoplasmic reticulum protein that binds SCAP and blocks export of sterol regulatory element-binding proteins. *Proc. Natl. Acad. Sci. USA*, 99, 12753–12758.

Yang, T., P. J. Espenshade, M. E. Wright, D. Yabe, Y. Gong, R. Aebersold, J. L. Goldstein and M. S. Brown. 2002. Crucial step in cholesterol homeostasis: Sterols promote binding of SCAP to INSIG-1, a membrane protein that facilitates retention of SREBPs in ER. *Cell*, 110, 489–500.

Yu, S. G., A. M. Thomas, A. Gapor, B. Tan, N. Qureshi and A. A. Qureshi. 2006. Dose-response impact of various tocotrienols on serum lipid parameters in 5-week-old female chickens. *Lipids*, 41, 453–461.

Zhang, F. L. and P. J. Casey. 1996. Protein prenylation: Molecular mechanisms and functional consequences. *Annu. Rev. Biochem.*, 65, 241–269.

19 Tocotrienols in Cardiometabolic Diseases

Barrie Tan and Anne M. Mueller

CONTENTS

19.1 INTRODUCTION

The commercialization of natural soy- and corn-derived tocopherols in the 1950s brought about an era of increasing popularity of alpha-tocopherol (alpha-T), making it synonymous to vitamin E. With an RDA escalating from 30 IU to more than 2,000 IU for daily supplemental use, alpha-T has far exceeded its original purpose as a vitamin for protection against fetal resorption (Evans and Bishop, 1922), for the red blood cell (Horwitt, 1960) or even as an antioxidant (Olcott and Emerson, 1937). The null effects of numerous alpha-T trials could have signaled the lack of alpha-T's benefits from large doses earlier. Disappointing as it may seem, alpha-T has most recently been proposed as a mere antioxidant and nothing more (Traber and Atkinson, 2007). Independently, recent publications on vitamin E continually expand the dossier of research marked by the benefits of tocotrienols—and especially desmethyl tocotrienols—over alpha-T. In the 1980s, tocotrienols were shown to uniquely lower endogenous synthesis of cholesterol and caught the attention of the scientific public (Qureshi et al., 1986). Since alpha-T does not have the benefits tocotrienol exhibits and has been shown to attenuate or interfere with the effects of tocotrienol (Qureshi et al., 1996), the usage and dosage of alpha-T should be reevaluated and more emphasis should be accorded to tocotrienols (Sen et al., 2007).

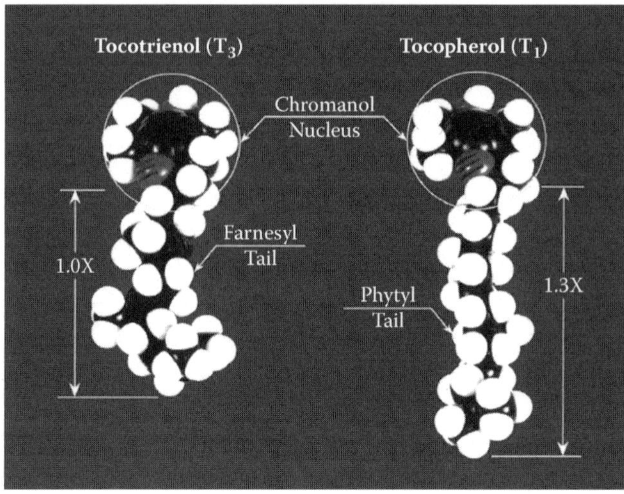

FIGURE 19.1 Structure of tocochromanol (Vitamin E) molecules.

Tocotrienol and tocopherol are chemically related compounds of vitamin E, with enough structural difference to distinguish their individual properties and functionalities (Figure 19.1). The focus of this chapter is on the cardiovascular benefits of tocotrienols, including its mechanism of action/interaction, as well as preclinical and clinical studies.

19.2 HMG COA REDUCTASE AND CHOLESTEROL SYNTHESIS PATHWAY

19.2.1 Mechanisms of Action

HMG CoA reductase (HMGR) is an important rate-limiting enzyme that is at the center of cholesterol synthesis. It is part of the lengthy pathway from which some 80% of all our body cholesterol is synthesized. Cholesterol, although often frowned upon in today's fast-food nation, is a necessary component of our bodies, giving cells their flexibility/fluidity and making biosynthesis of vitamin D, steroid hormones and bile salts possible. Other essential isoprenoids are produced via the cholesterol synthesis pathway, including ubiquinone (also known as coenzyme Q10 or CoQ10), dolichol, heme, farnesylated and geranylgeranylated groups, all of which play an important role in the synthesis of cellular proteins and energy production.

It is believed that tocotrienols (T3), which contain a unique farnesyl moiety, disphosphorates the farnesyl pyrophosphate; the thus-freed farnesol down-regulates the HMGR (Mo and Elson, 2004) (Figure 19.2). Tocotrienols also degrade the protein HMGR, a mechanism of action that was elucidated in the early 1990s (Pearce et al., 1992; Parker et al., 1993). Fifteen years later, this original study carried out by Bristol-Myers Squibb was recently revalidated, where researchers elucidate the biochemical mechanism for the hypocholesterolemic effect of tocotrienols on HMGR (Song and DeBose-Boyd, 2006). In both earlier and recent studies, only desmethyl tocotrienols (namely, delta- and gamma-isomers) had this effect on HMGR. Tocotrienol was found to act like a sterol, creating a feedback mechanism that causes a decrease of HMGR activity by increase of sterol-sensing, including inhibition of gene transcription, blocking translation of mRNA and accelerating degradation of HMGR protein. However, in the more recent study, tocotrienol's mechanism of action goes further.

Tocotrienol was found to block processing of sterol regulatory element-binding proteins (SREBPs), membrane-bound transcription factors that modulate transcription of genes encoding cholesterol biosynthetic enzymes and low-density lipoprotein (LDL) receptor. With increased sterol-sensing, the configuration of HMGR changes, which in turn promotes binding of Insig (an

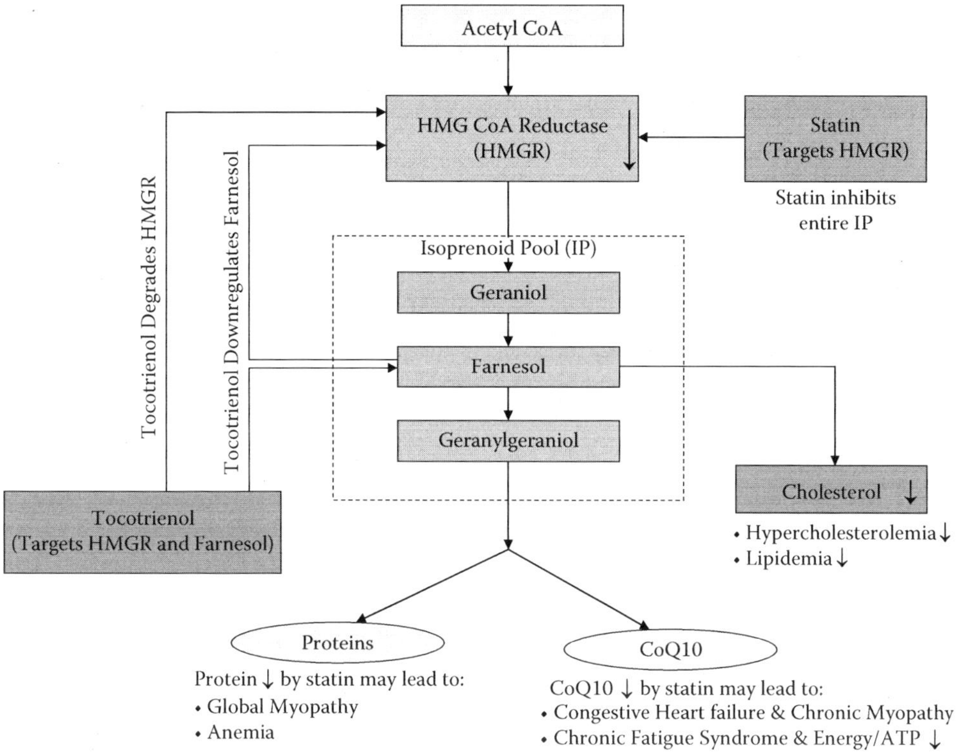

FIGURE 19.2 Tocotrienol mechanism in cholesterol synthesis pathway.

insulin-induced protein found in the endoplasmic reticulum [ER]) to the sterol-sensing domain of SREBP cleavage-activating protein (SCAP). Binding of Insig to SCAP prevents SCAP from binding SREBP and escorting the complex to the Golgi, where SREBP is proteolitically processed to generate transcription factors that activate lipid synthesis. Only gamma-T3 and delta-T3 stimulate the ubiquitination and degradation of the HMGR and delta-T3 uniquely blocks processing of sterol SREBPs (Song and DeBose-Boyd, 2006). Blocking SREBP processing may specifically reduce triglyceride synthesis with importance in prediabetic and diabetic conditions (see "Hypertriglyceridemia" section). Other forms of vitamin E (all four tocopherols and alpha-T3 and beta-T3) do not degrade, down-regulate, or block SREBP processing (Song and DeBose-Boyd, 2006).

In short, delta-T3 and gamma-T3 inhibit the *cholesterol synthesis* via down-regulation and ubiquitination of HMGR and inhibit *triglyceride synthesis* via the sterol-mimic blocking of SREBP processing.

19.2.2 Structure-Analysis, Metabolism and Bioavailability

Tocotrienol and tocopherol, the two forms of the vitamin E family, are similar in that both have the same head (chromanol nucleus), which is the site of their well-known antioxidant activities. Tocotrienol and tocopherol differ in the molecule's tail. Tocotrienol has a shorter farnesyl tail containing double bonds that down-regulate HMGR, the rate-limiting enzyme of cholesterol synthesis. Tocopherol, on the other hand, has a longer phytyl tail without double bonds. Alpha, beta, delta and gamma are among the common isomers of tocotrienol as well as tocopherol. Besides these eight common isomers, other tocopherols and tocotrienols have been identified, although their occurrence is rare (Qureshi et al., 2000; Yamamoto et al., 2001). For tocotrienol, the potency of cholesterol inhibition by these isomers is as follows: delta>gamma>>alpha>beta.

The isomers of tocotrienol differ depending on the substitution and location of methyl groups at the head region of the molecule. Desmethyl tocotrienols (tocotrienols with fewer methyl groups) are more active, especially in the absence of a methyl group at C5 position on the chromanol (Tan, 2005). Delta-T3 and gamma-T3 are the only two common isomers that fit this C5 unsubstituted molecular formula.

Delta-T3 is monomethylated at C8 position of the chromanol, making it the least substituted and therefore the most potent isomer of the four tocotrienol compounds. Gamma-T3, which is dimethylated at C8 and C7 positions of the chromanol is the second most potent isomer.

Tocopherols do not have the cholesterol-lowering ability that tocotrienols do. In fact, alpha-T has been shown to attenuate or interfere with the cholesterol-lowering action of tocotrienols (Qureshi et al., 1996). The majority of vitamin E supplements contain mostly tocopherols (and for that, mostly alpha-T) with traces of tocotrienols. Large clinical studies on alpha-T's benefits to cardiovascular health have been equivocal at best. Use of alpha-T will need to be reassessed and this question has been raised elsewhere (Sen et al., 2007; Traber and Atkinson, 2007).

Preparations effective in cholesterol lowering consist of less than 15–20% alpha-T and more than 60% gamma-T3 and delta-T3, whereas less effective or ineffective preparations consist of more than 30% alpha-T and less than 45% of gamma-T3 and delta-T3 (Qureshi et al., 1996). This has been supported by clinical studies in which tocotrienol supplements with high alpha-T content did not contribute to the lowering of cholesterol, whereas tocotrienol supplements containing low amounts of alpha-T and high amounts of gamma-T3 and delta-T3 led to a significant decrease in total and LDL cholesterol. Interestingly, alpha-T by itself has been shown to up-regulate HMGR synthesis. In addition, tocotrienols absorbed better than tocopherols and alpha-T (if present with other E vitamers) has been shown to prevent absorption of tocopherols and tocotrienols (Ikeda et al., 2003) while increasing the catabolism of tocotrienols (Sontag and Parker, 2007).

Tocotrienols, although found in low amounts in the American diet (naturally in oils and fats, whole foods and some processed foods) are most abundant in palm, rice and annatto (Tan, 2005). *Rice* contains about 50% tocotrienols (mainly alpha-T3 and gamma-T3) and 50% tocopherols (mainly alpha-T), whereas *palm* contains 75% tocotrienols (mainly alpha-T3 and gamma-T3) and 25% tocopherols (mainly alpha-T). *Annatto* contains only desmethyl tocotrienols (mainly delta-T3 and gamma-T3) and it is virtually tocopherol-free (Figure 19.3).

Tocotrienol's tail is about 30% shorter than tocopherol's tail. The longer tocopherol tail anchors deeply into lipid membranes and become less mobile, while tocotrienols anchor less deeply and have greater intra- and inter-membrane mobility, enabling them to cross from one membrane to the next (Packer et al., 2001; Yoshida et al., 2003). This may explain why tocotrienol is 40- to 60-fold more powerful as an antioxidant (free radical scavenger) than tocopherol (Serbinova et al., 1991) and 70-fold more bioavailable for cellular absorption/distribution (Saito et al., 2004). Tocotrienols also accumulate approximately 25–95-fold greater than alpha-T in human aortic endothelial cells due to higher intracellular concentration/distribution (Naito et al., 2005). Other studies have also

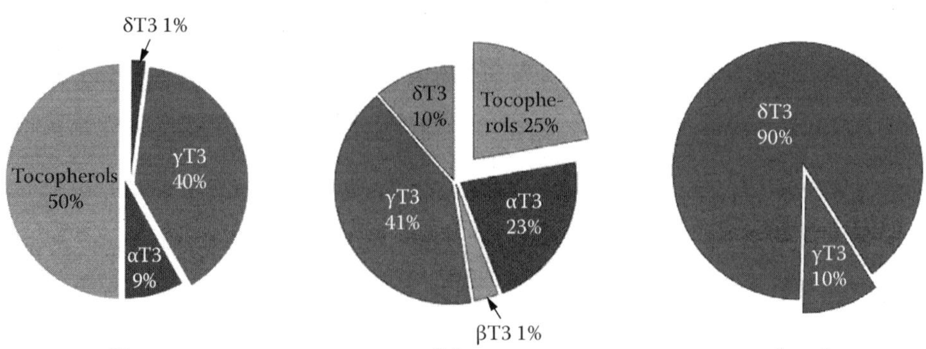

FIGURE 19.3 Tocotrienol compositions in rice bran, palm oil and annatto bean. Desmethyl tocotrienol (i.e., delta-T3 and gamma-T3) contents are annatto > palm > rice.

suggested the difference in the tail to be responsible for the difference in functionalities (Sylvester and Theriault, 2003; Yu et al., 2005). In sum, the functional characteristics of tocotrienol are dependent on the head-group chromanol substitution (e.g., desmethyl isomers) and the tail length (e.g., unsaturated, farnesylated).

Tocotrienol and tocopherol are both metabolized via side chain catabolism. This involves an initial omega-oxidation, followed by repeated cycles of beta-oxidation for the shortening of the phytyl tail to yield the water-soluble urinary carboxyethylhydroxychroman (CEHC) metabolites of the corresponding tocotrienol and tocopherol isomers (Brigelius-Flohe and Traber, 1999; Lodge et al., 2001; You et al., 2005; Sontag and Parker, 2007). However, only the desmethyl CEHCs have benefits of sodium excretion, reduction of body fluid retention and hypertension (Wechter et al., 1996; Murray et al., 1997), inhibition of prostate cancer (Galli et al., 2004) and suppression of TNF-alpha-induced activation of microglial cells (Hensley et al., 2004). This natriuretic factor was first discovered from CEHCs of desmethyl tocopherols in 1996 (Wechter et al., 1996). Since the CEHCs of desmethyl tocotrienol have just been shown to be identical to that from desmethyl tocopherols, it is summarily expected that *desmethyl* tocochromanols have natriuretic effects.

Tocotrienols and tocopherols also differ in their cellular uptake and bioavailability following intestinal absorption. Tocotrienols are mainly transported in triglyceride-rich particles (TRP) (Fairus et al., 2006), consisting of chylomicrons, chylomicron remnants and very low density lipoprotein (VLDLs). Tocopherols are mainly transported in LDL (Mardones and Rigotti, 2004). Tocotrienols have a "small window" from gut absorption to tissue deposition. In the blood, tocotrienol appears at 2 hrs, diminishes at 8 hrs and peaks at 4–6 hrs (Figure 19.4) (Yap et al., 2001; Fairus et al., 2006). Once the tocotrienol reaches the small intestine and is absorbed (1–2 hr), it will be transported by chylomicrons to the lymphatic system, where it may remain 2–4 hr. During the lymphatic passage, chylomicrons are processed into smaller particles, such as chylomicron remnants and VLDL. From the lymph, the tocotrienol-containing chylomicron is transferred to the arteries,

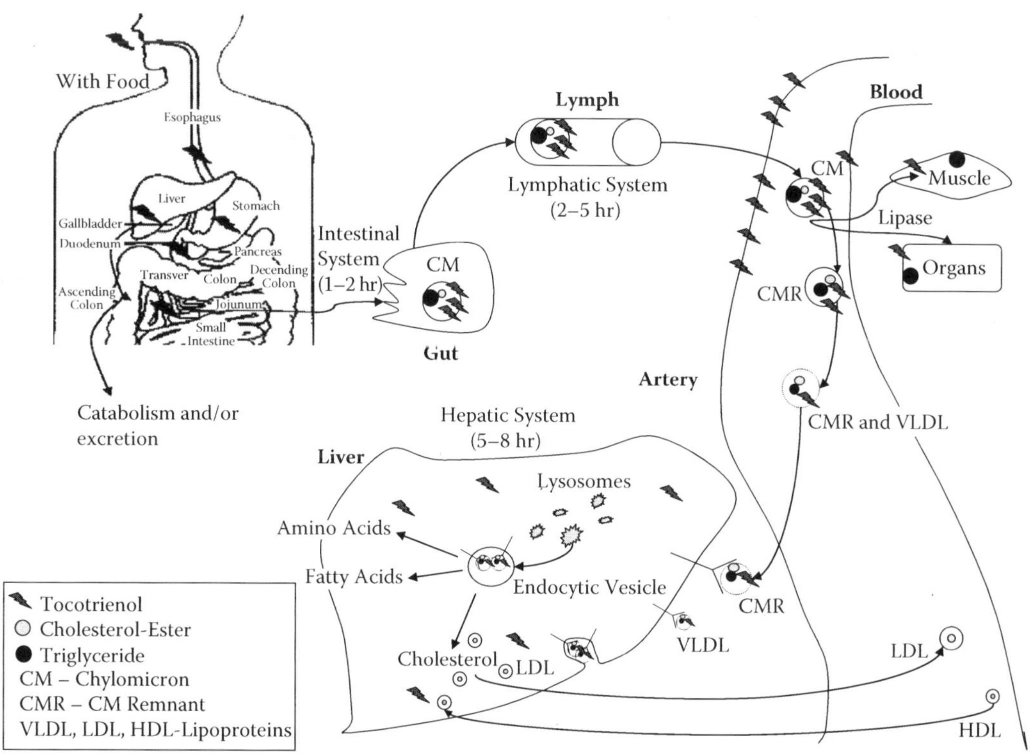

FIGURE 19.4 Absorption and disposal of tocotrienol.

where some of the tocotrienol is deposited in the artery wall during transfer (Naito et al., 2005). Along the artery, some chylomicrons are digested by lipoprotein lipase, an enzyme that mediates transfer of TG to various organs such as the muscle. During this process, tocotrienol and TG are simultaneously deposited in the various organs (Hayes et al., 1993). The remainder of the tocotrienol in blood is then transported to the liver via chylomicron remnants and VLDL, which are taken up into the liver by receptor-mediated endocytosis.

Much of the tocotrienol deposits in the liver, where it will remain 5–8 hr, while very little may be repackaged to exit the liver (Pearson and Barnes, 1970; Sontag and Parker, 2007). In the liver, tocotrienol assists in the down-regulation and degradation of HMGR, therefore reducing cholesterol and fatty acid synthesis (see earlier section). After hepatic metabolism and biodiscrimination, most of the tocotrienol will not appear in the plasma after 8 hrs, while the predominant alpha-T chaperoned by the alpha-tocopherol transport protein (ATTP) and transported by LDL, can be found in the blood (Hayes et al., 1993; Traber, 2007). In animal studies, the distribution kinetics of tocotrienol are mirrored in organ tissues such as the liver and spleen (4–8 hrs), as well as the muscle and heart (4–16 hrs) (Pearson and Barnes, 1970). The liver has the highest deposition, with the other tissues as distant second.

As opposed to tocotrienols, alpha-T is found in high concentrations in the plasma following hepatic biodiscrimination. This is mostly attributed to the ATTP, which has the greatest affinity for alpha-T, but little to no affinity for other forms of vitamin E (Traber, 2007). The function of ATTP is to facilitate secretion of alpha-T from the liver to the plasma by acquiring it from endosomes, transporting it to the plasma membrane and releasing it to uptake by lipoproteins (Horiguchi et al., 2003). High doses of alpha-T are thought to prevent excess of cytochrome P-450-mediated metabolism (Traber, 2007) and as such, high concentrations of this vitamin E form remain in plasma circulation. This in turn creates interference with other isomers of vitamin E, in particular those that exhibit cardiovascular benefits beyond alpha-T's antioxidant activity. In addition, alpha-T accelerated the degradation and catabolism of tocotrienol (Sontag and Parker, 2007).

Research has shown that alpha-T interferes with tocotrienol's ability to lower cholesterol (Qureshi et al., 1996), inhibits tocotrienol absorption (Ikeda et al., 2003), up-regulates HMGR (Qureshi et al., 1996) and up-regulates human Supernatant Protein Factor (SPF) (Stocker, 2004)—cholesterol biosynthesis increases when HMGR and SPF are up-regulated.

In sum, tocotrienol delivery occurs in two phases. First, it is delivered to various organs (lymphatic processing) during the postprandial stage (1–5 hr). Second, after liver uptake and catabolism, it is delivered to various organs (hepatic packaging) during the fasting stage (8–12 hr). Third, tocotrienol that remains in the liver reduces the synthesis of cholesterol and fatty acids/triglycerides. Fourth, an undetermined amount of tocotrienol is metabolized or excreted (Traber and Kayden, 1989; Schultz et al., 1995; Sontag and Parker, 2007). Future pharmacokinetic and bioavailability studies will help clarify tocotrienol disposal in the body.

19.2.3 Drug Interactions and Influence on Cholesterol Synthesis Pathway

Prescription drugs such as the widely used statins for hyperlipidemia and bisphosphonates for osteoporosis have a direct impact on the cholesterol synthesis pathway. Statins act as competitive inhibitors on HMGR, therefore preventing not only biosynthesis of cholesterol, but also many other essential isoprenoids and proteins, resulting in side effects (Figure 19.5) (Blanco-Colio et al., 2002; Johnson et al., 2004). In effect, statins are *indiscriminate* cholesterol reducers, affecting downstream products, especially isoprenoids. For example, failure to produce CoQ10 may lead to lower energy levels and decreased ATP synthesis and may eventually result in chronic fatigue syndrome. Lack of CoQ10 is also linked to increased incidence of congestive heart failure and chronic myopathy (Hargreaves et al., 2005). Statins also prevent isoprenylation (farnesylation and geranylgeranylation) of proteins necessary for the production of hemes, dolichols and other important proteins, which may lead to non-iron-induced anemia, cell signal/nerve damage and skeletal/global myopathy (Johnson et al., 2004).

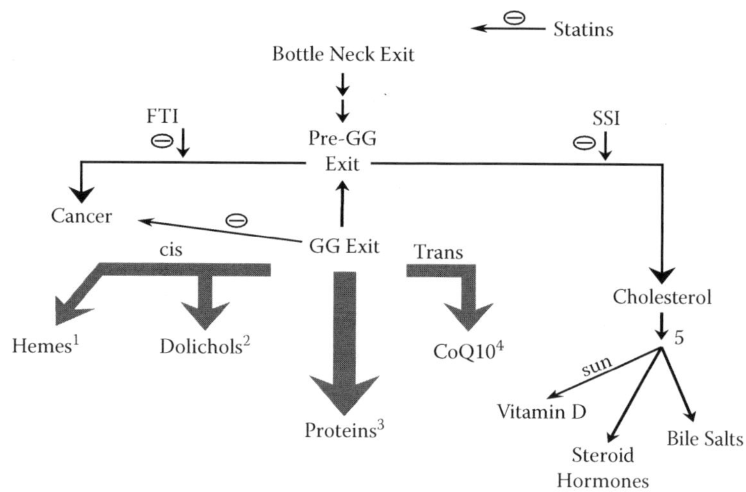

[1]Non iron induced anemia
[2]Cell signal/nerve damage
[3]Skeletal & global myopathy and rhabdomyolysis
[4]Cardiomyopathy, congestive heart failure, and CFS
[5]Cholesterol-derived metabolites

FIGURE 19.5 Drug interactions with cholesterol synthesis pathway.

As opposed to the competitive HMGR inhibitor statin, tocotrienol is a *discriminate* cholesterol reducer. Figure 19.2 identifies the critical junctures in the HMGR pathways where the role of cholesterol reduction by statins is indiscriminate and that by tocotrienol is discriminate. Most of the side effects of statins can be traced to the systemic decimation of the isoprenoid pool products, only one of which is the desired cholesterol reduction. Specific downstream isoprenoid-derived products and potential clinical symptoms have been identified (Figure 19.5).

Like statins, bisphosphonates used for the treatment of post-menopausal osteoporosis interfere with the HMGR pathway. Nitrogenous bisphosphonates act on bone metabolism by binding and blocking farnesyl diphosphate synthase (van Beek et al., 2003), an intermediate enzyme in the HMGR pathway. This prevents formation of the farnesol and geranylgeraniol isoprenoids essential for protein prenylation and sub-cellular protein trafficking (van Beek et al., 1999). The inhibition of geranylgeranylated-protein prevents bone loss, the molecular basis of this bisphosphonate class of drugs. Therefore, the side effects of this drug may be similar to that of the statin drugs.

19.3 CARDIOVASCULAR AND CARDIOMETABOLIC BENEFITS OF TOCOTRIENOL

19.3.1 Overview of Benefits

19.3.1.1 Hypercholesterolemia

Animal studies supported results found in earlier cell line studies. Animals whose diet was supplemented with gamma-T3 and delta-T3 showed the greatest decrease in cholesterol levels (32% total and 66% LDL cholesterol), whereas alpha-T had no effect on cholesterol-lowering (Yu et al., 2006). In this study, HDL/LDL cholesterol ratios were improved by 123–150%. The safe dose of various tocotrienols for human consumption is estimated to be 1,000 mg/day.

In humans, two open studies measured fasting blood lipids before and after 2 months of 75mg annatto tocotrienol (approximately 67mg delta-T3 and 8mg gamma-T3) via daily supplementation. In both groups, total cholesterol levels dropped 13%, whereas LDL cholesterol dropped 9–15% and

HDL cholesterol increased by 4–7%. The LDL/HDL ratio was reduced by 12–21% (Tan, 2005). Among others, a study conducted by Bristol-Myers Squibb found that after 4-weeks' supplementation with gamma-T3 and delta-T3 (100mg/day), total cholesterol was reduced by 15–22% and LDL cholesterol was decreased by 10–20%. The delta-T3 group had 10–15% better lipid control than the gamma-T3 group (Qureshi and Qureshi, 1993).

19.3.1.2 Hypertriglyceridemia

An estimated 16% of U.S. residents, some 47 million, have metabolic syndrome (American Heart Association, 2006). Some of the defining hallmarks of metabolic syndrome include increased waist circumference (apple-shaped), increased serum triglyceride levels, elevated blood pressure (hypertension), elevated serum glucose (prediabetes) and insulin resistance. Tocotrienols, especially gamma-T3 and delta-T3, increase vascular and cardiometabolic integrity and lead to improved management of metabolic syndrome.

Studies on rats in which diabetes was induced showed a significant decrease of cardiometabolic events. Increase of serum-advanced glycosylation end-products (AGE) was prevented, while a decrease in blood glucose and glycated hemoglobin were observed (Wan Nazaimoon and Khalid, 2002). In addition, rice bran oil containing tocotrienols lowered plasma triglyceride levels, LDL cholesterol and hepatic triglyceride concentration, therefore suppressing hyperlipidemic and hyperinsulinemic responses in diabetic rats (Chen and Cheng, 2006).

In several clinical studies with metabolic syndrome patients or patients with diabetes, even small amounts of tocotrienol derived from rice bran were shown to reduce the symptoms associated with the disease. Rice bran water solubles reduced hyperglycemia, glycosylated hemoglobin and increased insulin levels, while rice bran fiber reduced hyperlipidemia in both type 1 and type 2 diabetics (Qureshi et al., 2002). In another large clinical study, vitamin E intake from diet was associated with reduced risk of type 2 diabetes (Montonen et al., 2004). In patients with type 2 diabetes, progression of atherosclerosis is more rapid and two out of three patients die of atherosclerotic events (American Diabetes Association, 2007). In addition, LDL-lowering therapies prescribed for patients with diabetes (who are already on diabetes medications) have higher side-effect risks, creating a need for alternative treatment. Tocotrienols, which have no known side effects, were shown to decrease serum total lipids by 23%, total cholesterol by 30% and LDL cholesterol by 42% (from 179mg/dL to 104mg/dL) within 60 days in type 2 diabetics (Baliarsingh et al., 2005).

Tocotrienols may have uses in treating diabetes, especially in patients with hypertriglyceridemia. This underscores the mechanism proposed, where delta-T3 uniquely blocks SREBP processing (Song and DeBose-Boyd, 2006). This was previously overlooked because of tocotrienol's role in hypercholesterolemia.

19.3.1.3 Atherosclerosis

Atherosclerosis develops perhaps haphazardly dependent on a variety of pathologies working in concert or directed by one or more dominant factors. Among the known atherosclerosis factors are accumulation of cholesterol in arterial walls, release of chemotaxis factors/cytokines, injury and chronic inflammation, altered lipoprotein metabolism, proliferation of smooth muscle cells, migration of monocytes and macrophages and, in some cases, bacterial involvement (see Chapter 25 in this book). An early step of atherogenesis is fatty streak formation in the arteries, which begins with the adherence of circulating monocytes tethering onto the endothelium. Tocotrienols have been shown to reduce cellular adhesion molecule expression and monocytic cell adherence (Theriault et al., 2002). In particular, delta-T3 showed the most profound inhibitory effect on monocytic cell adherence as compared with tocopherols and other tocotrienol isomers (Chao et al., 2002). This is an exceptional finding because delta-T3 was 60–90-fold more potent than the other tocotrienols. The potency of tocotrienols in descending order is delta-T3>gamma-T3>>alpha-T3>beta-T3. It has

TABLE 19.1
Inhibit Atherosclerotic Lesions

Diets (Months)	Alpha-T (0% DMT3*)	71% DMT3	100% DMT3
High Fat (4.5)	19%	28%	33%
High Fat (6)	23%	36%	57%
Low Fat (3.5)	11%	42%	47%

* Desmethyl tocotrienols (gamma- and delta-tocotrienol)
Source: Black, et al., 2000. Qureshi, et al., 2001.

been suggested that this phenomenon occurs via inhibition of vascular cell adhesion molecule, VCAM-1 expression by delta-T3 (Naito et al., 2005).

A later step in atherogenesis is the formation of unstable plaques, which occurs when platelets aggregate at the plaque site of blood vessel walls to seal tears and cuts and to repair the damaged plaque, forming clots and inadvertently blocking the blood flow through arteries. In a human double-blind crossover study, delta-T3 was shown to be significantly more potent in the inhibition of platelet aggregation than the other tocotrienol isomers, giving an overall inhibition of 71%, as compared with 5–37% with other tocotrienols (Holub, 1989).

The effects of tocotrienols on atheroma formation have also been compared in animals. Mice fed an atherogenic diet and given desmethyl tocotrienols had 60% lower plasma cholesterol than the control group on the same diet without supplementation; the size of atherosclerotic lesions was reduced 10-fold. Alpha-T, on the other hand, had no effect (Black et al., 2000). This finding was further corroborated in a similar independent study, where desmethyl tocotrienols inhibited atherosclerotic lesions in hyperlipidemic mice. Atherosclerotic lesion size in mice supplemented with desmethyl tocotrienols was decreased by 57% if mice were on a high-fat diet and 47% if mice were on a low-fat diet, whereas with alpha-T, lesion size was decreased to a lesser extent, by 23% on the high-fat and 11% on the low-fat diet (Table 19.1) (Qureshi et al., 2001). Similarly, following supplementation with palm-derived tocotrienols, the size of atherosclerotic lesions in mice fed an atherogenic diet was dramatically 92–98% smaller than in the control groups. Decrease in lesion size with alpha-T supplementation was insignificant (Black et al., 2000). In the same study, the control group had large lakes of lipid accumulation with clefts due to cholesterol crystals in liver histology, while the tocotrienol-supplemented group showed normal histology.

It has been shown that crystalline cholesterol (as part of the plaque composition) expands, protrudes and pierces the membrane wall, providing a physical mechanism by which the lipid crystals themselves may cause mechanical plaque rupture (Abela and Aziz, 2005; Abela and Aziz, 2006). The idea that tocotrienol decreases the occurrence of cholesterol clefts and crystals is a novel hypothesis and may be responsible for the prevention of atherosclerotic plaque rupture.

A 4-year study on patients with carotid artery arteriosclerosis, the blocking of the artery supplying oxygen to the brain, showed that tocotrienol supplementation caused regression of carotid atherosclerosis. In 88% of patients who took the supplement, carotid artery stenosis was regressed or stabilized. Of the control group receiving a placebo, 60% deteriorated and only 8% improved (Tomeo et al., 1995; Kooyenga et al., 2001). Interestingly, total cholesterol decreased 14% and LDL cholesterol fell 21% in the third and fourth year of the study (Watkins et al., 1999).

19.3.1.4 Lipid Peroxidation

Antioxidants play an important role in slowing the process of atherosclerosis, especially by preventing oxidation of LDL. Vitamin E is widely known for its antioxidant properties. The antioxidant efficiency of tocotrienols was evaluated as the ability of the compounds to inhibit lipid peroxidation, reactive oxygen species (ROS) production and heat shock protein expression. Delta-tocotrienol was found to have the most potent antioxidant properties among the tocotrienol isomers (Palozza et al., 2006), which in part is due to the decreased methylation on the chromanol ring that allows the molecule to be more easily incorporated into cell membranes (Tan, 2005). A comparative *in vitro* study showed that gamma-T3 and delta-T3 was fourfold more efficient as a scavenger of peroxyl radicals than other tocotrienol isomers. Tocopherols were relatively less efficient than tocotrienols, especially in complex systems (Qureshi et al., 2000). Therefore, the superior antioxidant properties of tocotrienols, especially the gamma- and delta-isomers, may contribute to cardiovascular benefits by inhibiting lipid oxidation in cell membranes that influence the progress of atherosclerosis or hypertension. A recent randomized, double-blind placebo-controlled trial showed that tocotrienol prevented ROS damage to DNA in older adults. Participants used 118 mg/day of tocotrienols (and 42 mg alpha-T) for 6 months. Of the 118mg tocotrienols, approximately 80 mg/day consumed were gamma-T3 and delta-T3 (Chin et al., 2007).

19.3.1.5 Hypertension

In our general circulation, red blood cells (RBCs) travel 30,000 miles of arteries to deliver oxygen and nutrients to all organs and extremities. The 75 trillion cells depend on the oxygen and nutrients that RBCs carry, as well as on the integrity of the arterial network that permits such delivery.

RBCs and arteries are subjected to great and unrelenting pressure. The heart beats 100,000 times per day in order to deliver 1.5 gallons (about 5.5–6.0 L) of blood through the body. This blood pressure remains constant so that the RBCs can deliver their goods, provided that the integrity of the artery is maintained.

Arterial integrity is a systemic requirement of general circulation. This integrity depends on active modulations of the endothelial surface (e.g., nitric oxide, adhesion molecules, oxidative events, inflammatory proteins) and lipid processing (e.g., postprandial triglyceride-rich particles, various lipoproteins).

Hypertension, elevated blood pressure, can cause damage to arterial walls and loss of arterial integrity, making them more susceptible to plaque formation. In recent animal studies tocotrienols were shown to lower blood pressure. When hypertensive rats were treated with gamma-T3 for 3 months, plasma and blood vessel lipid peroxides were reduced and total antioxidant status was improved (Newaz and Nawal, 1999). Gamma-T3 was shown to reduce systolic blood pressure significantly and improve nitric oxide synthase activity (NOS), both of which play a critical role in the pathogenesis of hypertension (Newaz et al., 2003). Tocotrienol's impact on hypertension was confirmed in humans, where tocotrienol-rich vitamin E supplementation resulted in significant reductions in their aortic systolic blood pressure, as well as a 9.2% improvement in total antioxidant status (Rasool et al., 2006). In addition, the natriuretic properties of desmethyl tocotrienols may also contribute to the reduction of hypertension.

19.3.2 Tocotrienols in Dyslipidemia and Metabolic Syndrome (Clinical Study)

Two open clinical studies were conducted on hypercholesterolemic subjects using a tocopherol-free annatto-sourced tocotrienol containing predominantly delta-T3.

Annatto tocotrienol is composed typically of 90% delta-T3 and 10% gamma-T3, the two most active constituents of vitamin E. Two open studies (A and B) were conducted, each involving five subjects. The volunteers were given 75 mg of annatto tocotrienols in three softgels per day, to be taken with a meal. Fasting blood lipids were measured prior to supplementation and 2 months after the supplementation. Each softgel contained 25 mg of tocotrienols (typically 22.5 mg delta-T3 and 2.5 mg gamma-T3) mixed with rice bran oil to 300 mg fill-weight to assist in intestinal absorption.

TABLE 19.2
Lipid and CoQ10 profile of Hypercholesterolemic Subjects on Annatto Tocotrienols

	1	2	3	4	5
			Study A*		
TC	230(209)**	215(203)	237(208)	269(197)	243(217)
LDL	123(104)	121(104)	156(134)	175(126)	151(145)
HDL	67(70)	51(55)	44(56)	57(60)	54(52)
TG	166(96)	242(132)	218(184)	298(218)	234(206)
TG/HDL***	2.48(1.37)	4.75(2.40)	4.95(3.29)	5.23(3.63)	4.33(3.96)
			Study B*		
TC	295(267)**	226(211)	241(204)	280(246)	230(184)
LDL	175(146)	174(159)	205(209)	187(180)	175(140)
HDL	33(35)	42(40)	54(55)	75(78)	60(66)
TG	228(203)	92(100)	164(96)	180(176)	276(205)
TG/HDL***	6.91(5.80)	2.19(2.50)	3.04(1.75)	2.40(2.26)	4.60(3.11)
CoQ10	1.03(1.21)	1.09(1.34)	0.97(1.06)	1.12(1.35)	0.86(1.06)

* TC, LDL, and HDL levels are given in mg/dl and CoQ10 in μg/ml.
** Levels before (after) two-month supplementation of 75mg tocotrienols/day.
*** TG/HDL ratios calculated from data.

The 75 mg tocotrienol/day dosage was chosen based on an earlier dose-dependent human study that approximated the optimal range to be 50–100 mg (Qureshi et al., 2002).

19.3.2.1 Lipids

The lipid and CoQ10 profiles of hypercholesterolemic subjects on annatto tocotrienol are documented in Table 19.2. Tocotrienols lowered blood lipids in both studies. On average, total cholesterol and LDL dropped by 12–13%, triglyceride by 23%, and HDL rose by 6% at a dosage of 75 mg/day (Figure 19.6).

These results are comparable to past palm TRF (tocotrienol-rich-fractions) studies that employed a much higher dosage of 200 mg/day (Qureshi et al., 1995; Qureshi and Bradlow, 1997). TRF from palm and rice consists of alpha T, gamma-T3, alpha-T3 and small amounts of delta-T3 (Figure 19.3). Annatto tocotrienols are predominantly in the form of delta-T3. Animal and cell line studies consistently show that delta-T3 ≥ gamma-T3 > TRF > alpha-T3 for lipid reduction while alpha-T has no effect on lowering cholesterol (Pearce et al., 1992; Qureshi et al., 1996; Yu et al., 2006). It is interesting to note that, when tested in combination, only delta-T3 and gamma-T3 were synergistic in cholesterol reduction (Pearce et al., 1992). The combined effects perhaps underscore why the dosage of annatto-based tocotrienol is about half that of palm-based tocotrienol in treatment for hypercholesterolemia.

19.3.2.2 Insulin Resistance

Although simplistic, the clinical endpoint of diabetes is hyperglycemia. Hypertriglyceridemia, as part of the metabolic syndrome (MS) cluster, also characterizes diabetes and prediabetes. The idea of fatty acid–sugar connection is about 40 years old (Randle et al., 1963), but the development of the concept and clinical proofs came some two decades later, much through the efforts of Stanford's Gerald Reaven and his Syndrome X concept (Fraze et al., 1985; Swislocki et al., 1987). In

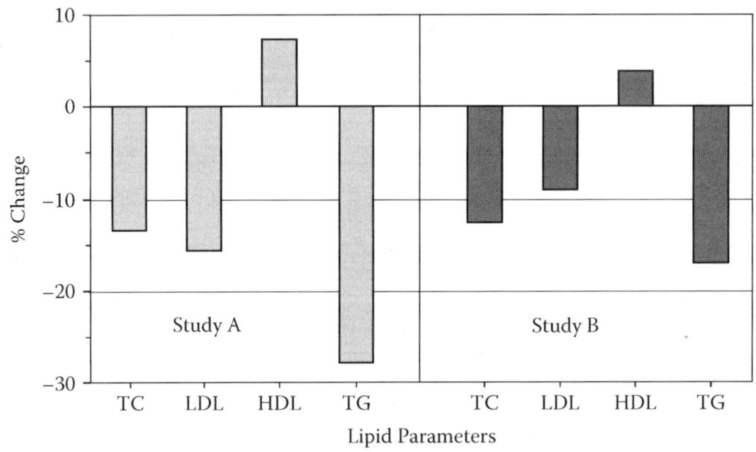

FIGURE 19.6 Effect of annatto tocotrienol on human lipid parameters.

the present understanding of diabetes, the state of hypertriglyceridemia precedes hyperglycemia (McLaughlin et al., 2003). This seemingly simple fatty acid–sugar connection means that diabetes is not just a sugar problem but it is initially a triglyceride problem (Carpentier et al., 1999). Today, some two decades after "Syndrome X" was first identified, elevated triglyceride control (with a disease named "hypertriglyceridemia") is now a drug target for the treatment of obesity and Type 2 diabetes (Boden and Shulman, 2002).

According to the U.S. government's publication of clinical identification, triglyceride and glucose are prominent markers for MS (NIH, 2001). The main indicator of MS is insulin resistance. However, the current tests for insulin measurements are unreliable because they are not standardized across clinical laboratories and measurement is not always practical since it requires a whole day's participation by the patient. Gerald Reaven, who identified Syndrome X in the 1980s and subsequently forwarded much understanding of MS, recently proposed powerful yet simple surrogate markers for MS and insulin resistance (McLaughlin et al., 2003). According to this surrogate marker criteria, a person is insulin resistant when triglyceride (TG) > 130 mg/dl and/or TG/HDL ≥ 3.0; these numbers are approximately 12–15% lower than the U.S. government's criteria (NIH, 2001).

Subjects on tocotrienols saw improvement in surrogate markers of approximately 20–30%. Based on these markers, nine of ten subjects have decreased triglyceride and TG/HDL, showing greater insulin sensitivity (Table 19.2). Decrease in triglycerides with tocopherol-free tocotrienol interventions support the idea of a mechanistic involvement of tocotrienol in blocking SREBP processing discussed earlier. The surrogate markers also suggest that two of ten subjects who were insulin resistant prior to annatto tocotrienol supplementation reversed back to being insulin sensitive after the supplementation. The annatto tocotrienols' ability in reducing cardiovascular events may be summarized by reductions in cardiovascular risk index (TC/HDL and LDL/HDL) and metabolic risk index (TG/HDL) of approximately 10–20% and 20–30%, respectively (Figure 19.7). This was a small study and the ideas proposed are tantalizing. Larger controlled studies will be needed to confirm current findings.

19.3.2.3 CoQ10

Statins are widely used for treatment of elevated cholesterol. Well-documented side effects of statin drugs are suppression of CoQ10 production (Bliznakov, 2002) and protein syntheses (Flint, Masters et al., 1997; Flint, Masters et al., 1997). Deficiency in CoQ10 may lead to congestive heart failure and chronic fatigue while reduced protein syntheses may lead to myalgia, myopathy, skeletal muscle wasting and, in extreme cases, rhabdomyolysis (Graveline, 2004; Johnson et al., 2004). Statins have

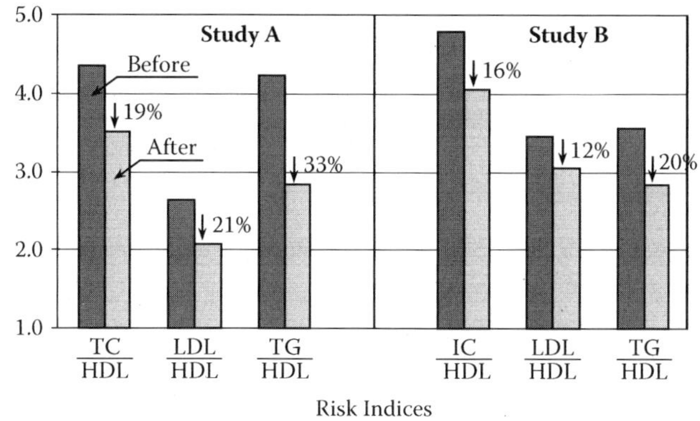

FIGURE 19.7 Annatto tocotrienol reduces cardiovascular and cardiometabolic risk index.

other major adverse reactions and readers are encouraged to consult the *Physicians' Desk Reference*, 2nd ed. or www.PDR.net, or statin drugs' fact sheet for further information.

CoQ10 and cholesterol share the same bio-pathway in the early steps of their syntheses. The question was asked if annatto tocotrienol also lowered CoQ10 while it lowered cholesterol. In Study B, subjects were given a daily dose of 75 mg of tocotrienols and the fasting CoQ10 level was measured after 2 months of supplementation. On average, the endogenous CoQ10 rose from 1.01 to 1.20 μg/ml, a 19% increase (Figure 19.8). Interestingly, this increase in plasma CoQ10 level is equivalent to an estimated 20–30 mg/day supplementation of exogenous CoQ10 (Judy, 2004). It may be possible that annatto tocotrienol extract upregulates the liver's *de novo* CoQ10 synthesis, thereby causing cell-to-blood CoQ10 rise. This is an interesting finding and further research will shed light on the tocotrienol–CoQ10 connection. It is possible that the disphosphorylation of the FPP to farnesol may avail the synthesis of GG (see Figures 19.2 and 19.4), the pathway for the synthesis of CoQ10. If the tocotrienol upregulation of endogenous biosynthesis of CoQ10 can be proven, it would be a significant finding in nutritional biochemistry and medicine, in light of the critical role that CoQ10 plays in mitochondria and in the body.

Tocotrienols may offer early protection in dyslipidemia, triglyceridemia and atherogenic inflammation that could lead to clinical outcomes of cardiovascular and diabetes-related diseases. The present open studies provide evidence that annatto tocotrienols at lower dosages (e.g., 75–100mg/day) could reduce cardiovascular and metabolic indices significantly. Tocopherol-free tocotrienol supplementation of 75 mg/day reduced TC and LDL in hypercholesterolemic subjects by 13%, TG

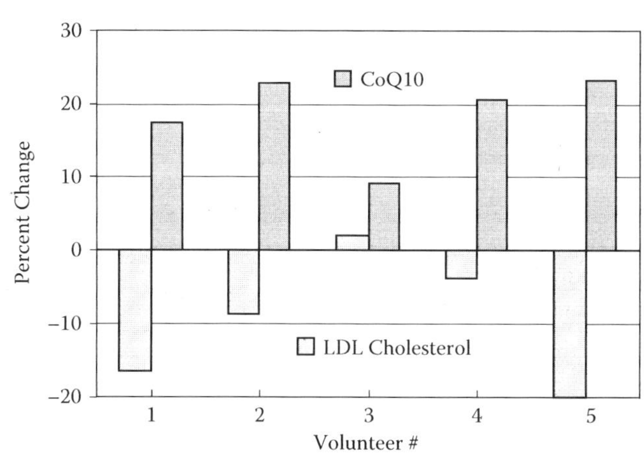

FIGURE 19.8 Annatto tocotrienol increases endogenous CoQ10 in humans.

by 23% and raised HDL by 6%. Based on the metabolic syndrome surrogate marker (TG/HDL), 20% of subjects reverted from being insulin resistant to insulin sensitive and 90% showed improved insulin sensitivity. Unlike statin drugs, tocotrienol supplementation does not lower plasma CoQ10 but increases endogenous CoQ10 by 19%. Tocotrienol supplementation is compatible and complementary with patients on statins.

19.4 CONCLUSION

Tocotrienols possess cholesterol-lowering properties that are not shared by tocopherols (Sen et al., 2006). Research also shows that high levels of alpha-T may attenuate the bioavailability and functional activity of other vitamin E isomers. Desmethyl tocotrienols such as delta-T3 and gamma-T3 were found to be much more bioactive than fully methylated tocotrienols and tocopherols. Delta-T3 and gamma-T3 are powerful heterogeneous antioxidants working at the cellular surfaces. Loss of vascular integrity and hypercoagulability (e.g. adhesion molecules↑, platelet aggregation↑, ROS↑ and NOS↓) is responsible for a plethora of cardiometabolic disorders (e.g. cholesterol↑, triglyceride↑, glucose↑) that are characteristic of prediabetes and diabetes. Delta-T3 and gamma-T3 (compositionally matched by annatto tocotrienols) improve vascular and cardiometabolic integrity, which may result in managing hypertension, diabetes, metabolic syndrome (prediabetes) and atherosclerosis.

REFERENCES

Abela, G. S. and K. Aziz. 2005. Cholesterol crystals cause mechanical damage to biological membranes: A proposed mechanism of plaque rupture and erosion leading to arterial thrombosis. *Clin Cardiol* 28(9): 413–20.

Abela, G. S. and K. Aziz. 2006. Cholesterol crystals rupture biological membranes and human plaques during acute cardiovascular events—a novel insight into plaque rupture by scanning electron microscopy. *Scanning* 28(1): 1–10.

American Diabetes Association. 2007.

American Heart Association. 2006.

Baliarsingh, S., Z. H. Beg, et al. 2005. The therapeutic impacts of tocotrienols in type 2 diabetic patients with hyperlipidemia. *Atherosclerosis* 182(2): 367–74.

Black, T. M., P. Wang, et al. 2000. Palm tocotrienols protect ApoE +/- mice from diet-induced atheroma formation. *J Nutr* 130(10): 2420–6.

Blanco-Colio, L. M., A. Villa, et al. 2002. 3-Hydroxy-3-methyl-glutaryl coenzyme A reductase inhibitors, atorvastatin and simvastatin, induce apoptosis of vascular smooth muscle cells by down-regulation of Bcl-2 expression and Rho A prenylation. *Atherosclerosis* 161(1): 17–26.

Bliznakov, E. G. 2002. Lipid-lowering drugs (statins), cholesterol and coenzyme Q10. The Baycol case—a modern Pandora's box. *Biomed Pharmacother* 56(1): 56–9.

Boden, G. and G. I. Shulman. 2002. Free fatty acids in obesity and type 2 diabetes: defining their role in the development of insulin resistance and beta-cell dysfunction. *Eur J Clin Invest* 32 Suppl 3: 14–23.

Brigelius-Flohe, R. and M. G. Traber. 1999. Vitamin E: Function and metabolism. *Faseb J* 13(10): 1145–55.

Carpentier, A., S. D. Mittelman, et al. 1999. Acute enhancement of insulin secretion by FFA in humans is lost with prolonged FFA elevation. *Am J Physiol* 276(6 Pt 1): E1055–66.

Chao, J. T., A. Gapor, et al. 2002. Inhibitory effect of delta-tocotrienol, a HMG CoA reductase inhibitor, on monocyte-endothelial cell adhesion. *J Nutr Sci Vitaminol. Tokyo)* 48(5): 332–7.

Chen, C. W. and H. H. Cheng. 2006. A rice bran oil diet increases LDL-receptor and HMG-CoA reductase mRNA expressions and insulin sensitivity in rats with streptozotocin/nicotinamide-induced type 2 diabetes. *J Nutr* 136(6): 1472–6.

Chin, S. F., N. A. Hamid, et al. 2007. Reduction of DNA damage in older healthy adults by Tri E((R)) Tocotrienol supplementation. *Nutrition.*

Evans, H. M. and K. S. Bishop. 1922. On the existence of a hitherto unrecognized dietary factor essential for reproduction. *Science* 56: 650–651.

Fairus, S., R. M. Nor, et al. 2006. Postprandial metabolic fate of tocotrienol-rich vitamin E differs significantly from that of alpha-tocopherol. *Am J Clin Nutr* 84(4): 835–42.

Flint, O. P., B. A. Masters, et al. 1997. HMG CoA reductase inhibitor-induced myotoxicity: pravastatin and lovastatin inhibit the geranylgeranylation of low-molecular-weight proteins in neonatal rat muscle cell culture. *Toxicol Appl Pharmacol* 145(1): 99–110.

Flint, O. P., B. A. Masters, et al. 1997. Inhibition of cholesterol synthesis by squalene synthase inhibitors does not induce myotoxicity in vitro. *Toxicol Appl Pharmacol* 145(1): 91–8.

Fraze, E., C. C. Donner, et al. 1985. Ambient plasma free fatty acid concentrations in noninsulin-dependent diabetes mellitus: evidence for insulin resistance. *J Clin Endocrinol Metab* 61(5): 807–11.

Galli, F., A. M. Stabile, et al, 2004. The effect of alpha- and gamma-tocopherol and their carboxyethyl hydroxychroman metabolites on prostate cancer cell proliferation. *Arch Biochem Biophys* 423(1): 97–102.

Graveline, D. 2004. *Lipitor: Theif of memory: Statin drugs side effects and the misguided war on cholesterol.* Self-published.

Hargreaves, I. P., A. J. Duncan, et al. 2005. The effect of HMG-CoA reductase inhibitors on coenzyme Q10: possible biochemical/clinical implications. *Drug Saf* 28(8): 659–76.

Hayes, K. C., A. Pronczuk, et al. 1993. Differences in the plasma transport and tissue concentrations of tocopherols and tocotrienols: Observations in humans and hamsters. *Proc Soc Exp Biol Med* 202(3): 353–9.

Hensley, K., E. J. Benaksas, et al. 2004. New perspectives on vitamin E: Gamma-tocopherol and carboxyelthylhydroxychroman metabolites in biology and medicine. *Free Radic Biol Med* 36(1): 1–15.

Holub, B. 1989. Inhibition of platelet aggregation by tocotrienols. Ontario, Canada, University of Guelph. PORIM presentation, Kuala Lumpur, Malaysia.

Horiguchi, M., M. Arita, et al. 2003. pH-dependent translocation of alpha-tocopherol transfer protein. Alpha-TTP) between hepatic cytosol and late endosomes. *Genes Cells* 8(10): 789–800.

Horwitt, M. K. 1960. Vitamin E and lipid metabolism in man. *Am J Clin Nutr* 8: 451–61.

Ikeda, S., T. Tohyama, et al. 2003. Dietary alpha-tocopherol decreases alpha-tocotrienol but not gamma-tocotrienol concentration in rats. *J Nutr* 133(2): 428–34.

Johnson, T. E., X. Zhang, et al. 2004. Statins induce apoptosis in rat and human myotube cultures by inhibiting protein geranylgeranylation but not ubiquinone. *Toxicol Appl Pharmacol* 200(3): 237–50.

Judy, W. 2004. Personal communication.

Kooyenga, D. K., T. R. Watson, et al. 2001. Antioxidants modulate the course of carotid atherosclerosis: A four-year report. *Micronutrients and Health.* K. Nesaretnam and L. Packer. Urbana, Illinois, AOCS Press 366–375.

Lodge, J. K., J. Ridlington, et al. 2001. Alpha- and gamma-tocotrienols are metabolized to carboxyethyl-hydroxychroman derivatives and excreted in human urine. *Lipids* 36(1): 43–8.

Mardones, P. and A. Rigotti. 2004. Cellular mechanisms of vitamin E uptake: relevance in alpha-tocopherol metabolism and potential implications for disease. *J Nutr Biochem* 15(5): 252–60.

McLaughlin, T., F. Abbasi, et al. 2003. Use of metabolic markers to identify overweight individuals who are insulin resistant. *Ann Intern Med* 139(10): 802–9.

Mo, H. and C. E. Elson. 2004. Studies of the isoprenoid-mediated inhibition of mevalonate synthesis applied to cancer chemotherapy and chemoprevention. *Exp Biol Med. Maywood)* 229(7): 567–85.

Montonen, J., P. Knekt, et al. 2004. Dietary antioxidant intake and risk of type 2 diabetes. *Diabetes Care* 27(2): 362–6.

Murray, E. D., Jr., W. J. Wechter, et al. 1997. Endogenous natriuretic factors 7: Biospecificity of a natriuretic gamma-tocopherol metabolite LLU-alpha. *J Pharmacol Exp Ther* 282(2): 657–62.

Naito, Y., M. Shimozawa, et al. 2005. Tocotrienols reduce 25-hydroxycholesterol-induced monocyte-endothelial cell interaction by inhibiting the surface expression of adhesion molecules. *Atherosclerosis* 180(1): 19–25.

Newaz, M. A. and N. N. Nawal. 1999. Effect of gamma-tocotrienol on blood pressure, lipid peroxidation and total antioxidant status in spontaneously hypertensive rats. SHR. *Clin Exp Hypertens* 21(8): 1297–313.

Newaz, M. A., Z. Yousefipour, et al. 2003. Nitric oxide synthase activity in blood vessels of spontaneously hypertensive rats: Antioxidant protection by gamma-tocotrienol. *J Physiol Pharmacol* 54(3): 319–27.

Olcott, H. S. and O. H. Emerson. 1937. Antioxidants and autoxidation of fats: the antioxidant properties of tocopherols. *J Amer Chem Soc* 59: 1008–1009.

Packer, L., S. U. Weber, et al. 2001. Molecular aspects of alpha-tocotrienol antioxidant action and cell signalling. *J Nutr* 131(2): 369S–73S.

Palozza, P., S. Verdecchia, et al. 2006. Comparative antioxidant activity of tocotrienols and the novel chromanyl-polyisoprenyl molecule FeAox-6 in isolated membranes and intact cells. *Mol Cell Biochem* 287(1–2): 21–32.

Parker, R. A., B. C. Pearce, et al. 1993. Tocotrienols regulate cholesterol production in mammalian cells by post-transcriptional suppression of 3-hydroxy-3-methylglutaryl-coenzyme A reductase. *J Biol Chem* 268(15): 11230–8.

Pearce, B. C., R. A. Parker, et al. 1992. Hypocholesterolemic activity of synthetic and natural tocotrienols. *J Med Chem* 35(20): 3595–606.

Pearson, C. K. and M. M. Barnes. 1970. The absorption and distribution of the naturally occurring tocochromanols in the rat. *Br J Nutr* 24(2): 581–7.

Qureshi, A. A. and B. A. Bradlow. 1997. Novel tocotrienols of rice bran modulate cardiovascular disease risk parameters of hypercholesterolemic humans. *J Nutr Biochem*(8): 290–298.

Qureshi, A. A., B. A. Bradlow, et al. 1995. Response of hypercholesterolemic subjects to administration of tocotrienols. *Lipids* 30(12): 1171–7.

Qureshi, A. A., W. C. Burger, et al. 1986. The structure of an inhibitor of cholesterol biosynthesis isolated from barley. *J Biol Chem* 261(23): 10544–50.

Qureshi, A. A., H. Mo, et al. 2000. Isolation and identification of novel tocotrienols from rice bran with hypocholesterolemic, antioxidant and antitumor properties. *J Agric Food Chem* 48(8): 3130–40.

Qureshi, A. A., B. C. Pearce, et al. 1996. Dietary alpha-tocopherol attenuates the impact of gamma-tocotrienol on hepatic 3-hydroxy-3-methylglutaryl coenzyme A reductase activity in chickens. *J Nutr* 126(2): 389–94.

Qureshi, A. A. and N. Qureshi. 1993. Tocotrienols: Novel hypocholesterolemic agents with antioxidant properties. *Vitamin E in Health and Disease*. L. Packer and J. Fuchs (Eds.). New York, Marcel Dekker, 247–267.

Qureshi, A. A., W. A. Salser, et al. 2001. Novel tocotrienols of rice bran inhibit atherosclerotic lesions in C57BL/6 ApoE-deficient mice. *J Nutr* 131(10): 2606–18.

Qureshi, A. A., S. A. Sami, et al. 2002. Effects of stabilized rice bran, its soluble and fiber fractions on blood glucose levels and serum lipid parameters in humans with diabetes mellitus types I and II. *J Nutr Biochem* 13(3): 175–187.

Qureshi, A. A., S. A. Sami, et al. 2002. Dose-dependent suppression of serum cholesterol by tocotrienol-rich fraction. TRF25) of rice bran in hypercholesterolemic humans. *Atherosclerosis* 161(1): 199–207.

Randle, P. J., P. B. Garland, et al. 1963. The glucose fatty-acid cycle. Its role in insulin sensitivity and the metabolic disturbances of diabetes mellitus. *Lancet* 1: 785–9.

Rasool, A. H., K. H. Yuen, et al. 2006. Dose dependent elevation of plasma tocotrienol levels and its effect on arterial compliance, plasma total antioxidant status and lipid profile in healthy humans supplemented with tocotrienol rich vitamin E. *J Nutr Sci Vitaminol Tokyo)* 52(6): 473–8.

Saito, Y., Y. Yoshida, et al. 2004. Characterization of cellular uptake and distribution of vitamin E. *Ann N Y Acad Sci* 1031: 368–75.

Schultz, M., M. Leist, et al. 1995. Novel urinary metabolite of alpha-tocopherol, 2,5,7,8-tetramethyl-2(2'-carboxyethyl)-6-hydroxychroman, as an indicator of an adequate vitamin E supply? *Am J Clin Nutr* 62(6 Suppl): 1527S–1534S.

Sen, C. K., S. Khanna, et al. 2007. Tocotrienols: The emerging face of natural vitamin E. *Vitam Horm* 76: 203–61.

Sen, C. K., S. Khanna, et al. 2006. Tocotrienols: Vitamin E beyond tocopherols. *Life Sci* 78(18): 2088–98.

Sen, C. K., S. Khanna, et al. 2007. Tocotrienols in health and disease: The other half of the natural vitamin E family. *Mol Aspects Med.*

Serbinova, E., V. Kagan, et al. 1991. Free radical recycling and intramembrane mobility in the antioxidant properties of alpha-tocopherol and alpha-tocotrienol. *Free Radic Biol Med* 10(5): 263–75.

Song, B. L. and R. A. DeBose–Boyd. 2006. Insig-dependent ubiquitination and degradation of 3-hydroxy-3-methylglutaryl coenzyme a reductase stimulated by delta- and gamma-tocotrienols. *J Biol Chem* 281(35): 25054–61.

Sontag, T. J. and R. S. Parker. 2007. Influence of major structural features of tocopherols and tocotrienols on their omega-oxidation by tocopherol-omega-hydroxylase. *J Lipid Res* 48(5): 1090–8.

Stocker, A. 2004. Molecular mechanisms of vitamin E transport. *Ann N Y Acad Sci* 1031: 44–59.

Swislocki, A. L., C. C. Donner, et al. 1987. Can insulin resistance exist as a primary defect in noninsulin-dependent diabetes mellitus? *J Clin Endocrinol Metab* 64(4): 778–82.

Sylvester, P. and A. Theriault. 2003. Role of tocotrienols in the prevention of cardiovascular disease and breast cancer. *Curr Top in Nutra Res* 1(2): 121–136.

Tan, B. 2005. Appropriate spectrum vitamin E and new perspectives on desmethyl tocopherols and tocotrienols. *JANA* 8(1): 35–42.

Theriault, A., J. T. Chao, et al. 2002. Tocotrienol is the most effective vitamin E for reducing endothelial expression of adhesion molecules and adhesion to monocytes. *Atherosclerosis* 160(1): 21–30.

Tomeo, A. C., M. Geller, et al. 1995. Antioxidant effects of tocotrienols in patients with hyperlipidemia and carotid stenosis. *Lipids* 30(12): 1179–83.

Traber, M. G. 2007. Vitamin E regulatory mechanisms. *Annu Rev Nutr* 27: 347–62.

Traber, M. G. and J. Atkinson. 2007. Vitamin E, antioxidant and nothing more. *Free Radic Biol Med* 43(1): 4–15.

Traber, M. G. and H. J. Kayden. 1989. Alpha-tocopherol as compared with gamma-tocopherol is preferentially secreted in human lipoproteins. *Ann N Y Acad Sci* 570: 95–108.

van Beek, E., C. Lowik, et al. 1999. The role of geranylgeranylation in bone resorption and its suppression by bisphosphonates in fetal bone explants in vitro: A clue to the mechanism of action of nitrogen-containing bisphosphonates. *J Bone Miner Res* 14(5): 722–9.

van Beek, E. R., L. H. Cohen, et al. 2003. Differentiating the mechanisms of antiresorptive action of nitrogen containing bisphosphonates. *Bone* 33(5): 805–11.

Wan Nazaimoon, W. M. and B. A. Khalid. 2002. Tocotrienols-rich diet decreases advanced glycosylation end-products in non-diabetic rats and improves glycemic control in streptozotocin-induced diabetic rats. *Malays J Pathol* 24(2): 77–82.

Watkins, T. R., M. Geller, et al. 1999. Hypocholesterolemic and antioxidant effect of rice bran oil non-saponifiables in hypercholesterolemic subjects. *Env and Nutr Int* 3: 115–122.

Wechter, W. J., D. Kantoci, et al. 1996. A new endogenous natriuretic factor: LLU-alpha. *Proc Natl Acad Sci U S A* 93(12): 6002–7.

Yamamoto, Y., A. Fujisawa, et al. 2001. An unusual vitamin E constituent (alpha-tocomonoenol) provides enhanced antioxidant protection in marine organisms adapted to cold-water environments. *Proc Natl Acad Sci U S A* 98(23): 13144–8.

Yap, S. P., K. H. Yuen, et al. 2001. Pharmacokinetics and bioavailability of alpha-, gamma- and delta-tocotrienols under different food status. *J Pharm Pharmacol* 53(1): 67–71.

Yoshida, Y., E. Niki, et al. 2003. Comparative study on the action of tocopherols and tocotrienols as antioxidant: Chemical and physical effects. *Chem Phys Lipids* 123(1): 63–75.

You, C. S., T. J. Sontag, et al. 2005. Long-chain carboxychromanols are the major metabolites of tocopherols and tocotrienols in A549 lung epithelial cells but not HepG2 cells. *J Nutr* 135(2): 227–32.

Yu, F. L., A. Gapor, et al. 2005. Evidence for the preventive effect of the polyunsaturated phytol side chain in tocotrienols on 17beta-estradiol epoxidation. *Cancer Detect Prev* 29(4): 383–8.

Yu, S. G., A. M. Thomas, et al. 2006. Dose–response impact of various tocotrienols on serum lipid parameters in 5-week-old female chickens. *Lipids* 41(5): 453–61.

20 Tocotrienols in Hyperlipidemic Conditions

Jahangir Iqbal and Mohammad Minhajuddin

Lipids are essential for numerous aspects of cellular biology, including energy homeostasis, reproductive and organ physiology. The major plasma lipids are cholesterol and triglycerides. Cholesterol is a constituent of membranes and triglycerides are an energy source. The human body has evolved a sophisticated lipoprotein transport system to deliver cholesterol and triglycerides to a variety of tissues in order to meet the different demands. Lipoproteins contain a hydrophobic core of cholesterol ester and triglycerides and an amphiphilic coat consisting of phospholipids, free cholesterol and apolipoproteins. They are classified into four major subtypes depending on the size, density, protein and lipid content (Lindgren et al. 1972). The apoproteins, the protein components of the lipoproteins, serve as membrane stabilizers. They also serve as cofactors in the activation of enzymes that modify the lipoproteins and interact with specific receptors that remove lipoproteins from the circulation. In addition, they are required for synthesis and secretion of certain lipoproteins.

Dietary lipids initially enter the circulation in the form of chylomicron particles. Chylomicrons are the least dense lipoproteins exclusively synthesized by the intestine after the consumption of a lipid-rich meal and may provide peripheral tissues with an important source of energy through the β-oxidation of fatty acids. In the post-prandial period, a proportion of these dietary lipids reenter the circulation in the form of very low density lipoprotein (VLDL) particles, which are synthesized and secreted by the liver (Heath et al. 2003). VLDL also transports non-dietary lipids formed from the catabolism of dietary carbohydrate, the recycling of cellular membranes and the esterification of free fatty acids that may derive from adipose tissue (Wiggins and Gibbons 1996; Parks and Hellerstein 2000; Haemmerle et al. 2003).

While circulating through the peripheral tissues, both the chylomicrons and VLDL are acted upon by the enzyme lipoprotein lipase, which removes triglyceride from these particles for storage in fat or energy consumption in muscle (Nilsson-Ehle P 1982). The action of lipoprotein lipases transforms the chylomicrons and VLDL into cholesterol-rich remnant particles that are removed from the circulation by the liver through the action of a specific remnant receptor (Goldstein and Brown and Goldstein 1976; Brown 1977). VLDL can be further metabolized to the more cholesterol rich LDL particle by the action of hepatic lipase, which is then taken up by a specific LDL receptor (Goldstein and Brown 1977). Metabolized VLDL, after the action of lipoprotein lipases, is left with excess surface coat as its core diminishes in size. In exchange for surface coat, cholesterol ester transfer protein (CETP) transfers cholesterol esters from HDL to VLDL and this exchanged surface coat allows the HDL particle to continue to absorb cholesterol and grow in size. The exchanged cholesterol ester can then be taken up by the liver as the VLDL remnant particles. This represents a very important mechanism by which nascent HDL, which is synthesized and secreted by the intestine and liver, can remove cholesterol from extrahepatic tissues, including macrophages and foam cells (Chinetti et al. 2000; Brewer, Jr. and Santamarina-Fojo 2003) and is known as reverse cholesterol transport (Bruce et al. 1998). The excess cholesterol from the extrahepatic tissues can be recycled or catabolized to bile acid by the liver (Russell 1992; Rader 2003). Any disturbance in this system leads to many pathological processes such as obesity, diabetes and heart disease.

Hyperlipidemia is a pathological condition that arises due to an excess of lipids, largely cholesterol and triglycerides, in the blood. Hyperlipidemia, in general, can be divided into two subcategories: hypercholesterolemia, in which there is a high level of cholesterol, and hypertriglyceridemia, in which there is a high level of triglycerides. When hyperlipidemia is defined in terms of a class or classes of elevated lipoproteins in the blood, the term hyperlipoproteinemia is used. There are several types of hyperlipidemia (types I, IIA, IIB, III, IV and V), which are differentiated by the types of lipids that are elevated in the blood (Fredrickson et al. 1967). Some types of hyperlipidemia may be caused by a primary disorder such as a familial hyperlipidemia. Familial combined hyperlipidemia is an inherited disorder of high serum cholesterol or high blood triglycerides (Goldstein et al. 1973). People with this condition have an increased risk of cardiovascular disease (Austin et al. 2000; Voors-Pette and de Bruin 2001; Hopkins et al. 2003). The types of elevated lipoproteins may vary between affected family members. This disorder predisposes the person to greater risk of early coronary artery disease and therefore, heart attacks (Austin et al. 1988). People with this condition have a higher rate of obesity and glucose intolerance and it is worsened by diabetes, alcoholism and hypothyroidism (Carmena et al. 2001; Denke 2001; Nieves et al. 2003). The rare person who gets two defective genes is at much higher risk for early heart attack due to very high blood lipid (cholesterol or triglyceride) levels. Most hyperlipidemia is the result of secondary causes such as lifestyle habits or treatable medical conditions. Lifestyle contributors include obesity, smoking and not exercising. Medical conditions that cause hyperlipidemia include diabetes, kidney disease, pregnancy and an underactive thyroid gland (Assmann et al. 1999).

The cholesterol in the body is derived from either synthesis by the liver and extrahepatic tissues or absorption by the intestine. There is very little change in the pool of cholesterol within the body. This is mainly because cholesterol input is balanced by cholesterol output via excretion in bile/feces. The liver plays a central role in balancing cholesterol from all sources. Cholesterol produced by the liver is either secreted in bile or incorporated into lipoproteins and secreted into plasma. Cholesterol biosynthesis is regulated by the rate-limiting enzyme HMG-CoA reductase (Goldstein and Brown 1990) and represents the single therapeutic target for statins. These statins work by reducing the production of cholesterol within the body (Maron et al. 2000). The most commonly used statins to treat high LDL cholesterol levels are atorvastatin (Lipitor) or simvastatin (Mevacor). Although safe and effective, statins very rarely cause muscle damage, typically when used in combination with other medications (Thompson et al. 2003).

Another major route for the entry of cholesterol into the body is intestinal absorption. The cholesterol pool in the intestine comes from cholesterol in the diet and biliary excretion. Intestinal cholesterol absorption significantly contributes to blood cholesterol levels and therefore may contribute to atherosclerosis (Kesaniemi and Miettinen 1987; McGill 1979; Wilson and Rudel 1994). Despite many years of study, detailed mechanistic understanding of cholesterol absorption and its regulation is sketchy. Until now, it was believed that all of the absorbed cholesterol in the intestine is packaged with apoB-containing lipoproteins (LDL) and secreted into blood to be carried to different tissues in the body. But recently, we provided evidence for multiple independently regulated pathways of cholesterol transport across the intestinal epithelial cells (Iqbal et al. 2003a; Hussain et al. 2005; Brunham et al. 2006; Iqbal and Hussain 2005). Recently, scientists at Schering-Plough Research Institute identified a new protein, namely Niemann-Pick C1-like 1 protein (NPC1L1), in the small intestine, which functions in absorption of cholesterol (Davis et al. 2004; Altmann et al. 2004). Inhibition of cholesterol absorption with novel agents such as ezetimibe has thus become an important and attractive therapeutic target, particularly since postprandial lipoproteins (cholesterol-rich chylomicron remnants) appear to be particularly atherogenic, with the ability to enter the arterial wall and promote atherogenesis. In the past few years, an innovative progression in cholesterol-lipid lowering therapy has occurred by co-administering ezetimibe together with any dose of statin. This results in superior LDL-C lowering efficacy by inhibiting cholesterol production in the liver and absorption in the intestine (Davis, Jr. et al. 2001; Stone 2002; Gagne et al. 2002; Stein 2002; Kosoglou et al. 2002).

Currently, research has been focused on finding the alternate means of reducing the plasma lipid levels. In this regard, development of new cholesterol-lowering agents has been given more and more attention. One of the compounds that have attracted great attention is tocotrienol. Tocotrienols are fat-soluble vitamins related to the family of tocopherols. Nowadays, the term vitamin E is used as a generic name describing both the tocopherols and tocotrienols. Tocotrienols and tocopherols are sometimes collectively called tocols. However, tocotrienols differ from the tocopherols in the chemical nature of the side chain. While tocopherols have a saturated phytyl tail, tocotrienols have an unsaturated isoprenoid or farnesyl side chain possessing three double bonds. Depending on the number and position of methyl substitution on the chromanol ring, tocopherols and tocotrienols are further separated into individual compounds namely, alpha-, beta-, gamma- and delta (Dormann 2007). The major source of tocotrienols is plant oils, with the richest source being the palm oil, rice bran oil, palm kernel oil and coconut oil (Sundram et al. 2003). Several cereal grains such as oat, barley and rye have also been shown to contain some tocotrienols. On the other hand, vegetable oils, such as those from canola, cottonseed, olive, peanut, safflower, soybean and sunflower, contain little to no tocotrienols. However, these vegetable oils do contain tocopherols (Horvath et al. 2006).

Tocotrienols are absorbed from the lumen of the intestine and the efficiency of absorption is lower on an empty stomach than with meals (Yap et al. 2001). Similar to the dietary fats, tocotrienols are emulsified with the aid of bile salts prior to the absorption. This results in the formation of micelles with dietary fats and products of lipid hydrolysis. In rat studies (Ikeda et al. 1996; Yap et al. 2003), absorption of α-tocotrienol was preferentially higher than absorption of γ- and δ-tocotrienols (Ikeda et al. 1996). This has been suggested to result from the differences in the number of methyl groups in the chromanol rings of the tocotrienol molecules, which affect the lipophilicity of the molecule and transportation to the lymphatic system via biological membranes (Yap et al. 2003). After absorption, tocotrienols are secreted by the enterocytes into the lymphatics in the form of chylomicrons. The chylomicrons are transported by the lymphatics to the circulation, where they are acted upon by lipoprotein lipases to form chylomicron remnants. Tocotrienols in the circulation are transferred from the chylomicrons to HDL which, in turn, transfers them to LDL and VLDL. Apolipoprotein E present in these remnant particles directs them and the tocotrienols they contain to the liver for further metabolism. Tocotrienols do not bind very well to the hepatic α-tocopherol transfer protein that is involved in the secretion of α-tocopherol in VLDLs (Kaempf-Rotzoll et al. 2003). Hence, very little tocotrienol is secreted by the liver to the circulation in VLDLs. Some tocotrienols are transported to several extrahepatic tissues such as adipose tissue, muscle and possibly the brain (Hosomi et al. 1997). Some tocotrienol is also metabolized and excreted in the urine. However, fecal excretion is the main route of excretion of non-absorbed tocotrienols and tocotrienols that may be excreted by the biliary route.

All of the tocotrienols, as well as the tocopherols, are fat-soluble, water-insoluble oils that possess chain-breaking, peroxyl radical scavenging activities (Serbinova and Packer 1994). Tocotrienols, but not tocopherols, inhibit the rate-limiting enzyme of the cholesterol biosynthetic pathway, HMG-CoA reductase (Pearce et al. 1992; Pearce et al. 1994). Farnesol, which is derived from mevalonate and analogues of farnesol have been proposed as post-mevalonate regulators of HMG-CoA reductase (Bradfute and Simoni 1994; Correll and Edwards 1994; Correll et al. 1994; Giron et al. 1994). The cholesterol lowering effect of tocotrienols, which are the natural farnesylated analogues of tocopherols, was attributed to repression of hepatic HMG-CoA reductase through a post-transcriptional mechanism that involved accelerated degradation of the enzyme (Song and DeBose-Boyd 2006). This mechanism is different from that of the statin hypocholesterolemic drugs, which are competitive inhibitors of the enzyme. Tocotrienols, by virtue of their unsaturated isoprenoid side chains, accelerate reductase degradation by mimicking the action of nonsterol end-products of mevalonate metabolism (Parker et al. 1993). On the other hand, tocopherols, which contain a saturated phytyl side chain, neither accelerate reductase degradation nor lower blood cholesterol. The possible anti-atherogenic activity of tocotrienols can also be accounted for by a few other mechanisms. These include inhibition of LDL oxidation, inhibition of platelet aggregation, reduction of plasma apolipoprotein B-100 levels, reduction of lipoprotein (a) plasma levels and inhibition of adhesion molecule (e.g., ICAM-1 and VCAM-1) expression and monocyte cell adherence (Theriault et al. 2002).

Tocotrienols, but not tocopherols, have also shown significant tumor-inhibition activity in several *in vitro* studies (Komiyama et al. 1989; Sundram et al. 1989; Yano et al. 2005; He et al. 1997; Mo and Elson 1999). In one of these studies, a tocotrienol-rich fraction of palm oil significantly inhibited the growth of a human breast cancer cell line, whereas α-tocopherol did not (Gould et al. 1991). Additional *in vitro* studies have demonstrated that tocotrienols inhibit the growth of human breast cancer cells in culture irrespective of the estrogen receptor status of the cells (Nesaretnam et al. 1998). We have demonstrated that the tocotrienol-rich fraction from rice bran oil significantly reduces the DMBA induced mammary (Iqbal et al. 2003b) and DEN/AAF induced hepatic carcinogenesis in rats (Iqbal et al. 2004).

As demonstrated in animal and human studies, tocotrienols have been shown to lower cholesterol concentrations in the blood (Qureshi et al. 1986; Qureshi et al. 1991a; Qureshi et al. 1991b; Qureshi et al. 1995; Qureshi 2000; Qureshi et al. 2001a; Qureshi et al. 2002; Tan et al. 1991; Qureshi et al. 1997; Khor et al. 1995; Hood 1995). This involves inhibition of cholesterol biosynthesis by a mechanism that differs from that of the statin drugs (Goldstein and Brown 1990; Parker et al. 1993); indeed, synergy in the inhibition of cholesterol biosynthesis between a statin (lovastatin) and a tocotrienol-rich fraction of rice bran oil has been reported, reinforcing the assertion that tocotrienols act via a different mechanism(s) (Qureshi et al. 2001b; Qureshi and Peterson 2001). It was demonstrated in human hepatoma HepG2 cells that tocotrienols reduced HMG-CoA reductase protein synthesis rate and increased its degradation rate (Parker et al. 1993). We have also shown previously that tocotrienols lower plasma lipid levels by decreasing the HMG-CoA reductase activity and protein mass in the liver of high cholesterol fed rats (Minhajuddin et al. 2005).

Several studies have also shown that different tocotrienol subtypes possess various degrees of hypocholesterolemic activity, with δ- and γ-tocotrienol being more active than α-tocotrienol, whereas β-tocotrienol is least active (Raederstorff et al. 2002; Yu et al. 2006). *In vitro*, γ-tocotrienol is 30 times more active in inhibiting cholesterol biosynthesis than α-tocotrienol (Pearce et al. 1992). A study done in cholesterol-fed rabbits found that γ-tocotrienols lowered plasma cholesterol levels by 22% after 6 weeks of treatment (Hasselwander et al. 2002). This decrease in plasma cholesterol level was mainly due to a reduction of 23% in LDL cholesterol. In one study conducted by Qureshi et al. (1991a), both total and LDL-cholesterol levels were significantly reduced in swine by 44% and 60%, respectively. Another study done by the same group showed that serum cholesterol levels were significantly lowered in hypercholesterolemic chickens fed a tocotrienol-enriched diet (Qureshi et al. 2000).

In a long series of studies, Qureshi and co-workers have reported that tocotrienols have favorable effects in lowering blood lipids in hypercholesterolemic humans (Qureshi et al. 1991b; Qureshi et al. 2002; Qureshi et al. 1997; Qureshi et al. 1995). A double-blind, crossover study of hypercholesterolemic subjects who used a dose of 200 milligrams of tocotrienol-enriched fraction of palm oil daily for 4 weeks significantly lowered total cholesterol, LDL-cholesterol, Apo B, thromboxane, platelet factor 4 and glucose (Qureshi et al. 1991a). The study done on tocotrienols from palm oil by Tan et al. (1991) demonstrated that daily ingestion of a tocotrienol-rich fraction from palm oil resulted in lowered serum concentrations of LDL cholesterol in both normocholesterolemic and hypercholesterolemic men and women. However, in this study, no change was found in serum triglyceride concentrations.

Another double-blind, crossover, 8-week study done by Qureshi et al. (Qureshi et al. 1991b) examined the effects of tocotrienols in 25 hypercholesterolemic men and women. The study drug was a mixture of tocotrienol-rich fraction (30–40 mg of α-tocopherol, 24–30 mg of α-tocotrienol, 70–80 mg of γ-tocotrienol and 50–60 mg of δ-tocotrienol) from palm oil called Palmvitee supplied by the Palm Oil Research Institute of Malaysia. Subjects were randomly assigned to receive either Palmvitee or corn oil (placebo) for 4 weeks and crossed to the other regimen for another 4 weeks. This treatment resulted in a reduction of serum LDL cholesterol concentrations by only 8%. However, out of 15 participants in the tocotrienol group, three patients responded poorly to the tocotrienol-rich fraction. When these poor responders were excluded from the statistical analysis, a significant 28% decrease in serum cholesterol level was found. In a substudy, these investigators gave the three poor responders and four new hypercholesterolemic subjects a daily supplementation of 200 mg of the specific γ-tocotrienol instead of the Palmvitee for 4 weeks. The supplementation of γ-tocotrienol fraction, instead of a mixture of tocopherols and tocotrienols, decreased the LDL cholesterol by 27% in these subjects. These observations led the authors to conclude that α-tocotrienol might be the most effective cholesterol-lowering compound in palm oil. The additional antihypercholesterolemic effect with γ-tocotrienol alone was later attributed to the absence of α-tocopherol, as α-tocopherol was shown to attenuate the impact of the tocotrienols on HMG-CoA reductase activity (Qureshi et al. 1996). Therefore, additional dietary supplementation with vitamin E should be avoided since it may augment the antihyperlipidemic effects of tocotrienols. Another trial performed by the same group in hypercholesterolemic subjects consuming an AHA step I diet also demonstrated a 13% decline in serum LDL cholesterol concentrations after the daily supplementation with a tocotrienol-rich fraction (40 mg of α-tocopherol, 48 mg α-tocotrienol, 112 mg of γ-tocotrienol and 60 mg of δ-tocotrienol) from palm oil for 4 weeks (Qureshi et al. 1995).

Despite good results in humans as well as animals coupled with *in vitro* and epidemiological data suggesting that high tocotrienol status reduces hyperlipidemia, some recent small studies have not been quite as promising. In contrast to the above studies, various other research groups found no significant change in the serum lipid and lipoprotein profile after supplementation with tocotrienols from palm oil. In the study of Wahlqvist et al. (1992), increased doses of up to 240 mg/d of tocotrienol-rich fraction (30% of α-tocopherol, 23% of α-tocotrienol, 31% of γ-tocotrienol and 16% of δ-tocotrienol) to men and women with hypercholesterolemia for 4 weeks had no changes in serum concentrations of total, LDL and HDL cholesterol, or triglycerides. Similarly, Tomeo et al. (1995) confirmed the above observations by examining the effects of daily supplementation of tocotrienol-rich fraction (29% α-tocopherol and 71% γ- plus α-tocotrienols) from palm oil in increasing doses of up to 336 mg for 18 months on serum lipids and lipoproteins in hyperlipidemic men and women with carotid atherosclerosis. Although these patients showed no lipid-lowering effect upon treatment with α-tocopherol and γ-tocotrienol, compared with controls receiving placebo, there was a significant improvement in terms of ultrasonigraphically measured rate of progression. In some cases regression of carotid stenosis was also observed.

Another randomized, double-blind, placebo-controlled study found no lipid effects from a supplement containing 35 milligrams of tocotrienols and 20 milligrams of α-tocopherol in 20 men with slightly elevated lipid concentrations. One of the reasons for this could be that the dose of tocotrienols used for this trial was not enough to elicit any hypolipidemic effect (Mensink et al. 1999). Furthermore, O'Byrne et al. (2000) found no changes in serum lipid and lipoprotein concentrations in hypercholesterolemic subjects who received supplements containing tocotrienyl acetates from palm oil for 8 weeks. The controversial effects of tocotrienols in the tocotrienol-rich fraction from palm oil were attributed to the presence of α-tocopherol, which was shown to attenuate the effect of the cholesterol-lowering action of tocotrienols in chickens (Qureshi et al. 1996). Qureshi et al. (1996) suggested that the most effective supplements in terms of cholesterol lowering action provided 15–20% α-tocopherol and ~60% γ- (and δ-) tocotrienol, whereas the less effective supplements consisted of ≥30% α-tocopherol and 45% γ- (and δ-) tocotrienol.

Like palm oil, rice bran oil is a rich source of tocotrienols, especially γ- and δ-tocotrienols, which have been shown to possess the most hypocholesterolemic activity (Qureshi et al. 1995; Qureshi et al. 1996; Raederstorff et al. 2002; Yu et al. 2006; Rukmini and Raghuram 1991). The cholesterol-lowering effect of tocotrienols from rice bran oil (Qureshi et al. 1997) are more pronounced than the effects seen in tocotrienols from palm oil (Qureshi et al. 1991b; Qureshi et al. 1995). Qureshi et al. (2000; 2001a; 2002) attributed these promising effects to two new types of tocotrienols isolated from rice bran oil. These tocotrienols were identified and named as desmethyl (P_{21}) and didesmethyl (P_{25}) tocotrienols (Qureshi et al. 2000). In a study conducted in hypercholesterolemic subjects who were consuming a NCEP step I diet, daily consumption of ~200 mg of tocotrienol-rich fraction (12 mg of α-tocopherol, 25 mg of α-tocotrienol, 42 mg of γ-tocotrienol, 20 mg of δ-tocotrienol, 9 mg of P_{21}-tocotrienol, 34 mg of P_{25}-tocotrienol, 36 mg of unidentified tocopherols and tocotrienols and 20 mg of sterols and triacylglycerol) from rice bran oil for 4 weeks reduced serum LDL cholesterol concentrations by 23% (Qureshi et al. 2002). In a clinical study done by Baliarsing et al. (2005), 19 hyperlipidemic type 2 diabetic subjects were supplemented daily with 6 mg/kg body weight of tocotrienol-rich fraction from rice bran oil for 60 days. The subjects had been withdrawn from statin use 3 weeks before the study and were eating a diet recommended for diabetics. At the end of the trial, significant reductions in serum total lipids, total cholesterol and LDL-cholesterol were seen in the hyperlipidemic type 2 diabetic subjects compared with placebo.

In a research article published by Song and DeBose-Boyd (2006), the authors provided a biochemical mechanism for the hypocholesterolemic effects of tocotrienols that have been observed in animals and humans. They have shown evidence that γ- and δ-tocotrienols mimic sterols, rather than nonsterol isoprenoids in stimulating ubiquitination/degradation of HMG-CoA reductase. They suggested that a mevalonate-derived nonsterol product must combine with either γ- or δ-tocotrienol to maximally stimulate degradation of HMG-CoA reductase via the ubiquitination pathway. These authors also demonstrated that the tocotrienol-dependent ubiquitination and degradation of endogenous reductase was mediated through the Insigs. A mutant form of HMG-CoA reductase was resistant to tocotrienol-stimulated degradation when either it was defective in Insig binding or lacked the two lysine residues necessary for Insig-mediated ubiquitination. It was shown that tocotrienols themselves trigger Insig binding and lead to the ubiquitination and subsequent degradation of HMG-CoA reductase.

Tocopherols, on the other hand, were unable to stimulate reductase degradation (Gil et al. 1985; Parker et al. 1993). These findings indicate that the isoprenoid-like phytyl side chain of tocotrienols is a crucial determinant of activity and may stimulate the binding of HMG-CoA reductase to Insigs. The specificity of the action of tocotrienols appears to be depending on the substitution of a methyl group to the chroman ring. Presence of a methyl group at R2 position in α- and β-tocotrienols diminishes its action of HMG-CoA reductase degradation (Gil et al. 1985). On the other hand, a methyl group at R1 position in γ-tocotrienol or hydrogen at the R1 and R2 positions, instead of a methyl group, in δ-tocotrienol enhances their action of HMG-CoA reductase degradation.

Song and DeBose-Boyd (2006) postulated that tocotrienols mediate sterol-stimulated degradation of reductase through binding to an accessory protein. Alternatively, tocotrienols may trigger a conformational change in the reductase by directly binding to the sterol-sensing domains which in turn allows Insig binding. However, the exact mechanism by which tocotrienols mediate the degradation of HMG-CoA reductase still needs further investigation. Thus, understanding the mechanistic action of tocotrienols on Insig-mediated degradation of HMG-CoA reductase may provide insights into the development of new cholesterol-lowering drugs that treat or prevent coronary heart disease.

REFERENCES

Altmann, S.W., Davis, H.R., Jr., Zhu, L.J., Yao, X., Hoos, L.M., Tetzloff, G., Iyer, S.P., Maguire, M., Golovko, A., Zeng, M., Wang, L., Murgolo, N. and Graziano, M.P. 2004. Niemann-Pick C1 Like 1 protein is critical for intestinal cholesterol absorption. *Science* 303: 1201–1204.

Assmann, G., Cullen, P., Jossa, F., Lewis, B. and Mancini, M. 1999. Coronary heart disease: reducing the risk: the scientific background to primary and secondary prevention of coronary heart disease. A worldwide view. International task force for the prevention of coronary heart disease. *Arterioscler. Thromb. Vasc. Biol.* 19: 1819–1824.

Austin, M.A., Breslow, J.L., Hennekens, C.H., Buring, J.E., Willett, W.C. and Krauss, R.M. 1988. Low-density lipoprotein subclass patterns and risk of myocardial infarction. *JAMA* 260: 1917–1921.

Austin, M.A., McKnight, B., Edwards, K.L., Bradley, C.M., McNeely, M.J., Psaty, B.M., Brunzell, J.D. and Motulsky, A.G. 2000. Cardiovascular disease mortality in familial forms of hypertriglyceridemia: A 20-year prospective study. *Circulation* 101: 2777–2782.

Baliarsingh, S., Beg, Z.H. and Ahmad, J. 2005. The therapeutic impacts of tocotrienols in type 2 diabetic patients with hyperlipidemia. *Atherosclerosis* 182: 367–374.

Bradfute, D.L. and Simoni, R.D. 1994. Non-sterol compounds that regulate cholesterogenesis. Analogues of farnesyl pyrophosphate reduce 3-hydroxy-3-methylglutaryl-coenzyme A reductase levels. *J. Biol. Chem.* 269: 6645–6650.

Brewer, H.B., Jr. and Santamarina-Fojo, S. 2003. Clinical significance of high-density lipoproteins and the development of atherosclerosis: Focus on the role of the adenosine triphosphate-binding cassette protein A1 transporter. *Am. J. Cardiol.* 92: 10K–16K.

Brown, M.S. and Goldstein, J.L. 1976. Receptor-mediated control of cholesterol metabolism. *Science* 191: 150–154.

Bruce, C., Chouinard, R.A., Jr. and Tall, A.R. 1998. Plasma lipid transfer proteins, high-density lipoproteins and reverse cholesterol transport. *Annu. Rev. Nutr.* 18: 297–330.

Brunham, L.R., Kruit, J.K., Iqbal, J., Fievet, C., Timmins, J.M., Pape, T.D., Coburn, B.A., Bissada, N., Staels, B., Groen, A.K., Hussain, M.M., Parks, J.S., Kuipers, F. and Hayden, M.R. 2006. Intestinal ABCA1 directly contributes to HDL biogenesis *in vivo*. *J. Clin. Invest.* 116: 1052–1062.

Carmena, R., Ascaso, J.F. and Real, J.T. 2001. Impact of obesity in primary hyperlipidemias. *Nutr. Metab Cardiovasc. Dis.* 11: 354–359.

Chinetti, G., Gbaguidi, F.G., Griglio, S., Mallat, Z., Antonucci, M., Poulain, P., Chapman, J., Fruchart, J.C., Tedgui, A., Najib-Fruchart, J. and Staels, B. 2000. CLA-1/SR-BI is expressed in atherosclerotic lesion macrophages and regulated by activators of peroxisome proliferator-activated receptors. *Circulation* 101: 2411–2417.

Correll, C.C. and Edwards, P.A. 1994. Mevalonic acid-dependent degradation of 3-hydroxy-3-methylglutaryl-coenzyme A reductase in vivo and in vitro. *J. Biol. Chem.* 269: 633–638.

Correll, C.C., Ng, L. and Edwards, P.A. 1994. Identification of farnesol as the non-sterol derivative of mevalonic acid required for the accelerated degradation of 3-hydroxy-3-methylglutaryl-coenzyme A reductase. *J. Biol. Chem.* 269: 17390–17393.

Davis, H.R., Jr., Pula, K.K., Alton, K.B., Burrier, R.E. and Watkins, R.W. 2001. The synergistic hypocholesterolemic activity of the potent cholesterol absorption inhibitor, ezetimibe, in combination with 3-hydroxy-3-methylglutaryl coenzyme a reductase inhibitors in dogs. *Metabolism* 50: 1234–1241.

Davis, H.R., Jr., Zhu, L.J., Hoos, L.M., Tetzloff, G., Maguire, M., Liu, J., Yao, X., Iyer, S.P., Lam, M.H., Lund, E.G., Detmers, P.A., Graziano, M.P. and Altmann, S.W. 2004. Niemann-Pick C1 Like 1 (NPC1L1) is the intestinal phytosterol and cholesterol transporter and a key modulator of whole-body cholesterol homeostasis. *J. Biol. Chem.* 279: 33586–33592.

Denke, M.A. 2001. Connections between obesity and dyslipidaemia. *Curr. Opin. Lipidol.* 12: 625–628.

Dormann, P. 2007. Functional diversity of tocochromanols in plants. *Planta* 225: 269–276.

Fredrickson, D.S., Levy, R.I. and Lees, R.S. 1967. Fat transport in lipoproteins—an integrated approach to mechanisms and disorders. *N. Engl. J. Med.* 276: 34–42.

Gagne, C., Gaudet, D., Bruckert, E. and for the Ezetimibe Study Group. 2002. Efficacy and safety of ezetimibe coadministered with atorvastatin or simvastatin in patients with homozygous familial hypercholesterolemia. *Circulation* 105: 2469–2475.

Gil, G., Faust, J.R., Chin, D.J., Goldstein, J.L. and Brown, M.S. 1985. Membrane-bound domain of HMG CoA reductase is required for sterol-enhanced degradation of the enzyme. *Cell* 41: 249–258.

Giron, M.D., Havel, C.M. and Watson, J.A. 1994. Mevalonate-mediated suppression of 3-hydroxy-3-methylglutaryl coenzyme A reductase function in alpha-toxin-perforated cells. *Proc. Natl. Acad. Sci. USA* 91: 6398–6402.

Goldstein, J.L. and Brown, M.S. 1977. The low-density lipoprotein pathway and its relation to atherosclerosis. *Annu. Rev. Biochem.* 46: 897–930.

Goldstein, J.L. and Brown, M.S. 1990. Regulation of the mevalonate pathway. *Nature* 343: 425–430.

Goldstein, J.L., Schrott, H.G., Hazzard, W.R., Bierman, E.L. and Motulsky, A.G. 1973. Hyperlipidemia in coronary heart disease. II. Genetic analysis of lipid levels in 176 families and delineation of a new inherited disorder, combined hyperlipidemia. *J. Clin. Invest.* 52: 1544–1568.

Gould, M.N., Haag, J.D., Kennan, W.S., Tanner, M.A. and Elson, C.E. 1991. A comparison of tocopherol and tocotrienol for the chemoprevention of chemically induced rat mammary tumors. *Am. J. Clin. Nutr.* 53: 1068S–1070S.

Haemmerle, G., Zimmermann, R. and Zechner, R. 2003. Letting lipids go: Hormone-sensitive lipase. *Curr. Opin. Lipidol.* 14: 289–297.

Hasselwander O., Kramer K., Hoppe P.P., Oberfrank U., Baldenius K., Schroder H., Kaufmann W., Bahnemann R. and Nowakowsky B. 2002. Effects of feeding various tocotrienol sources on plasma lipids and aortic atherosclerotic lesions in cholesterol-fed rabbits. *Food Res. Int.* 35: 245–251.

He, L., Mo, H., Hadisusilo, S., Qureshi, A.A. and Elson, C.E. 1997. Isoprenoids suppress the growth of murine B16 melanomas *in vitro* and *in vivo*. *J. Nutr.* 127: 668–674.

Heath, R.B., Karpe, F., Milne, R.W., Burdge, G.C., Wootton, S.A. and Frayn, K.N. 2003. Selective partitioning of dietary fatty acids into the VLDL TG pool in the early postprandial period. *J. Lipid Res.* 44: 2065–2072.

Hood, R.L. 1995. Tocotrienols and cholesterol metabolism. In A.S.M.Ong, E.Niki and L.Packer, Eds. *Nutrition, lipids, health and diseases.* AOCS Press, Champaign, Illinois, pp 96–103.

Hopkins, P.N., Heiss, G., Ellison, R.C., Province, M.A., Pankow, J.S., Eckfeldt, J.H. and Hunt, S.C. 2003. Coronary artery disease risk in familial combined hyperlipidemia and familial hypertriglyceridemia: A case-control comparison from the National Heart, Lung and Blood Institute Family Heart Study. *Circulation* 108: 519–523.

Horvath, G., Wessjohann, L., Bigirimana, J., Jansen, M., Guisez, Y., Caubergs, R. and Horemans, N. 2006. Differential distribution of tocopherols and tocotrienols in photosynthetic and non-photosynthetic tissues. *Phytochemistry* 67: 1185–1195.

Hosomi, A., Arita, M., Sato, Y., Kiyose, C., Ueda, T., Igarashi, O., Arai, H. and Inoue, K. 1997. Affinity for alpha-tocopherol transfer protein as a determinant of the biological activities of vitamin E analogs. *FEBS Lett.* 409: 105–108.

Hussain, M.M., Fatma, S., Pan, X. and Iqbal, J. 2005. Intestinal lipoprotein assembly. *Curr. Opin. Lipidol.* 16: 281–285.

Ikeda, I., Imasato, Y., Sasaki, E. and Sugano, M. 1996. Lymphatic transport of alpha-, gamma- and delta-tocotrienols and alpha-tocopherol in rats. *Int. J. Vitam. Nutr. Res.* 66: 217–221.

Iqbal, J., Anwar, K. and Hussain, M.M. 2003a. Multiple, independently regulated pathways of cholesterol transport across the intestinal epithelial cells. *J. Biol. Chem.* 278: 31610–31620.

Iqbal, J. and Hussain, M.M. 2005. Evidence for multiple complementary pathways for efficient cholesterol absorption in mice. *J. Lipid Res.* 46: 1491–1501.

Iqbal, J., Minhajuddin, M. and Beg, Z.H. 2003b. Suppression of 7, 12-dimethylbenz[alpha]anthracene-induced carcinogenesis and hypercholesterolaemia in rats by tocotrienol-rich fraction isolated from rice bran oil. *Eur. J. Cancer Prev.* 12: 447–453.

Iqbal, J., Minhajuddin, M. and Beg, Z.H. 2004. Suppression of diethylnitrosamine and 2-acetylaminofluorene-induced hepatocarcinogenesis in rats by tocotrienol-rich fraction isolated from rice bran oil. *Eur. J. Cancer Prev.* 13: 515–520.

Kaempf-Rotzoll, D.E., Traber, M.G. and Arai, H. 2003. Vitamin E and transfer proteins. *Curr. Opin. Lipidol.* 14: 249–254.

Kesaniemi, Y.A. and Miettinen, T.A. 1987. Cholesterol absorption efficiency regulates plasma cholesterol level in the Finnish population. *Eur. J. Clin. Invest.* 17: 391–395.

Khor, H.T., Chieng, D.Y. and Ong, K.K. 1995. Tocotrienols inhibit liver HMG CoA reductase activity in the guinea pig. *Nutr. Res.* 15: 537–544.

Komiyama, K., Iizuka, K., Yamaoka, M., Watanabe, H., Tsuchiya, N. and Umezawa, I. 1989. Studies on the biological activity of tocotrienols. *Chem. Pharm. Bull.* (Tokyo) 37: 1369–1371.

Kosoglou, T., Meyer, I., Veltri, E.P., Statkevich, P., Yang, B., Zhu, Y., Mellars, L., Maxwell, S.E., Patrick, J.E., Cutler, D.L., Batra, V.K. and Affrime, M.B. 2002. Pharmacodynamic interaction between the new selective cholesterol absorption inhibitor ezetimibe and simvastatin. *Br. J. Clin. Pharmacol.* 54: 309–319.

Lindgren, F.T., Jensen LC and Hatch FT 1972. The isolation and quantitative analysis of serum lipoproteins. In Nelson GJ., Ed. *Blood lipids and lipoproteins: Quantification, composition and metabolism.* John Wiley and Sons, New York, pp 181.

Maron, D.J., Fazio, S. and Linton, M.F. 2000. Current perspectives on statins. *Circulation* 101: 207–213.

McGill, H.C., Jr. 1979. The relationship of dietary cholesterol to serum cholesterol concentration and to atherosclerosis in man. *Am. J. Clin. Nutr.* 32: 2664–2702.

Mensink, R.P., van Houwelingen, A.C., Kromhout, D. and Hornstra, G. 1999. A vitamin E concentrate rich in tocotrienols had no effect on serum lipids, lipoproteins, or platelet function in men with mildly elevated serum lipid concentrations. *Am. J. Clin. Nutr.* 69: 213–219.

Minhajuddin, M., Beg, Z.H. and Iqbal, J. 2005. Hypolipidemic and antioxidant properties of tocotrienol rich fraction isolated from rice bran oil in experimentally induced hyperlipidemic rats. *Food Chem. Toxicol.* 43: 747–753.

Mo, H. and Elson, C.E. 1999. Apoptosis and cell-cycle arrest in human and murine tumor cells are initiated by isoprenoids. *J. Nutr.* 129: 804–813.

Nesaretnam, K., Stephen, R., Dils, R. and Darbre, P. 1998. Tocotrienols inhibit the growth of human breast cancer cells irrespective of estrogen receptor status. *Lipids* 33: 461–469.

Nieves, D.J., Cnop, M., Retzlaff, B., Walden, C.E., Brunzell, J.D., Knopp, R.H. and Kahn, S.E. 2003. The atherogenic lipoprotein profile associated with obesity and insulin resistance is largely attributable to intra-abdominal fat. *Diabetes* 52: 172–179.

Nilsson-Ehle, P. 1982. Regulation of lipoprotein lipase: Triacylglycerol transport in plasma. In Carlson, L.A. and Pernow, B. (Eds). *Metabolic risk factors in ischemic cardiovascular disease.* Raven Press, New York, pp 49.

O'Byrne, D., Grundy, S., Packer, L., Devaraj, S., Baldenius, K., Hoppe, P.P., Kraemer, K., Jialal, I. and Traber, M.G. 2000. Studies of LDL oxidation following alpha-, gamma-, or delta-tocotrienyl acetate supplementation of hypercholesterolemic humans. *Free Radic. Biol. Med.* 29: 834–845.

Parker, R.A., Pearce, B.C., Clark, R.W., Gordon, D.A. and Wright, J.J. 1993. Tocotrienols regulate cholesterol production in mammalian cells by post-transcriptional suppression of 3-hydroxy-3-methylglutaryl-coenzyme A reductase. *J. Biol. Chem.* 268: 11230–11238.

Parks, E.J. and Hellerstein, M.K. 2000. Carbohydrate-induced hypertriacylglycerolemia: Historical perspective and review of biological mechanisms. *Am. J. Clin. Nutr.* 71: 412–433.

Pearce, B.C., Parker, R.A., Deason, M.E., Dischino, D.D., Gillespie, E., Qureshi, A.A., Volk, K. and Wright, J.J. 1994. Inhibitors of cholesterol biosynthesis. 2. Hypocholesterolemic and antioxidant activities of benzopyran and tetrahydronaphthalene analogues of the tocotrienols. *J. Med. Chem.* 37: 526–541.

Pearce, B.C., Parker, R.A., Deason, M.E., Qureshi, A.A. and Wright, J.J. 1992. Hypocholesterolemic activity of synthetic and natural tocotrienols. *J. Med. Chem.* 35: 3595–3606.

Qureshi, A.A., Bradlow, B.A., Brace, L., Manganello, J., Peterson, D.M., Pearce, B.C., Wright, J.J., Gapor, A. and Elson, C.E. 1995. Response of hypercholesterolemic subjects to administration of tocotrienols. *Lipids* 30: 1171–1177.

Qureshi, A.A., Burger, W.C., Peterson, D.M. and Elson, C.E. 1986. The structure of an inhibitor of cholesterol biosynthesis isolated from barley. *J. Biol. Chem.* 261: 10544–10550.

Qureshi, A.A., Mo, H., Packer, L. and Peterson, D.M. 2000. Isolation and identification of novel tocotrienols from rice bran with hypocholesterolemic, antioxidant and antitumor properties. *J. Agric. Food Chem.* 48: 3130–3140.

Qureshi, A.A., Pearce, B.C., Nor, R.M., Gapor, A., Peterson, D.M. and Elson, C.E. 1996. Dietary alpha-tocopherol attenuates the impact of gamma-tocotrienol on hepatic 3-hydroxy-3-methylglutaryl coenzyme A reductase activity in chickens. *J. Nutr.* 126: 389–394.

Qureshi, A.A. and Peterson, D.M. 2001. The combined effects of novel tocotrienols and lovastatin on lipid metabolism in chickens. *Atherosclerosis* 156: 39–47.

Qureshi, A.A., Peterson, D.M., Hasler-Rapacz, J.O. and Rapacz, J. 2001a. Novel tocotrienols of rice bran suppress cholesterogenesis in hereditary hypercholesterolemic swine. *J. Nutr.* 131: 223–230.

Qureshi, A.A., Qureshi, N., Hasler-Rapacz, J.O., Weber, F.E., Chaudhary, V., Crenshaw, T.D., Gapor, A., Ong, A.S., Chong, Y.H., Peterson, D. and . 1991a. Dietary tocotrienols reduce concentrations of plasma cholesterol, apolipoprotein B, thromboxane B2 and platelet factor 4 in pigs with inherited hyperlipidemias. *Am. J. Clin. Nutr.* 53: 1042S–1046S.

Qureshi, A.A., Qureshi, N., Wright, J.J., Shen, Z., Kramer, G., Gapor, A., Chong, Y.H., DeWitt, G., Ong, A., Peterson, D.M. 1991b. Lowering of serum cholesterol in hypercholesterolemic humans by tocotrienols (palmvitee). *Am. J. Clin. Nutr.* 53: 1021S–1026S.

Qureshi, A.A., Sami, S.A., Salser, W.A. and Khan, F.A. 2001b. Synergistic effect of tocotrienol-rich fraction (TRF(25)) of rice bran and lovastatin on lipid parameters in hypercholesterolemic humans. *J. Nutr. Biochem.* 12: 318–329.

Qureshi, A.A., Sami, S.A., Salser, W.A. and Khan, F.A. 2002. Dose-dependent suppression of serum cholesterol by tocotrienol-rich fraction (TRF25) of rice bran in hypercholesterolemic humans. *Atherosclerosis* 161: 199–207.

Qureshi, A.A., Bradlow, B.A., Salser, W.A. and Brace, L.D. 1997. Novel tocotrienols of rice bran modulate cardiovascular disease risk parameters of hypercholesterolemic humans. *J. Nutr. Biochem.* 8: 290–298.

Rader, D.J. 2003. Regulation of reverse cholesterol transport and clinical implications. *Am. J. Cardiol.* 92: 42J–49J.

Raederstorff, D., Elste, V., Aebischer, C. and Weber, P. 2002. Effect of either gamma-tocotrienol or a tocotrienol mixture on the plasma lipid profile in hamsters. *Ann. Nutr. Metab.* 46: 17–23.

Rukmini, C. and Raghuram, T.C. 1991. Nutritional and biochemical aspects of the hypolipidemic action of rice bran oil: A review. *J. Am. Coll. Nutr.* 10: 593–601.

Russell, D.W. 1992. Cholesterol biosynthesis and metabolism. Cardiovasc. *Drugs Ther.* 6: 103–110.

Serbinova, E.A. and Packer, L. 1994. Antioxidant properties of alpha-tocopherol and alpha-tocotrienol. *Meth. Enzymol.* 234: 354–366.

Song, B.L. and DeBose-Boyd, R.A. 2006. Insig-dependent ubiquitination and degradation of 3-hydroxy-3-methylglutaryl coenzyme a reductase stimulated by delta- and gamma-tocotrienols. *J. Biol. Chem.* 281: 25054–25061.

Stein, E.A. 2002. An investigative look: selective cholesterol absorption inhibitors—embarking on a new standard of care. *Am. J. Manag. Care* 8: S36–S39.

Stone, N. 2002. Combination therapy: Its rationale and the role of ezetimibe. *Eur. Heart J.* Suppl 4: J19–J22.

Sundram, K., Khor, H.T., Ong, A.S. and Pathmanathan, R. 1989. Effect of dietary palm oils on mammary carcinogenesis in female rats induced by 7, 12-dimethylbenz(a)anthracene. *Cancer Res.* 49: 1447–1451.

Sundram, K., Sambanthamurthi, R. and Tan, Y.A. 2003. Palm fruit chemistry and nutrition. Asia Pac. *J. Clin. Nutr.* 12: 355–362.

Tan, D.T., Khor, H.T., Low, W.H., Ali, A. and Gapor, A. 1991. Effect of a palm-oil-vitamin E concentrate on the serum and lipoprotein lipids in humans. *Am. J. Clin. Nutr.* 53: 1027S-1030S.

Theriault, A., Chao, J.T. and Gapor, A. 2002. Tocotrienol is the most effective vitamin E for reducing endothelial expression of adhesion molecules and adhesion to monocytes. *Atherosclerosis* 160: 21–30.

Thompson, P.D., Clarkson, P. and Karas, R.H. 2003. Statin-associated myopathy. *JAMA* 289: 1681–1690.

Tomeo, A.C., Geller, M., Watkins, T.R., Gapor, A. and Bierenbaum, M.L. 1995. Antioxidant effects of tocotrienols in patients with hyperlipidemia and carotid stenosis. *Lipids* 30: 1179–1183.

Voors–Pette, C. and de Bruin, T.W. 2001. Excess coronary heart disease in familial combined hyperlipidemia, in relation to genetic factors and central obesity. *Atherosclerosis* 157: 481–489.

Wahlqvist, M.L., Krivokuca-Bogetic, Z., Lo, C.S., Hage, B., Smith, R. and Lukito, W. 1992. Differential serum responses of tocopherols and tocotrienols during vitamin supplementation in hypercholesterolaemic individuals without change in coronary risk factors. *Nutr. Res.* 12: S181–S201.

Wiggins, D. and Gibbons, G.F. 1996. Origin of hepatic very-low-density lipoprotein triacylglycerol: The contribution of cellular phospholipid. *Biochem. J.* 320 (Pt 2): 673–679.

Wilson, M.D. and Rudel, L.L. 1994. Review of cholesterol absorption with emphasis on dietary and biliary cholesterol. *J. Lipid Res.* 35: 943–955.

Yano, Y., Satoh, H., Fukumoto, K., Kumadaki, I., Ichikawa, T., Yamada, K., Hagiwara, K. and Yano, T. 2005. Induction of cytotoxicity in human lung adenocarcinoma cells by 6-O-carboxypropyl-alpha-tocotrienol, a redox-silent derivative of alpha-tocotrienol. *Int. J. Cancer* 115: 839–846.

Yap, S.P., Yuen, K.H. and Lim, A.B. 2003. Influence of route of administration on the absorption and disposition of alpha-, gamma- and delta-tocotrienols in rats. *J. Pharm. Pharmacol.* 55: 53–58.

Yap, S.P., Yuen, K.H. and Wong, J.W. 2001. Pharmacokinetics and bioavailability of alpha–, gamma- and delta-tocotrienols under different food status. *J. Pharm. Pharmacol.* 53: 67–71.

Yu, S.G., Thomas, A.M., Gapor, A., Tan, B., Qureshi, N. and Qureshi, A.A. 2006. Dose-response impact of various tocotrienols on serum lipid parameters in 5-week-old female chickens. *Lipids* 41: 453–461.

21 Vitamin E Isomers, Tocotrienols, in Cardioprotection

Samarjit Das, Manika Das and Dipak K. Das

CONTENTS

21.1 INTRODUCTION

Tocotrienols and tocopherols together compose the vitamin E family. Tocotrienols offer many health benefits of vitamin E including the ability to lower cholesterol levels and provide anticancer and tumor-suppressive activities. Dietary tocotrienols reduce the concentration of plasma cholesterol and apolipoprotein B, platelet factor 4, and thromboxane B_2, indicating their ability to protect against platelet aggregation and endothelial dysfunction (Qureshi, Qureshi et al. 1991a, 1991b). Red palm oil is one of the richest sources of carotenoids, tocotrienols and ascorbic acid. Thus, this oil represents a powerful network of antioxidants that can protect tissues and cells from oxidative damage (Edem 2002; Krinsky 1992; Pacer 1992). For rat hearts, α-tocotrienol were more proficient in the protection against oxidative stress induced by ischemia-reperfusion than α-tocopherol (Serbinova et al. 1992). Tocotrienols are found to be more effective in the protection of the central nervous system than α-tocopherol (Sen et al. 2004). In another study, TRF (tocotrienol rich fraction) was found to inhibit the glutamate-induced pp60 c-src kinase activation in HT4 neuronal cells (Sen et al. 2000). One study indicated that TRF was able to reduce myocardial infarct size, improve postischemic ventricular dysfunction and reduce the incidence of ventricular arrhythmias (Das et al. 2005). TRF was also shown to stabilize 20S and 26S proteasome activities and reduce the ischemia-reperfusion-induced increase in c-Src phosphorylation (Das et al. 2005).

The growing interest in tocotrienols among all other vitamin E isoforms is the focus of this chapter.

21.2 A BRIEF HISTORY OF VITAMIN E

In 1922 at Berkeley University in California, Dr. Herbert M. Evans, a physician-scientist, and his assistant Katherine S. Bishop, discovered a fat-soluble alcohol that functioned as an antioxidant, which they named "Factor X" (Papas 1999). Evans and Bishop were feeding rats a semi-purified diet when they noticed that the female rats were unable to produce offspring because the pups died in the womb. They then fed the female rats lettuce and wheat germ, and observed that healthy offspring were produced. During their research, Evans and Bishop discovered that Factor X was contained in the lipid extract of the lettuce and concluded that this Factor X was fat-soluble (Papas 1999).

In 1924, Dr. Bennet Sure renamed Factor X vitamin E. The first component identified was α-tocopherol. It was named as such from the Greek *tokos* (offspring) and *pheros* (to bear) and the *ol* ending was added to indicate the alcoholic properties of the molecules. For more than 30 years, it was believed that vitamin E existed in only one form, α-tocopherol. As a result, vitamin E was named α-tocopherol. It is the most abundant form of vitamin E found in blood and tissues. But in 1956, a scientist by the name of J. Green discovered the eight isoforms of vitamin E, four tocopherol isomers (α-, β-, γ-, and δ-) and four tocotrienol isomers (α-, β-, γ-, and δ-), split into two different categories: tocopherols and tocotrienols, which are corresponding stereoisomers. Tocopherols and tocotrienols are very similar, except for the fact that tocopherols have a saturated phytyl tail, and tocotrienols have an isoprenoid tail with three unsaturated points. In addition, on the chromanol nucleus, the various isoforms differ in their methyl substitutions (Figure 21.1). Tocotrienols were initially named ζ, ε or η-tocopherols. The δ-form has one methyl group, the γ- and β- forms have two methyl groups, and the α-form contains three methyl groups on its chromanol head. Tocopherols and tocotrienols share a common chromanol head and a side chain at the C-2 position (Theriault et al. 1999). Very recently, two new isomers of tocotrinols have been found and are present in TRF of rice bran oil, desmethyl (D-P_{21}-T3) and didesmethyl (D-P_{25}-T3) tocotrienols (Das et al. 2007).

The therapeutic application of vitamin E was first shown by Kamimura (1997). The inhibitory effect of the unsaturated fatty acid by α-tocopherol was well established by Tappel (Tappel 1953; 1954; 1955). This observation was repeated in humans with the same result by Horwitt et al., the very next year when Tappel et al. concluded that the deficiency of α-tocopherol might lead to high levels of oxidative lipid damage (Horwitt et al. 1956). The antioxidative effect of vitamin E could be seen in both *in vitro* and *in vivo* studies, due to the equal contribution of phenolic head as well as the phytyl tails (Burton and Ingold 1989). Since α-tocopherol is the most abundant vitamin E in the body, its activity as antioxidant and its role in protection from oxidative stress have been studied more extensively than other forms of vitamin E. Studies show that α-tocopherols are protective against atherosclerosis. In a study of α-tocopherol (Devaraj and Jialal 2005), the effect on important proinflammatory cytokine, tumor necrosis factor-alpha (TNFα), released from human monocytes, found that α-tocopherols inhibited the release of TNFα via inhibition of 5-lipoxygenase. Inhibition of 5-lipoxygenase significantly reduced TNFα mRNA and NFκB binding activity. Other studies (Meydani 2004) show how α-tocopherol inhibits the activation of endothelial cells stimulated by high levels of low-density lipoprotein cholesterol and pro-inflammatory cytokines. This inhibition is associated with the suppression of chemokines, the expression of cell surface adhesion molecules, and the adhesion of leukocytes to endothelial cells, all of which contribute to the development of lesions in the arterial wall. While the benefits of tocopherols have been studied for years, health benefits of the other seven forms of vitamin E are only recently being explored. Just like cholesterol, tocopherols also influence biophysical membrane characteristics such as fluidity (Sen et al. 2006).

During the last few years, research on tocotrienols is receiving more attention than tocopherols because tocotrienols have more potent antioxidative property than α-tocopherols (Serbinova et al. 1991; Serbinova and Packer 1994). However, the amount of tocotrienol research is still far less than the extensive work done on tocopherols.

21.3 COMPARISON OF TOCOTRIENOLS AND TOCOPHEROLS

There are at least eight isoforms commonly found to possess vitamin E's activity: α-, β-, γ-and δ-tocopherol; α-, β-, γ- and δ-tocotrienol (Figure 21.1). Tocotrienols differ from tocopherols by hav-

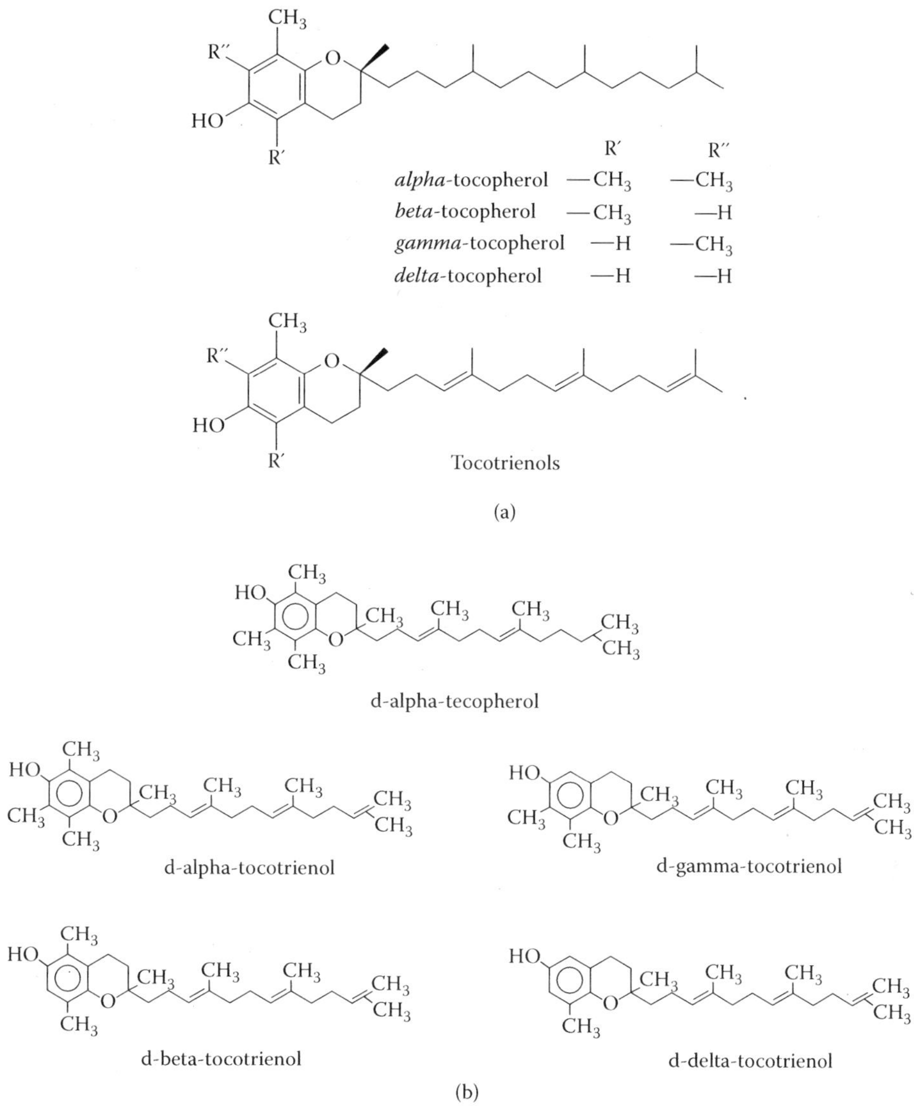

FIGURE 23.1 (a) Chemical structures of two different isoforms of vitamin E: tocopherol and tocotrienols. (b) Four different isoforms of tocotrienols: α, β, γ and δ, different by their methyl group position in their respective ring structure.

ing a farnesyl (isoprenoid) structure compared with a saturated phytyl side chain. The abundance of α-tocopherol in the living cells compared with other isoforms, and the maximum half life period of the same isoform may be the major cause of its importance among the various disciplines of clinical and basic research. It is well established that the antioxidative power of tocotrienols is 1600 times more potent than that of α-tocopherol (Serbinova and Packer 1994). The reason for tocotrienol's superior antioxidant power lies in the unsaturation in the aliphatic tail, which facilitates easier penetration into the tissue (Suzuki et al. 1993). These important findings make tocotrienols better therapeutic agents than tocopherols. It has already been proven by various research groups that tocotrienols possess neuroprotective, anti-cancer and also cholesterol lowering properties as compared with its other isoform, tocopherols.

Only tocotrienols at nanomolar (nM) concentration protect the neuronal cells from glutamate-induced cell death (Sen et al. 2000; Roy et al. 2002; Khanna et al. 2003). In a very interesting study,

Sen et al. showed that tocotrienols, but not tocopherols, inhibit the activation of pp60 (c-Src), which is a key regulator of glutamate-induced neuronal cell death (Sen et al. 2000). In another study, it was found that tocotrienols and not tocopherols protect the neurons from glutamate-induced 12-lipoxygenase (12-Lox) activation (Khanna et al. 2005). This 12-Lox plays an important role in the signal transduction pathway to kill the neurons. The molecular target for the neuroprotective effect of tocotrienols (mainly α-tocotrienol) is cytosol, and not the nucleus (Sen et al. 2000; Khanna et al. 2003). It is now well established that tocotrienols (mainly α-tocotrienol), and not tocopherols, possess potent neuroprotective properties (Khanna et al. 2005).

The anti-carcinogenic property of tocotrienols has been established. Many studies have shown that tocotrienols provide better protection against cancer than tocopherols do. In a mouse model, tocotrienols were compared with tocopherols, and interestingly, it was found that intraperitoneal (ip) administration of α- and γ- tocotrienols, and not the tocopherols, showed a slight life-prolonging effect in mice with transplanted tumors (Komiyama et al. 1989). Similar observation was found by Gould et al. in rats (Gould et al. 1991) for chemoprevention of chemically induced mammary tumors. Also, in a human study, it was shown that tocotrienols significantly suppressed growth of breast cancer cells in culture, whereas tocopherols failed to show similar action under identical conditions (Nesaretnam et al. 1995). In another study, it was shown that the anti-carcinogenic property of tocotrienols might be a better option than tamoxifen for breast cancer prevention (Guthrie et al. 1997). γ- and δ-tocotrienols are considered the most effective isoforms among the all eight isoforms of vitamin E, for a physiological role in modulating normal mammary gland growth, function and remodeling (McIntyre et al. 2000). Relative to tocopherols, tocotrienols are more potent suppressors of EGF-dependent normal mammary epithelial cell growth, the mechanism of which is by the deactivation of PKC-α, than tocopherols (Sylvester et al. 2002).

The hypocholesterolemic effect of tocotrienols is also found to be more potent than that of tocopherols. Due to the presence of three double bonds in the isoprenoid chain, tocotrienols can lower cholesterol levels much more effectively than tocopherols (Qureshi, Burger et al. 1986). Tocotrienols significantly reduced the concentration of plasma cholesterol and apolipoprotein B, platelet factor 4, and thromboxane B_2, indicating its ability to protect against platelet aggregation and endothelial dysfunction (Qureshi et al. 1991a; Qureshi et al. 1991b). It was found that tocotrienols and not tocopherols, suppress the HMG-CoA reductase, which directly inhibits the biosynthesis of cholesterol (Parker et al. 1993; Pearce et al. 1992; Pearce et al. 1994). Later on, the significant hypocholesterolemic effect of tocotrienols was compared with tocopherols in humans (Qureshi, Peterson et al. 2001; Qureshi, Sami et al. 2002), chicken (Qureshi and Peterson 2001), hypercholesterolemic rat (Iqbal et al. 2003), swine (Qureshi, Peterson et al. 2001) and as well as hamster's plasma (Raederstorff et al. 2002). In conclusion, researchers have shown that for lowering the cholesterol, tocotrienols are a better option than tocopherols.

21.3.1 Natural Sources of Tocotrienols

Tocotrienols are mainly found in the seed endosperm of almost all the monocots, such as wheat, rice, barley, oat, rye and sour cherry. Some dicots endosperm also contains tocotrienols in some Apiaceae species and in some Solanaeceae species, such as tobacco (Sen et al. 2006). But tocotrienols are not the only member of vitamin E present in the endosperm; they are always present as a mixture of tocopherol and tocotrienols. That is why tocotrienols are generally referred to as tocotrienols-rich factor (TRF). The ratio of tocotrienols to tocopherols in rice bran oil is 90:10, the maximum so far identified. In this particular oil, apart from the normal four isoforms of tocotrienols, two new isoforms are also found: desmo- and didesmo-tocotrienols. Crude palm oil extract from the fruit of Elaeis guineensis also contains a very high ratio of tocotrienol to tocopherol, almost 80:20. Normally, the major components of palm-derived TRF extract contain mainly 36% γ-tocotrienol, 26–30% α-tocotrienol and 20–22% α-tocopherol and 12% δ-tocotrienol (Kamat et al. 1997). See also Table 21.1.

TABLE 23.1
Tocopherol and Tocotrienol Contents (mg/Kg) in Some Seed Oils

	α–T*	β–T	γ–T	δ–T	α–TT*	β–TT	γ–TT	δ–TT
palm	89	–	18	–	128	–	323	72
soybean	100	8	1021	421	–	–	–	–
maize	282	54	1034	54	49	8	161	6
sunflower	670	27	11	1	–	–	–	–
rapeseed	202	65	490	9	–	–	–	–

* *T = tocopherol; TT = tocotrienol*

Data from: Gunstone, F.D., Harwood, J.L. and Padley, F.B. 1994. *The Lipid Handbook* (Second Edition), London: Chapman & Hall.

21.3.2 Cardioprotective Effects of Tocotrienols

Since cardiovascular diseases contribute to the major cause of morbidity and mortality, they are becoming a strain on the economy of many countries worldwide. Various factors have been identified as possible causes of different cardiac diseases such as heart failure and ischemic heart disease. However, although there are very few reports about the cardioprotective abilities of tocotrienol compared with the tocopherols, several recent studies indicate that tocotrienols can be used as potent cardioprotective agents (Das et al. 2006).

21.4 TOCOTRIENOLS AGAINST ATHEROSCLEROSIS

Atherosclerosis is the process by which the depositions of cholesterol plaque on the wall of blood vessels cause those vessels to become narrower and ultimately blocked by the fatty deposits. Atherosclerosis finally renders ischemic insult to the heart muscle and causes extensive damage to the heart tissue. The complete blockages of the arteries lead to myocardial infraction (MI). According to the World Health Organization, the major cause of death worldwide by the year 2020 will be acute coronary occlusion (Murray and Lopez 1997).

As mentioned earlier, the tocotrienols differ from tocopherols only in three double bonds in the isoprenoid chain, which appear to be essential for the inhibition of cholesterogenesis by higher cell penetration followed by better interaction with the deposited plaques (Qureshi, Burger et al. 1986). In some clinical trials with hyper-cholesterolemic patients, tocotrienols significantly reduced the serum cholesterols (Qureshi, Peterson et al. 2001). In another related clinical trial, tocotrienols lowered both the serum cholesterols, total cholesterol (TC), and, more interestingly the low-density-lipoprotein cholesterols (LDL) (Tan et al. 1991).

In the late 80s, it was found that the one of the major causes of lipid oxidation was the oxidation of low-density-lipoprotein. Therefore, Tan et al.'s (1991) observation drew many researchers' attention toward tocotrienols as a better anti-lipid oxidative agent. Later on, a diet rich in tocotrienols, especially dietary tocotrienols from a TRF of palm oil, reduced the concentration of plasma cholesterol and apolipoprotein B, platelet factor 4, and thromboxane B_2, indicating its ability to protect against platelet aggregation and endothelial dysfunction (Qureshi, Qureshi et al. 1991a; Qureshi, Peterson et al. 2001).

In mammalian cells, 3-hydroxy-3-methylglutaryl Coenzyme A (HMG CoA) reductase regulates the cholesterol production. Tocotrienols, mainly γ-isoform or the tocotrienols mixture, significantly suppressed the secretion of HMG CoA reductase, which ultimately lowered the production of cholesterols in the cells (Parker et al. 1993; Pearce et al. 1992; Pearce et al. 1994).). Another possible mechanism of protection from lipid peroxidation by tocotrienols was found from isoprenoid-mediated suppression of mevalonate synthesis depleting tumor tissues of two intermediate products, farnesyl pyrophosphate and geranylgeranyl pyrophosphate, which were incorporated post-translationally into growth control-associated proteins (Elson and Qureshi 1995). These observations led the researcher to compare tocotrienols with the statins group of medicines.

In one of the studies, Qureshi and Patterson (2001) showed that, when tocotrienols were applied with lovastatin or when lovastatin was compared with tocotrienol, there were no differences in terms of cholesterol-lowering power in chickens. Interestingly, apart from these two mechanisms of action, tocotrienols can also protect from the hypercholesterolemic phase by activating the conversion of low-density-lipoprotein (LDL) to high-density-lipoprotein (HDL) through inter phase VLDL-LDL and finally HDL (Qureshi and Patterson 2001a; Qureshi et al. 2001). In the hypercholesterolemic phase, it was also observed that either γ-tocotrienol or the tocotrienols mixture increased the level of HDL, which then interacts with LDL to reduce the concentration of LDL in the plasma (Qureshi et al. 2001a). HDL may also be converted by phagocytosis to lower the LDL. In a clinical trial, 100 mg/day of TRF derived from rice bran oil effectively lowered the serum cholesterol in hypercholesterolemic patients (Qureshi and Peterson 2001). In the same study, it was also shown that α-tocopherol induced the HMG CoA reductase and, for this reason, in higher doses of TRF, the opposite effect was observed compared with 100 mg/day of TRF (Qureshi and Peterson 2001). This study clearly shows that it is only tocotrienols that are responsible for lowering the serum cholesterol, and this cannot be achieved with tocopherols. In this study, tocopherols increased the cholesterol level by inducing HMG CoA reductase.

21.5 TOCOTRIENOLS AGAINST ISCHEMIC HEART DISEASE

Ischemia is a stage when there is no blood flow in tissue; as blood is the only carrier of air or oxygen, the under-supplied cell undergoes a lot of stress. When this situation arises in the heart, the tissues suffer from ischemic insult.

Apart from atherosclerotic plaque deposition, oxidative stress is also considered one of the major causes of ischemic heart disease. TRF has excellent free radical scavenging capacity (Kamat et al. 1997). Numerous studies (Kamat et al. 1997; Ikeda et al. 2003) show that it is a potent inhibitor of lipid peroxidation and protein peroxidation in rat microsomes and mitochondria. Among the different isomers of tocotrienols, γ-tocotrienol and, to a lesser extent α- and δ-tocotrienols, significantly inhibited oxidative damage to both lipids and proteins in rat brain mitochondria. Studies on the effect of γ-tocotrienols on endothelial nitric oxide synthase (eNOS) activity in spontaneously hypertensive rats have shown that upon treatment with antioxidant, γ-tocotrienol increased the nitric oxide (NO) activity and concomitantly reduced the blood pressure and enhanced total antioxidant status in plasma and blood vessels (Ikeda et al. 2003).

In general, TRF has significantly higher antioxidant activity than tocopherols. This can be explained by the structural difference between the saturated side chain of tocopherols and the unsaturated side chain of tocotrienols. The molecular mobility of polyenoic lipids in the membrane bilayer (composed mainly of unsaturated fatty acid) is much higher than that of saturated lipids, and hence tocotrienols are more mobile and less restricted in their interaction with lipid radicals in membranes than tocopherols. This is further supported by the higher effectiveness of tocotrienols in processes of oxidative stress such as in red blood cells where tocotrienols have more potency against oxidative haemolysis than α-tocopherols (Kamat et al. 1997). In an *in vitro* study, the potency of the free radical scavenging property of α-tocotrienol was found to be 1600 times more than for α-tocopherol (Serbinova and Packer 1994). In another study, such antioxidative property of γ-tocotrienols was responsible for protection of the heart in spontaneously hypertensive rats (Newaz et al. 2003).

Gamma-tocotrienols are found to activate the endothelial nitric oxide synthase (eNOS) expression (Ikeda et al. 2003). eNOS is considered to be one of the major sources of intracellular NO generation. NO effects vasodilatation and protects the heart from the ischemic phase. Due to the eNOS regulating property, γ-tocotrienol is now considered an important pharmacological preconditioning agent (Newaz et al. 2003).

In a fairly recent study, it was shown for the first time that the beneficial effects of tocotrienol derived from palm oil were due to its ability to reduce c-Src activation, which was linked with the stabilization of proteasomes, mainly 20S and 26S (Das et al. 2005). Tocotrienols have extremely short half-lives; after oral ingestion, they are not recognized by γ-tocotrienol transport protein, which also accounts for their low bioavailability. For this reason, TRF was used in an acute experiment to determine its immediate effects on the ischemic-reperfused myocardium. The results indicate that tocotrienol readily blocks the ischemia-reperfusion-mediated increase in Src kinase activation and proteasome inactivation, thereby providing cardioprotection (Das et al. 2005). After this observation, in a continuing study with gavaging (oral dosing) of the TRF (derived from palm oil) for 15 days showed protection of the heart from ischemia-reperfusion injury in rats (Das et al. 2005). In this chronic experiment, the key mechanism of action was shown as the inhibition of Src activation by TRF. Myocardial ischemia/reperfusion caused an induction of the expression of cSrc protein (Hattori et al. 2001), and inhibition of cSrc with PPI reduced the extent of cellular injury. The ability of TRF to block the increased phosphorylation of cSrc appears to play a crucial role in its ability to protect the heart from ischemia reperfusion injury.

21.5 CONCLUSION

It should be clear from the preceding discussion that tocotrienols can provide cardioprotection not only by their cholesterol lowering property or by their reducing oxidative stress but also through their ability to perform redox signaling by potentiating an anti-death signal through the reduction of proapototic factor. So, c Src has been found to play an important role in stabilization of proteasome and cardioprotection. Ischemia/reperfusion reduces both 20S- and 26S- proteasome activities, an effect prevented by tocotrienol pretreatment. Out of four different isoforms of tocotrienols, α-tocotrienols and γ-tocotrienols are considered to be the effective isoforms that possess cardioprotective abilities. Apart from the anti-atherosclerotic property of tocotrienols, they could reverse ischemia/reperfusion-mediated cardiac dysfunction. Overall observations warrant that tocotrienol isomers can be used as cardioprotective drugs in the near future.

REFERENCES

Burton, G.W. and Ingold, K.U. 1989. Vitamin E as an *in vitro* and *in vivo* antioxidant. *Ann NY Acad Sci*, 570, 7–22.

Das, S., Nesaretnam, K. and Das, D.K. 2007. Tocotrienols in cardioprotection. *Vitam Horm*, 75, 285–299.

Das, S., Powell, S.R., Wang, P., Divald, A., Nasaretnam, K., Tosaki, A., Cordis, G.A., Maulik, N. and Das, D.K. 2005. Cardioprotection with palm tocotrienol: Antioxidant activity of tocotrienol is linked with its ability to stabilize proeasomes. *Am J Physiol Heart Circ Physiol*, 289, H361–H367.

Devaraj, S. and Jialal, I. 2005. Alpha-tocopherol decreases tumor necrosis factor-alpha mRNA and protein from activated human monocytes by inhibition of 5-lipoxygenase. *Free Radic Biol Med*, 38, 1212–1220.

Edem, D.O. 2002. Palm oil: Biochemical, physiological, nutritional, hematological, and toxicological aspects: A review. *Plant Foods Hum Nutr*, 57, 319–41.

Elson, C.E. and Qureshi, A.A. 1995. coupling the cholesterol- and tumor-suppressive actions of palm oil to the impact of its minor constituents on 3-hydroxy-3-methylglutaryl coenzyme A reductase activity. *Prostaglandins, Leukotrienes and Essential Fatty Acids*, 52, 205–207.

Gould, M.N., Haag, J.D., Kennan, W.S., Tanner, M.A. and Elson, C.E. 1991. A comparison of tocopherol and tocotrienol for the chemoprevention of chemically induced rat mammary tumors. *Am J Clin Nutr*, 53(4 Suppl), 1068S–1070S.

Gunstone, F.D., Harwood, J.L. and Padley, F.B. 1994. *The Lipid Handbook (Second Edition)*, London: Chapman & Hall.

Guthrie, N., Gapor, A., Chambers, A.F. and Carroll, K.K. 1997. Inhibition of proliferation of estrogen receptor negative MDA-MB-435 and positive MCF-7 human breast cancer cells by palm oil tocotrienols and tamoxifen, alone and in combination. *J Nutr*, 127, 544S–548S.

Hattori, R., Otani, H., Uchiyama, T., Imamura, H., Cui, J., Maulik, N., Cordis, G.A., Zhu, L. and Das, D.K. 2001. Src tyrosine kinase is the trigger but not the mediator of ischemic preconditioning. *Am J Physiol Heart Circ Physiol*, 281, H1066–H1074.

Horwitt, M.K., Harvey, C.C., Duncan, G.D. and Wilson, W.C. 1956. Effects of limited tocopherol intake in man with relationships to erythrocyte hemolysis and lipid oxidations. *Am J Clin Nutr*, 4, 408–419.

Ikeda, S., Tohyama, T., Yoshimura, H., Hamamura, K., Abe, K. and Yamashita, K. 2003. Dietary alpha-tocopherol decreases alpha-tocotrienol but not gamma-tocotrienol concentration in rats. *J Nutr*, 133, 428–434.

Iqbal, J., Minhajuddin, M and Beg, Z.H. 2003. Suppression of 7,12-dimethylbenz[alpha] anthracene-induced carcinogenesis and hypercholesterolemia in rats by tocotrienol-rich fraction isolated from rice bran oil. *Eur J Cancer Prev*, 12, 447–453.

Kamat, J.P., Sarma, H.D., Devasagayam, T.P., Nesaretnam, K. and Basiron, Y. 1997. Tocotrienols from palm oil as effective inhibitors of protein oxidation and lipid peroxidation in rat liver microsomes. *Mol Cell Biochem*,170, 131–137.

Kamimura, M. 1977. Physiology and clinical use of vitamin E (author's transl), *Hokkaido Igaku Zasshi*, 52, 185–188.

Khanna, S., Roy, S., Ryu, H., Bahadduri, P., Swaan, P.W., Ratan, R.R. and Sen, C.K. 2003. Molecular basis of vitamin E action: Tocotrienol modulates 12-lipoxygenase, a key mediator of glutamate-induced neurodegeneration. *J Biol Chem*, 278, 43508–43515.

Khanna, S., Roy. S., Slivka, A., Craft, T.K., Chaki, S., Rink, C., Notestine, M.A., DeVries, A.C., Parinandi, N.L. and Sen, C.K. 2005. Neuroprotective properties of the natural vitamin E alpha-tocotrienol. *Stroke*, 36, 2258–2264.

Komiyama, K., Iizuka, K., Yamaoka, M., Watanabe, H., Tsuchiya, N. and Umezawa, I. 1989. Studies on the biological activity of tocotrienols. *Chem Pharm Bull* (Tokyo), 37, 1369–1371.

Krinsky, N.I. 1992. Mechanism of action of biological antioxidants. *Proc Soc Exp Biol Med*, 200, 248–254.

McIntyre, B.S., Briski, K.P., Tirmenstein, M.A., Fariss, M.W., Gapor, A. and Sylvester, P.W. 2000. Antiproliferative and apoptotic effects of tocopherols and tocotrienols on normal mouse mammary epithelial cells. *Lipids*, 35, 171–180.

Meydani, M. 2004. Vitamin E modulation of cardiovascular disease. *Ann N Y Acad Sci*, 1031, 271–279.

Murray, C.J. and Lopez, A.D. 1997. Alternate projections of mortality and disability by cause 1990–2020: Global burden of disease study. *Lancet*, 349, 1498–1504.

Nesaretnam, K., Guthrie, N., Chambers, A.F. and Carroll, K.K. 1995. Effect of tocotrienols on the growth of a human breast cancer cell line in culture. *Lipids*, 30, 1139–1143.

Newaz, M.A., Yousefipour, Z., Nawal, N. and Adeeb, N. 2003. Nitric oxide synthase activity in blood vessels of spontaneously hypertensive rats: Antioxidant protection by gamma–tocotrienol. *J Physiol Pharmacol*, 54, 319–327.

Packer, L. 1992. Interactions among antioxidants in health and disease. Vitamin E and the redox cycle. *Proc Soc Exp Biol Med*, 200, 271–276.

Papas, A. 1999. *The vitamin E Factor: The miraculous antioxidant for the prevention and treatment of heart disease, cancer, and aging*. New York: Harper Collins.

Parker, R.A., Pearce, B.C., Clark, R.W., Gordon, D.A. and Wright, J.J. 1993. Tocotrienols regulate cholesterol production in mammalian cells by post–transcriptional suppression of 3-hydroxy-3-methylglutarylco-enzyme-A reductase. *J Biol Chem*, 268, 11230–11238.

Pearce, B.C., Parker, R.A., Deason, M.E., Dischino, D.D., Gillespie, E., Qureshi, A.A., Volk, K. and Wright, J.J. 1994. Inhibitors of cholesterol biosynthesis. 2. Hypocholesterolemic and antioxidant activities of benzopyran and tetrahydronaphthalene analogues of the tocotrienols. *J Medicinal Chem*, 37, 526–541.

Pearce, B.C., Parker, R.A., Deason, M.E., Qureshi, A.A. and Wright, J.J. 1992. Hypocholesterolemic activity of synthetic and natural tocotrienols. *J Medicinal Chem*, 35, 3595–3606.

Qureshi, A.A. and Peterson, D.M. 2001. The combined effects of novel tocotrienols and lovastatin on lipid metabolism in chickens. *Atherosclerosis*, 156, 39–47.

Qureshi, A.A., Burger, W.C., Peterson D.M. and Elson C.E. 1986. The structure of an inhibitor of cholesterol biosynthesis isolated from barley. *J Biol Chem*, 261, 10544–10550.

Qureshi, A.A., Peterson, D.M., Hasler-Rapacz, J.O. and Rapacz, J. 2001. Novel tocotrienols of rice bran suppress cholesterogenesis in hereditary hypercholesterolemic swine. *J Nutr*, 131, 223–230.

Qureshi, A.A., Qureshi, N., Hasler-Rapacz, J.O., Weber, F.E., Chaudhary, V., Crenshaww, T.D., Gapor, A., Ong, A.S., Chong, Y.H., Peterson, D. and Rapacz, J. 1991. Dietary tocotrienols reduce concentrations of plasma cholesterol, apolipoprotein B, thromboxane B_2, and platelet factor 4 in pigs with inherited hyperlipidemias. *Am J Clin Nutr*, 53(4), 1042S–1046S.

Qureshi, A.A., Qureshi, N., Wright, J.J., Shen, Z., Kramer, G., Gapor, A., Chong, Y.H., DeWitt, G., Ong, A. and Peterson, D.M. 1991. Lowering of serum cholesterol in hypercholesterolemic humans by tocotrienols (palmvitee). *Am J Clin Nutr.*, 53, 1021S–1026S.

Qureshi, A.A., Sami, S.A., Salser, W.A. and Khan, F.A. 2002. Dose-dependent suppression of serum cholesterol by tocotrienol-rich fraction (TRF25) of rice bran in hypercholesterolemic humans. *Atherosclerosis*, 161, 199–207.

Qureshi, A.A., Sami, S.A., Salser, W.A. and Khan, F.A. 2001. Synergistic effect of tocotrienol-rich fraction (TRF(25)) of rice bran and lovastatin on lipid parameters in hypercholesterolemic humans. *J Nutr Biochem*, 12, 318–329.

Raederstorff, D., Elste, V., Aebischer, C. and Weber, P. 2002. Effect of either gamma-tocotrienol or a tocotrienol mixture on the plasma lipid profile in hamsters. *Ann Nutr Metab*, 46, 17–23.

Roy, S., Lado, B.H., Khanna, S. and Sen, C.K. 2002. Vitamin E sensitive genes in the developing rat fetal brain: A high-density oligonucleotide micro array analysis. *FEBS Lett*, 530, 17–23.

Sen, C.K., Khanna, S. and Roy, S. 2004. Tocotrienol: The natural vitamin E to defend the nervous system? *Ann NY Acad Sci*, 1031, 127–142.

Sen, C.K., Khanna, S. and Roy, S. 2006. Tocotrienols: Vitamin E beyond tocopherols. *Life Sci*, 78, 2088–2098.

Sen, C.K., Khanna, S., Roy, S. and Packer, L. 2000. Molecular basis of vitamin E action. Tocotrienol potently inhibits glutamate-induced pp60(c-Src) kinase activation and death of HT4 neuronal cells. *J Biol Chem*, 275, 13049–13055.

Serbinova, E., Kagan, V., Han, D. and Packer, L. 1991. Free radical recycling and intramembrane mobility in the antioxidant properties of alpha-tocopherol and alpha-tocotrienol. *Free Radic Biol Med*, 10, 263–275.

Serbinova, E., Khwaja, S. and Catudioc, J. 1992. Palm oil vitamin E protects against ischemia/reperfusion injury in the isolated perfused Langendorff heart. *Nutr Res*, 12, S203–S215.

Serbinova, E.A. and Packer, L. 1994. Antioxidant properties of alpha-tocopherol and alpha-tocotrienol. *Meth Enzymol*, 234, 354–366.

Suzuki, Y.J., Tsuchiya. M., Wassall. S.R., Choo, Y.M., Govil, G., Kagan, V.E. and Packer, L. 1993. Structural and dynamic membrane properties of alpha-tocopherol and alpha-tocotrienol: Implication to the molecular mechanism of their antioxidant potency. *Biochemistry*, 32, 10692–10699.

Sylvester, P.W., Nachnani, A., Shah, S. and Briski, K.P. 2002. Role of GTP-binding proteins in reversing the antiproliferative effects of tocotrienols in preneoplastic mammary epithelial cells. *Asia Pacif J Clin Nutr*, 11(7), S452–S459.

Tan, D.T., Khor, H.T., Low, W.H., Ali, A. and Gapor, A. 1991. Effect of a palm-oil–vitamin E concentrate on the serum and lipoprotein lipids in humans. *Am J Clin Nutr*, 53(4), 1027S–1030S.

Tappel, A. L. 1954. Studies of the mechanism of vitamin E action. II. Inhibition of unsaturated fatty acid oxidation catalyzed by hematin compounds. *Arch Biochem Biophys*, 50, 473–485.

Tappel, A L. 1955. Studies of the mechanism of vitamin E action. III. *In vitro* copolymerization of oxidized fats with protein. *Arch Biochem*, 54, 266–280.

Tappel, A.L. 1953. The inhibition of hematin-catalyzed oxidations by alpha-tocopherol. *Arch Biochem Biophys*, 47, 223–225.

Theriault, A., Chao, J.T., Wang, Q., Gapor, A. and Adeli, K. 1999. Tocotrienol: A review of its therapeutic potential. *Clin Biochem*, 32, 309–319.

Part G

Metabolism and Absorption

22 Absorption and Disposition of Tocotrienols

Kah-Hay Yuen, Bee-Hong Ng and Jia-Woei Wong

CONTENTS

22.1 INTRODUCTION

In most instances, except in cases where the drug can be applied directly to the affected tissues, such as a skin infection, drug therapy entails using the blood as a transport medium to deliver the drug to its site of action. Therefore, the absorption of the administered drug into the systemic blood circulation can be an important determinant of its therapeutic efficacy. It cannot be assumed that anything taken orally is well absorbed. This applies to the drugs, nutraceutical compounds or the foods we eat. Indeed, it is a case of we are what we absorb rather than what we eat.

Studies have shown that some molecules, including those from natural products, are inherently poorly bioavailable via the oral route. For example, the oral bioavailability of 9-methoxycanthin-6-one from the Malaysian herbal plant *Eurycoma longifolia* J. was found to be less than 1% in studies using rats (Tan et al. 2002). Such poor oral bioavailability was also observed with andrographolide from the herb *Andrographis paniculata* (unpublished data). A similar rat study on sinensitin from another herbal plant, *Orthosiphon stamineus*, also showed that its oral bioavailability was less than 20% (Loon et al. 2005). Considering the results of these studies, therefore, it cannot be overemphasized that the absorption characteristics of a potentially useful compound, whether synthesized in the laboratory or of herbal origin, must be carefully assessed before being made available as a oral product for human use. In studies, particularly those using cultured cells or where the drug is administered intravenously without involving an absorption step, a compound may show potential therapeutic benefits. However, if its oral bioavailability is poor, similar results might not be attainable if the study is repeated in whole-animal or human experiments by giving the compound via the oral route.

22.2 FACTORS AFFECTING ABSORPTION AND BIOAVAILABILITY OF THE TOCOTRIENOLS

22.2.1 Route of Administration

Despite the recent interest in tocotrienols, there is a paucity of information regarding their absorption, especially via different routes of administration. Tocotrienols, like α-tocopherol, exist as an oily liquid. Due to poor aqueous solubility and miscibility, their bioavailability can be poor and erratic.

Yap et al. conducted a study to evaluate the absorption of α-, γ- and δ-tocotrienols administered as an oily mixture via the oral, intraperitoneal and intramuscular routes in rats. It was found that all the three tocotrienols were negligibly absorbed via the intramuscular and intraperitoneal routes, with levels essentially similar to baseline concentrations. (Yap et al. 2003) The negligible absorption could be due to a lack of partitioning of the compounds out of the lipidic vehicle for absorption in the peritoneal compartment or muscle. These two routes of administration should therefore be avoided in animal studies of the tocotrienols. However, a review of the literature revealed that the intraperitoneal route has been used in some studies. For example, in a study to evaluate the HMG-CoA reductase activity of the tocotrienols in hamsters, Khor and Ng (1999) administered the compounds intraperitoneally. It is thus not surprising that they could not determine the tocotrienols in the serum and liver. In a subsequent study in which the tocotrienols were also given intraperitoneally to hamsters, Khor et al. (2000) reported that the inhibitory effect of the tocotrienols on the HMG-CoA reductase activity tended to decline with increase in the dose level. This somewhat unusual inverse activity versus dose relationship might be an artifact, since the tocotrienols are essentially not absorbed via the intraperitoneal route.

Compared with the intraperitoneal and intramuscular routes, the tocotrienols appeared to be better absorbed orally (Figure 22.1a and Figure 22.1b). Following oral administration to the rats, plasma concentrations of the tocotrienols showed a rapid increase, reaching peak concentration at approximately 3 hours after dosing and then declining gradually thereafter (Yap et al. 2003). However, the oral absorption of the three tocotrienols was found to be incomplete. The absolute oral bioavailability of α-tocotrienol was found to be approximately 27.7%, while that of δ- and γ-tocotrienols was even lower, being approximately 9.1% and 8.5% respectively. These values were estimated by comparing the plasma levels (more specifically, the area under the plasma concentration versus time curve) obtained after oral administration with those obtained after intravenous injection of the tocotrienols as an emulsion.

22.2.2 Influence of Food and Biodiscrimination in Oral Absorption of Tocotrienols

It is well established that the oral bioavailability of lipophilic drugs can be significantly increased when administered with food, especially fat-rich meals. Hence, it is recommended that fat-soluble vitamins (A, D, E, K) should be taken after a meal to ensure better absorption.

In a study conducted on healthy human volunteers, Yap et al. (2001) reported that the bioavailability of α-, γ- and δ-tocotrienols was increased approximately 3-fold when administered with a high-fat breakfast, according to the recommendations of USP23-NF18, supplement 5. Moreover, the bioavailability of the tocotrienols tended to be more variable when taken in the fasted state than in taking them with food. Interestingly, a secondary peak was observed in the plasma concentration profiles of the tocotrienols in the fed state, suggesting that they exhibit entero-hepatic cycling.

Lipophilic drugs administered orally are known to undergo intraluminal processing to form mixed micelles with bile salts, a process essential for their absorption (MacGregor et al. 1997). Since food can stimulate the secretion of bile salts, their absorption will be increased when taken with a meal. Such processing is absent in intramuscular and intraperitoneal administrations, which may explain the negligible absorption of the tocotrienols administered via these two routes.

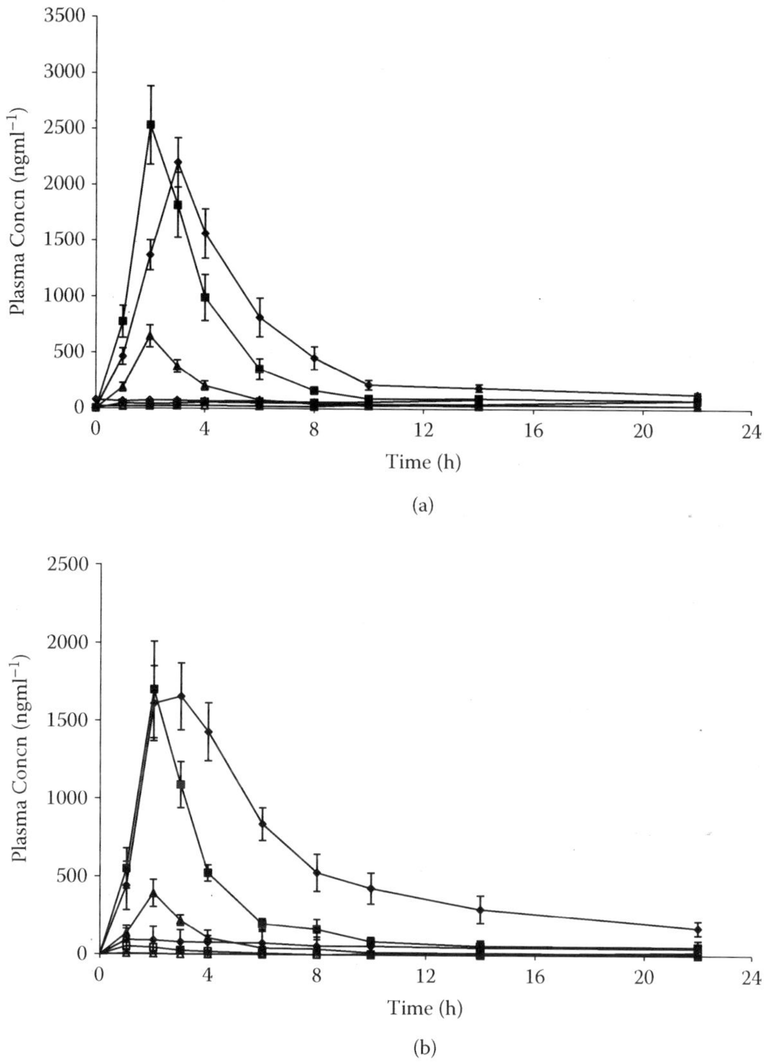

FIGURE 22.1 Plasma concentration–time profiles (mean ± s.e.m., n=6) of α-, γ- and δ-tocotrienols after (a) intraperitoneal and oral and (b) intramuscular and oral administration of a single dose of 5 mg mixed tocotrienols (approx. 1.50, 2.75 and 0.75 mg of α, γ and δ-tocotrienol, respectively). ◇ = intraperitoneal α-tocotrienol, ◆ = oral α-tocotrienol, □ = intraperitoneal γ-tocotrienol, ■ = oral γ-tocotrienol, △ = intraperitoneal δ-tocotrienol, ▲ = oral δ-tocotrienol.

Yap et al. (2001) also noted that, while the dose of γ-tocotrienol was almost twice that of α-tocotrienol, the plasma levels obtained were essentially comparable in both the fasted and fed states (Figure 22.2). This could be attributed to γ-tocotrienol's having a larger distribution volume or lower oral bioavailability or a combination of both. However, referring to the later study by Yap et al. (2003) conducted in rats, γ-tocotrienol was found to have a lower oral absolute bioavailability of approximately 9.1% compared with 27.7% observed with α-tocotrienol. Thus, it appears that there is biodiscrimination in the absorption of the tocotrienols. The absolute oral bioavailability of δ-tocotrienol was also reported to be low, being quite similar to that of γ-tocotrienol, with a value of about only 8.5%.

From studies using thoracic duct-cannulated rats, Ikeda and coworkers demonstrated that not only were the tocotrienols transported via the lymphatic system after oral absorption, but α-tocotri-

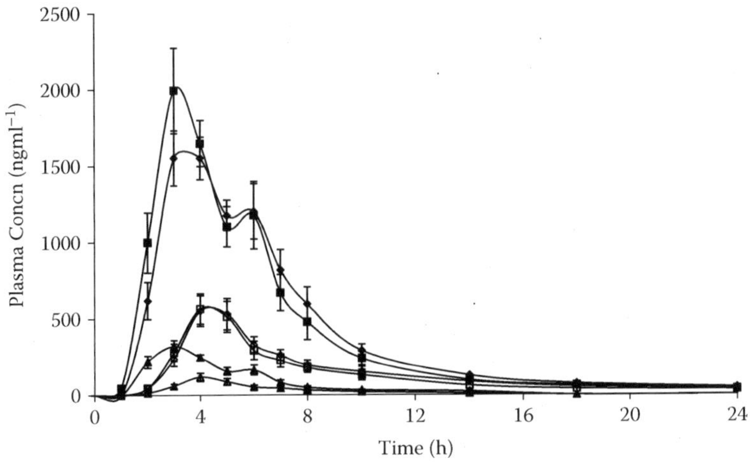

FIGURE 22.2 Plasma concentration–time profiles (mean ± s.e.m., n=8) of α-, γ- and δ-tocotrienols after oral administration of a single dose of 300 mg mixed tocotrienols. ◇ = α-tocotrienol without food, ◆ = α-tocotrienol with food, □ = γ-tocotrienol without food, ■ = γ-tocotrienol with food, △ = δ-tocotrienol without food, ▲ = δ-tocotrienol with food.

enol was preferentially absorbed over γ- and δ-tocotrienols (Ikeda et al. 1996). The authors suggested that the mechanism of preferential absorption of the tocotrienols might be attributed to differences in their micellar solubility, affinity for the intestinal brush border membranes, their incorporation into chylomicrons or a combination of these processes, which in turn are related to the lipophilicity of the molecules. Of the three tocotrienols studied, the α-isoform has three methyl groups on the chromanol ring structure, whereas the γ- and δ-isoforms have two and one each respectively. Thus, α-tocotrienol is most lipophilic followed by γ- and δ-tocotrienols. Since lipophilicity can affect the passage of a molecule across biological membranes and its transport into the intestinal lymphatic system, the higher lipophilicity of the α-tocotrienol might in part explain the higher bioavailability obtained with α-tocotrienol compared with γ- and δ-isomers.

Such biodiscrimination has also been reported with the tocopherols. Plasma and tissue concentrations of α-tocopherol were observed to be two to three times higher than those of γ-tocopherol, even though the diet of the subjects studied contained more γ- than α-tocopherol (Bieri and Evarts, 1973). This discrepancy was attributed to the presence of α-tocopherol transfer protein (ATTP), which has high selectivity in regulating the secretion of α-tocopherol from the liver as well as maintaining its plasma concentrations (Kayden and Traber, 1993). It was demonstrated that the methyl group at position 5 of the chromanol ring structure of the α-tocopherol was important for recognition by this regulatory protein (Hosomi et al. 1997).

The importance of ATTP in regulating the absorption and distribution of α-tocopherol is borne out by observations that ATTP-deficient mice are infertile (Terasawa et al. 2000) and suffer from α-tocopherol deficiency even in the presence of dietary α-tocopherol (Jishage et al. 2001). However, ATTP has approximately eightfold lower binding affinity for α-tocotrienol (Hosomi et al. 1997) and its role in the absorption and distribution of α-tocotrienol and its other isoforms remains unclear. Interestingly, supplementation of ATTP knockout female mice with α-tocotrienol was able to restore their fertility (Khanna et al. 2005), suggesting that the absorption and distribution of α-tocotrienol are not dependent on ATTP. In a study to investigate the postprandial fate of the tocotrienols, Fairus (2006) was able to determine the presence of α-, δ- and γ-tocotrienols in various circulating lipoprotein fractions in the plasma. The concentrations of the tocotrienols in the circulating triacylglycerol-rich particles, low density lipoproteins and high density lipoproteins were observed to increase with an increase in the dose of the tocotrienols. These lipoprotein fractions may play a role in the distribution of the tocotrienols to various tissues and organs.

22.2.3 Influence of Transporters and Metabolic Enzymes in the Gastrointestinal Tract

Oral absorption of drugs can also be influenced by specific counter transporters and enzymes present in the endothelial cells lining the gastrointestinal tract. A glycoprotein called P-gp, found on the apical surface of the endothelial cells, functions like a extrusion pump that will counter-transport absorbed molecules back into the gastrointestinal lumen. Also present in the endothelial cells is a phase 1 metabolic enzyme, CYP3A4, which can metabolize the absorbed molecules. Hence, both P-gp and CYP3A4 act synergistically as a barrier to the absorption of drugs (Mizuno et al. 2003; Benet et al. 2004) They share many common substrates with diverse chemical structures and pharmacological activities. However, both are saturable, with potential for drug interaction when two or more common substrates are given concomitantly. For example, ketoconazole is a well known substrate for both P-gp and CYP3A4. When given with another common substrate, the bioavailability of both compounds can be mutually enhanced. In a study using rats, the bioavailability of α-, γ- and δ-tocotrienols was found to be increased when co-administered with ketoconazole, providing evidence that the tocotrienols might also be a substrate of P-gp and/or CYP3A4 (Yap et al. 2003).

22.3 DISPOSITION AND DISTRIBUTION OF THE TOCOTRIENOLS

22.3.1 Pharmacokinetics

Few studies have specifically addressed the fate of the tocotrienols after their administration or absorption into the body. In a study to investigate the influence of the route of administration on the absorption and disposition of α-, δ- and γ-tocotrienols in rats, Yap et al. (2003) reported that intravenous administration of the compounds (in an emulsion form) yielded a biphasic log concentration versus time plot for all three tocotrienols, being better described by a classic two-compartment pharmacokinetic model (Figure 22.3). There was an initial rapid decline in the plasma concentrations due to redistribution of the compounds from the plasma compartment to other tissues and organs. This was followed by a gradual decline in the plasma levels after an equilibrium has been achieved between the compounds in the plasma compartment and the tissues or organs. The biological half-lifes of the three tocotrienols calculated from this terminal log-linear part of the plots were quite comparable, being 7.5 hours for α-tocotrienol, 7.0 hours for γ-tocotrienol and 7.4 hours for δ-tocotrienol.

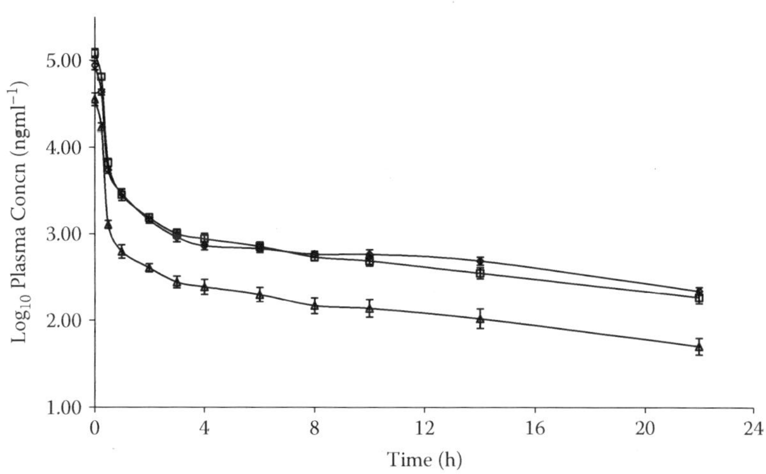

FIGURE 22.3 Log_{10} plasma concentration–time profiles (mean ± s.e.m., n=6) of α-, γ- and δ-tocotrienols after intravenous administration of a single dose of 5 mg mixed tocotrienols (approx. 1.50, 2.75 and 0.75 mg of α-, γ- and δ-tocotrienol, respectively). ◇ = α-tocotrienol, □ = γ-tocotrienol, △ = δ-tocotrienol.

In another study conducted on eight human volunteers to investigate the pharmacokinetics and bioavailability of the tocotrienols under fed and fasted conditions, the estimated biological half-lifes of the tocotrienols reported were relatively shorter than those of the rat study (Yap et al. 2001; Yap et al. 2003). The half-lifes for α-, δ- and γ-tocotrienols estimated from the human subjects were 4.4, 2.3 and 4.3 hours, respectively.

22.3.2 Distribution of Tocotrienols in Various Tissues

Several papers have been published on the tissue distribution of the tocotrienols in animal studies. However, discrepancies were observed among the few published studies, which could partly be attributed to the different animal models being employed and the preparations used.

Various studies suggested that the distribution of tocotrienols was tissue-specific. In the study by Cheng (2005) that involved oral administration of 18.8 mg mixed-tocotrienols to 10 male Sprague-Dawley rats for 15 consecutive days, the distribution of total tocotrienols was highest in the heart. A 28-fold increase in the α-tocotrienol alone was observed as compared with the control group, achieving a concentration of 4.62 ± 2.22 μg/g while the concentrations of γ- and δ-tocotrienols were 2.23 ± 0.56 and 0.52 ± 0.29 μg/g, respectively. This was followed by the skin, liver, muscle and eyeball, while the brain contained the least amount of total tocotrienols. As for the skin, the concentrations of α- and γ-tocotrienols achieved were 4.24 ± 2.54 μg/g and 2.43 ± 1.07μg/g after supplementation, recording a respective 28 and 26 folds increase compared to the control group. The concentration of δ-tocotrienol was 0.67 μg/g. Feeding the rats with mixed tocotrienols also caused a marked increase in the concentrations of α-, γ- and δ-tocotrienols in the liver, achieving values of approximately 4.85 ± 1.57 μg/g, 1.21 ± 0.52 μg/g and 0.38 ± 0.14 μg/g, respectively. Accumulation of higher amounts of tocotrienols to the heart and liver could be attributed to both tissues being highly perfused and hence more tocotrienols preferentially accumulated in these tissues. Okabe and coworkers (2002) reported a similar observation, that is, intragastric administration of an emulsion containing 200 mg of mixed tocotrienols showed the highest accumulation in these two tissues.

On the other hand, the findings by Ikeda and coworkers (2001) were different to a certain extent in terms of the relative tissue distribution. Negligible amounts of tocotrienols were detected in the liver and heart, while the highest accumulation was observed in the skin. The results pertaining to the distribution of tocotrienols to the skin are consistent with those reported by Podda et al. (1996), Ikeda et al. (2000), and Ikeda et al. (2003). Significant accumulation of tocotrienols in the skin was reported by Podda after feeding hairless mice with standard mouse chow which contained tocopherols and tocotrienols (Podda et al. 1996). In comparison, negligible accumulation was observed in the brain, heart, kidney and liver. Although poorly perfused, the skin still received significant amount of tocotrienols and this could be attributed to its role as a storage site for lipid-soluble drugs such as tocotrienols. Moreover, Ikeda et al. (2003) suggested that the tocotrienols were transferred primarily from chylomicrons by lipoprotein lipase to be deposited in the skin before selection by α-tocopherol transfer protein in the liver for subsequent distribution. The transfer of tocotrienols from chylomicrons was further enhanced by the inherent molecular structure of tocotrienols, that is, possessing an unsaturated phytyl chain (Ikeda et al. 2003).

Adipose tissue has also been shown to be the target tissue for tocotrienol accumulation (Hayes et al. 1993; Ikeda et al. 2001; Kawakami et al. 2007). Hayes et al. (1993) reported that tocotrienols accumulated mainly in the adipose tissue of hamsters after supplementation with a purified diet containing 223 ppm of tocotrienols for 11 to 15 weeks (Hayes et al. 1993). Distribution of tocotrienols in other tissues such as heart, liver, brain, retina, spleen, kidney, pancreas, muscle and testes was very low. The low accumulation in various organs was not unexpected in view of the preparation used by Hayes (1993), which contained a high percentage of tocopherol, being approximately 24% or 70 ppm in comparison with that used in the study by Cheng (2005), which contained only 4.3%. Khanna et al. (2005) reported that co-supplementation of α-tocopherols and α-tocotrienols would compromise tissue delivery of α-tocotrienol due to the competition between both compounds for binding to α-tocopherol transfer protein and subsequent distribution into various tissues (Khanna et al. 2005; Ikeda et al. 2003). Moreover, Hosomi and coworkers (1997) reported that the relative affinity of α-tocotrienol for α-tocopherol transfer protein was approximately 12% of that of α-tocopherol. Hence, distribution of α-tocotrienol to tissue would be lower when it was administered with α-tocopherol compared to when it was given alone. Kawakami et al. (2007) even suggested that the distribution of tocotrienol is dependent on its affinity for α-tocopherol transfer protein and based on the cytochrome P450 expression level in each organ. In their study conducted in rats using rice bran tocotrienol, which contained approximately 23% of tocopherol, γ-tocotrienol was predominantly accumulated in adipose tissue and was found at comparatively high level in the skin, lung, kidney and muscle. In comparison, little γ-tocotrienol was found in the liver, spleen and aorta.

In the study by Cheng (2005), the brain of the supplemented rats received the lowest tocotrienol distribution among the organs and tissues studied. The concentration of α-tocotrienol in the brain of rats supplemented with tocotrienols was increased by fourfold in comparison with the non-supplemented group, while, for other tissues, the increase was at least tenfold. The observation with regards to the distribution of tocotrienols to the brain is consistent among most published studies whereby the brain accumulated one of the lowest concentrations of tocotrienols (Cheng, 2005; Hayes et al. 1993; Okabe et al. 2002; Podda et al. 1996; Ikeda et al. 2001; Ikeda et al. 2003; Kawakami et al. 2007). This could be attributed to the blood brain barrier that separates the brain parenchyma from the systemic circulation and may act as a barrier to limit the penetration of drugs across the tight junction into the brain. Moreover, P-gp lining the apical surface of the endothelial cells of the brain capillaries may limit uptake of tocotrienols from blood circulation into the brain by acting as an efflux pump as mentioned previously.

Until recently, little has been known about distribution of tocotrienols into the eyeballs, as it has not been reported except for the study by Hayes, which reported no tocotrienol was present in the retina of hamsters after supplementation (Hayes et al. 1993). This is in contrast with the results obtained by Cheng (2005). The concentration of α-tocotrienol was increased by 22-fold, with a value of 1.09 ± 0.26 μg/g, while the concentrations of γ- and δ- were 0.18 ± 0.05 μg/g and 0.05 μg/g, respectively, after supplementation with 18.8 mg of mixed tocotrienols.

As for the individual isomer of tocotrienol, Cheng (2005) observed that α-tocotrienol was preferentially accumulated in the tissues compared with the other isomers of tocotrienols, although the dose of γ-tocotrienol administered to the rats was higher than the α-tocotrienol. This could be attributed to the higher lipophilicity of the α-isomer as mentioned previously. The concentrations of α-tocotrienol in all six tissues investigated (liver, heart, skin, muscle, eyeballs, brains) were relatively higher than γ- and δ-tocotrienols.

22.4 DELIVERY SYSTEMS FOR TOCOTRIENOLS

22.4.1 Lipid Absorption and Lipid-Based Formulation

Tocotrienols are highly lipophilic compounds, as evidenced by their natural occurrence in an oily liquid form; their absorption is believed to be similar to that of lipids and other lipophilic substances. Therefore, lipid-based formulations can be useful delivery systems for tocotrienols. Moreover, like many fat-soluble substances, tocotrienols would have a high log P value of more than 5, which indicates their high lipophilicity; thus, they are good candidates for lipid-based formulations, as they could be taken up into the intestinal lymphatic system. Intestinal lymphatic uptake of compounds with high log P value (more than 5) has always been associated with the stimulation of enterocyte chylomicron synthesis as a result of lipid ingestion followed by partitioning of these compounds into the chylomicrons (Porter and Charman 1997). Lipid-based formulations can range from pure medium- or long-chain triglyceride oils, medium- or long-chain mixed mono- and diglyceride oils, mixed glyceride oils with lipophilic or hydrophilic surfactants, to a mixture of glyceride oils, lipophilic or hydrophilic surfactants with hydrophilic co-solvent (Pouton 2000). Thus, lipid-based formulations can exist in the form of an oily suspension or solution or an emulsion.

Tocotrienols, being an oily liquid, can be formulated into an oily solution, the simplest form of lipid-based formulation. This can be achieved by dissolving tocotrienols in a chosen lipid/oil, often called a vehicle. With the recent advances in pharmaceutical engineering leading to more affordable encapsulation facilities, the oily solution can be encapsulated in the form of soft gelatin capsules, which provide better ease and convenience of administration. Besides the simple formulation of oily solution, there are more advanced lipid-based formulation techniques such as the use of emulsions and self-emulsifying systems (SESs) which are also feasible delivery systems for tocotrienols.

An emulsion is a thermodynamically unstable two-phase system consisting of at least two immiscible liquids (or two liquids that are saturated with each other), one of which is dispersed as globules (internal or dispersed phase) within the other liquid phase (external or continuous phase), generally stabilized by emulsifying agent(s). These emulsifying agent(s) will form a monolayer around the emulsion droplets and hence reduce the interfacial energy between the two immiscible phases, as well as providing a barrier to coalescence. Apart from formulation consideration in terms of drug characteristics and choice of oily vehicles and surfactants as well as their concentrations used, production of stable conventional emulsion also requires input of energy. Using suitable surfactants and oily vehicles, tocotrienols can be delivered in the form of an emulsion, such as Scott's Emulsion of Cod Liver Oil. Nevertheless, formulation of tocotrienols in the form of the conventional emulsion may encounter problems of transportation due to its bulkiness as well as problems in physical and chemical stability.

The emergence of self-emulsifying drug delivery systems (SEDDSs) has offered a new alternative for efficient oral dosing of lipophilic substances via an *in vivo* administration of emulsions, thereby overcoming the limitations of conventional emulsions. An SES is a mixture of oil and surfactant, sometimes including co-solvents, which emulsifies spontaneously or under conditions of gentle agitation upon contact with an aqueous medium (Pouton, 1985; 1997). The mixture, either in the form of solution or suspension, can be encapsulated in soft or hard gelatin capsules. After oral administration, the content of the capsule will be liberated upon dissolution of the capsule shell. After coming into contact with the gastrointestinal fluids, the self-emulsifying (SE) formulation spreads readily within the gastrointestinal tract and self-emulsification will be initiated by the gentle agitation resulting from the digestive motility of the stomach and the small intestine (Shah et al. 1994).

Like conventional emulsions, emulsifying agents are still needed in an SES to stabilize the two immiscible phases. The key difference between an SES and a conventional emulsion system is that the former requires very low and positive or negative free energy to form an emulsion (Craig et al. 1995), whereas the latter requires energy input to create a new surface between the two immiscible phases.

Various formulation aspects in the development of SESs as well as factors affecting their *in vivo* performance has been well studied and documented (Bachynsky et al. 1997; Pouton 1997, 2000, 2006; Gershanik and Benita 2000; Wasan 2001; Gursoy and Benita 2004). To obtain good oral bioavailability for the contained substance, the droplet sizes of the emulsion products should be as fine as possible, preferably in colloidal dimensions (Pouton 2000; Gursoy and Benita 2004). For example, the newer SE formulation of cyclosporine A, Sandimune Neoral®, which could produce emulsion droplets in the colloidal dimensions, exhibited better bioavailability enhancement of the drug than the earlier SE formulation, Sandimune®, which produced a coarser emulsion product (Mueller et al. 1994). Furthermore, Yap and Yuen (2004), as well as de Smidt et al. (2004), also reported that the droplet size of the emulsion product was an important determinant for achieving significant improvement in oral drug bioavailability in their investigations. Should a coarse emulsion product be formed, these workers reported that the dispersed oil droplets should then be amenable to lipolysis, so that the droplet sizes would be further reduced to colloidal dimension. On the other hand, if a lipid-based formulation is non-self-emulsifying, then its susceptibility to digestion or solubilization by mixed micelles of bile salts and phospholipids in the gastrointestinal tract is important to produce the required colloidal dispersion for absorption, on provision that the contained substances is not precipitated during the digestion process (MacGregor et al. 1997, Pouton, 2000).

In view of the extensive information on SE formulation, tocotrienols being a suitable candidate for lipid-based formulation, can be formulated into a SES in either hard or soft gelatin capsules. In summary, the formulation aspects of a successful SES for tocotrienols would include consideration of the type and amount of oil as well as emulsifying agents/surfactants used, the droplet size of the emulsion product and the susceptibility of the system to digestion/lipolysis. As mentioned earlier, a Malaysian pharmaceutical company, Hovid Bhd, Malaysia, has introduced a patented formulation (Ho et al. 2003) for the tocotrienols in which can increase the extent of bioavailability of the three tocotrienols by approximately 300%.

22.4.2 Solid Dispersion

Besides entailing the use of lipid-based formulations, tocotrienols (in an oily form) can also be formulated into a dry powder form using the solid dispersion technique. This can be achieved by dispersing the tocotrienols into a hydrophilic carrier matrix via complexation or simple surface adsorption. When the solid dispersion is exposed to the aqueous medium, the carrier dissolves and the contained compound is released as fine colloidal particles or oily globules. The resulting enhanced surface area produces a higher dissolution rate and improved bioavailability of poorly water-soluble compounds (Karanth et al. 2006). Examples of the hydrophilic carrier matrix used in solid dispersion are polyethylene glycols (PEGs), poloxamers, complex forming agents such as cyclodextrins etc. Tocotrienols in a dry powder form have been successfully commercialized as Tocomax™ (a 20% water dispersible tocopherol/tocotrienol complex powder) by Carotech Berhad, Malaysia, using a hydrophilic carrier matrix in the solid dispersion formulation.

Apart from using hydrophilic carrier matrix, lipid-based excipients such as Gelucire® have also been used in solid dispersion formulation. Gelucire is a family of semi-solid waxy, glyceride-based excipients that has been widely used as controlled release matrices and also for enhancing the oral bioavailability of lipophilic substances. Barker et al. (2003) successfully prepared a dispersion of α-tocopherol in Gelucire 44/14 (one of the Gelucire grade found to be useful in SE formulations) which could improve the bioavailability of the α-tocopherol. Since tocotrienols also appear in an oily form like α-tocopherol and they are members of the natural vitamin E, Gelucire can also be used to prepare tocotrienols in solid dispersion formulation.

REFERENCES

Bachynsky, M.O., N.H. Shah, O.I. Patel, A.W. Malick. 1997. Factors affecting the efficiency of a self-emulsifying oral delivery system. *Drug Dev. Ind. Pharm., 23(8)*, 809–816.

Barker, S.A., S.P. Yap, K.H. Yuen, C.P. McCoy, J.R. Murphy, D.Q.M Craig. 2003. An investigation into the structure and bioavailability of α-tocopherol dispersion in Gelucire® 44/14. *J. Control. Release, 91*, 477–488.

Benet L.Z., C.L. Cummins, C.Y. Wu. 2004. Unmasking the dynamic interplay between efflux transporters and metabolic enzymes. *Int. J. Pharm., 277*, 3–9.

Bieri J.G. and R.P. Evarts. 1973. Tocopherols and fatty acids in American diets. *J. Am. Diet Assoc., 62*, 147–151.

Cheng C.K. 2005. Absorption and Disposition of α-, γ- and δ-tocotrienol in rat organs and tissues. MSc thesis., Universiti Sains Malaysia.

Craig, D.Q.M., S.A. Barker, D. Banning, S.W. Booth. 1995. An investigation into the mechanisms of self-emulsification using particle size analysis and low frequency dielectric spectroscopy. *Int. J. Pharm., 114*, 103–110.

de Smidt, P.C., M.A. Campanero, I.F. Trocóniz. 2004. Intestinal absorption of penclomedine from lipid vehicles in the conscious rat: Contribution of emulsification versus digestibility. *Int. J. Pharm., 270*, 109–118.

Fairus A.B. 2006. The postprandrial metabolic fate and antioxidant potential of vitamin E (alpha-tocopherol and tocotrienols) in humans. PhD thesis., University of Malaya.

Gershanik, T., S. Benita. 2000. Self-dispersing lipid formulations for improving oral absorption of lipophilic drugs. *Eur. J. Pharm. Biopharm.*, *50*, 179–188.

Gursoy, R.N., S. Benita. 2004. Self-emulsifying drug delivery systems (SEDDS) for improved oral delivery of lipophilic drugs. *Biomed. Pharmacother. 58*, 173–182.

Hayes K.C., A. Pronczuck, J.S. Liang. 1993. Differences in the plasma transport and tissue concentrations of tocopherols and tocotrienols: observations in humans and hamsters. *Proc. Soc. Exp. Biol. Med.*, *202*, 353–360.

Ho, D.S.S, K.H. Yuen, S.P. Yap. 2003. Drug delivery system: formulation for fat-soluble drugs. *US Patent, 6,596,306.*

Hosomi A., M. Arita, Y. Sato, C. Kiyose, T. Ueda, O. Igarashi, H. Arai, K. Inoue. 1997. Affinity for α-tocopherol transfer protein as a determinant of the biological activities of vitamin E analogs. *FEBS Lett.*, *409*, 105–108.

Ikeda I., Y. Imasato, E. Sasaki, M. Sugano. 1996. Lymphatic transport of α-, γ- and δ-tocotrienols and α-tocopherol in rats. *Int. J. Vitam. Nutr. Res.*, *66*, 217–221.

Ikeda S., K. Toyoshima, K. Yamashita. 2001. Dietary sesame seeds elevate α- and γ-tocotrienol concentrations in skin and adipose tissue of rats fed the tocotrienol–rich fraction extracted from palm oil. *J. Nutr.*, *131*, 2892–2897.

Ikeda S., T. Niwa, K. Yamashita. 2000. Selective uptake of dietary tocotrienols into rat skin. *J Nutr. Sci. Vitaminol.*, *46(3),* 141–143.

Ikeda S., T. Tohyama, H. Yoshimura, K. Hamamura, K. Abe, K. Yamashita. 2003. Dietary α-tocopherol decreases α-tocotrienol but not γ-tocotrienol concentration in rats. *J. Nutr.*, *133*, 428–434.

Jishage K., M. Arita, K. Igarashi, T. Iwata, M. Watanabe, M. Ogawa, O. Ueda, N. Kamada, K. Inoue, H. Arai et al. 2001. Alpha–tocopherol transfer protein is important for the normal development of placental labyrinthine trophoblasts in mice. *J. Biol. Chem.*, *276(3),* 1669–1672.

Karanth, H., V.S. Shenoy, R.S. Murthy. 2006. Industrially feasible alternative approach in the manufacture of solid dispersions: a technical report. *AAPS Pharm. Sci. Tech.*, *7(4)*, Article 87, E1–E8 (http://www.aapspharmscitech.org)

Kawakami Y., T. Tsuzuki, K. Nakagawa, T. Miyazawa. 2007. Distribution of Tocotrienols in Rats Fed a Rice Bran Tocotrienol Concentrate. *Biosci. Biotechnol. Biochem.*, *71*(2), 464–471.

Kayden H.J. and M.G. Traber. 1993. Absorption, lipoprotein transport and regulation of plasma concentrations of vitamin E in humans. *J. Lipid Res.*, *34*, 343–358.

Khanna S., V. Patel, C. Rink, S. Roy, C.K. Sen. 2005. Delivery of orally supplemented alpha-tocotrienol to vital organs of rats and tocopherol–transport protein deficient mice. *Free Radical Biol. Med.*, *39*(10), 1310–1319.

Khor H.T. and T.T. Ng. 1999. Effects of adminstration of α-tocopherol and tocotrienols on serum lipids and liver HMG–CoA reductase activity. PORIM International Palm Oil Congress (PIPOC), Nutrition Conference, Kuala Lumpur, Malaysia. 1–6 February 1999, 177–186.

Khor H.T., T.T. Ng, R. Raajeswari. 2000. Palm oil tocotrienols and the regulatory enzymes of cholesterol metabolism. Proceedings of the Oils and Fats International Congress, Kuala Lumpur, Malaysia. 4–8 September 2000, 4–11.

Loon Y.H., J.W. Wong, S.P. Yap, K.H. Yuen. 2005. Determination of flavonoids from *Orthosiphon stamineus* in plasma using a simple HPLC method with ultraviolet detection. *J. Chromatogr. B*, *816*, 161–166.

MacGregor K. J., J.K. Embleton, J.E. Lacy, E.A. Perry, L.J. Solomon, H. Seager, C.W. Pouton. 1997. Influence of lipolysis on drug absorption from the gastro–intestinal tract. *Adv. Drug Deliv. Rev.*, *25*, 33–46.

Mizuno N., T, Niwa, Y. Yotsumoto, Y. Sugiyama, Y. 2003. Impact of drug transporters studies on drug discovery and development. *Pharmacol. Rev.*, *55*, 425–461.

Mueller, E.A., J.M. Kovarik, J.B. van Bree, W. Tetzloff, J. Grevel, K. Kutz. 1994. Improved dose linearity of cyclosporine pharmacokinetics from a microemulsion formulation. *Pharm. Res.*, *11(2),* 301–304.

Okabe M., M. Oji, I. Ikeda, H. Tachinbana, K. Yamada. 2002. Tocotrienols levels in various tissues of Sprague-Dawley rats after intragastric administration of tocotrienols. *Biosci. Biotechnol. Biochem.*, *66(8),* 1768–1771.

Podda M., C. Weber, M. G. Traber, L. Packer. 1996. Simultaneous determination of tissue tocopherols, tocotrienols, ubiquinols and ubiquinones. *J. Lipid Res.*, *37*, 893–901.

Porter, C.J.H., W.N. Charman. 1997. Uptake of drugs into the intestinal lymphatics after oral administration. *Adv. Drug Deliv. Rev.*, *25*, 71–89.

Pouton, C.W. 2006. Formulation of poorly water-soluble drugs for oral administration: Physicochemical and physiological issues and the lipid formulation classification system. *Eur. J. Pharm. Sci.*, *20*, 278–287.

Pouton, C.W. 1997. Formulation of self-emulsifying drug delivery systems. *Adv. Drug. Deliv. Rev.*, *25*, 47–58.

Pouton, C.W. 2000. Lipid formulation for oral administration of drugs: non–emulsifying, self-emulsifying and 'self-microemulsifying' drug delivery systems. *Eur. J. Pharm. Sci.*, *11(suppl. 2)*, S93–S98.

Pouton, C.W. 1985. Self-emulsifying drug delivery systems: assessment of the efficiency of emulsification. *Int. J. Pharm.*, *27*, 335–348.

Shah, N.H., M.T. Carvajal, C.I. Patel, M.H. Infeld, A.W. Malick. 1994. Self-emulsifying drug delivery systems (SEDDS) with polyglycolyzed glycerides for improving *in–vitro* dissolution and oral absorption of lipophilic drugs. *Int. J. Pharm.*, *106*, 15–23.

Tan S., K.H. Yuen, K.L. Chan. 2002. HPLC analysis of plasma 9–methoxycanthin–6–one from *Eurycoma longifolia*, Jack and its application in a bioavailability/pharmacokinetic study. *Planta medica*, *68*, 355–358.

Terasawa Y., Z. Ladha, S.W. Leonard, J.D. Morrow, D. Newland, D. Sanan, L. Packer, M.G. Traber, R.V. Farese Jr. 2000. Increased atheroslcerosis in hyperlipidemic mice deficient in alpha-tocopherol transfer protein and vitamin E. *Proc. Natl. Acad. Sci. USA*, *97*(25), 13830–13834.

Wasan, K.M. 2001. Formulation and physiological biopharmaceutical issues in the development of oral lipid–based drug delivery systems. *Drug Dev. Ind. Pharm.*, *27(4)*, 267–276.

Yap S.P. and K.H. Yuen. 2004. Influence of lipolysis and droplet size on tocotrienol absorption from self-emulsifying formulations. *Int. J. Pharm.*, *281*, 67–78.

Yap S.P. 2003. Biopharmaceutic and pharmacokinetic studies of δ-, γ- and α- tocotrienol. PhD thesis, Universiti Sains Malaysia.

Yap S.P., K.H. Yuen, A.B. Lim. 2003. Influence of route of administration on the absorption and disposition of α-, γ- and δ-tocotrienols in rats. *J. Pharm. Pharmacol.*, *55(1)*, 53–58.

Yap S.P., K.H. Yuen, J.W. Wong. 2001. Pharmacokinetics and bioavailability of α-, γ- and δ-tocotrienols under different food status. *J. Pharm. Pharmacol.*, *53(1)*, 67–71.

Yap, S.P., K.H. Yuen. 2004. Influence of lipolysis and droplet size on tocotrienol absorption from self-emulsifying formulations. *Int. J. Pharm.*, *281*, 67–68.

23 The Metabolism of Tocopherols and Tocotrienols and Novel Functions of Their Metabolites

Qing Jiang

CONTENTS

23.1 INTRODUCTION

Natural forms of vitamin E are composed of eight membrane-soluble antioxidants, i.e., α-, β-, γ-, or δ-tocopherol (α-, β-, γ-, or δ-T) and α-, β-, γ-, or δ-tocotrienol (α-, β-, γ-, or δ-TE) (Figure 23.1). All these molecules have a chromanol ring and a 16-carbon hydrophobic side chain, which are, respectively, responsible for the potent antioxidant activity and lipophilic property. Tocopherols

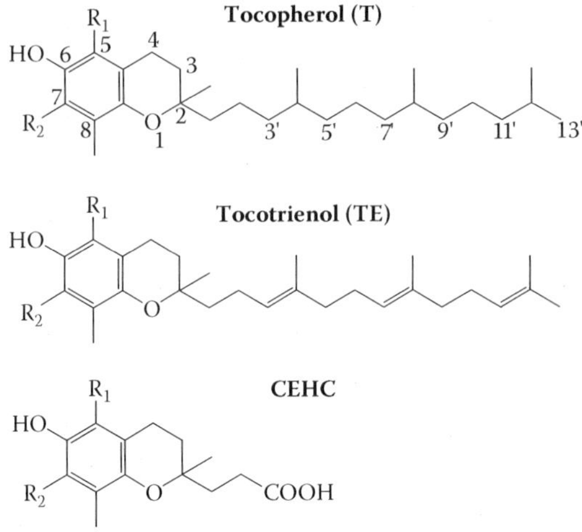

α-T, α-TE or α-CEHC, R1 = CH_3, R2 = CH_3
β-T, β-TE or β-CEHC, R1 = CH_3, R2 = H
γ-T, γ-TE or γ-CEHC, R1 = H, R2 = CH_3
δ-T, δ-TE or δ-CEHC, R1 = H, R2 = H

FIGURE 23.1 Structures of tocopherols, tocotrienols and their terminal urinary-excreted metabolites, CEHCs (carboxyethyl hydroxychroman).

have a saturated side chain, while tocotrienols have an unsaturated side chain that contains three double bonds at 3', 7' and 11' position (Figure 23.1). Despite structural similarity, different forms of vitamin E appear to have distinct bioactivity and be distinctively metabolized (Brigelius-Flohe and Traber 1999; Jiang et al. 2001). Alpha-T, the predominant form of vitamin E in tissues, is preferentially retained by the body. On the other hand, non-α forms of vitamin E are likely to be readily metabolized or excreted via the bile (Kayden and Traber 1993), because they do not appear to be accumulated to the same extent as α-T in most tissues. Not only does the metabolism play a role in the bioavailability, it also has an impact on the bioactivities of vitamin E forms. This chapter reviews the current knowledge of vitamin E metabolism including its historical discovery and recent advance in the understanding of how vitamin E is metabolized and how the metabolic pathway is regulated. Potential novel biological functions of the metabolites are also discussed.

23.2 OVERVIEW OF ABSORPTION, METABOLISM AND EXCRETION OF VITAMIN E

Plants are the only species capable of making vitamin E. Alpha-T is mainly found in green leaves and plant seeds, but γ-T is usually the most prevalent form of vitamin E in plant seeds and plant oils (McLaughlin and Weihrauch 1979). Vegetable oils such as corn, soybean and sesame oil, as well as nuts such as walnuts, pecans and peanuts, are rich sources of γ-T and δ-T (McLaughlin and Weihrauch 1979). Due to the widespread use of these plant products, γ-T and δ-T represent ~50–60 % and ~20% of the vitamin E consumed in the typical U.S. diet (McLaughlin and Weihrauch 1979). Tocotrienols, less prevalent than tocopherols, are mostly found in palm oil, and some cereal grains (McLaughlin and Weihrauch 1979; Theriault et al. 1999).

The absorption and metabolism of natural forms of vitamin E are summarized in Figure 23.2. Tocopherols and tocotrienols appear to be similarly taken up along with dietary fat by the intestine and secreted in chylomicron particles together with triacylglycerol and cholesterol. The nearly identical incorporation of α-T and γ-T in chylomicrons following supplementation with equal amounts of the two tocopherols indicates that their absorption is not selective (Bieri and Evarts 1974; Traber

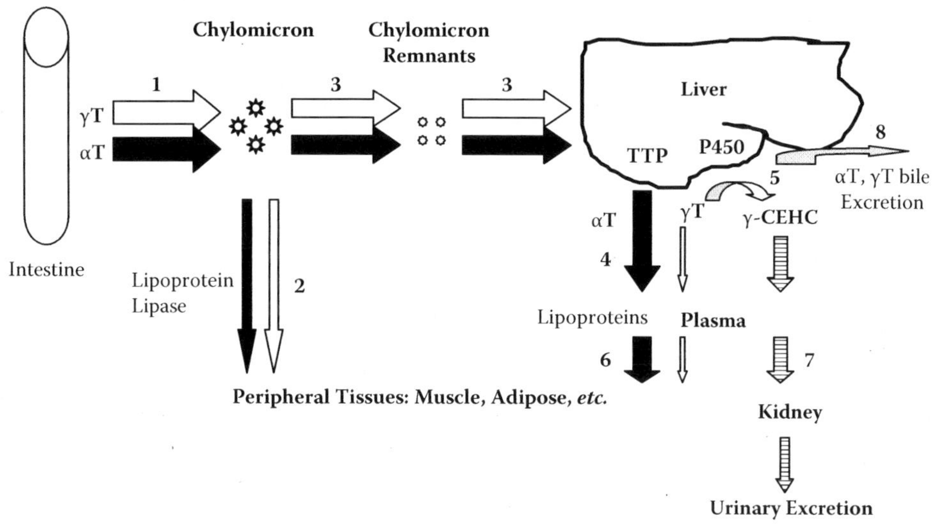

FIGURE 23.2 Absorption, transport, metabolism and excretion of tocopherols and tocotrienols. This is modified from a review by Jiang et al. (2001). γ-T represents non-alpha-form of vitamin E. Both α-T and γ-T (other vitamin E forms) are similarly absorbed by the intestine along with dietary fat, and secreted into chylomicron particles (1). Some of the chylomicron-bound vitamin E is transported to peripheral tissues with the aid of lipoprotein lipase (2). The resulting chylomicron remnants are subsequently taken up by the liver (3). In the liver, most of the remaining α-T but only a small fraction of γ-T is reincorporated into nascent VLDL by TTP (4). Plasma vitamin E is further delivered to tissues by LDL and HDL (6). Substantial amounts of γ-T are probably degraded by a cytochrome P450 3A mediated reaction to γ-CEHC (5), which is then excreted into urine (7). Excess amounts of tocopherols and tocotrienols may also be excreted via bile (8).

et al. 1992). During the subsequent lipoprotein lipase-mediated catabolism of chylomicron particles, some of the chylomicron-bound vitamin E appears to be transported and transferred to peripheral tissues including muscle and adipose (and possibly also brain) (Traber et al. 1985). Chylomicron-associated tissue uptake of vitamin E, which occurs prior to liver metabolism, may be important for the accumulation of non-alpha forms of vitamin E such as γ-T in skin, adipose and muscle tissue. This could explain the strong correlation in humans between dietary γ-T uptake and γ-T concentration in these tissues (Burton et al. 1998). The resulting chylomicron remnants are subsequently taken up by the liver, where α-T is preferentially reincorporated into nascent very-low-density lipoprotein (VLDL) by α-tocopherol-transfer protein (α-TTP) (Traber et al. 1992). The absolute requirement of VLDL for α-T distribution in the body was questioned by a recent study that showed that absence of VLDL secretion in mice that lack microsomal triglyceride transfer protein (MTTP) has little effect on the stores of α-T in peripheral tissues (Minehira-Castelli et al. 2006).

Although α-T is protected by α-TTP, other forms of vitamin E appear to be degraded largely to the hydrophilic CEHCs by a cytochrome P450-dependent process (Brigelius-Flohe and Traber 1999; Jiang et al. 2001), and are then primarily excreted into urine. Catabolism of α-T by this route, compared with the rest of the vitamin E forms, appears to be quantitatively much less important, because urinary excretion of α-CEHC is lower than that of γ-CEHC (Traber et al. 1998; Stahl et al. 1999).

In addition to urinary excretion (as CEHCs), biliary excretion is an alternative route to eliminate excess tocopherols and tocotrienols (Traber and Kayden 1989). Excretion of excess hepatic vitamin E into the bile has been shown to be mediated by the ABC transporter P-glycoprotein (MDR2) (Mustacich et al. 1998). Liver may also preferentially excrete γ-T compared with α-T, which is supported by the fact that the biliary ratio of γ-T to α-T is several-fold higher than that in plasma (Traber and Kayden 1989; Stone et al. 1998; Yamashita et al. 2000). Excess γ-T secreted into feces during supplementation may play a role in eliminating fecal mutagens and thus reduce colon cancer (Stone and Papas 1997; Stone et al. 1998).

23.3 DISCOVERY OF URINARY METABOLITES OF VITAMIN E

The understanding of how vitamin E is metabolized was initiated by the identification of their urinary-excreted metabolites. In 1956, working with Eisengart, Simon (Eisengart et al. 1956; Gross et al. 1956) identified two metabolites of α-T as α-tocopheronic acid and the lactone derivative from the urine of rabbits and humans given larges doses of α-T. Based on the structural characteristics of these so-called Simon metabolites, these investigators proposed a mechanism of α-T metabolism that includes a radical mediated oxidation of the hydroxyl group on the chromanol ring to form α-tocopherylquinone and then β-oxidation of the hydrophobic side chain to generate α-tocopheronic acid (Figure 23.3A). The Simon metabolites, resulting from the oxidation of the chromanol ring, were commonly believed to indicate the function of α-T as an antioxidant. However, only relatively recently did it become clear that the Simon metabolites are likely to be generated from oxidation of the un-modified chromanol-ring metabolites from α-T (2,5,7,8-tetramethyl 2-(β-carboxyethyl)-6-hydroxychroman or α-CEHC) during sample processing, which involves prolonged incubation during acid hydrolysis.

Almost 30 years after the Simon metabolites were identified, in 1984, Chiku, Hamamura and Nakamura isolated a new metabolite from the urine of rats that were injected intravenously with the radiolabeled d-3,4-[^{3}H2]-δ-tocopherol. The structure of this metabolite was determined by infrared spectra, nuclear magnetic resonance (NMR) and mass spectrometry (MS) and identified as [7, 8-dimethyl 2-(β-carboxyethyl)-6-hydroxychroman] (δ-CEHC). The proposed structure was also confirmed by comparing the analytical results with those of a synthetically derived compound. In addition, this study indicated that most urinary δ-CEHC is in the sulfate-conjugated form, as the non-conjugated form was released by sulfatase but not glucuronidase digestion. Based on the structure of δ-CEHC, which has an intact chromanol ring and short side chain with a carboxylate end, these researchers proposed a mechanism of δ-T metabolism that is different from the pathway leading to the generation of the Simon metabolites from α-T; the new mechanism includes a direct ω-hydroxylation and β-oxidation of the side chain followed by sulfate conjugation of hydroxyl group on the chromanol ring to form sulfated derivative (similar to the metabolism of α-T, as shown in Figure 23.3). This pathway, although not fully recognized at that time, turns out to be the common mechanism of how other vitamin E forms are metabolized, which was confirmed and then unambiguously elucidated more than a decade later.

In 1995, Schultz, Leist and Petrzika reported a metabolite from α-T that was isolated from human urine samples after subjects were supplemented with up to 800 mg of α-T. Using gas chromatography mass spectrometry (GC-MS), these investigators identified the metabolite as α-CEHC (2,5,7,8-tetramethyl 2-(β-carboxyethyl)-6-hydroxychroman), which, like δ-CEHC, has an intact chromanol ring. α-CEHC was the major metabolite resulted from a mild sample-processing procedure that included a brief digestion using sulfatase and glucoronidase at room temperature in the absence of oxygen. In a series of elegant *in vitro* experiments, these investigators showed that α-CEHC is converted to α-tocopheronolactone, one of the Simon metabolites, during acid hydrolysis with 0.1M HCl in the presence of oxygen (Figure 23.3A). On the other hand, formation of the Simon metabolites was prevented by the removal of oxygen. This study therefore provides evidence that the Simon metabolites likely resulted from *in vitro* oxidation of α-CEHC but not the physiological metabolite. Therefore, similar to δ-T metabolism, the degradation of the hydrophobic side chain via β-oxidation was proposed for α-T (Figure 23.3B). In addition, these authors also concluded that most α-CEHC exists as sulfate conjugate, as the non-conjugated CEHC is generated by incubation of urine samples with sulfatase instead of glucoronidase.

In 1996, γ-CEHC (2,7,8-tetramethyl 2-(β-carboxyethyl)-6-hydroxychroman), the third metabolite in vitamin E family, was discovered by Wechter and his coworkers in the pursuit of identifying a long-sought endogenous natriuretic factor in human urine. The structure of γ-CEHC was identified by NMR and was confirmed by comparison with the synthetic compound. Like δ-CEHC and α-CEHC, γ-CEHC is likely derived from β-oxidation which catabolizes the hydrophobic side chain

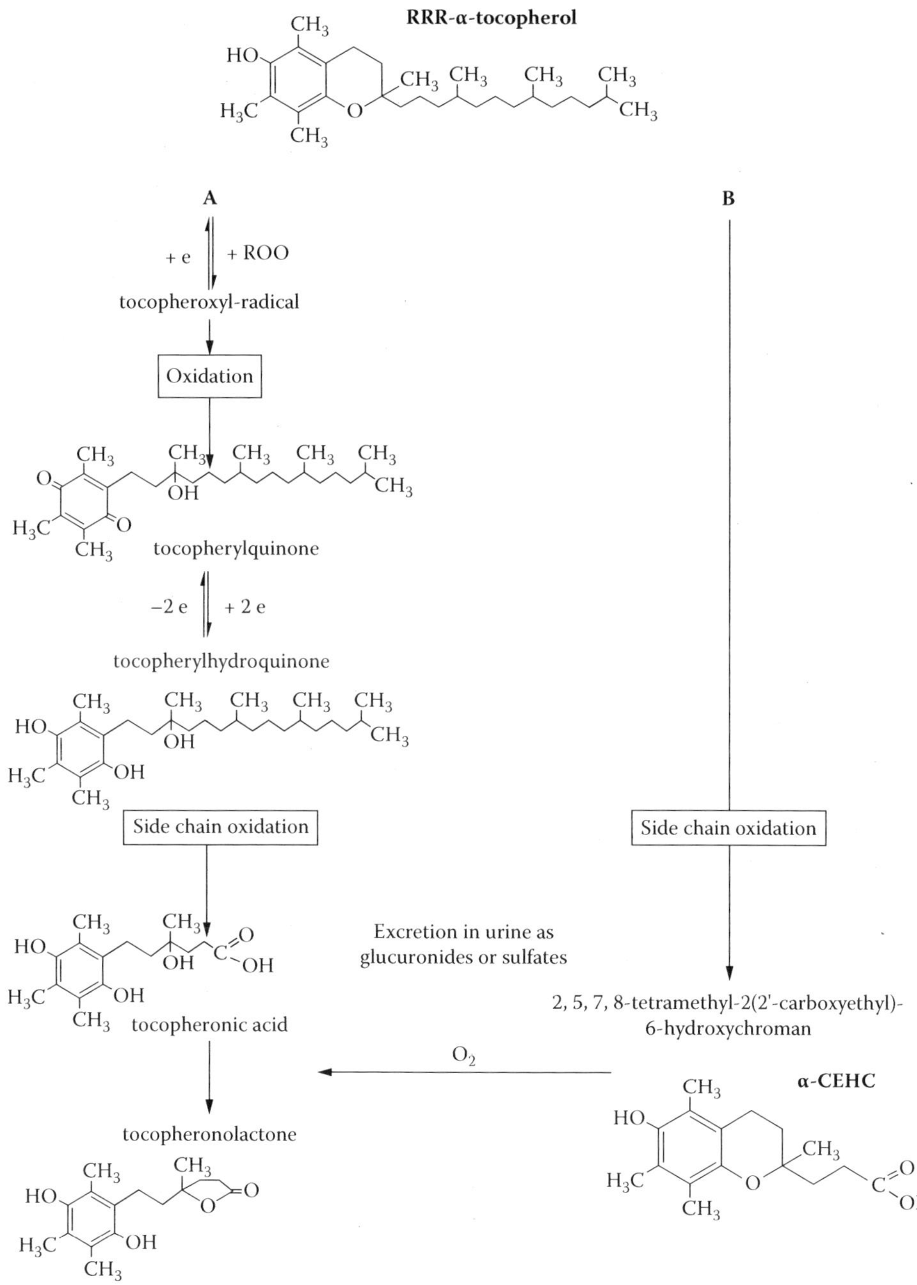

FIGURE 23.3 Proposed vitamin E metabolism based on the Simon metabolites (A) and an alternative mechanism based on the structures of δ-CEHC or α-CEHC (B). This figure is from an original article by Schultz et al. (1995).

of γ-T without oxidation of the chromanol ring. In a radio-isotope tracing study, the same group of investigators unambiguously established that γ-CEHC is derived from naturally occurring RRR-γ-T. Using x-ray crystallographic analysis, they demonstrated that γ-CEHC has an S(+) stereochemistry at the C-2 position, indicating that racemization does not occur during side-chain degradation by β-oxidation of RRR-γ-T (Kantoci et al. 1997).

23.4 MECHANISTIC ELUCIDATION OF THE METABOLIC PATHWAY

23.4.1 Elucidation of the Metabolic Pathway in HepG2 Cells

Although the structural characteristic of CEHCs suggests that vitamin E metabolism may involve oxidation of the hydrophobic side chain via cytochrome P-450 catalyzed reactions and leave the chromanol ring unmodified, direct experimental evidence to support this mechanism was not presented until 2002. In culture media obtained after human liver carcinoma HepG2 cells were incubated with γ-T, Sontag and Parker (2002) identified, by GC-MS, a series of various-length side chain carboxychromanols and hydroxychromanol, which include 13'-hydroxychromanol, 13'-, 11'-, 9'-, 7'-, 5'- and 3'-carboxychromanol (Figure 23.4A). 13'-carboxychromanol and 13'-hydroxychromanol were also formed by incubation of rat liver microsomes with γ-T. These intermediate metabolites support the notion that vitamin E forms are metabolized via cytochrome P-450 mediated ω-hydroxylation and oxidation of 13'-carbon, followed by stepwise β-oxidation to cut off a two- or three-carbon moiety each cycle from the side chain. Consistently, the formation of these metabolites was inhibited by cytochrome P-450 inhibitors including ketoconazole and sesamin (Parker, Sontag and Swanson 2000).

In an effort to determine which CYP isoform(s) might be involved, Sontag and Parker (2002) studied the metabolism of vitamin E in fibroblasts stably expressing human liver CYP2E1 and in insect microsomes selectively expressing various recombinant human CYP enzymes. These studies revealed that tocopherol-ω-hydroxylase activity is associated only with CYP4F2 but not other isoforms including CYP3A, which was previously proposed to metabolize vitamin E based on the experiments with cytochrome P450 inhibitors (Parker, Sontag and Swanson 2000). CYP4F2 has been known to also catalyze ω-hydroxylation of leukotriene B4 and arachidonic acid (Jin et al. 1998). These data also suggest that sesamin appears to be a specific inhibitor of CYP4F2 rather than CYP3A, but ketoconazole seems to inhibit both. Consistently, human lung epithelial A549 cells that express CYP4F2 also metabolize tocopherols and tocotrienols to long-chain carboxychromanols with 9'-carboxychromanol as the most abundant metabolites (You et al. 2005). The enrichment of long-chain carboxychromanols in culture media of these cells is caused by their insufficient conversion of 7'-carboxychromanols relative to HepG2 cells (You et al. 2005).

Birringer et al. (2002) compared the metabolism of tocotrienols and tocopherols in HepG2 cells. They identified a series of similar intermediate metabolites by GC-MS in the culture medium, which included 11'-, 9'-, 7'-, 5'- and 3'-carboxychromanol. Compared with tocopherols, the predominant 9'-carboxychromanol from γ-TE was two mass units greater than the predicted product generated from direct β-oxidation, i.e., dienoic acid (Figure 23.4B). This suggests that 9'-carboxychromanol may not have an α, β-unsaturated double bond which are conjugated with the carboxylic acid group, but is rather an enoic acid (Figure 23.4B). The mass of 11' indicates a dienoic acid, a typical product via β-oxidation from 13'-carboxychromanol. These metabolites suggest that in addition to ω-hydroxylation and β-oxidation, auxiliary enzymes are likely to be involved in acting on pre-existing double bonds for tocotrienols during the second and fourth round of β-oxidation (Birringer et al. 2002). Specifically, similar to the well-established oxidation of unsaturated fatty acids, e.g. oxidation of linoleate (18):2), reductases and isomerases have to be included to modify the intermediate with two conjugated double bonds at 7'- and 9'-carboxychromanol, which are not a substrate for the enoyl CoA hydratase or the β-hydroxyacyl CoA dehydrogenase (Kunau et al. 1995; Mukherji et al. 2003). Consistently, You et al. (2005) reported that 13'-carboxychromanol derived

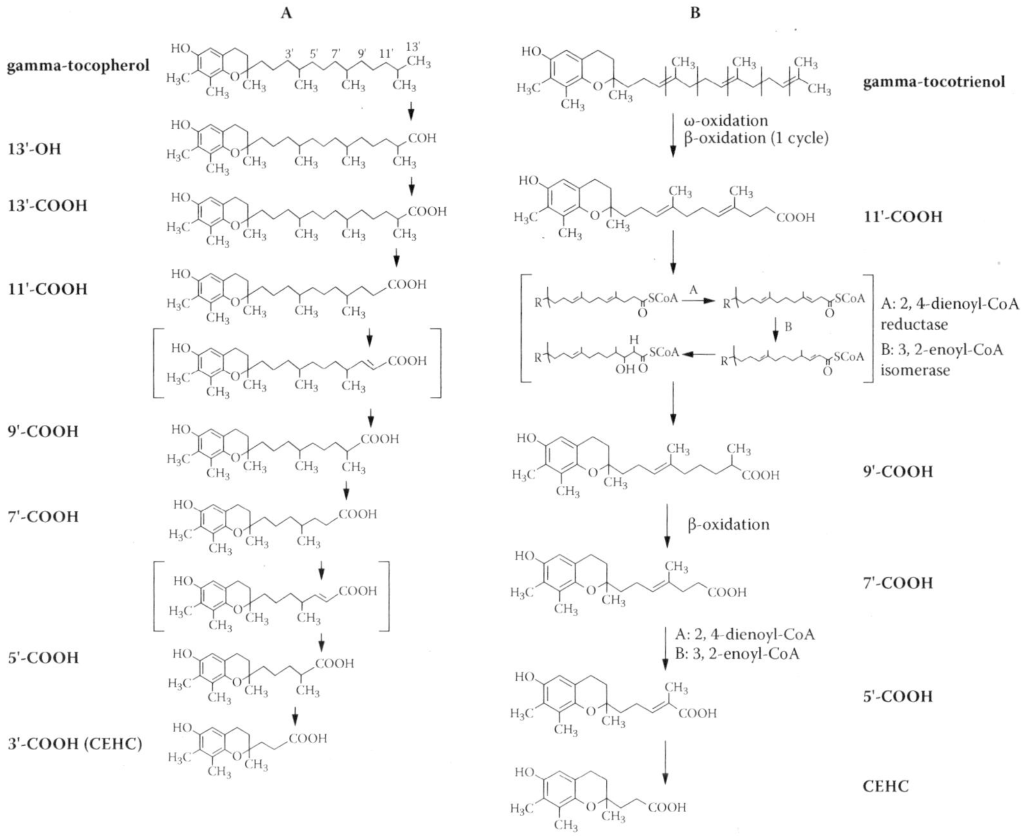

FIGURE 23.4 Proposed mechanism of the metabolism of tocopherols (A) and tocotrienols (B). For the metabolites from tocopherols, 9'-, 11'- and 13'-carboxychromanol (or 9'-, 11'- and 13'-COOH) are the abbreviations of 9-(6-hydroxy-2, 7, 8,-trimethyl-chroman-2-yl)-2,6-dimethyl-nomanoic acid, 11-(6-hydroxy-2, 7, 8,-trimethyl-chroman-2-yl)-4, 8-dimethyl-undecanoic acid, and 13-(6-hydroxy-2, 7, 8,-trimethyl-chroman-2-yl)-2, 6, 10-trimethyl-tridecanoic acid, respectively. For the metabolites from tocotrienols, 9'-, 11'-carboxychromanol (9'- and 11'-COOH) stands for (4E,8E)-11-(6-hydroxy-2,7,8-trimethylchroman-2-yl)-4,8-dimethylundeca-4,8-dienoic acid, and (6E,10E)-13-(6-hydroxy-2,7,8-trimethylchroman-2-yl)-2,6,10-trimethyltrideca-6,10-dienoic acid, respectively. Modified from Sontag and Parker (2002) and Birringer et al. (2002), respectively.

from δ-TE in A549 cells appears to be a dienoic acid instead of trienoic acid. The mechanism of how this intermediate is formed needs to be further determined. The involvement of the specific reductases and isomerases also waits to be identified.

23.4.2 Novel Discovery of Sulfated Long-Chain Carboxychromanols

Recently, Jiang et al. (2007) discovered that γ-tocopherol and δ-tocopherol are metabolized to novel metabolites, sulfated 9'-, 11'- and 13'-carboxychromanols, in human lung epithelial A549 cells. Incubation of confluent A549 cells with tocopherols resulted in a release of various metabolites including 9'-, 11'- and 13'-carboxychromanols, as revealed by an HPLC fluorescent detection and identified by electrospray ionization mass spectrometry (ESI-MS) (Figure 23.5). In addition to the long-chain carboxychromanols, three additional metabolites were present in culture media, each of which is 80 mass units more than 9'-, 11' and 13'-carboxychromanol. These results suggest a potential phosphorylation (HPO_3) or sulfation (SO_3) of carboxychromanols. Consistently, the tandem MS/MS of the phosphorylated/sulfated carboxychromanols $[M-H]^-$ gave a predominant peak corresponding to a loss of 80 mass units. Sulfation rather than phosphorylation was revealed by the

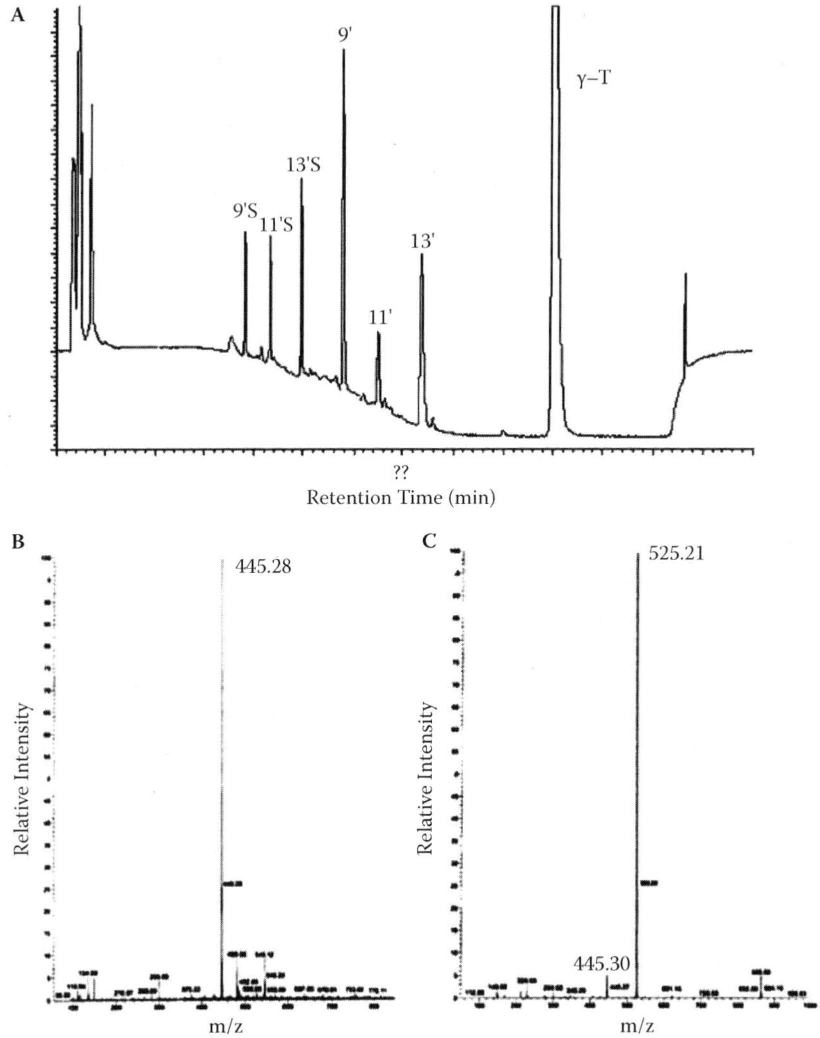

FIGURE 23.5 Identification of metabolites from γ-T in cultured A549 cells. Panel A shows a HPLC chromatograph (with fluorescent detection) of γ-T metabolites accumulated in the cell-culture medium after A549 cells were incubated with 50 μM of γ-T for 72 h. 9', 11', and 13' represent 9'-COOH, 11'-COOH and 13'-COOH, and 9'S, 11'S and 13'S stand for sulfated 9'-COOH, sulfated 11'-COOH and sulfated 13'-COOH, respectively. Panel B and Panel C show ESI-MS of 13'-COOH and sulfated 13'-COOH, respectively.

following observations. First, the isotope pattern from the ESI-MS strongly suggests sulfation rather than phosphorylation. Second, inductively coupled plasma mass spectrometry (ICP-MS) of isolated sulfated/phosphorylated 9'-carboxychromanol showed an increase in sulfur (^{34}S) ion but not phosphorous (^{31}P) ion signal compared with the blank control. In addition, digestion of isolated sulfated 9'-carboxychromanol with sulfatase resulted in a marked decrease in this sulfated metabolite, and a simultaneous increase in non-conjugated 9'-carboxychromanol. This also suggests that sulfation is likely to occur at the hydroxyl group on the chromanol ring based on the substrate specificity of sulfatases. Sulfation at the hydroxyl group was further confirmed by comparison of the relative redox activity between sulfated and unsulfated carboxychromanols. Thus, although 9'-carboxychromanol is readily oxidized, sulfated carboxychromanols are resistant to electrochemical oxidation, which supports the notion that conjugation takes place in the hydroxyl group and the sulfated metabolites appear to lack antioxidant activities (Jiang et al. 2007).

Using a sensitive HPLC-fluorescent assay, Jiang et al. (Jiang et al. 2007) studied the formation of intermediate metabolites in A549 cells. The amount of total metabolites increased proportionally with incubation time. The generation of sulfated metabolites lagged behind unsulfated carboxychromanols, suggesting that carboxychromanols are likely the primary targets for sulfation. The presence of sesamin, an inhibitor of tocopherol-ω-hydroxylase, almost completely abolished the formation of all metabolites. The total amount of metabolites from δ-T was higher than that of γ-T, while more sulfated long-chain carboxychromanols were found from γT; thus, after 72 h incubation, about 45% metabolites from γ-T, but only 10% from δ-T, were sulfated.

To test whether the long-chain carboxychromanols and their sulfated metabolites are present in tissues, Jiang et al. (2007) conducted animal experiments in which Wistar rats were orally administered with various doses of γ-T, i.e., 9, 45 or 90 mg/kg of body weight, respectively. Control rats received tocopherol-stripped corn oil, which was used as the vehicle to deliver γ-T. Six hours after supplemented with γ-T, rats had elevated tissue levels of sulfated 9'-, 11'- and 13'-carboxychromanols, 13'-hydroxychromanol, 13'-carboxychromanol and γ-CEHC. The plasma concentrations of combined sulfated long-chain metabolites were comparable to or exceeded those of CEHCs, and increased proportionally with the supplement dosages of γ-tocopherol. In the liver, 13'-hydroxychromanol, 13'-carboxychromanol, and sulfated 13'-carboxychromanol were detected in rats supplemented with γ-T. Liver concentrations of these metabolites were three- to five-fold higher than those in the plasma.

The formation of conjugated metabolites including sulfated or glucuronidated esters, were previously reported in the urine (Chiku, Hamamura and Nakamura 1984; Schultz et al. 1995; Traber, Elsner and Brigelious-Flohe 1998; Stahl et al. 1999; Swanson et al. 1999; Pope et al. 2002) and in tissues (Leonard et al. 2005). However, studies on conjugated metabolites were confined to the terminal CEHCs. For example, Schultz et al. (1995) concluded that α-CEHC sulfate but not glucuronide conjugate was predominantly present in human urines. Pope et al. (2002) showed that both glucuronidated and sulfated α-CEHC were detectable in human urines. On the other hand, Chiku Hamamura and Nakamura (1984) reported that δ-CHEC sulfate was the major conjugate excreted in rat's urine. The findings of sulfated long-chain metabolites call attention to further investigation of potential formation of conjugated (both glucuronide and sulfate) long-chain carboxychromanols following vitamin E supplementation in humans. In addition, the detection of sulfated 9'-, 11' and 13'-carboxychromanol, as well as 13'-hydroxychromanol and 13'-carboxychromanol in rat plasma and liver, together with other literatures documenting intermediate metabolites including 5'-carboxychromanol (Parker et al. 2000) and 13'-hydroxychromanol in tissues (Leonard et al. 2005; Mustacich et al. 2006), provides direct evidence for tissue existence of intermediate metabolites as a result of ω-hydroxylation and β-oxidation.

The formation of novel sulfated long-chain carboxychromanols from vitamin E metabolism suggests that sulfation may occur parallel with β-oxidation, as shown in Figure 23.6, in addition to its role in conjugation of terminal CEHCs. Sulfation of intermediate long-chain metabolites is likely to facilitate the metabolism and may be particularly important under supplementation conditions. The fact that the extent of sulfated metabolites formed varies among different forms of vitamin E suggests a possible distinct substrate specificity of sulfotransferase(s) (Chapman et al. 2004), and that sulfation may play distinctive roles in the metabolism of different vitamin E forms. In addition, the current evidence suggests that sulfated long-chain carboxychromanols may be novel excreted metabolites, especially under supplementation conditions.

23.5 MEASUREMENT OF CEHCS IN ANIMALS AND HUMANS

23.5.1 Methods for Detection of Metabolites

Several methods, such as GC-MS, HPLC electrochemical detection, HPLC fluorescent detection and LC-MS, have been used to measure the metabolites from vitamin E. All these methods include

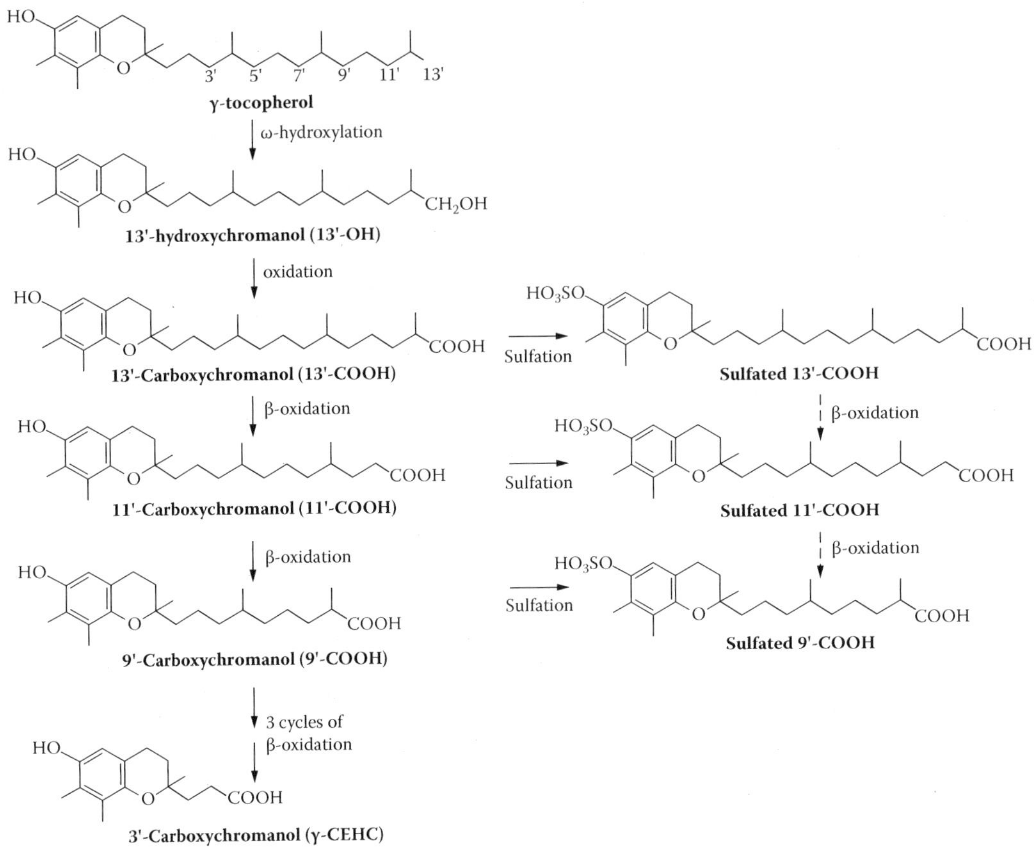

FIGURE 23.6 The metabolic pathway of tocopherols based on novel sulfated metabolites. The study suggests that sulfation is a parallel processing with β-oxidation. Dash-line arrows indicate hypothesized reaction pathways which need to be further characterized.

a sample processing procedure to extract metabolites from the biological matrix to organic solvents (ethyl acetate or ether) after samples are acidified to make the carboxylate group protonated. GC-MS method generally involves derivation of the hydroxyl and carboxylate group. This method can be used to detect non-conjugate carboxychromanols but not sulfated carboxychromanols, because carboxychromanol cannot be derived due to the block of the phenolic group. Similarly, HPLC electrochemical detection is limited to the unconjugated metabolites because sulfated carboxychromanols lack redox activity. For both methods, sulfatase has been used to unblock the phenolic group during sample preparation. However, the efficiency of the enzyme digestion has not been demonstrated. It is therefore premature to use these methods to quantify conjugated metabolites. In addition, enzyme digestion adds extra steps to the method.

Jiang et al. (2007) have developed a sensitive HPLC-fluorescent assay, which allows a simultaneous analysis of sulfated and non-conjugated intermediate metabolites that differ greatly in hydrophobicity. This assay made use of the fact that chromanol rings have strong fluorescent signals, regardless of the length of the side chain. Both sulfated and unconjugated carboxychromanols are fluorescent active. Based on the observation that the fluorescent signal of sulfated carboxychromanols is suppressed by a factor of 1.4 compared with their unconjugated counterparts, sulfated carboxychromanols can be directly quantified even without authentic compounds as external standards (Jiang et al. 2007). In addition, LC-MS could be an alternative approach for conjugated and non-conjugated metabolites. A LC-MS method for non-conjugated metabolites were recently reported by Leonard et al. (Leonard et al. 2005). The advantage of these latter two methods is that both sulfated and unconjugated metabolites can be simultaneously measured without the requirement of sulfatase digestion.

23.5.2 Metabolites in the Plasma and Tissues

Since CEHCs were identified as the major urinary metabolites of different forms of vitamin E, many studies have been conducted to measure γ-CEHC and α-CEHC in the urine and plasma. Schultz et al. (Schultz et al. 1995) were the first to show that α-CEHC is predominantly present in the sulfated form in human urine. Using d3-RRR-α-tocopherol and d6-all rac-α-tocopherol, Traber et al. (Traber et al. 1998) demonstrated that plasma is enriched with d3-RRR-α-T, while urine is enriched with α-CEHC derived from all rac-α-T, which indicates that compared with natural vitamin E, synthetic form is preferentially metabolized and excreted. There are substantial data in humans showing that more γ-CEHC than α-CEHC is excreted in urine (Traber et al. 1998; Swanson et al. 1999; Lodge et al. 2001), consistent with the fact that γ-T or γ-TE are more readily metabolized than α-T and α-TE. Leonard et al. (2005) showed that an 80-fold increase of α-CEHC is detected in the liver after rats are given high doses of α-T. Interestingly, the increase of γ-CEHC seems to be much more moderate in response to the supplementation with γ-T.

Although 5'-carboxychroman was also identified as another metabolite in cell culture supernatant and human urine, γ-CEHC appears to be quantitatively far more important (Parker and Swanson 2000). Plasma concentrations of γ-CEHC were reported to be 50-100 nmol/L in humans (Stahl et al. 1999) and > 300 nmol/L in rats (Hattori et al. 2000). Swanson et al. 1999) reported that in human urine, γ-CEHC exists predominantly as a glucuronide conjugate with concentrations ranging from 4 to 33 μmol/L, which increase to >100 μmol/L after supplementation with γ-T (Parker and Swanson 2000).

23.6 REGULATION OF METABOLISM

Although tocopherols and tocotrienols are similarly metabolized by cytochrome P-450 catalyzed ω-hydroxylation and β-oxidation, the relative extent that individual vitamin E forms are metabolized varies markedly. The metabolism appears to be mainly regulated by tocopherol binding proteins such as α-tocopherol transfer protein (TTP), and cytochrome P-450s that are responsible for the degradation.

23.6.1 Alpha-Tocopherol Transfer Protein

Alpha-TTP belongs to the CRAL-TRIO family, which consists of a small group of lipid-binding proteins responsible for intracellular trafficking of hydrophobic ligands. Other members in this family include the cellular retinaldehyde binding protein, yeast phosphatidylinositol transfer protein (Sec14p), and supernatant protein factor (SPF), a protein involved in cholesterol biosynthesis (Panagabko et al. 2003). α-TTP showed strong affinity for α-T, exhibiting a K(d) of 25 nM, but all other homologous proteins bind α-T with much weaker affinities (10-fold) than α-T. α-TTP has markedly distinct affinity for different forms of vitamin E in the following order): α-T (100%) > β-T (50%) > α-TE (12%) > γ-T (9%) >> δ-T, γ-TE. This differential binding affinity parallels the relative bioavailability of different forms of vitamin E, and the bioactivity shown in the rat fetal resorption assays. Among stereoisomers of α-T, α-TTP preferentially recognizes RRR-α-T compared with, for example, SRR-α-T. α-TTP binding affinity is therefore an important determining factor for tissue retention of vitamin E. The crystal structure of α-TTP revealed that this protein has a hinge and a cover that entraps α-T in the binding pocket which is enriched with hydrophobic amino acids (Meier et al. 2003; Min et al. 2003). α-TTP mRNA has been detected in various tissues including liver, spleen, lung, brain and kidney (Copp et al. 1999; Gohil et al. 2004). In addition, α-TTP has been reported to be present in pregnant mouse uterus and placenta (Kaempf-Rotzoll et al. 2002; Kaempf-Rotzoll et al. 2003).

Alpha-TTP-mediated α-T binding and transfer is key to the preferential enrichment of α-T in most tissues. α-TTP maintains α-T levels not only by facilitating its re-incorporation into nascent VLDL, but also by preventing it from being degraded (Traber et al. 1990a; Traber et al. 1990b; Traber et al. 1992). Therefore, patients with a defect in TTP have substantially reduced plasma levels of α-T compared with normal individuals. Schuelke et al. (2000) reported that patients who have a defect in α-TTP have enhanced urinary excretion of α-CEHC despite their much reduced plasma αT concentrations, as compared with normal controls. In some of these patients, the re-incorporation of RRR-αT into VLDL is not preferred compared with other stereoisomers, such as SRR-αT (Traber et al. 1993), in contrast to healthy individuals who preferentially enrich RRR-αT, presumably by hepatic α-TTP (Traber et al. 1992). Besides humans, α-TTP knockout mice have greatly reduced plasma and tissue concentrations of α-T (Terasawa et al. 2000).

It is well documented that plasma and tissue γT levels are suppressed by the supplementation of α-T (Bieri and Evarts 1974; Handelman et al. 1985). In sharp contrast, γ-T supplementation can lead to a marked increase in both tocopherols (Clement and Bourre 1997). The observation that supplementation of α-T depletes plasma and tissue γ-T may be partially rooted in TTP's preferential affinity for α-T. This is because an increase in α-T may further reduce γ-T's incorporation into VLDL, which consequently leaves more γ-T to be degraded by cytochrome P-450. It is interesting to note that α-TTP knockout mice not only have lowered α-T, but also have reduced γ-T (Traber et al. 2005). This unexpected observation suggests that α-TTP may also play a role in preventing γ-T from being degraded. On the other hand, supplementation of γ-T may spare α-T from being degraded, which can explain the fact that γ-T supplementation results in an increase in α-T (Clement and Bourre 1997).

23.6.2 Tocopherol ω-Hydroxylase

In contrast to the preferential protection of α-T from being degraded by α-TTP, hepatic catabolism of other forms of vitamin E appears to be responsible for the relatively low preservation of non-alpha forms of vitamin E in plasma and tissues. Sontag and Parker (2002) showed that CYP4F2 is responsible for the ω-hydroxylation, based on the study using fibroblasts stably expressing human liver CYP2E1 and in insect microsomes selectively expressing various recombinant human CYP enzymes. More recently, Sontag and Parker (2007) investigated the influence of the structural features of tocopherols and tocotrienols on their ω-oxidation by tocopherol-ω-hydroxylase in the similar recombination systems and liver microsomes. They showed that methylation at C5 of the chromanol ring, such as α-T and β-T, is associated with markedly low hydroxylase activity, while higher enzyme activity is observed for γ-T and δ-T which lack methylation at C5. Tocotrienols exhibited much higher Vmax than their tocopherol counterparts. On the other hand, side chain stereochemistry appears to have no effect on ω-hydroxylation of α-T. In another study, these investigators showed that *Drosophila* which lacks α-TTP exhibits similar tocopherol selectivity via cytochrome P450 (Parker and McCormick 2005). These observations indicate that although α-TTP is important for the retention of vitamin E, tocopherol-ω-hydroxylase plays an important role in selective degradation of different forms of vitamin E, and that methylation at C5 seems to be a key determinant factor. Consistently, α-TTP-knockout mice preferentially enrich α-T vs. γ-T, despite total tocopherol levels that are greatly reduced relative to the wild type (Terasawa et al. 2000).

The importance of cytochrome P450 in tocopherol metabolism is also evident from the study using cytochrome P450 inhibitors. Sesamin, a major lignan in sesame seeds, has been shown to inhibit the metabolism of tocopherols and tocotrienols in cultured cells (Parker et al. 2000; Sontag and Parker 2002). Supplementation with sesamin or sesame seed led to an increase of tissue levels of γ-T and γ-TE in animals (Kamal-Eldin et al. 1995; Yamashita et al. 2000; Ikeda et al. 2001). Consistently, consumption of moderate amounts of sesame seeds significantly increased plasma concentrations of γ-T in humans (Cooney et al. 2001). In addition, other plant products may enhance the tissue levels of vitamin E forms via the similar mechanism. For examples, genistein has long been known to inhibit cytochrome P450 activity (Foster et al. 2003; Roberts et al. 2004). Our preliminary data showed that genistein at 5-10μM inhibited metabolite generation from γ-T in cultured cells (Jiang et al. unpublished observations).

Cytochrome P450 activity seems to vary with species. The observation that rodents and humans often have substantially different P-450 activity (Turesky et al. 1999) may partially explain the findings that rats have lower concentrations of γ-T (Behrens and Madere 1987) but higher γ-CEHC in the plasma (Hattori et al. 2000) than humans (Stahl et al. 1999). In addition to the plasma, γ-T concentrations are substantially higher in tissues of humans than those of rodents. For example, concentrations of γ-T in human skin and muscle, i.e., 180 and 107 nmol per gram of tissues, respectively, are 20–50-fold higher than those measured in rodents (Handelman et al. 1994; Weber et al. 1997; Burton et al. 1998). The hypothesis that the different retention of tocopherols between humans and rodents is due to differential activity of cytochrome P450 warrants further investigation.

23.6.3 Alpha-T Regulates the Metabolism of Other Forms of Vitamin E and Drugs by Modulating the Expression of Cytochrome P-450 and p-Glycoprotein

Alpha-T appears to play a role in regulation of the metabolism of other forms of vitamin E as well as pharmaceutical drugs. This may be at least partially due to its ability to affect expression of xenobiotic enzymes and ABC transporters. Mustacich et al. (2006) reported that a high dose of α-T resulted in an up-regulation of cytochrome P450 proteins, including CYP3A and CYP2P, as well as a protein involved in biliary xenobiotic excretion, p-glycoprotein. On the other hand, high doses of γ-T did not show a similar effect (Traber et al. 2005). The effect of α-T on CYP expression is likely rooted in its activation of the pregnane X receptor (PXR) (Traber 2004). In an *in vitro* system, Landes et al. (2003) showed that both α-T and rifampicin, a known stimulator of xenobiotic metabolism, activated the PXR, an orphan nuclear receptor (Brigelius-Flohe 2003; Landes et al. 2003). PXR as a heterodimer with the retinoid X receptor (RXR), binds to specific cis-elements in the promoter regions of genes. PXR/RXR regulates cytochrome P450 (CYP), CYP3A, involved in the hepatic detoxification of more than 50% of prescription drugs. Interestingly, among all the vitamin E forms tested, α-TE and γ-TE are the strongest activators of PXR-RXR, and α-T is the most moderate, while γ-T is the least active (Landes et al. 2003).

Increases in xenobiotic metabolism and excretion pathways by α-T may lead to acceleration of the metabolism of vitamin E forms and alterations in the efficacy of some pharmaceutical drugs. This action of α-T may partially account for the observation that α-T supplementation causes depletion of γ-T, in addition to the above-mentioned competition between α-T and γ-T for α-TTP. The potentiation of cytochrome P-450 and p-glycoprotein may be an explanation of the adverse effects caused by supplementation of pharmaceutical doses of α-T in patients with multi-drug treatment as reported in recent studies (Miller et al. 2005).

23.6.4 The Role of Sulfation

Jiang et al. (2007) recently showed that significant amounts of sulfated metabolites are formed in cultured cells and in rats supplemented with γ-T. The presence of sulfated long-chain carboxychromanols suggests that sulfation may be a parallel processing with β-oxidation. It is currently not clear how sulfation plays a role in regulation of vitamin E metabolism. When different forms of vitamin E are incubated in A549 cells, the amounts of sulfated carboxychromanols formed varied markedly. The reason for the different extent of sulfation is currently not clear. However, these results suggest a possible distinct substrate specificity of sulfotransferase(s) (Chapman et al. 2004), and a potentially distinct role of sulfation among different forms of vitamin E. It is conceivable that inhibitors of sulfotransferases including phenolic compounds (Wang and James 2006) would be able to modulate the extent of sulfation and therefore affect the metabolism. Future study in this area may provide information regarding how botanical compounds have an effect on the bioavailability of vitamin E and their metabolites.

23.7 NOVEL FUNCTIONS OF VITAMIN E METABOLITES

23.7.1 Natriuretic Activity of γ-CEHC

Wechter et al. (1996; Murray et al. 1997) showed that γ-CEHC, which was originally named LLU-α, possesses natriuretic activity by inhibition of the 70 pS potassium channel in the thick ascending limb cells of the kidney, whereas α-CEHC does not exhibit any appreciable activity. In the *in vivo* natriuresis/diuresis/kaliuresis/blood pressure assay, these investigators found that infusion of 4-8 μg/kg γ-CEHC led to significant natriuresis, which is indicated by an enhanced excretion of sodium ion, and mild diuresis with no evidence of kaliuresis in male Harlan Sprague Dawley rats. On the other hand, the treatment shows no effect on mean arterial pressure. In addition, γ-CEHC does not inhibit the Na^+/K^+-ATPase when evaluated in Madin-Darby bovine kidney cells. In line with the natriuretic effect of γ-CEHC, supplementation of γ-T or γ-TE, which leads to an increase of γ-CEHC excretion to the urine, was found to increase urinary sodium excretion (Saito et al. 2003; Uto et al. 2004). Saito et al. (2003) showed that supplementation with 10 mg of γ-TE by gastric tube over 3 days leads to an acceleration and increase of sodium excretion only in rats given a high-NaCl diet. γ-TE supplementation also increases urine volume in the high-NaCl group but has no effect on potassium excretion. Similarly, oral administration of 20 mg γ-T results in an increase of urine volume and sodium excretion in rats given a high-NaCl diet compared with animals given control diet supplemented with γ-T (Uto et al. 2004).

23.7.2 Protection Against Nephrotoxicity by γ-CEHC

Appenroth et al. (2001) examined the protective effect of synthetic γ-CEHC in comparison with the effect of α-T and γ-T on metal nephrotoxicity induced by sodium dichromate (Cr) or thallium sulfate (Tl) in rats. Pretreatment with γ-CEHC resulted in lower chromate nephrotoxicity than α-T and γ-T, but did not affect Cr concentration in renal tissue. The protective effect of γ-CEHC against Cr toxicity seemed to be caused by its stronger antioxidant activity in comparison to α-T and γ-T. Consistently, when tested by iron stimulated lipid peroxidation, the ranking of antioxidant activity was determined in the following order: α-T < γ-T < γ-CEHC. Pretreatment with γ-CEHC resulted in lower thallium-induced proteinuria, a lower concentration of Tl in the renal medulla, and higher urinary Tl excretion. Unlike γ-CEHC, which has been shown to inhibit K(+) channels in the apical membrane of the thick ascending limb of Henle's loop, γ-T did not have this effect. These investigators assumed that the protective effect of γ-CEHC against Tl nephrotoxicity is caused by its antioxidant effect and, at least in part, by its ability to decrease Tl concentration as a consequence of inhibited Tl(+) uptake through K(+) channels.

23.7.3 Anti-Inflammatory Activity of CEHC: Inhibition of Cyclooxygenase-Catalyzed Proinflammatory Eicosanoid Formation

Inflammatory diseases afflict millions of people worldwide. Chronic inflammation contributes to the development of cancers, cardiovascular diseases and neurodegenerative disorders (Coussens and Werb 2002; Libby 2002; Perry et al. 2007). Cyclooxygenases (COX) catalyze enzymatic oxidation of arachidonic acid (AA) to prostaglandin H_2 (PGH_2), the common precursor to prostaglandins and thromboxane, which are important lipid mediators for regulation of inflammatory response and other physiological as well as pathophysiological processes (Vane 1976; Dubois et al. 1998). Two COX isoforms have been identified. COX-1 is a constitutive form that regulates homeostasis in many tissues, and COX-2 is an inducible form that is mainly responsible for the generation of pro-inflammatory eicosanoids, including prostaglandin E_2 (PGE_2) under acute inflammatory conditions (Vane et al. 1998). COX inhibitors, which belong to non-steroidal anti-inflammatory drugs (NSAIDs), have been used for the relief of fever, pain and inflammation (Vane and Botting 1998a; Vane and Botting 1998b), as well as treatment for chronic diseases. It is now well established that

NSAIDs are effective and useful chemoprevention agents for colon cancer (Giovannucci et al. 1995; Gupta and Dubois 2001) and possibly other types of cancer (Thun et al. 1993; Fulton et al. 2006).

Gamma-CEHC appears to have anti-inflammatory activity by inhibition of COX-catalyzed reactions. Jiang et al. (Jiang et al. 2000) showed that, similar to γ-T, γ-CEHC inhibits pro-inflammatory PGE_2 in lipopolysacharide-activated macrophages and interlukin-1β-stimulated human epithelial cells. The apparent IC50s in these cells are 30-40 μM. Like γ-T, γ-CEHC does not affect COX-2 expression or the substrate availability, and the inhibition is independent of antioxidant activity. Instead, γ-CEHC directly inhibits the enzyme activity, as indicated in intact cell assays. The inhibitory potency, however, is diminished with an increased concentration of arachidonic acid, the physiological substrate of COXs. The reason for this observation is not fully understood, but may be explained by the possibility that γ-CEHC serves as a weak competitive inhibitor of COX. Consistently, we recently found that γ-CEHC inhibits the activity of purified COX-1 and COX-2 but the IC50s are much higher than that shown in cellular environments (Jiang et al. unpublished data). The selective inhibition of cyclooxygenase in cells over purified enzymes supports the notion that γ-CEHC is a weak inhibitor of cyclooxygenases, similar to classic weak cyclooxygenase inhibitors like acetaminophen and salicylate (Mitchell et al. 1997; Boutaud et al. 2002; Aronoff et al. 2003). Grammas et al. (2004) reported that both α-CEHC and γ-CEHC inhibit PGE_2 in rat aortic endothelial cells and mouse microglial cultures, showing apparent IC50 of 70–80 μM. Neither α-T nor γ-T is inhibitory in these cells.

In addition to the studies in cultured cells, Jiang and Ames (2003) demonstrated that γ-CEHC has an anti-inflammatory effect in a rat model in which inflammation is induced by injection of carrageenan in the intrascapular area. This model is believed to mimic joint diseases. In this model, administration of γ-CEHC led to a significant reduction of carrageenan-induced PGE_2 and leukotriene B_4 at the site of inflammation. Although the potential anti-inflammatory activity of γ-CEHC has not been directly tested in humans, Himmelfarb and colleagues (2003) reported that in chronic hemodialysis patients, supplementation with γT-enriched mixed tocopherols, which contain 60% RRR-γT, 28% RRR-δT and 10% RRR-αT, at doses of 300 mg for 2 weeks, led to a significant reduction (>50%) of C-reactive protein, an excellent marker of inflammation. On the other hand, in the five hemodialysis patients, supplementation of αT-enriched tocopherols, which contain 99% RRR-αT, at doses of 300 mg for 2 weeks, had no effect on C-reactive protein, but caused a significant increase in IL-6, a pro-inflammatory cytokine (Himmelfarb et al. 2003). In this study, these investigators reported that plasma concentrations of γ-CEHC increase four- to five-fold in subjects given γ-T supplementation, in contrast to less than two-fold increase of γ-T after 1 to 6 days of supplementation. These investigators believe that the observed anti-inflammatory effect from supplementation is at least partially rooted in γ-CEHC.

23.7.4 Long-Chain Carboxychromanols as Potent Inhibitors of Cyclooxygenases

Jiang et al. (unpublished data) have investigated the effect of different forms of vitamin E and their metabolites, including long-chain carboxychromanols and sulfated carboxychromanols, on cyclooxygenase-catalyzed reactions. In interleukin-1β-activated A549 cells, vitamin E forms differentially inhibited PGE_2 formation but did not have an effect on COX-2 expression. Among vitamin E forms, γ-tocotrienol, δ-tocopherol and γ-tocopherol inhibited PGE_2 at physiologically relevant concentrations. On the other hand, α-, β-tocopherol and α-tocotrienol are much less to not effective. The cellular inhibition of PGE_2 was partially diminished by sesamin that prevents vitamin E from being metabolized in A549 cells. This observation suggests that long-chain carboxychromanols or their sulfated counterparts may contribute to the inhibitory effect of PGE_2. To investigate whether long-chain carboxychromanols inhibit COX-2 activity, we examined the effect of conditioned media that contain vitamin E metabolites generated by A549 cells. Conditioned media enriched with long-chain carboxychromanols dose-dependently reduced COX-2 activity in intact-cell assays. On the other hand, conditioned media containing predominantly sulfated carboxychromanols do not appear to be effective.

These results suggests that long-chain carboxychromanols are effective inhibitors of cyclooxygenases, but vitamin E forms are weak inhibitors, which are likely to be effective in cellular environments (Mitchell et al. 1997; Boutaud et al. 2002; Aronoff et al. 2003). One important implication of these findings is that different bioactivity among vitamin E forms such as α-T and γ-T may be partially rooted in their distinct metabolism. Specifically, long-chain carboxychromanols may in part account for *in vivo* anti-inflammatory effect of γ-T (Reiter et al. 2007). On the other hand, compared with γ-T, carboxychromanols generated from α-T are likely to be quantitatively much less important because α-T is preferentially protected from being degraded by tocopherol transfer protein (Brigelius-Flohe and Traber 1999; Jiang et al. 2001). To this end, we and others have demonstrated that γ-T administration inhibits proinflammatory eicosanoids at the inflammatory site and attenuates inflammation-caused damage in various animal models (Jiang et al. 2002; Jiang and Ames 2003; Takahashi et al. 2006; Yoshida et al. 2006; Wagner et al. 2007). Himmelfard et al. reported that γ-T enriched but not α-T-enriched mixed tocopherols inhibit proinflammatory C-reactive protein and IL-6 in kidney-dialysis patients (Himmelfarb et al. 2003). We recently showed that 13'-carboxychromanol is detected in the plasma and liver in rats supplemented with γ-T (Jiang et al. 2007). While pharmacokinetics of 13'-carboxychromanol formation need to be further established, our preliminary data revealed that relatively large amounts of 13'-carboxychromanol are found in rat feces 24 hours after γ-T supplementation (Jiang and Freiser, unpublished observation). This suggests that long-chain carboxychromanols, inhibitors of cyclooxygenases and potentially accumulated in colon tissues, may also contribute to the impressive anticancer effect of mixed tocopherols enriched with γ-T and δ-T on aberrant crypt foci in azoxymethane-induced colon cancer in rodents (Newmark et al. 2006).

23.7.5 Sulfated Compounds

Sulfated CEHCs and long-chain carboxychromanols are formed in the liver and found in the plasma in animals or humans supplemented with tocopherols and tocotrienols. Sulfated metabolites do not have antioxidant activity because of their conjugated phenolic group. Unlike unconjugated carboxychromanols, sulfated counterparts are resistant to electrochemical oxidation (Jiang et al. 2007). Recent studies suggest that sulfation is not just a simple modification involved in detoxification, but could play a role in regulation of specific biological activities (Strott and Higashi 2003; Totta et al. 2005). For example, daidzein-sulfate metabolites affect transcriptional and antiproliferative activities of estrogen receptor-beta in cultured human cancer cells (Totta et al. 2005). Accumulating evidence has demonstrated a regulatory function for cholesterol sulfate (Strott and Higashi 2003); it protects erythrocytes from osmotic lysis, regulates sperm capacitation and the activity of serine proteases, and supports platelet adhesion. Cholesterol sulfate appears to be also involved in signal transduction, as indicated by its ability to regulate the activity of selective protein kinase C isoforms and modulate the specificity of phosphatidylinositol 3-kinase. It is tempting to speculate that some of the non-antioxidant bioactivities observed from supplementation of certain vitamin E forms were performed or shared by the sulfated metabolites. Future studies are needed to investigate potentially interesting activity of these conjugated carboxychromanols.

23.8 SUMMARY

Although vitamin E has been known for approximately 85 years, its function and metabolism are only partially elucidated. The fact that vitamin E consists of eight structurally related molecules has certainly complicated the issue. Because of the structural similarity, all eight molecules are potent membrane-soluble antioxidants *in vitro*. However, these molecules have very distinct bioactivity and bio-availability *in vivo*. In this regard, current evidence strongly suggests that the metabolism of vitamin E is not only important for determination of their bioavailability but also plays a role in regulation of the biological functions. It is now established that the metabolism of vitamin E involves ω-hydroxylation and oxidation of the 13'-carbon of the hydrophobic side chain, and then β-oxidation to cut off a two- to three-carbon moiety each cycle via the formation of various-length side chain carboxychromanols to finally generate terminal urinary-excreted metabolites, CEHCs. During this process, sulfation of intermediate carboxychromanols may occur parallel to β-oxidation, in addition to formation of the terminal conjugated CEHCs. The sulfation may be particularly important under supplementation conditions, and may play distinct roles for different forms of vitamin E, which warrants further investigation.

Because of its potential importance to the bioactivity and availability of vitamin E, the metabolism is highly regulated. α-TTP appears to play a key role in the protection of α-T from being metabolized and may also facilitate intracellular traffic of vitamin E forms. The mechanism regarding how α-TTP facilitates vitamin E transport in cells has not been elucidated. Besides α-T, TTP seems also to help maintain the tissue levels of other forms of vitamin E. While α-TTP is important to tissue retention of tocopherols, tocopherol hydroxylase appears to be a determining factor for the selectivity of vitamin E metabolism. Methylation of C5 such as α-T or β-T decreases the hydroxylase activity, but vitamin forms lacking methylation at C5 are more readily degraded due to high hydroxylase activity. It remains to be established whether CYP4F2 is the sole isotype of cytochrome P-450 for vitamin E degradation. Future studies using knockout/transgenic mice will not only elucidate the importance of CYP4F2 in vitamin E metabolism, but also will answer the question whether other CYPs are involved in the metabolism. In addition, other dietary factors may modulate vitamin E bioavailability and metabolism via modulation of CYP activity, which warrants further investigation.

To completely elucidate the functions of vitamin E, studies are also needed to investigate the functional bioactivity of the metabolites. This is particularly important for non-alpha forms due to their higher rate of metabolism and potentially high accumulation of the metabolites in tissues.

ACKNOWLEDGMENT

This work was supported in part by National Institute of Health Grants R01AT001821 and P01 AT002620.

REFERENCES

Appenroth, D., E. Karge, G. Kiessling, et al. 2001. LLU-alpha, an endogenous metabolite of gamma-tocopherol, is more effective against metal nephrotoxicity in rats than gamma-tocopherol. *Toxicol Lett* 122(3): 255–65.

Aronoff, D.M., O. Boutaud, L.J. Marnett, et al. 2003. Inhibition of prostaglandin H2 synthases by salicylate is dependent on the oxidative state of the enzymes. *J Pharmacol Exp Ther* 304(2): 589–95.

Behrens, W.A. and R. Madere. 1987. Mechanisms of absorption, transport and tissue uptake of RRR-alpha-tocopherol and d-gamma-tocopherol in the white rat. *J Nutr* 117(9): 1562–9.

Bieri, J.G. and R.P. Evarts. 1974. Gamma tocopherol: Metabolism, biological activity and significance in human vitamin E nutrition. *Am J Clin Nutr* 27(9): 980–986.

Birringer, M., P. Pfluger, D. Kluth, et al. 2002. Identities and differences in the metabolism of tocotrienols and tocopherols in HepG2 cells. *J Nutr* 132(10): 3113–8.

Boutaud, O., D.M. Aronoff, J.H. Richardson, et al. 2002. Determinants of the cellular specificity of acetaminophen as an inhibitor of prostaglandin H(2 synthases. *Proc Natl Acad Sci U S A* 99(10): 7130–5.

Brigelius-Flohe, R. 2003. Vitamin E and drug metabolism. *Biochem Biophys Res Commun* 305(3): 737–40.

Brigelius-Flohe, R. and M.G. Traber. 1999. Vitamin E: Function and metabolism. *Faseb J* 13(10): 1145–55.

Burton, G.W., M.G. Traber, R.V. Acuff, et al. 1998. Human plasma and tissue alpha-tocopherol concentrations in response to supplementation with deuterated natural and synthetic vitamin E [see comments]. *Am J Clin Nutr* 67(4): 669–684.

Chapman, E., M.D. Best, S.R. Hanson, et al. 2004. Sulfotransferases: Structure, mechanism, biological activity, inhibition, and synthetic utility. *Angew Chem Int Ed Engl* 43(27): 3526–48.

Chiku, S., K. Hamamura and T. Nakamura. 1984. Novel urinary metabolite of d-delta-tocopherol in rats. *J Lipid Res* 25(1): 40–8.

Clement, M. and J.M. Bourre. 1997. Graded dietary levels of RRR-gamma-tocopherol induce a marked increase in the concentrations of alpha- and gamma-tocopherol in nervous tissues, heart, liver and muscle of vitamin-E-deficient rats. *Biochim Biophys Acta* 1334(2–3): 173–81.

Cooney, R.V., L.J. Custer, L. Okinaka, et al. 2001. Effects of dietary sesame seeds on plasma tocopherol levels. *Nutr Cancer* 39(1): 66–71.

Copp, R.P., T. Wisniewski, F. Hentati, et al. 1999. Localization of alpha-tocopherol transfer protein in the brains of patients with ataxia with vitamin E deficiency and other oxidative stress related neurodegenerative disorders. *Brain Res* 822(1–2): 80–7.

Coussens, L.M. and Z. Werb. 2002. Inflammation and cancer. *Nature* 420(6917): 860–7.

Dubois, R.N., S.B. Abramson, L. Crofford, et al. 1998. Cyclooxygenase in biology and disease. *Faseb J* 12(12): 1063–73.

Eisengart, A., A.T. Milhorat, E.J. Simon, et al. 1956. The metabolism of vitamin E. II. Purification and characterization of urinary metabolites of alpha-tocopherol. *J Biol Chem* 221(2): 807–17.

Foster, B.C., S. Vandenhoek, J. Hana, et al. 2003. *In vitro* inhibition of human cytochrome P450-mediated metabolism of marker substrates by natural products. *Phytomedicine* 10(4): 334–42.

Fulton, A.M., X. Ma and N. Kundu. 2006. Targeting prostaglandin E EP receptors to inhibit metastasis. *Cancer Res* 66(20): 9794–7.

Giovannucci, E., K.M. Egan, D.J. Hunter, et al. 1995. Aspirin and the risk of colorectal cancer in women. *N Engl J Med* 333(10): 609–614.

Gohil, K., R. Godzdanker, E. O'Roark, et al. 2004. Alpha-tocopherol transfer protein deficiency in mice causes multi-organ deregulation of gene networks and behavioral deficits with age. *Ann N Y Acad Sci* 1031): 109–26.

Grammas, P., L. Hamdheydari, E.J. Benaksas, et al. 2004. Anti-inflammatory effects of tocopherol metabolites. *Biochem Biophys Res Commun* 319(3): 1047–52.

Gross, C.S., A.T. Milhorat and E.J. Simon. 1956. The metabolism of vitamin E. I. The absorption and excretion of d-alpha-tocopheryl-5-methyl-C14-succinate. *J Biol Chem* 221(2): 797–805.

Gupta, R.A. and R.N. Dubois. 2001. Colorectal cancer prevention and treatment by inhibition of cyclooxygenase-2. *Nat Rev Cancer* 1(1): 11–21.

Handelman, G.J., W.L. Epstein, J. Peerson, et al. 1994. Human adipose alpha-tocopherol and gamma-tocopherol kinetics during and after 1 y of alpha-tocopherol supplementation. *Am J Clin Nutr* 59(5): 1025–1032.

Handelman, G.J., L.J. Machlin, K. Fitch, et al. 1985. Oral alpha-tocopherol supplements decrease plasma gamma-tocopherol levels in humans. *J Nutr* 115(6): 807–813.

Hattori, A., T. Fukushima and K. Imai. 2000. Occurrence and determination of a natriuretic hormone, 2,7,8-trimethyl-2-(beta-carboxyethyl-6-hydroxy chroman), in rat plasma, urine, and bile. *Anal Biochem* 281(2): 209–15.

Himmelfarb, J., J. Kane, E. McMonagle, et al. 2003. Alpha and gamma tocopherol metabolism in healthy subjects and patients with end-stage renal disease. *Kidney Int* 64(3): 978–91.

Ikeda, S., K. Toyoshima and K. Yamashita. 2001. Dietary sesame seeds elevate alpha- and gamma-tocotrienol concentrations in skin and adipose tissue of rats fed the tocotrienol-rich fraction extracted from palm oil. *J Nutr* 131(11): 2892–7.

Jiang, Q. and B.N. Ames. 2003. Gamma-tocopherol, but not alpha-tocopherol, decreases proinflammatory eicosanoids and inflammation damage in rats. *Faseb J* 17(8): 816–22.

Jiang, Q., S. Christen, M.K. Shigenaga, et al. 2001. Gamma-tocopherol, the major form of vitamin E in the US diet, deserves more attention. *Am J Clin Nutr* 74(6): 714–22.

Jiang, Q., I. Elson–Schwab, C. Courtemanche, et al. 2000. gamma-tocopherol and its major metabolite, in contrast to alpha-tocopherol, inhibit cyclooxygenase activity in macrophages and epithelial cells. *Proc Natl Acad Sci USA* 97(21): 11494–9.

Jiang, Q., H. Freiser, K.V. Wood, et al. 2007. Identification and quantitation of novel vitamin E metabolites, sulfated long–chain carboxychromanols, in human A549 cells and in rats. *J Lipid Res* 48(5): 1221–30.

Jiang, Q., J. Lykkesfeldt, M.K. Shigenaga, et al. 2002. Gamma-tocopherol supplementation inhibits protein nitration and ascorbate oxidation in rats with inflammation. *Free Radic Biol Med* 33(11): 1534–42.

Jin, R., D.R. Koop, J.L. Raucy, et al. 1998. Role of human CYP4F2 in hepatic catabolism of the proinflammatory agent leukotriene B4. *Arch Biochem Biophys* 359(1): 89–98.

Kaempf–Rotzoll, D.E., M. Horiguchi, K. Hashiguchi, et al. 2003. Human placental trophoblast cells express alpha-tocopherol transfer protein. *Placenta* 24(5): 439–44.

Kaempf–Rotzoll, D.E., K. Igarashi, J. Aoki, et al. 2002. Alpha-tocopherol transfer protein is specifically localized at the implantation site of pregnant mouse uterus. *Biol Reprod* 67(2): 599–604.

Kamal–Eldin, A., D. Pettersson and L.A. Appelqvist. 1995. Sesamin. A compound from sesame oil increases tocopherol levels in rats fed ad libitum. *Lipids* 30(6): 499–505.
Kantoci, D., W.J. Wechter, E.D. Murray, Jr., et al. 1997. Endogenous natriuretic factors 6: The stereochemistry of a natriuretic gamma-tocopherol metabolite LLU-alpha. *J Pharmacol Exp Ther* 282(2): 648–56.
Kayden, H.J. and M.G. Traber. 1993. Absorption, lipoprotein transport, and regulation of plasma concentrations of vitamin E in humans. *J Lipid Res* 34(3): 343–58.
Kunau, W.H., V. Dommes and H. Schulz. 1995. Beta-oxidation of fatty acids in mitochondria, peroxisomes, and bacteria): A century of continued progress. *Prog Lipid Res* 34(4): 267–342.
Landes, N., P. Pfluger, D. Kluth, et al. 2003. Vitamin E activates gene expression via the pregnane X receptor. *Biochem Pharmacol* 65(2): 269–73.
Leonard, S.W., E. Gumpricht, M.W. Devereaux, et al. 2005. Quantitation of rat liver vitamin E metabolites by LC-MS during high-dose vitamin E administration. *J Lipid Res* 46(5): 1068–75.
Libby, P. 2002. Inflammation in atherosclerosis. *Nature* 420(6917): 868–74.
Lodge, J.K., J. Ridlington, S. Leonard, et al. 2001. Alpha- and gamma-tocotrienols are metabolized to carboxyethyl-hydroxychroman derivatives and excreted in human urine. *Lipids* 36(1): 43–8.
McLaughlin, P.J. and J.L. Weihrauch. 1979. Vitamin E content of foods. *J Am Diet Assoc* 75(6): 647–65.
Meier, R., T. Tomizaki, C. Schulze-Briese, et al. 2003. The molecular basis of vitamin E retention: Structure of human alpha-tocopherol transfer protein. *J Mol Biol* 331(3): 725–34.
Miller, E.R., 3rd, R. Pastor-Barriuso, D. Dalal, et al. 2005. Meta-analysis: High-dosage vitamin E supplementation may increase all-cause mortality. *Ann Intern Med* 142(1): 37–46.
Min, K.C., R.A. Kovall and W.A. Hendrickson. 2003. Crystal structure of human alpha-tocopherol transfer protein bound to its ligand: Implications for ataxia with vitamin E deficiency. *Proc Natl Acad Sci U S A* 100(25): 14713–8.
Minehira-Castelli, K., S.W. Leonard, Q.M. Walker, et al. 2006. Absence of VLDL secretion does not affect alpha-tocopherol content in peripheral tissues. *J Lipid Res* 47(8): 1733–8.
Mitchell, J.A., M. Saunders, P.J. Barnes, et al. 1997. Sodium salicylate inhibits cyclo-oxygenase-2 activity independently of transcription factor. nuclear factor kappaB activation: Role of arachidonic acid. *Mol Pharmacol* 51(6): 907–12.
Mukherji, M., C.J. Schofield, A.S. Wierzbicki, et al. 2003. The chemical biology of branched-chain lipid metabolism. *Prog Lipid Res* 42(5): 359–76.
Murray, E.D., Jr., W.J. Wechter, D. Kantoci, et al. 1997. Endogenous natriuretic factors 7: Biospecificity of a natriuretic gamma-tocopherol metabolite LLU-alpha. *J Pharmacol Exp Ther* 282(2): 657–62.
Mustacich, D.J., S.W. Leonard, M.W. Devereaux, et al. 2006. Alpha-tocopherol regulation of hepatic cytochrome P450s and ABC transporters in rats. *Free Radic Biol Med* 41(7): 1069–78.
Mustacich, D.J., J. Shields, R.A. Horton, et al. 1998. Biliary secretion of alpha-tocopherol and the role of the mdr2 P-glycoprotein in rats and mice. *Arch Biochem Biophys* 350(2): 183–92.
Newmark, H.L., M.T. Huang and B.S. Reddy. 2006. Mixed tocopherols inhibit azoxymethane-induced aberrant crypt foci in rats. *Nutr Cancer* 56(1): 82–5.
Panagabko, C., S. Morley, M. Hernandez, et al. 2003. Ligand specificity in the CRAL-TRIO protein family. *Biochemistry* 42(21): 6467–74.
Parker, R.S. and C.C. McCormick. 2005. Selective accumulation of alpha-tocopherol in Drosophila is associated with cytochrome P450 tocopherol-omega-hydroxylase activity but not alpha-tocopherol transfer protein. *Biochem Biophys Res Commun* 338(3): 1537–41.
Parker, R.S., T.J. Sontag and J.E. Swanson. 2000. Cytochrome P4503A-dependent metabolism of tocopherols and inhibition by sesamin. *Biochem Biophys Res Commun* 277(3): 531–4.
Parker, R.S. and J.E. Swanson. 2000. A novel 5'-carboxychroman metabolite of gamma-tocopherol secreted by HepG2 cells and excreted in human urine. *Biochem Biophys Res Commun* 269(2): 580–3.
Perry, V.H., C. Cunningham and C. Holmes. 2007. Systemic infections and inflammation affect chronic neurodegeneration. *Nat Rev Immunol* 7(2): 161–7.
Pope, S.A., G.E. Burtin, P.T. Clayton, et al. 2002. Synthesis and analysis of conjugates of the major vitamin E metabolite, alpha-CEHC. *Free Radic Biol Med* 33(6): 807–17.
Reiter, E., Q. Jiang and S. Christen. 2007. Anti-inflammatory properties of alpha- and gamma-tocopherol. *Mol Aspects Med*: Jan 11; [Epub ahead of print].
Roberts, D.W., D.R. Doerge, M.I. Churchwell, et al. 2004. Inhibition of extrahepatic human cytochromes P450 1A1 and 1B1 by metabolism of isoflavones found in Trifolium pratense (red clover). *J Agric Food Chem* 52(21): 6623–32.

Saito, H., C. Kiyose, H. Yoshimura, et al. 2003. Gamma-tocotrienol, a vitamin E homolog, is a natriuretic hormone precursor. *J Lipid Res* 44(8): 1530–5.

Schuelke, M., A. Elsner, B. Finckh, et al. 2000. Urinary alpha-tocopherol metabolites in alpha-tocopherol transfer protein-deficient patients. *J Lipid Res* 41(10): 1543–51.

Schultz, M., M. Leist, M. Petrzika, et al. 1995. Novel urinary metabolite of alpha-tocopherol, 2,5,7,8-tetramethyl-2(2'-carboxyethyl)-6-hydroxychroman, as an indicator of an adequate vitamin E supply? *Am J Clin Nutr* 62(6 Suppl): 1527S–1534S.

Sontag, T.J. and R.S. Parker. 2002. Cytochrome P450 omega-hydroxylase pathway of tocopherol catabolism. Novel mechanism of regulation of vitamin E status. *J Biol Chem* 277(28): 25290–6.

Sontag, T.J. and R.S. Parker. 2007. Influence of major structural features of tocopherols and tocotrienols on their {omega}-oxidation by tocopherol-{omega-hydroxylase. *J Lipid Res* 48(5): 1090–8.

Stahl, W., P. Graf, R. Brigelius-Flohe, et al. 1999. Quantification of the alpha- and gamma-tocopherol metabolites 2,5,7, 8-tetramethyl-2-(2'-carboxyethyl)-6-hydroxychroman and 2,7, 8-trimethyl-2-(2'-carboxyethyl)-6-hydroxychroman in human serum. *Anal Biochem* 275(2): 254–9.

Stone, W.L. and A.M. Papas. 1997. Tocopherols and the etiology of colon cancer. *J Natl Cancer Inst* 89(14): 1006–14.

Stone, W.L., A.M. Papas, I.O. LeClair, et al. 1998. The influence of dietary iron and tocopherols on oxidative stress in the colon. *Cancer Detect Prev* 22: S110.

Strott, C.A. and Y. Higashi. 2003. Cholesterol sulfate in human physiology: What's it all about? *J Lipid Res* 44(7): 1268–78.

Swanson, J.E., R.N. Ben, G.W. Burton, et al. 1999. Urinary excretion of 2,7, 8-trimethyl-2-(beta-carboxyethyl)-6-hydroxychroman is a major route of elimination of gamma-tocopherol in humans. *J Lipid Res* 40(4): 665–671.

Takahashi, K., T. Komaru, S. Takeda, et al. 2006. Gamma-tocopherol, but not alpha-tocopherol, potently inhibits neointimal formation induced by vascular injury in insulin resistant rats. *J Mol Cell Cardiol* 41(3): 544–54.

Terasawa, Y., Z. Ladha, S.W. Leonard, et al. 2000. Increased atherosclerosis in hyperlipidemic mice deficient in alpha-tocopherol transfer protein and vitamin E. *Proc Natl Acad Sci U S A* 97(25): 13830–4.

Theriault, A., J.T. Chao, Q. Wang, et al. 1999. Tocotrienol: A review of its therapeutic potential. *Clin Biochem* 32(5): 309–19.

Thun, M.J., M.M. Namboodiri, E.E. Calle, et al. 1993. Aspirin use and risk of fatal cancer. *Cancer Res* 53(6): 1322–1327.

Totta, P., F. Acconcia, F. Virgili, et al. 2005. Daidzein-sulfate metabolites affect transcriptional and antiproliferative activities of estrogen receptor-beta in cultured human cancer cells. *J Nutr* 135(11): 2687–93.

Traber, M.G. 2004. Vitamin E, nuclear receptors and xenobiotic metabolism. *Arch Biochem Biophys* 423(1): 6–11.

Traber, M.G., G.W. Burton, L. Hughes, et al. 1992. Discrimination between forms of vitamin E by humans with and without genetic abnormalities of lipoprotein metabolism. *J Lipid Res* 33(8): 1171–82.

Traber, M.G., G.W. Burton, K.U. Ingold, et al. 1990a. RRR- and SRR-alpha-tocopherols are secreted without discrimination in human chylomicrons, but RRR-alpha-tocopherol is preferentially secreted in very low density lipoproteins. *J Lipid Res* 31(4): 675–85.

Traber, M.G., A. Elsner and R. Brigelius-Flohe. 1998. Synthetic as compared with natural vitamin E is preferentially excreted as alpha-CEHC in human urine: Studies using deuterated alpha-tocopheryl acetates. *FEBS Lett* 437(1–2): 145–8.

Traber, M.G. and H.J. Kayden. 1989. Preferential incorporation of alpha-tocopherol vs. gamma-tocopherol in human lipoproteins. *Am J Clin Nutr* 49(3): 517–26.

Traber, M.G., T. Olivecrona and H.J. Kayden. 1985. Bovine milk lipoprotein lipase transfers tocopherol to human fibroblasts during triglyceride hydrolysis *in vitro*. *J Clin Invest* 75(5): 1729–34.

Traber, M.G., L.L. Rudel, G.W. Burton, et al. 1990b. Nascent VLDL from liver perfusions of cynomolgus monkeys are preferentially enriched in RRR compared with SRR-alpha-tocopherol: Studies using deuterated tocopherols. *J Lipid Res* 31(4): 687–94.

Traber, M.G., L.K. Siddens, S.W. Leonard, et al. 2005. Alpha-tocopherol modulates Cyp3a expression, increases gamma-CEHC production, and limits tissue gamma-tocopherol accumulation in mice fed high gamma-tocopherol diets. *Free Radic Biol Med* 38(6): 773–85.

Traber, M.G., R.J. Sokol, A. Kohlschutter, et al. 1993. Impaired discrimination between stereoisomers of alpha-tocopherol in patients with familial isolated vitamin E deficiency. *J Lipid Res* 34(2): 201–10.

Turesky, R.J., A. Constable, L.B. Fay, et al. 1999. Interspecies differences in metabolism of heterocyclic aromatic amines by rat and human P450 1A2. *Cancer Lett* 143(2): 109–12.

Uto, H., C. Kiyose, H. Saito, et al. 2004. Gamma-tocopherol enhances sodium excretion as a natriuretic hormone precursor. *J Nutr Sci Vitaminol (Tokyo)* 50(4): 277–82.

Vane, J.R. 1976. Prostaglandins as mediators of inflammation. *Adv Prostaglandin Thromboxane Res* 2: 791–801.

Vane, J.R., Y.S. Bakhle and R.M. Botting. 1998. Cyclooxygenases 1 and 2. *Annu Rev Pharmacol Toxicol* 38: 97–120.

Vane, J.R. and R.M. Botting. 1998a. Mechanism of action of antiinflammatory drugs. *Int J Tissue React* 20(1): 3–15.

Vane, J.R. and R.M. Botting. 1998b. Mechanism of action of nonsteroidal anti-inflammatory drugs. *Am J Med* 104(3A): 2S–8S; discussion 21S–22S.

Wagner, J.G., Q. Jiang, J.R. Harkema, et al. 2007. Ozone enhancement of lower airway allergic inflammation is prevented by gamma-tocopherol. *Free Radic Biol Med,* in press.

Wang, L.Q. and M.O. James. 2006. Inhibition of sulfotransferases by xenobiotics. *Curr Drug Metab* 7(1): 83–104.

Weber, C., M. Podda, M. Rallis, et al. 1997. Efficacy of topically applied tocopherols and tocotrienols in protection of murine skin from oxidative damage induced by UV- irradiation. *Free Radic Biol Med* 22(5): 761–769.

Wechter, W.J., D. Kantoci, E.D. Murray, Jr., et al. 1996. A new endogenous natriuretic factor: LLU-α. *Proc Natl Acad Sci USA* 93(12): 6002–6007.

Yamashita, K., N. Takeda and S. Ikeda. 2000. Effects of various tocopherol-containing diets on tocopherol secretion into bile. *Lipids* 35(2): 163–70.

Yoshida, E., T. Watanabe, J. Takata, et al. 2006. Topical application of a novel, hydrophilic gamma-tocopherol derivative reduces photo-inflammation in mice skin. *J Invest Dermatol* 126(7): 1633–40.

You, C.S., T.J. Sontag, J.E. Swanson, et al. 2005. Long-chain carboxychromanols are the major metabolites of tocopherols and tocotrienols in A549 lung epithelial cells but not HepG2 cells. *J Nutr* 135(2): 227–32.

24 Tocotrienols Activate the Steroid and Xenobiotic Receptor SXR to Modulate Small Molecule Metabolism

Kameran R. Johnson, Tiffany Hsu, and Bruce Blumberg

CONTENTS

24.1 BACKGROUND

Vitamin E, a known antioxidant and commonly used dietary supplement, occurs naturally in eight different forms: α, β, γ and δ tocopherols and α, β, γ and δ tocotrienols. These differ in the saturation of their side chains and the number and position of methyl groups around the chromanol head structure. Both tocopherols and tocotrienols share this chromanol ring, but tocopherols have a completely saturated phytol tail side chain whereas tocotrienols have double bonds at the 3', 7' and 11' positions of the tail (Figure 24.1) (Kamat et al. 1997; Saito et al. 2003). The Greek letter designates the position at which methyl groups are located on the ring. The most biologically active form of vitamin E is considered to be α-tocopherol, due to its relatively slow metabolism and consequent high bioavailability (Brigelius-Flohe and Traber, 1999). α-tocopherol also has the highest level of antioxidant activity among the vitamins E (Brigelius-Flohe and Traber, 1999).

Tocotrienols are less biologically accessible than tocopherols because they are quickly metabolized (Landes et al. 2003a). Once absorbed from the intestine, tocotrienols are transported by chylomicrons into the circulatory system. Chylomicrons are then transferred from the lymph into the liver, where the tocotrienols undergo an initial side chain ω-oxidation, followed by sequential β-oxidation reactions (Brigelius-Flohe, 2003). This first ω-oxidation is catalyzed by cytochrome P4503A4 (CYP3A4) proteins (Brigelius-Flohe, 2003) which are transcriptionally regulated by the steroid and xenobiotic receptor, SXR (Blumberg et al. 1998).

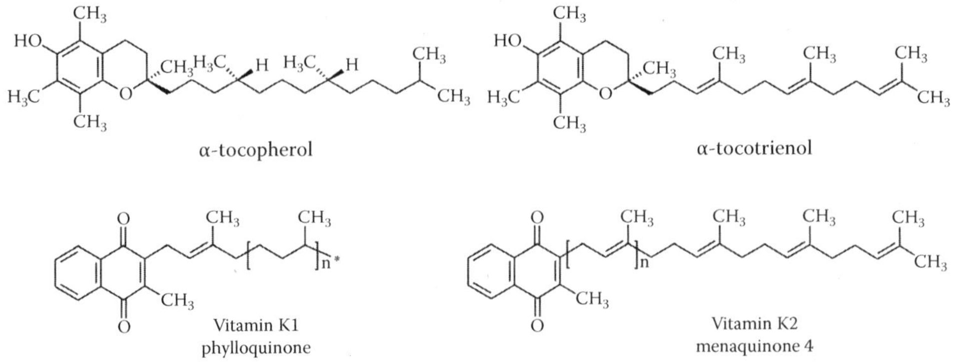

FIGURE 24.1 Structures of representative vitamins E and vitamins K. Vitamins E differ primarily in the position and number of methyl groups around the chromanol ring. Vitamin K1 and vitamin K2 are each families of molecules differing in the number of repeating units on the side chain. For vitamin K1, a generic phylloquinone structure is shown. The most common form of dietary vitamin K1 has 7 repeating units. The most common and active form of vitamin K2, menaquinone 4, is shown.

24.2 THE STEROID AND XENOBIOTIC RECEPTOR SXR

SXR (Blumberg et al. 1998), also known as PXR (Kliewer et al. 1998), PAR (Bertilsson et al. 1998), and NR1I2 (Nuclear Receptor Nomenclature Committee, 1999) is an orphan nuclear receptor that regulates the breakdown of a large number of steroids, hormones and other compounds. Orphan nuclear receptors are those members of the nuclear receptor superfamily that do not have known physiological ligands, although they may be activated by one or more compounds. To date, no physiological ligand has been identified for SXR. Rather, it is activated by numerous endogenous steroids and bile acids (endobiotics), prescription drugs (e.g., rifampicin, taxol), dietary compounds (e.g., hyperforin, vitamin K2) and a variety of synthetic (xenobiotic) chemicals (reviewed in Kliewer et al. 2002; Willson and Kliewer, 2002). Classically, steroid receptors bind to DNA as homodimers to activate their target genes (Beato et al. 1995). In contrast, SXR is unable to bind DNA as a homodimer and instead forms heterodimers with the retinoid 'X' receptor (RXR) to bind DNA. The RXR-SXR heterodimer is expressed at high levels in the small intestine and liver (Blumberg et al. 1998; Kliewer et al. 1998), where it activates expression of cytochrome p450 genes, such as CYP3A4 and CYP2B6, that are involved in detoxifying and eliminating endogenous, dietary and xenobiotic compounds (reviewed in Kliewer et al. 2002; Willson and Kliewer, 2002). SXR was further shown to be a master regulator of drug and xenobiotic metabolism and to regulate genes involved in all three phases of metabolism of endo- and xenobiotic compounds: oxidation by cytochrome p450 enzymes (phase I), conjugation to glutathione, sulfates and sugars (phase II), and transport out of the cell by ABC family transporters (phase III) (reviewed in Dussault and Forman, 2002; Kliewer et al. 2002; Orans et al. 2005; Timsit and Negishi, 2007; Willson and Kliewer, 2002).

24.3 TOCOTRIENOLS BIND TO AND ACTIVATE SXR

The observations that CYP3A4 catalyzed the initial ω-oxidation of vitamins E (Birringer et al. 2002; Brigelius-Flohe, 2005) and that SXR is a key regulator of CYP3A4 (Blumberg et al. 1998; Kliewer et al. 1998; Lehmann et al. 1998), led to the hypothesis that one or more vitamin E congeners might be SXR activators. Several groups have demonstrated activation of SXR by forms of vitamin E. Brigelius-Flohé and colleagues first showed that tocopherol and tocotrienol forms of vitamin E could activate a reporter gene containing two copies of the SXR response element from the rat CYP3A1 gene in transfected HepG2 cells (Landes et al. 2003b). They found that α-, γ-, and δ-tocopherols and α- and γ-tocotrienols were able to activate the reporter in HepG2 cells (Landes et al. 2003b). β- and δ- tocotrienols were not tested. The rank order of potency for these compounds as

SXR activators was γ-tocotrienol ≈ α-tocotrienol > rifampicin > δ-tocopherol > RRR α-tocopherol ≥ γ-tocopherol (Landes et al. 2003b).

In contrast to these results, we showed that tocotrienols, but not tocopherols were bona fide activators of SXR in human primary hepatocytes, HepG2, and LS-180 cells (Zhou et al. 2004). Moreover, we found that tocotrienols were considerably less active (about 1/5 as active) than the potent SXR activator rifampicin (Zhou et al. 2004), whereas Landes and colleagues found that tocotrienols were approximately as active as rifampicin in SXR activation (Landes et al. 2003b). We employed a highly sensitive scintillation proximity assay to show that tocotrienols bind directly to SXR, displacing the high-affinity SXR ligand SR12813 (Zhou et al. 2004). In contrast, tocopherols did not show detectable binding to SXR. In addition, tocotrienols were able to modulate co-repressor release from SXR, whereas tocopherols were not (Zhou et al. 2004). Thus, it was concluded that only tocotrienol forms of vitamin E were significant SXR activators (Zhou et al. 2004).

24.4 ARE TOCOPHEROLS BONA FIDE SXR ACTIVATORS?

The differences between the Landes (2003b) and Zhou (2004) studies are difficult to reconcile since they come to opposing conclusions regarding the ability of tocopherols to activate SXR. Landes et al. used transient transfection assays with a human receptor and reporter from a mouse CYP3 gene to show that both tocopherols and tocotrienols activated SXR, although tocopherols were less active than tocotrienols (Landes et al. 2003b). In contrast, Zhou et al. employed a human receptor and reporter from the human CYP3A4 gene to show that only tocotrienols were significant activators of SXR (Zhou et al. 2004). Moreover, they used human primary hepatocytes and intestinal LS-180 cells without the addition of overexpressed SXR to confirm the ability of tocotrienols alone to activate SXR. In vitro ligand binding assays demonstrated that only tocotrienols were able to compete effectively for SXR ligand binding or to mediate co-repressor release when tested on native response elements. One notable point is that Zhou et al. found a cell-type specific induction of reporter genes by tocotrienols (Zhou et al. 2004). This could suggest that differences in the cell type and/or reporter gene combinations employed by the different groups contributed to the divergent results observed.

24.5 TISSUE SPECIFIC INDUCTION OF CYP GENES BY TOCOTRIENOLS

SXR is expressed at different levels in liver and intestine, prompting Zhou and colleagues (Zhou et al. 2004) to ask whether there were any significant differences in the induction of SXR target genes in these tissues. All four tocotrienols were able to up-regulate expression of CYP3A4 mRNA (phase I) but not UGT1A1 (phase 2) or MDR1 (phase 3) mRNAs in primary hepatocytes. Tocopherols were inactive. Remarkably, tocotrienols induced expression of UGT1A1 and MDR1, but not CYP3A4 in intestinal LS-180 cells. Rifampicin induced all 3 genes in both cell types, suggesting that the ligand, and not the cell type, was the determining factor in which target genes were induced. This established tocotrienols as the first selective SXR response mediators (Zhou et al. 2004).

The identification of tocotrienols as tissue-specific modulators of SXR response leads naturally to the question of what molecular mechanisms underlie the specificity. Transcriptional regulation of target gene expression by nuclear receptors is achieved, in part, by the specific interaction of nuclear receptors with a variety of co-regulators. These include co-repressors and co-activators, which recruit histone deacetylase or histone acetyl transferase complexes respectively to regulate the accessibility of chromatin to the transcriptional machinery (Mahajan and Samuels, 2005; Nettles and Greene, 2005). SXR can interact with co-repressors such as silencing mediator for retinoid and thyroid receptor (SMRT) and nuclear receptor co-repressor (NCoR) in the absence of ligands. The presence of ligands triggers a conformational change in the receptor, which reduces the affinity of the receptor for co-repressors and facilitates co-activator interactions (Blumberg et al. 1998). The receptor:co-repressor complex exists in a dynamic equilibrium with receptor:co-activator complexes in any given cell type. Therefore, the ratio of co-repressors to co-activators can alter the sensitivity of the receptor to ligands.

It was shown that the differential ability of tocotrienols to activate intestinal phase 2 and phase 3 gene expression resided in the relatively higher ratios of the co-repressor NCoR to co-activators in LS-180 cells compared with hepatocytes (Zhou et al. 2004). Overexpression of a dominant negative form of NCoR (which blocks the ability of the endogenous co-repressor to inhibit transcription) rescued the ability of tocotrienols to induce CYP3A4 in LS-180 cells, whereas overexpression of co-activators did not alter the response of CYP3A4 to tocotrienols. This suggests that tocotrienols are protected from inducing their own degradation in the intestine because intestinal epithelial cells lack the ability to induce CYP3A4 in response to tocotrienol levels. In contrast, tocotrienols are robust inducers of hepatic CYP3A4 which is likely to be a primary site of metabolism. This possibility is further suggested by the presence of the tocotrienol metabolites, carboxyethyl hydroxychromans, in the liver (Brigelius-Flohe, 2003).

24.6 VITAMINS AS ACTIVATORS OF NUCLEAR RECEPTORS

The demonstration that an orphan nuclear receptor (HAP) was a high-affinity ligand for the vitamin A derivative, all-*trans* retinoic acid provided the first demonstration that vitamins could act through transcription factors to modulate gene expression (Giguere et al. 1987; Petkovich et al. 1987). This identification of the retinoic acid receptor (RAR) was an important advance, linking nutrition to gene expression. In the subsequent years, a second class of nuclear receptors responsive to retinoic acid was identified (Mangelsdorf et al. 1990). This retinoid "X" receptor (RXR) proved to be responsive to 9-*cis* retinoic acid. Perhaps the most important link between nutrition and gene expression came with the identification of SXR in 1998 (Bertilsson et al. 1998; Blumberg et al. 1998; Kliewer et al. 1998). We and others showed that SXR was activated by vitamin K2 (Landes et al. 2003a; Tabb et al. 2003), which further solidified the important link between diet and the genetic regulation of small molecular metabolism. We showed that menaquinone forms of vitamin K2 activated SXR to promote the activation of genes important for the development and function of osteoblasts such as bone alkaline phosphatase, osteoprotogerin, and matrix Gla protein (Tabb et al. 2003). We went on to show that vitamin K2 activated SXR to stimulate the deposition of collagen and that SXR was a direct regulator of the small matrix proteoglycans tsukushi, the extracellular matrix protein matrilin-2, and extracellular CD14 antigen (Ichikawa et al. 2006). Phylloquinone forms of vitamin K (vitamin K1) were inactive on SXR. Similarly, Landes and colleagues showed that menaquinones, but not phylloquinones, activated SXR in transient transfection assays (Landes et al. 2003a).

A second link between vitamins and SXR came with the identification of tocotrienol forms of vitamin E as SXR activators (Landes et al. 2003a; Landes et al. 2003b; Zhou et al. 2004). As described above, tocotrienols are robust inducers of hepatic CYP3A4, suggesting that ingestion of high levels of vitamin E may lead to induction of enzymes that degrade drugs and other chemicals. Interestingly, there are structural parallels between the forms of vitamin E and vitamin K that activate SXR. Tocotrienols and menaquinones, both of which activate SXR, contain unsaturated side chains (Figure 24.1) (Landes et al. 2003a; Landes et al. 2003b; Tabb et al. 2003; Zhou et al. 2004). In contrast, the inactive tocopherols and phylloquinones contain saturated side chains (Figure 24.1) (Landes et al. 2003a; Landes et al. 2003b; Tabb et al. 2003; Zhou et al. 2004). It is likely that the more rigid 3-D structure of the unsaturated side chains is an important contributing factor to SXR activation.

24.7 INTERACTIONS BETWEEN NUTRACEUTICALS AND PRESCRIPTION DRUGS

Although drug–drug interactions are known to be a common problem in pharmacology, drug–nutrient interactions were, until recently, rarely considered when prescribing medications. The identification of SXR as a key regulator of steroid, drug and xenobiotic metabolism has provided a molecular test with which to predict and identify such interactions. Among the first examples was the discovery that hyperforin, the active component of the herbal antidepressant St. John's wort, activates SXR, which, in turn, induces enzymes in the xenobiotic metabolism pathway (Moore et al. 2000; Wentworth et al. 2000). Activation of SXR and the consequent induction of key metabolic enzymes such as CYP3A4 and MDR1 have the potential to alter the metabolism of prescription drugs being taken concurrently (e.g., oral contraceptives). Activation of SXR by tocotrienols has a similar potential for inducing drug interactions.

The field of drug–nutrient interactions is currently much less developed than the clinical pharmacology of drug interactions. There is some evidence to suggest that vitamin supplements can affect the absorption and effectiveness of drugs (Brown and Dickerson, 1999; Miller, 1998; Trovato et al. 1991). It is interesting to note that more than 35 million people in the United States consume vitamin E supplements daily (Traber, 2004). Vitamin K2 is rarely utilized as a dietary supplement in the U.S. and is, therefore, not considered to be a risk. Vitamins E and K are present in foods and it is formally possible that individuals can consume sufficient quantities to affect xenobiotic metabolism. Natto (fermented soybeans) is very high in vitamin K2. Vitamins E are abundant in foods such as vegetable oils, nuts, green leafy vegetables, and fortified cereals. Tocotrienols are found in aleurone and subaleurone layers of cereal seeds and in palm oils (Yoshida et al. 2003). Tocopherols occur in the germ of cereal seeds and in polyunsaturated vegetable oils. Dietary supplements containing vitamin E vary considerably in their composition. It is ironic that so-called natural vitamin E supplements may contain tocotrienols together with mixed tocopherols and thereby have a greater potential for modulating drug and xenobiotic metabolism via SXR. In contrast, our data suggest that synthetic α-tocopherols would not cause such effects.

One reasonable question to be considered is whether one can consume sufficient doses of tocotrienols to achieve levels capable of activating SXR. Tocotrienols can bind to and activate SXR at low micromolar concentrations and mediate the induction of SXR target genes (Landes et al. 2003a; Zhou et al. 2004). Published pharmacokinetic studies suggest that plasma concentration of tocotrienols can exceed 2000 ng/ml (~5 μM) after oral administration of a single dose of 300 mg of mixed tocotrienols (Yap et al. 2001). While these blood levels of tocotrienols are already sufficient to activate SXR, it is probable that the hepatic levels are even higher. This suggests that dietary tocotrienols can induce hepatic CYP3A4 levels, together with phase 2 and phase 3 enzymes in the intestine. Therefore, it seems plausible that consumption of dietary supplements or foods containing high levels of tocotrienols could lead to the breakdown and loss of therapeutic efficacy of prescription drugs. This is a matter of some concern for the large number of people who take dietary megavitamin supplements. It is particularly troublesome for those who rely on daily pharmaceutical use, such as the elderly.

The recent findings regarding the induction of hepatic CYP3 enzymes by vitamin K2 and tocotrienol forms of vitamin E are consistent with previous reports that a variety of herbal supplements, natural foods and beverages can modulate drug metabolism by inducing CYP3A enzymes (Miller, 1998; Sorensen, 2002). The *in vivo* metabolism of tocotrienols remains incompletely understood. For example, the tissues required for vitamin E metabolism *in vivo* have not been identified (Traber, 2004). It has been reported that tocotrienols do not accumulate, even in the livers of rats maintained on a tocotrienol-rich diet (Ikeda et al. 2001). These authors showed that consumption of sesame seeds increased the concentrations of tocotrienols in skin and adipose tissues, but apparently not elsewhere in the body (Ikeda et al. 2001). In contrast, tocopherol levels were elevated in most tissues. This suggests that the absorption and metabolism of vitamin E isoforms is markedly different. Therefore, a more complete understanding of how dietary tocopherols and tocotrienols affect drug metabolism will require a molecular dissection of the *in vivo* pathways underlying vitamin E metabolism.

24.8 SXR AND TOCOTRIENOLS: BEYOND DRUG INTERACTIONS

Considering that SXR has been demonstrated to have functions in addition to its role in regulating xenobiotic metabolism, one might reasonably ask whether tocotrienol activation of SXR has any associated significant biological functions. Tocotrienols have been associated with decreased proliferation of a variety of breast cancer cell lines, irrespective of estrogen receptor status (Guthrie et al. 1997; Kline et al. 2004; Nesaretnam et al. 2000; Nesaretnam et al. 1995; Nesaretnam et al. 1998; Wali and Sylvester, 2007; Yu et al. 1999). α-, γ- and δ-tocotrienols were shown to be the most effective inhibitors of breast cancer cell growth and also induced apoptosis in these cells (Guthrie et al. 1997; Nesaretnam et al. 2000; Nesaretnam et al. 1998; Yu et al. 1999). It is intriguing that tocotrienols activate SXR because we have recently shown that activation of SXR inhibits the growth and promotes apoptosis in both estrogen receptor positive (ER^+) and estrogen receptor negative (ER^-) breast cancer cell lines (Verma et al. 2007). The mechanism in ER^+, p53 wild type cells appears to be through induction of inducible nitric oxide synthase, production of nitrous oxide, stabilization of p53 and induction of p53 target genes leading to cell cycle arrest and apoptosis (Verma et al. 2007). The mechanism in ER^-, p53 mutant cell lines remains to be determined, although SXR is involved (Verma et al. 2007). It will be interesting to determine whether tocotrienols act through SXR to inhibit the growth of breast cancer cells and if tocotrienols inhibit breast cancer growth *in vivo*.

Tocotrienols have also been associated with inhibition of tumor growth in intestinal (Agarwal et al. 2004), prostate (Conte et al. 2004; Srivastava and Gupta, 2006), hepatocellular (Sakai et al. 2006; Wada et al. 2005) and lung (Wada et al. 2005) cancers. This suggests that tocotrienols might be more broadly acting anticancer agents. It is also interesting to note that vitamin K2 inhibits the proliferation of hepatocellular carcinomas and induces apoptosis in hepatocarcinoma cell lines such as HepG3 (Kakizaki et al. 2007; Liu et al. 2007; Matsumoto et al. 2006; Mizuta et al. 2006; Nakamura et al. 2006; Otsuka et al. 2007; Ozaki et al. 2007). Taken together with the results noted above, one can infer that activation of SXR by vitamins E and K2 is protective against a variety of cancers. The molecular mechanisms underlying these effects remain to be explored, but offer great promise for the development of novel chemopreventive or chemotherapeutic targets.

Recent work has established a link between activation of SXR and the inhibition of inflammation (Gu et al. 2006; Xie and Tian, 2006; Zhou et al. 2006). Activation of SXR inhibits the activity of the key mediator of inflammation and immunity, NF-κB (Gu et al. 2006; Xie and Tian, 2006; Zhou et al. 2006). Loss of SXR function leads to increased expression of a variety of inflammatory cytokines and lymphokines that are NF-κB target genes (Zhou et al. 2006). Increased NF-κB activity is often associated with cell proliferation in cancers and its inhibition by SXR activators might offer potentially new therapeutic targets. At least one report links tocotrienols with inhibition of inflammation, independent of their antioxidant properties (Qureshi et al. 2001). While it remains to be shown that tocotrienols act through SXR to inhibit inflammation, the possibility is consistent with the function of SXR and should be explored further in the future.

24.9 SUMMARY

In summary, tocotrienols bind to and activate SXR with affinities in the low micromolar range. Tocotrienol-mediated activation of SXR induces the expression of enzymes involved in xenobiotic metabolism, which increases the possibility of drug interactions. This provides a cautionary example for those who advocate that nutraceuticals can be taken at high doses with few, if any, side effects. Indeed, the intake of supplements and nutraceuticals should be carefully considered when planning or prescribing drug therapies. Tocotrienols appear to have broad anti-tumor and anti-inflammatory activities that may be associated with their ability to activate SXR. Currently, the vast majority of research on vitamins E is focused on tocopherols and their antioxidant properties (Sen et al. 2006, 2007). Considering the results summarized above, further research on the biology of tocotrienols is required to establish the biological function of these understudied, yet important forms of vitamin E.

ACKNOWLEDGMENTS

Work in our laboratory was supported by grants from the National Institutes of Health (GM-60572, ES-015849), the U.S. Environmental Protection Agency (STAR-R830686), and the Department of Defense (DAMD17-02-1-0323) to BB. K.J. was the recipient of grants from the University of California at Irvine Interdisciplinary Summer Undergraduate Research Experience, Undergraduate Research Opportunities Program and Summer Undergraduate Research Opportunities Program. T.H. was an American Cancer Society summer research fellow.

REFERENCES

Agarwal, M.K., Agarwal, M.L., Athar, M., and Gupta, S. 2004. Tocotrienol–rich fraction of palm oil activates p53, modulates Bax/Bcl2 ratio and induces apoptosis independent of cell cycle association. *Cell Cycle* (Georgetown, TX) 3, 205–211.

Beato, M., Herrlich, P., and Schutz, G. 1995. Steroid hormone receptors: Many actors in search of a plot. *Cell* 83, 851–857.

Bertilsson, G., Heidrich, J., Svensson, K., Asman, M., Jendeberg, L., Sydow-Backman, M., Ohlsson, R., Postlind, H., Blomquist, P., and Berkenstam, A. 1998. Identification of a human nuclear receptor defines a new signaling pathway for CYP3A induction. *Proc Natl Acad Sci USA* 95, 12208–12213.

Birringer, M., Pfluger, P., Kluth, D., Landes, N., and Brigelius-Flohe, R. 2002. Identities and differences in the metabolism of tocotrienols and tocopherols in HepG2 cells. *J Nutr* 132, 3113–3118.

Blumberg, B., Sabbagh, W., Jr., Juguilon, H., Bolado, J., Jr., van Meter, C.M., Ong, E.S., and Evans, R.M. 1998. SXR, a novel steroid and xenobiotic-sensing nuclear receptor. *Genes Dev* 12, 3195–3205.

Brigelius-Flohe, R. 2003. Vitamin E and drug metabolism. *Biochem Biophys Res Commun* 305, 737–740.

Brigelius-Flohe, R. 2005. Induction of drug metabolizing enzymes by vitamin E. *J Plant Physiol* 162, 797–802.

Brigelius-Flohe, R., and Traber, M.G. 1999. Vitamin E: Function and metabolism. *Faseb J* 13, 1145–1155.

Brown, R.O., and Dickerson, R.N. 1999. Drug–nutrient interactions. *Am J Managed Care* 5, 345–352; quiz 353–345.

Conte, C., Floridi, A., Aisa, C., Piroddi, M., Floridi, A., and Galli, F. 2004. Gamma-tocotrienol metabolism and antiproliferative effect in prostate cancer cells. *Ann NY Acad Sci* 1031, 391–394.

Dussault, I., and Forman, B.M. 2002. The nuclear receptor PXR: A master regulator of "homeland" defense. *Crit Rev Eukaryot Gene Expr* 12, 53–64.

Giguere, V., Ong, E.S., Segui, P., and Evans, R.M. 1987. Identification of a receptor for the morphogen retinoic acid. *Nature* 330, 624–629.

Gu, X., Ke, S., Liu, D., Sheng, T., Thomas, P.E., Rabson, A.B., Gallo, M.A., Xie, W., and Tian, Y. 2006. Role of NF-kappaB in regulation of PXR-mediated gene expression: A mechanism for the suppression of cytochrome P-450 3A4 by proinflammatory agents. *J Biol Chem* 281, 17882–17889.

Guthrie, N., Gapor, A., Chambers, A.F., and Carroll, K.K. 1997. Inhibition of proliferation of estrogen receptor-negative MDA-MB-435 and -positive MCF-7 human breast cancer cells by palm oil tocotrienols and tamoxifen, alone and in combination. *J Nutr* 127, 544S–548S.

Ichikawa, T., Horie-Inoue, K., Ikeda, K., Blumberg, B., and Inoue, S. 2006. Steroid and xenobiotic receptor SXR mediates vitamin K2-activated transcription of extracellular matrix-related genes and collagen accumulation in osteoblastic cells. *J Biol Chem* 281, 16927–16934.

Ikeda, S., Toyoshima, K., and Yamashita, K. 2001. Dietary sesame seeds elevate alpha- and gamma-tocotrienol concentrations in skin and adipose tissue of rats fed the tocotrienol-rich fraction extracted from palm oil. *J Nutr* 131, 2892–2897.

Kakizaki, S., Sohara, N., Sato, K., Suzuki, H., Yanagisawa, M., Nakajima, H., Takagi, H., Naganuma, A., Otsuka, T., Takahashi, H., et al. 2007. Preventive effects of vitamin K on recurrent disease in patients with hepatocellular carcinoma arising from hepatitis C viral infection. *J Gastro Hepatol* 22, 518–522.

Kamat, J.P., Sarma, H.D., Devasagayam, T.P., Nesaretnam, K., and Basiron, Y. 1997. Tocotrienols from palm oil as effective inhibitors of protein oxidation and lipid peroxidation in rat liver microsomes. *Mol Cell Biochem* 170, 131–137.

Kliewer, S.A., Goodwin, B., and Willson, T.M. 2002. The nuclear pregnane X receptor: A key regulator of xenobiotic metabolism. *Endocr Rev* 23, 687–702.

Kliewer, S.A., Moore, J.T., Wade, L., Staudinger, J.L., Watson, M.A., Jones, S.A., McKee, D.D., Oliver, B.B., Willson, T.M., Zetterstrom, R.H., et al. 1998. An orphan nuclear receptor activated by pregnanes defines a novel steroid signaling pathway. *Cell* 92, 73–82.

Kline, K., Yu, W., and Sanders, B.G. 2004. Vitamin E and breast cancer. *J Nutr* 134, 3458S–3462S.

Landes, N., Birringer, M., and Brigelius-Flohe, R. 2003a. Homologous metabolic and gene activating routes for vitamins E and K. *Mol Aspects Med* 24, 337–344.

Landes, N., Pfluger, P., Kluth, D., Birringer, M., Ruhl, R., Bol, G.F., Glatt, H., and Brigelius-Flohe, R. 2003b. Vitamin E activates gene expression via the pregnane X receptor. *Biochem Pharmacol* 65, 269–273.

Lehmann, J.M., McKee, D.D., Watson, M.A., Willson, T.M., Moore, J.T., and Kliewer, S.A. 1998. The human orphan nuclear receptor PXR is activated by compounds that regulate CYP3A4 gene expression and cause drug interactions. *J Clin Invest* 102, 1016–1023.

Liu, W., Nakamura, H., Yamamoto, T., Ikeda, N., Saito, M., Ohno, M., Hara, N., Imanishi, H., Shimomura, S., Yamamoto, T., et al. 2007. Vitamin K2 inhibits the proliferation of HepG2 cells by up-regulating the transcription of p21 gene. *Hepatol Res* 37, 360–365.

Mahajan, M.A., and Samuels, H.H. 2005. Nuclear hormone receptor coregulator: Role in hormone action, metabolism, growth, and development. *Endocr Rev* 26, 583–597.

Mangelsdorf, D.J., Ong, E.S., Dyck, J.A., and Evans, R.M. 1990. Nuclear receptor that identifies a novel retinoic acid response pathway. *Nature* 345, 224–229.

Matsumoto, K., Okano, J., Nagahara, T., and Murawaki, Y. 2006. Apoptosis of liver cancer cells by vitamin K2 and enhancement by MEK inhibition. *Int J Oncol* 29, 1501–1508.

Miller, L.G. 1998. Herbal medicinals: Selected clinical considerations focusing on known or potential drug–herb interactions. *Arch Int Med* 158, 2200–2211.

Mizuta, T., Ozaki, I., Eguchi, Y., Yasutake, T., Kawazoe, S., Fujimoto, K., and Yamamoto, K. 2006. The effect of menatetrenone, a vitamin K2 analog, on disease recurrence and survival in patients with hepatocellular carcinoma after curative treatment: A pilot study. *Cancer* 106, 867–872.

Moore, L.B., Goodwin, B., Jones, S.A., Wisely, G.B., Serabjit-Singh, C.J., Willson, T.M., Collins, J.L., and Kliewer, S.A. 2000. St. John's wort induces hepatic drug metabolism through activation of the pregnane X receptor. *Proc Natl Acad Sci USA* 97, 7500–7502.

Nakamura, M., Nagano, H., Noda, T., Wada, H., Ota, H., Damdinsuren, B., Marubashi, S., Miyamoto, A., Takeda, Y., Doki, Y., et al. 2006. Vitamin K2 has growth inhibition effect against hepatocellular carcinoma cell lines but does not enhance anti-tumor effect of combination treatment of interferon–alpha and fluorouracil in vitro. *Hepatol Res* 35, 289–295.

Nesaretnam, K., Dorasamy, S., and Darbre, P.D. 2000. Tocotrienols inhibit growth of ZR-75-1 breast cancer cells. *Int J Food Sci Nutr* 51 Suppl, S95–103.

Nesaretnam, K., Guthrie, N., Chambers, A.F., and Carroll, K.K. 1995. Effect of tocotrienols on the growth of a human breast cancer cell line in culture. *Lipids* 30, 1139–1143.

Nesaretnam, K., Stephen, R., Dils, R., and Darbre, P. 1998. Tocotrienols inhibit the growth of human breast cancer cells irrespective of estrogen receptor status. *Lipids* 33, 461–469.

Nettles, K.W. and Greene, G.L. 2005. Ligand control of coregulator recruitment to nuclear receptors. *Annu Rev Physiol* 67, 309–333.

Nuclear Receptor Nomenclature Committee. 1999. A unified nomenclature system for the nuclear receptor superfamily. *Cell* 97, 161–163.

Orans, J., Teotico, D.G., and Redinbo, M.R. 2005. The Nuclear xenobiotic receptor PXR: Recent insights and new challenges. *Mol Endocrinol* 19, 2891–2900.

Otsuka, T., Hagiwara, S., Tojima, H., Yoshida, H., Takahashi, T., Nagasaka, K., Tomioka, S., Ando, T., Takeuchi, K., Kori, T., et al. 2007. Hepatocellular carcinoma with peritoneal dissemination which was regressed during vitamin K2 and vitamin E administration. *Int Med* (Tokyo, Japan) 46, 711–715.

Ozaki, I., Zhang, H., Mizuta, T., Ide, Y., Eguchi, Y., Yasutake, T., Sakamaki, T., Pestell, R.G., and Yamamoto, K. 2007. Menatetrenone, a vitamin K2 analogue, inhibits hepatocellular carcinoma cell growth by suppressing cyclin D1 expression through inhibition of nuclear factor kappaB activation. *Clin Cancer Res* 13, 2236–2245.

Petkovich, M., Brand, N.J., Krust, A., and Chambon, P. 1987. A human retinoic acid receptor which belongs to the family of nuclear receptors. *Nature* 330, 444–450.

Qureshi, A.A., Salser, W.A., Parmar, R., and Emeson, E.E. 2001. Novel tocotrienols of rice bran inhibit atherosclerotic lesions in C57BL/6 ApoE-deficient mice. *J Nutr* 131, 2606–2618.

Saito, H., Kiyose, C., Yoshimura, H., Ueda, T., Kondo, K., and Igarashi, O. 2003. Gamma-tocotrienol, a vitamin E homolog, is a natriuretic hormone precursor. *J Lipid Res* 44, 1530–1535.

Sakai, M., Okabe, M., Tachibana, H., and Yamada, K. 2006. Apoptosis induction by gamma-tocotrienol in human hepatoma Hep3B cells. *J Nutri Biochem* 17, 672–676.

Sen, C.K., Khanna, S., and Roy, S. 2006. Tocotrienols: Vitamin E beyond tocopherols. *Life Sci* 78, 2088–2098.

Sen, C.K., Khanna, S., and Roy, S. 2007. Tocotrienols in health and disease: The other half of the natural vitamin E family. *Mol Aspects Med* 28, 692–728.

Sorensen, J.M. 2002. Herb–drug, food–drug, nutrient–drug, and drug–drug interactions: Mechanisms involved and their medical implications. *J Alt Complement Med NY* 8, 293–308.

Srivastava, J.K., and Gupta, S. 2006. Tocotrienol-rich fraction of palm oil induces cell cycle arrest and apoptosis selectively in human prostate cancer cells. *Biochem Biophys Res Commun* 346, 447–453.

Tabb, M.M., Sun, A., Zhou, C., Grun, F., Errandi, J., Romero, K., Phåm, H., Inoue, S., Mallick, S., Lin, M., et al. 2003. Vitamin K2 regulation of bone homeostasis is mediated by the steroid and xenobiotic receptor SXR. *J Biol Chem* 278, 43919–43927.

Timsit, Y.E., and Negishi, M. 2007. CAR and PXR: The xenobiotic-sensing receptors. Steroids 72, 231–246.

Traber, M.G. 2004. Vitamin E, nuclear receptors and xenobiotic metabolism. *Arch Biochem Biophys* 423, 6–11.

Trovato, A., Nuhlicek, D.N., and Midtling, J.E. 1991. Drug–nutrient interactions. *Am Fam Phys* 44, 1651–1658.

Verma, S., Tabb, M.M., and Blumberg, B. 2007. Activation of the steroid and xenobiotic receptor, SXR, induces apoptosis in breast cancer cells. Submitted for publication.

Wada, S., Satomi, Y., Murakoshi, M., Noguchi, N., Yoshikawa, T., and Nishino, H. 2005. Tumor suppressive effects of tocotrienol *in vivo* and *in vitro*. *Canc Lett* 229, 181–191.

Wali, V.B., and Sylvester, P.W. 2007. Synergistic Antiproliferative Effects of gamma-tocotrienol and statin treatment on mammary tumor cells. *Lipids* 42, 1113–1123.

Wentworth, J.M., Agostini, M., Love, J., Schwabe, J.W., and Chatterjee, V.K. 2000. St John's wort, a herbal antidepressant, activates the steroid X receptor. *J Endocrinol* 166, R11–16.

Willson, T.M., and Kliewer, S.A. 2002. PXR, CAR and drug metabolism. *Nat Rev Drug Discov* 1, 259–266.

Xie, W., and Tian, Y. 2006. Xenobiotic receptor meets NF-kappaB, a collision in the small bowel. *Cell Metab* 4, 177–178.

Yap, S.P., Yuen, K.H., and Wong, J.W. 2001. Pharmacokinetics and bioavailability of alpha-, gamma- and delta-tocotrienols under different food status. *J Pharm Pharmacol* 53, 67–71.

Yoshida, Y., Niki, E., and Noguchi, N. 2003. Comparative study on the action of tocopherols and tocotrienols as antioxidant: Chemical and physical effects. *Chem Phys Lipids* 123, 63–75.

Yu, W., Simmons-Menchaca, M., Gapor, A., Sanders, B.G., and Kline, K. 1999. Induction of apoptosis in human breast cancer cells by tocopherols and tocotrienols. *Nutr Canc* 33, 26–32.

Zhou, C., Tabb, M.M., Nelson, E.L., Grun, F., Verma, S., Sadatrafiei, A., Lin, M., Mallick, S., Forman, B.M., Thummel, K.E., et al. 2006. Mutual repression between steroid and xenobiotic receptor and NF-kappaB signaling pathways links xenobiotic metabolism and inflammation. *J Clin Invest* 116, 2280–2289.

Zhou, C., Tabb, M.M., Sadatrafiei, A., Grun, F., and Blumberg, B. 2004. Tocotrienols activate the steroid and xenobiotic receptor, SXR, and selectively regulate expression of its target genes. *Drug Metab Dispos* 32, 1075–1082.

Part H

Health Promotion

25 Tocotrienols in the Potential Treatment of Infectious Disease

Anne M. Mueller, Barrie Tan and Elizabeth S. Stuart

CONTENTS

25.1 INTRODUCTION

Atherosclerosis, the hardening of arteries, is the process of fatty substance deposits in the inner lining of arteries, resulting in the build-up of a plaque. The known risk factors for atherosclerosis include hypercholesterolemia, hypertension, hyperglycemia, obesity and smoking. However, these risk factors account for only about 50% of the diseased population. Other factors may be involved and while many are still unaccounted for, the concept of an infectious basis for atherosclerosis has been researched for many years (Ngeh et al. 2002). Both viruses and bacteria have been implicated in atherosclerosis, but *Chlamydiophila pneumoniae* has provided the strongest evidence for an association of infection and atherosclerosis, especially in conjunction with other risk factors (Campbell and Kuo, 2004).

25.1.1 Background on *Chlamydia*

Chlamydia pneumoniae (Cpn), a species of the Chlamydiaceae family, are gram-negative, coccoid, non-motile, obligate intracellular organisms that lack several metabolic pathways and depend on host intermediates (e.g., cholesterol, amino acids) for survival. Other important species are *Chlamydia trachomatis* (Ctr) and *Chlamydia psittaci*. *Chlamydia psittaci* causes respiratory, urogenital and gastrointestinal tract diseases and is most common in birds, reptiles and mammals. Ctr is widespread among humans and is the primary cause of sexually transmitted disease (STD) by a bacterium. Persistent inflammation of the genital tract by Ctr has been linked to ectopic pregnancies and infertility (Paavonen and Eggert-Kruse, 1999; Schachter, 1999; Mpiga and Ravaoarinoro, 2006). In addition to Ctr's prevalence as an STD bacterium, it is also a leading cause of preventable blindness worldwide (Thylefors et al. 1995).

As opposed to Ctr, Cpn causes multiple respiratory tract infections and has been linked to chronic diseases such as asthma (Hahn, 2004; Webley et al. 2005), Alzheimer's disease (Balin et al. 1998; Sriram et al. 1999; Stratton and Sriram, 2003), multiple sclerosis (Stratton and Sriram, 2003) and, importantly, atherosclerosis (Byrne and Kalayoglu, 1999; Campbell and Kuo, 2004). Ctr and Cpn are notorious for their tendency to develop chronic infections. Treatment options are few, and antibiotics have been shown to drive the bacteria into a persistent non-cultivable state that invites recurrence of infection once treatment is discontinued (Malinverni et al. 1995; Malinverni et al. 1995). *Chlamydia* exists in at least two morphological forms, one of which is the infectious elementary body (EB) that is not susceptible to antibiotics due to its non-replicative nature (Campbell and Kuo, 2004). The other morphological form is the non-infectious reticulate body (RB), which is the replicative form.

25.1.2 Entry and Developmental Cycle

Cellular entry by chlamydial infectious EBs most likely occurs via a variety of pathways. One of the earlier findings suggests that *Chlamydia* may use a microfilament/microtubule-dependent zipper-like process of phagocytosis (Ward and Murray, 1984). Participation of actin and tubulin appear to be necessary for optimal growth (Escalante-Ochoa et al. 2000). Another mechanism involves receptor-mediated endocytosis via clathrin-coated pits (Hodinka et al. 1988).

The most pertinent proposed mechanism in regard to tocotrienol research, however, is chlamydial entry of host cells via lipid raft domains (Stuart et al. 2003). These lipid rafts are dynamic, detergent-resistant regions of the cell membrane that contain sphingolipids and are high in cholesterol. When lipid rafts were depleted of cholesterol by nystatin or filipin, infection by *Chlamydia* was reduced significantly, and entry by various Ctr strains (e.g., serovar K, E, F) and Cpn were shown to be dependent on intact lipid rafts (Stuart et al. 2003). As shown in Figure 25.1, after *Chlamydia* entry into the host cell, the EB containing vacuoles fuse or aggregate to become what is termed an inclusion, a segregated membrane-bound compartment that progressively enlarges due to the metabolically active *Chlamydia* replication within the host cell that occurs after the EB has transformed into the non-infectious RB. Chlamydial transport to the inclusion appears to be Golgi-dependent, while sphingomyelin and cholesterol are co-transported to the inclusion via a Golgi-dependent pathway (Hackstadt et al. 1996; Carabeo et al. 2003). In addition, host lipid remodeling is required for chlamydial replication (Fukuda et al. 2005).

Recently, *Chlamydia* has been shown to target host lipid droplets and lipid droplet-like structures accumulated at the periphery of the inclusion. This finding suggests that *Chlamydia* may alter intracellular host lipid homeostasis (Kumar et al. 2006). Researchers have noted that Ctr stimulates fat production in the host, ordering cells to produce lipid bodies, or fat "halos." Since prevention of lipid body formation inhibited bacterial reproduction, these researchers concluded that *Chlamydia* is living off the fat of the cell (Beckman, 2005). Following replication, RBs transform back into EBs and the mature inclusion ruptures, setting free EBs to repeat the cycle of re-infection. Chlamydial entry via host cell lipid rafts presents a strategic rationale for tocotrienol therapy.

25.1.3 Link to Tocotrienol, Inhibition of Entry

The lack of treatment options and the unique nature of the chlamydial developmental cycle suggest that new compounds with a potential to treat or prevent infection are needed. Tocotrienol has been shown to lower lipids (Pearce et al. 1992; Song and DeBose-Boyd, 2006; Yu et al. 2006) and may possibly rearrange lipid raft domains (Black et al. 2000; Qureshi et al. 2001). Since cholesterol and intact lipid raft membranes are a requirement for successful chlamydial infection, reduction of

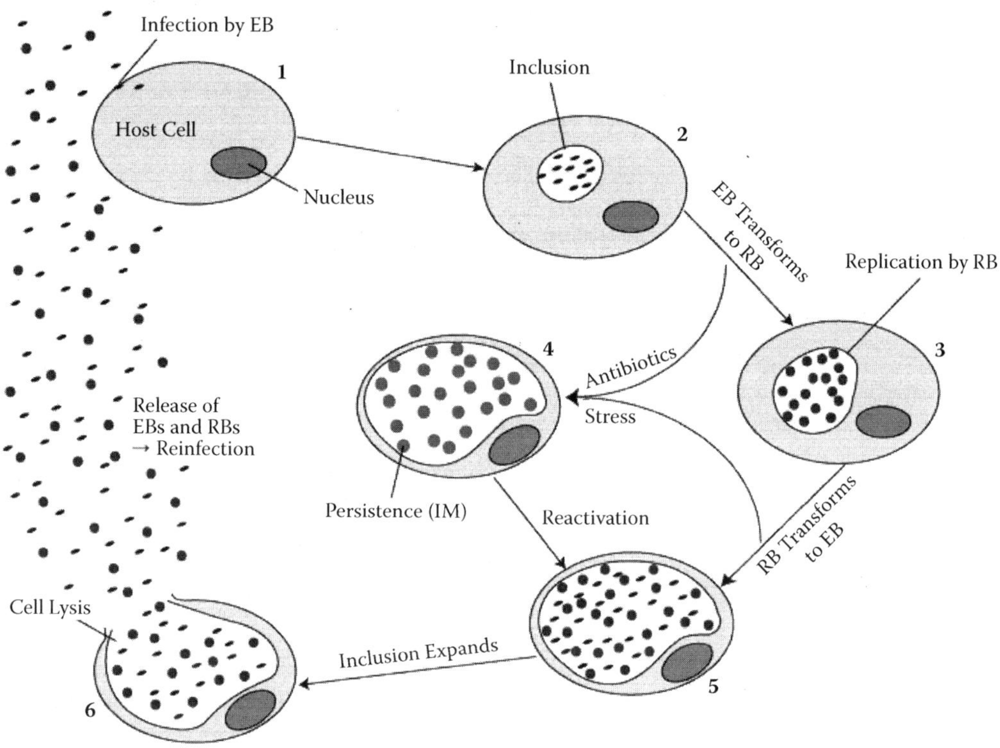

FIGURE 25.1 Chlamydial developmental cycle. In step (1), chlamydial elementary bodies (EBs) infect the host cell by a process similar to receptor-mediated endocytosis that may involve lipid rafts and proceed to form a vacuole-like structure called inclusion (2). The infectious EBs transform into non-infectious reticulate bodies (RBs) that are responsible for replication (3). If bacteria were treated with antibiotics or experienced some other form of stress, the infection may enter a persistent state (4), which could reactivate once conditions are more favorable. Following replication and growth, RBs transform back into EBs (5) and as the inclusion expands, it eventually ruptures the cell (6). EBs and RBs are released to infect surrounding cells.

cholesterol and interference with membrane rafts by tocotrienol may impair *Chlamydia's* ability to infect host cells. Tocotrienol may impact chlamydial infection in a variety of the developmental cycle phases. These include prevention of entry into host cells by reduction of cholesterol in membranes, as well as rearrangement of lipid raft regions during development if cholesterol reduction restricts chlamydial growth and inclusion fusion.

25.2 PRELIMINARY RESEARCH FINDINGS

25.2.1 Delta-Tocotrienol's Effect on Chlamydial Infection and Development

The potential for delta-tocotrienol to impact chlamydial infection and development was studied *in vitro*, using murine macrophages (J774A.1), human mammary tumor (MCF-7, TMX2-28), human B-lymphocyte (JY) and epithelial (HEp-2) cell lines incubated with delta-tocotrienol concentrations of 10-30 μmol/L for 6 h prior to infection by serovar K, a *C. trachomatis* strain of the sexually transmitted disease biovar. Controls were left untreated. At intervals between 24–72 h, monolayers were fixed and assessed for *Chlamydia* inclusions by immunofluorescent staining and fluoresence microscopy. Infection levels for delta-tocotrienol pretreated monolayers were decreased by >50% and confocal microscopy demonstrated the concomitant occurrence of aberrant inclusion development. For example, tocotrienol-treated infected human epithelial cells (HEp-2, Figure 25.2A) do not exhibit single large inclusions characteristically present at this time following *in vitro* infection with serovar

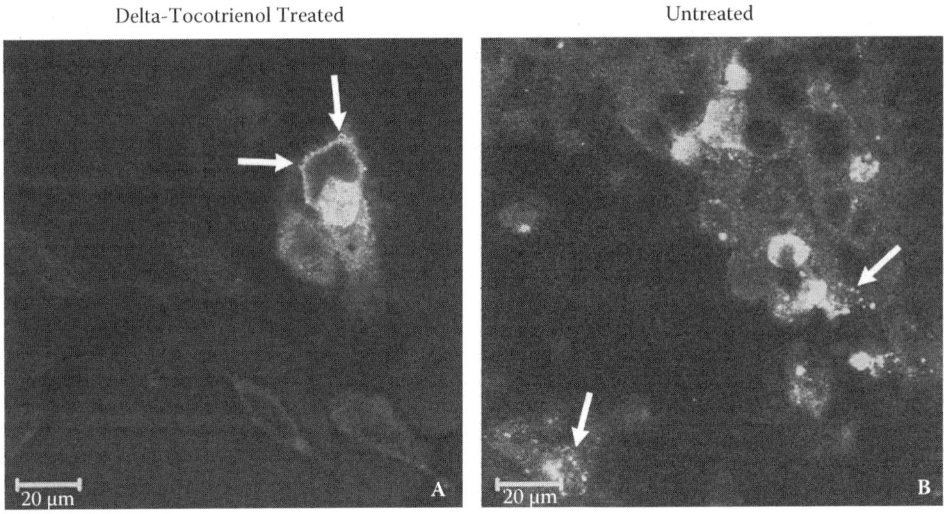

FIGURE 25.2 *Chlamydia*-infected human epithelial cells treated with delta-tocotrienol. Human epithelial cells (HEp-2 cells) were pretreated with a 30 µmol/L concentration of delta-tocotrienol in culture for 4 hours and infected with *C. trachomatis* serovar K EBs for 48 hours. At 630× magnification, the differences in the number of inclusions present in the tocotrienol-treated sample (A) and control (B) are readily visualized. There was no evidence of large, mature inclusions with tocotrienol treatment (A), whereas the level of *Chlamydia* infection in controls (B) was high. Inclusions in treated samples (A) have not fully fused and do not exhibit the morphology of mature inclusions. Arrows point to areas of unfused *Chlamydia*-positive vesicles surrounding the nucleus. In (B), inclusions are large, mature and solidly stained. Arrows point to areas where evidence of a second round of infection is present.

K, a biovar (strain) of Ctr. In contrast, the monolayers maintained in the control media (Figure 25.2B) show a large number of *Chlamydia* infected cells which have developed the large, classic inclusions characteristic of this stage in chlamydial development.

Clearly, in the delta-tocotrienol treated cells (Figure 25.2A) the *Chlamydia* positive material resides in numerous individual vesicles of varying size surrounding the entire nucleus, a distribution consistent with failure of normal vesicle fusion following intial chlamydial entry into the host cells. Importantly, in this field of view, a number of uninfected cells are present in delta-tocotrienol treated monolayers and these appear normal, indicating that tocotrienol toxicity is low if not absent. At 48 h post-infection (pi) infected cells in the control monolayers (Figure 25.2B) not only exhibit the characteristic large and solidly immunostained inclusions but also numerous *Chlamydia* positive "pin points" are evident. At this 48 h pi time, these likely represent early stages of *Chlamydia* EB entry to begin a second round of infection following their release from cells initially infected.

These results were successfully reproduced in other cell lines, including human mammary tumor, human B-lymphocyte and mouse macrophages (data not shown). In optical cross-sections of human mammary tumor cells (Figure 25.3), inclusions in the delta-tocotrienol treated cells appear less voluminous (Figure 25.3A) than inclusions of the controls cells (Figure 25.3B). These latter appeared much thicker and immunostain heavily for chlamydial antigens, suggesting that inclusions in treated monolayers contain less infectious material.

The findings presented above showed that, as compared with the controls, delta-tocotrienol treatment of HEp-2 monolayers and other cell lines was associated with a notable reduction in the number of large, classic chlamydial inclusions characteristically present at 48 or 72 h pi.

To obtain initial quantitative information, enumerations for each monolayer of a mouse macrophage cell line (J774A.1) were carried out and the numbers used to obtain the average of inclusions/cells counted in 100 fields of view at 40X magnification. Microscopic enumeration of large and small inclusions in the treated vs. control cells indicated decreases of three- and twofold, respec-

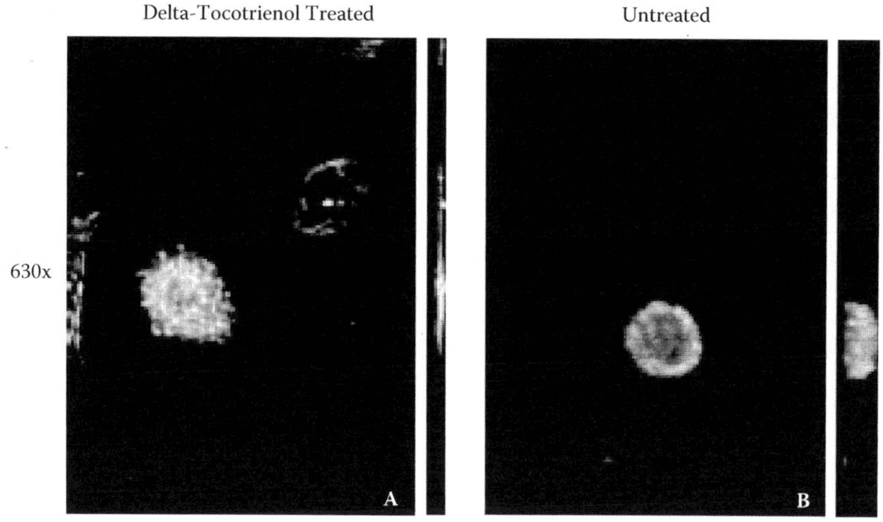

FIGURE 25.3 *Chlamydia*-infected mammary tumor cells treated with delta-tocotrienol. Mammary tumor cells (TMX2-28 cells) were pretreated with a 30 μmol/L concentration of delta-tocotrienol in culture for 4 hours and infected with *C. trachomatis* serovar K EBs for 72 hours. In cross-sections of monolayers at 630x magnification (A), the differences in volume of inclusions present in the tocotrienol-treated sample (A) and control (B) are readily visualized. Inclusions in tocotrienol-treated cells were flat and presumably contained less infectious material (A), whereas the level of *Chlamydia* infection in controls (B) was high, evident by the increased thickness of the cross-section.

tively. Several generations of serial passages of delta-tocotrienol treated supernatant containing EBs from the preceding infection showed notable decreases in inclusion formation, suggesting that with continued delta-tocotrienol treatment inhibition of infection would be augmented.

For the non-adherent human JY B-cells, flow cytometric quantification showed at least a two-fold decrease of *Chlamydia*-infected cells during an infection period of 72 h, with a 2.6-fold maximum at 36 h.

25.2.2 Delta-Tocotrienol and Other Tocotrienol Isomers: Potency in Effect on Chlamydia Infection

Although only delta-tocotrienol was studied in detail, the effect of the remaining tocotrienol isomers in the vitamin E family was assessed microscopically for their impact on inclusion formation *in vitro;* delta-tocotrienol is monomethylated, while the other tocotrienol isomers are di- or trimethylated, bulkier at the molecular level and potentially less readily internalized. In addition, delta-tocotrienol is more bioavailable than the other isomers (McIntyre et al. 2000; Naito et al. 2005). Thus, delta-tocotrienol might have a greater impact on *Chlamydia* infection levels. A series of J774A.1 cell monolayers were pretreated for 4 h with a 30 μmol/L concentration of alpha-, beta-, gamma- or delta-tocotrienol and were then infected with *C. trachomatis* serovar K EBs for 48 h using the methods outlined for delta-tocotrienol. Fixed treated and control samples were immunostained to detect *Chlamydia*, then examined microscopically. Enumeration of inclusions in isomer pretreated monolayers indicated that relative to the untreated controls, there were decreases in inclusion numbers of ~51% for the alpha-tocotrienol isomer and ~30% for the beta- and gamma- tocotrienol; the delta-tocotrienol isomer displayed the greatest decrease at 56.1% (Figure 25.4).

The isomers also affected inclusion formation. The alpha-, beta-, gamma- and delta-tocotrienol treated monolayers each contain few inclusion-like regions. Additionally, the beta- or gamma-T3 treatments result in aberrant but recognizable inclusions. In contrast, treatment with delta-tocotrienol shows a quite different appearance and only very small, unfused vesicles are present. Inclu-

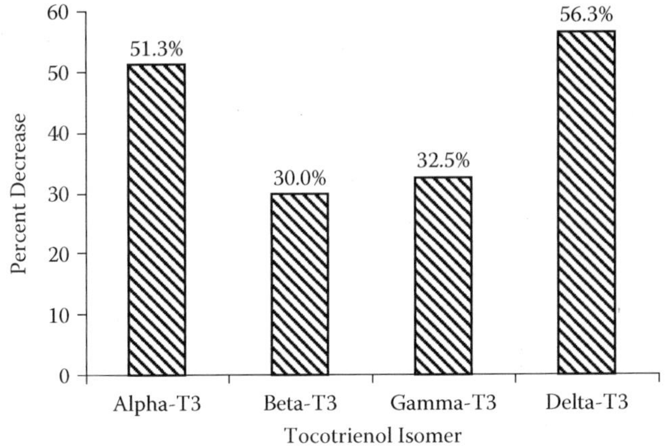

FIGURE 25.4 Summary of inclusion counts for *Chlamydia*-infected mouse macrophages treated with tocotrienol isomers. Mouse macrophages (J774A.1 cells) were pretreated with a 30μmol/L concentration of alpha-, beta-, gamma- and delta-tocotrienol in culture for 4 h and infected with *C. trachomatis* serovar K EBs for 48 h. Inclusion and cell counts were done for the average of 10 fields of view. The percent decrease of *Chlamydia* infection was calculated by comparing the tocotrienol-treated samples to the untreated control. The percent decrease of inclusion formation was highest in the sample treated with delta-tocotrienol and lowest for beta-tocotrienol. Surprisingly, gamma-tocotrienol treatment was less effective than anticipated. The high chlamydial inhibition by delta-tocotrienol and alpha-tocotrienol apparently did not fit our hypothesis that desmethyl tocotrienols as a class would be more potent. This may be due to the recognition of alpha-tocotrienol by alpha-tocopherol transport protein (ATTP).

sions of alpha-tocotrienol treated cells resembled those of untreated control cells and may therefore contain a larger number of infectious EBs despite the 51% decrease in total inclusion numbers. Therefore, since alpha-tocotrienol treated samples display inclusions resembling those of untreated control cells, this compound may be less effective in limiting repeat serial infections as compared to treatment of cells with the other isomers. These clearly induced abnormal inclusion formation and presumably had lower infectious *Chlamydia* carriage.

The high percent decrease in inclusion number in alpha-tocotrienol treated cells may be due to more efficient initial delivery of alpha-tocotrienol to the cell membrane via alpha-tocopherol transport protein (ATTP) present in the host cell.

25.3 PREVALENCE OF *C. PNEUMONIAE* IN HYPERCHOLESTEROLEMIC INDIVIDUALS

Since lipids and lipid levels could potentially impact carriage of *Chlamydia in vivo*, peripheral white blood cells from a small cohort (n = 29) of hyperlipidemic patients were also assessed. Immunostained blood smears indicated the *Chlamydia* carriage rate (58.6%) was approximately double in hyperlipidemic patients than that observed for normal blood donors (Cirino et al. 2006). Flow cytometric quantification of white cells from this cohort indicated an average *Chlamydia* infected white blood cell carriage level of 5054/10,000 +/– cells counted, meaning that at least half of the white cells in each sample were positive for *Chlamydia* (Figure 25.5).

25.4 OTHER CHOLESTEROL-REDUCERS AND *CHLAMYDIA*

There is strong previous evidence that antihyperlipidemic drugs such as statins reduce infection by *Chlamydia*, which supports the hypothesis that tocotrienol may have an effect on chlamydial infection through its hyperlipidemic properties. Depletion of cholesterol in lipid raft regions by filipin and nystatin use led to a significant decrease of infection by *Chlamydia* of several species, indicat-

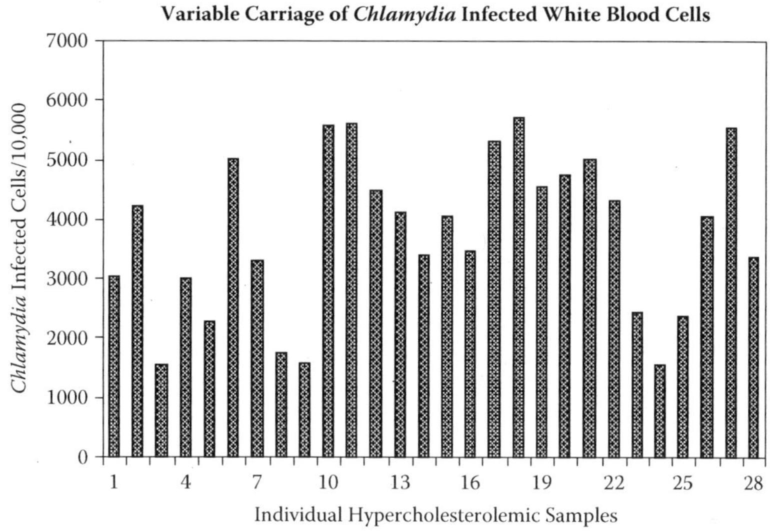

FIGURE 25.5 Carriage of *Chlamydia* in hypercholesterolemic individuals. Carriage of *Chlamydia* in white blood cells of hypercholesterolemic individuals (blood samples obtained from Vanderbilt University Medical Center) was assessed using quantitative flow cytometry. Of 29 patients, 58.6% were positive for *Chlamydia* carriage, while average carriage levels were 5054 infected cells / 10,000 cells counted.

ing that these are somewhat dependent on lipid raft-mediated entry (Stuart et al. 2003). Yamaguchi et al. showed that several antihyperlipidemic drugs, including statins and fibrates, may have an additional effect on prevention of atherosclerosis beyond cholesterol-lowering per se. Atherosclerosis-aggravating Cpn growth was inhibited by *in vitro* treatment with antihyperlipidemic drugs and this phenomenon was dose-dependent (Yamaguchi et al. 2004). In a more recent study, simvastatin was shown to decrease viable Cpn counts in mice, while increasing inflammatory cell infiltrates. The authors concluded that by disturbing intracellular trafficking of cholesterol, simvastatin inhibited replication of *Chlamydia* (Erkkila et al. 2005).

In vitro treatment of *Chlamydia*-infected cells with tea polyphenols, which are also thought to have hypocholesterolemic properties, completely inhibited both Ctr and Cpn without toxic effects (Yamazaki et al. 2005). Tea polyphenols are catechins found in green tea, such as epicatechin (EC), epigallocatechin (EGC), epichatechin-3-gallate (ECG) and epigallocatechin-3-gallate (EGCG). Among these phenolics, EGCG is known to be the most potent (Kuroda and Hara, 1999). These *in vitro* studies illustrate that agents that lower cholesterol may have a therapeutic effect vis-à-vis *Chlamydia* infection. In a clinical study, Cpn antibody level was associated with the cholesterol-lowering effect of statins. However, under these *in vivo* conditions for Cpn-positive patients who were taking statin medications, the lipid-lowering effect was decreased when compared with the Cpn negative group (Sawayama et al. 2003); the intake of cholesterol-lowering compounds thus might require adjustment. Therefore, statins may still be important in decreasing Cpn infections by creating a less favorable host environment for the pathogen. Other natural agents with the potential for a therapeutic effect on *Chlamydia* infection would include bioflavonoids, polymethoxylated flavones, plant sterols, oryzanol, policosanol, red yeast rice, soluble and insoluble fiber and gugul lipids (Mueller et al., 2006). These agents clearly affect cholesterol biosynthesis.

25.5 TOCOTRIENOL POTENTIAL IN PREVENTING INFECTION OF PATHOGENS WITH A REQUIREMENT FOR CHOLESTEROL

There are several bacteria, viruses and parasites that have a cholesterol requirement for successful infection of hosts, and some bacteria and viruses also use lipid rafts as the route of entry into host cells.

25.5.1 Bacteria

Similar to *Chlamydia*, species of the genera *Coxiella* and *Ehrlichia* are obligate intracellular organisms. *Coxiella burnetii* is the agent of Q fever and replicates in a parasitophorous vacuole derived from the host and modified by the bacterium to facilitate its survival and growth. A study in guinea pigs showed that liver lipids increased 3–4 days following infection with *C. burnetii* (Paretsky et al. 1964), implying that the pathogen may modify lipid synthesis in the host. This was confirmed years later, when *C. burnetii* was shown to increase host cell cholesterol by 1.75-fold and upregulate host genes involved in cholesterol metabolism (Howe and Heinzen, 2006). In addition, treatment with lovastatin and other cholesterol metabolism inhibitors significantly inhibited *C. burnetii* replication (Howe and Heinzen, 2005). This result is similar to findings obtained for *Chlamydia* when the same or analogous cholesterol inhibitors were used (Stuart et al. 2003; Erkkila et al. 2005). Another line of comparison is the cholesterol contained in the vacuole membranes of these organisms. Cholesterol is trafficked to the chlamydial inclusion membrane via the Golgi and is shown to associate with the inclusion membrane as well as individual EBs (Carabeo et al. 2003). *C. burnetii*, like *Chlamydia*, stained richly for the presence of cholesterol in the parasitophorous membrane (Howe and Heinzen, 2005). The above studies imply that host cholesterol is required for successful replication and infection of both *C. burnetii* and *Chlamydia* and may suggest that tocotrienol could have an effect on *C. burnetii* similar to the effect it had on *Chlamydia*.

Ehrlichia, another obligate intracellular organism that exhibits entry into host cells in association with cholesterol, causes monozytic ehrlichiosis with symptoms of fever and headaches and is transferred by ticks. *Ehrlichia chaffeensis* lacks genes for cholesterol synthesis, as does *Chlamydia*, and incorporation of cholesterol from its host is essential. Similarly, cholesterol depletion of host cells prevented cell entry of *E. chaffeensis* and resulted in pathogen death (Lin and Rikihisa, 2003). As with *Chlamydia, E. chaffeensis* entry into host cells was shown to involve lipid rafts (Lin and Rikihisa, 2003). Thus, modification of lipid rafts and cholesterol levels by tocotrienol could also potentially inhibit *E. chaffeensis* entry into host cells, thereby reducing infection levels.

Mycoplasma, a bacterium very different from the obligate intracellular *Chlamydia*, is unaffected by antibiotics such as penicillin because it lacks a cell wall. However, this lack makes incorporation of host cholesterol mandatory for this bacterium. *Mycoplasma* has been shown to exhibit a growth response to cholesterol (Razin and Tully, 1970) and tocotrienol reduction of cholesterol also may have an effect on this bacterium's survival.

Porphyromonas gingivalis, an anaerobic bacterium found in oral cavities, has implications in periodontal disease and shares the common association *Chlamydia* has with atherosclerosis and coronary heart disease (Triantafilou et al. 2007; Yamazaki et al. 2007). Depleting plasma membranes of cholesterol inhibited invasion of *P. gingivalis* into epithelial cells, suggesting that tocotrienol could have a similar, but less drastic effect. Interestingly, epithelial cells lacking caveolae, the small invaginations in the plasma membrane with which *Chlamydia* have also been associated, supported only limited invasion by *P. gingivalis* (Tamai et al. 2005).

25.5.2 Parasites

Cholesterol plays an important role in parasitic infections, where parasite enzymes may support degradation and subsequent consumption of lipids and cholesterol. Alternatively, certain parasites may induce significant changes in host lipid parameters (Bansal et al. 2005). An example of such a parasite is *Leishmania donovani*, which causes leishmaniasis accompanied by symptoms of skin sores, fever, damage to the spleen and liver and in some cases anemia. The parasite is spread by the sandfly and currently affects 12 million people in 88 countries. *L. donovani* is an obligate intracellular parasite that infects macrophages via lipid rafts. As noted for the intracellular bacteria discussed previously, cholesterol depletion from the macrophage plasma membrane resulted in significant reduction of leishmanial infection and this was reversed upon replenishment of membrane cholesterol (Pucadyil et al. 2004). This finding indicates a specific requirement of plasma membrane cholesterol in the efficient attachment and internalization of the parasite into host cells and could also be readily studied using tocotrienol to modify cholesterol levels.

Perkinsus marinus, a parasite of oysters, causes dermo—the proteolytic degradation of oyster tissue—and massive death of oyster populations. It thus poses a significant economic threat to the oyster industry. *P. marinus* cannot synthesize sterols and needs to acquire them from the host. In a recent study, *P. marinus* failed to proliferate in a cholesterol-free medium and alpha-tocopherol-substituted medium (Lund et al. 2007). Treatment of host cells with tocotrienol could modify lipid levels and reduce dermo in oyster populations.

Malaria is caused by the parasitic protozoa *Plasmodium* and may be fatal if left untreated. Each year 300–500 new cases occur worldwide and more than one million people die, particularly in poorer countries (Centers for Disease Control and Prevention, 2007). Although there is medication for malaria, drug resistance by *Plasmodium* is increasingly common (Chung et al. 2007). *P. yoelii* and *P. falciparum* demonstrate an involvement of host membrane cholesterol for invasion and cholesterol contributes to the organization of tetraspanin microdomains that facilitate *Plasmodium* entry (Silvie et al. 2006). An interesting observation is that *Plasmodium* flourished and grew most rapidly in hepatocytes, which are rich in cholesterol. The same study showed that *Plasmodium* modifies the permeability of the parasitophorous vacuole it inhabits to allow transfer of molecules, including cholesterol, from the host cytosol (Bano et al. 2007). The finding that host-derived cholesterol accumulates at the vacuole membrane is very reminiscent of the same phenomenon discussed earlier in the context of obligate intracellular bacteria.

Yet another parasitic protozoan, *Toxoplasma gondii*, infects cats, its main host, and also humans, on a less frequent basis. *T. gondii* causes toxoplasmosis, which can have serious side effects on the fetus in pregnant women and the immunocompromised. Like *Plasmodium*, *T. gondii* inhabits a parasitophorous vacuole that contains cholesterol incorporated from the host. Once again, depleting the host cell plasma membrane cholesterol blocks parasite internalization, thus indicating that host cholesterol controls entry of *T. gondii* (Coppens and Joiner, 2003). In contrast to *Chlamydia*, *T. gondii* does not obtain cholesterol through the host Golgi or ER, but scavenges it from the host endolysosomal compartments (Sehgal et al. 2005). Given their cholesterol-rich parasitophorous vacuole and a cholesterol requirement for host cell invasion, infection by both *Plasmodium* and *T. gondii*, like *Chlamydia*, might be impaired, or interdicted by tocotrienol.

25.5.3 Viruses

In addition to bacteria and parasites, several viruses have a cholesterol requirement, which is specific primarily due to their entry into the host cell via lipid rafts. Coronavirus causes upper respiratory and gastrointestinal tract infections, and strains of this virus are the agents of SARS and common colds. In a study with coronavirus murine hepatitis virus (MHV), cholesterol depletion reduced plaque development two- to twentyfold, while cholesterol supplementation increased susceptibility two- to tenfold. It therefore was concluded that cholesterol was an essential membrane fusion cofactor that promotes MHV entry into host cells (Thorp and Gallagher, 2004).

Human enteroviruses, including polio-, coxsackie- and echovirus, are the most common cause of aseptic meningitis. Some of the enteroviruses use the glycosylphosphatidylinositol (GPI)-anchored complement regulatory protein decay-accelerating factor (DAF) found in lipid rafts as a receptor during infection. These DAF-using enteroviruses are dependent on cholesterol for viral entry into host cells (Stuart et al. 2002).

Spread by mosquitoes, alphavirus, such as Semliki Forest virus, causes encephalitis in humans and animals. Alphavirus fusion is completely dependent on the presence of cholesterol in the target membrane (Stiasny et al. 2003) and budding is blocked in the absence of cholesterol (Lu and Kielian, 2000). Similar to the alphavirus, flavovirus causes encephalitis, as well as West Nile, dengue fever and yellow fever. The mechanism of flavovirus fusion was compared with that of alphavirus and research showed that in the tick-borne encephalitis virus (a flavovirus) cholesterol strongly promoted the membrane binding of fusion protein, as was found for the alphavirus (Stiasny et al. 2003).

The Newcastle disease virus (NDV), a paramyxovirus, causes sudden death in birds and, without available treatment options, it poses a serious threat to the poultry industry. Entry by NDV involves its direct fusion to the plasma membrane and the depletion of cholesterol reduced the extent of fusion, infectivity and virus-cell binding (Cantin et al. 2007). In the same study, blockage of caveolae-dependent endocytosis also reduced NDV fusion and infectivity. Comparison of NDV with *Chlamydia* discloses interesting similarities and these would support suggesting that tocotrienol could have a negative impact on infection by this virus.

The most common cause of severe diarrhea in children is the rotavirus, and in many cases, infection results in hospitalization and even death in poorer countries. Lipid rafts have been proposed as rotavirus receptors and, when tested, disorganization of these microdomains greatly inhibited infectivity (Arias et al. 2002). Due to its cholesterol-lowering activity, tocotrienol may rearrange lipid rafts and thus might also exhibit a blocking effect on infection by rotavirus.

There may be numerous other pathogens not mentioned here that have a requirement for host-derived cholesterol or use lipid rafts as their route of entry into host cells. A recent review suggests lipid rafts as a potential theraupeutic target to suppress propagation of a variety of pathogens (Hawkes and Mak, 2006). Previous hypotheses and results showing tocotrienol's inhibitory effect on chlamydial infection suggest that pathogens with similar routes of entry into host or replication also may be affected by the hypocholesterolemic compound. Therefore, further research should be conducted on the antibacterial and antiviral properties of tocotrienols. The cholesterol requirements of various pathogens and the potential interventions by tocotrienol are summarized in Table 25.1.

25.6 *CHLAMYDIA*, TOCOTRIENOL AND ATHEROSCLEROSIS—THE CONNECTION

Atherosclerosis, the clogging and hardening of the arteries, is characterized by fatty streaks followed by unstable plaque formation. Risk factors include high cholesterol, hypertension, metabolic syndrome, the lesser known chronic infections (such as Cpn) and others. While Cpn has been known as an exacerbator of atherogenic progression, tocotrienol was shown repeatedly to reduce several risk factors of atherosclerosis. Since the first publication that associated the presence of Cpn IgG with myocardial infarction and coronary heart disease (Saikku et al. 1988), there has been recurring evidence of the *Chlamydia*–atherosclerosis link. A summary of *Chlamydia*'s effect on atherosclerosis is depicted in Figure 25.6. Cpn is widespread, with 50% prevalence of antibodies found by age 20 and 70–80% in the elderly (Campbell and Kuo, 2004). Earlier *in vitro* studies showed that Cpn induced macrophages to accumulate excess cholesterol, leading to foam cell formation (Kalayoglu and Byrne, 1998) and release of proinflammatory cytokines (Blessing et al. 2002). Both of these features are contributing factors to atherosclerosis development. Further, the increased uptake of LDL occurred via an LDL-receptor-independent pathway (Kalayoglu et al. 1999). On the other hand, tocotrienol completely abolished tumor necrosis factor alpha (TNF)-induced NF-kappaB activation (Ahn et al. 2007).

Cpn was also repeatedly detected in atheromas (Shor et al. 1992; Kuo et al. 1993; Ramirez, 1996; Kuo and Campbell, 2000), while it is less commonly found in non-atherosclerotic tissue (Shor et al. 1992). Possibly the apo E deficiency in mice leads to an induction of hypercholesterolemia and atherosclerosis and may support development of persistent Cpn infections accompanied by foam cell formation that are not found in apo E mice (Nakashima et al. 1994; Reddick et al. 1994). In addition, mice with normal lipids had only transient Cpn infections (Blessing et al. 2000).

Interestingly, Cpn infection results in activation of an atherosclerosis-like signal transduction profile (Summersgill et al. 2000), while the histology of Cpn infection sites is typical of the chronic inflammatory response observed in atherosclerotic lesions (Ross, 1999). Cpn infection also resulted

TABLE 25.1
Pathogens with Cholesterol Requirements and Possible Effect of Tocotrienol on Infectivity

Pathogen	Manner of Cholesterol Usage	Effect by Tocotrienol
	Bacteria	
Coxiella burnetii	Modifies lipid synthesis, increases host cholesterol	Cholesterol metabolism modification may inhibit host cell entry and/or pathogen propagation
Ehrlichia chaffeensis	Lacks genes for cholesterol synthesis, incorporation of host cholesterol essential, lipid raft entry	Cholesterol depletion may prevent host cell entry and induce pathogen death
Mycoplasma	Lacks cell wall, host cholesterol incorporation mandatory	Cholesterol depletion may reduce pathogen growth
Porphyromonas gingivalis	Needs cholesterol to more effectively infect host cells	Cholesterol depletion may inhibit pathogen invasion into epithelial cells
	Parasites	
Leishmania donovani	Infects macrophages via lipid raft entry	Cholesterol depletion in lipid rafts may result in significant reduction of infection
Perkinsus marinus	Acquires sterols from host	Modification of lipid levels may reduce infection
Plasmodium	Involves host membrane cholesterol for invasion, host cholesterol accumulates in parasitophorous vacuole, flourishes in cholesterol-rich hepatocytes	Host cholesterol depletion may decrease infection and/or pathogen replication
Toxoplasma gondii	Incorporates host-derived cholesterol into parasitophorous vacuole	Host plasma membrane cholesterol depletion may block parasite internalization
	Viruses	
Coronavirus (MHV)	Uses cholesterol as essential membrane fusion cofactor	Cholesterol depletion may reduce viral plaque formation
Human enterovirus (DAF-using)	Depends on cholesterol for viral entry	Cholesterol depletion may decrease viral entry
Alphavirus (Semliki Forest Virus)	Depends on presence of cholesterol in target membrane for fusion	Cholesterol depletion in target membrane may block virus budding
Flavovirus	Uses cholesterol for membrane binding/ fusion protein	Cholesterol depletion may block fusion
Paramyxovirus (NDV)	Fuses direct to cholesterol-rich plasma membrane during entry	Cholesterol depletion may reduce fusion, infectivity, and virus-cell binding
Rotavirus	Uses lipid rafts as virus receptors	Disorganization of lipid rafts may reduce infectivity

in a 2.2-fold increase in total lesion size in mice (Ezzahiri et al. 2006). It is instructive to note here that tocotrienol supplemented in a high-fat diet decreased atherosclerotic lesion size by up to 57% in mice (Qureshi et al. 2001), a phenomenon that has been repeatedly noted in other studies (Black et al. 2000).

After demonstrating that viable Cpn reside in peripheral blood mononuclear cells of 18.5% of healthy blood donors, researchers suggested that the risk of developing atherosclerosis could increase in blood transfusion recipients (Yamaguchi et al. 2004). The finding that Cpn infection upregulates adhesion molecule expression, enhancing attachment of macrophages to the endothelium is important in regard to atherosclerosis development (Kaukoranta-Tolvanen et al. 1996; Kalayoglu et al. 2001). Increased adherence of macrophages to the endothelium would enhance their migration into

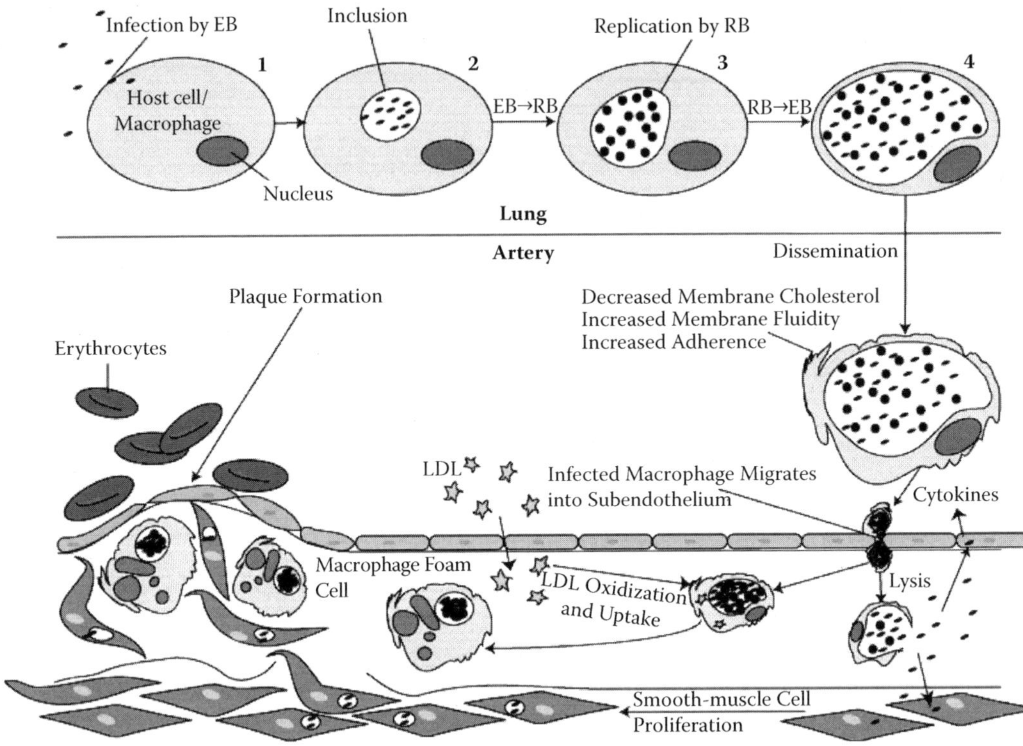

FIGURE 25.6 *Chlamydia*'s role in atherosclerosis. Following the first four steps of the chlamydial replication cycle within the host cell, infected macrophages may disseminate from the primary site of infection (lung) into the blood stream. As infection decreases membrane cholesterol and increases membrane fluidity, adherence to the endothelium of arteries is facilitated. The infected macrophage migrates into the subendothelium, where it could take one of two routes. First, the infected macrophage could take up oxidized LDL to create an environment which it flourishes in, forming foam cells. Secondly, the infected cell may burst, releasing EBs that proceed to infect endothelial cells and smooth-muscle cell, inducing smooth-muscle cell proliferation and cytokine production. All these factors increase the risk of unstable plaque formation, plaque rupture and thrombosis and contribute to the cause of angina and myocardial infarction.

the subendothelium, developing the earlier stages of plaque formation. This was confirmed by studies demonstrating accelerated plaque development correlated with *Chlamydia* infection (Moazed et al. 1999). Tocotrienol, on the other hand, has been shown to inhibit platelet aggregation up to 71%, with delta-tocotrienol being the most potent inhibitor (Holub, 1989; Qureshi et al. 1991). In Cpn infection, the heightened adherence of macrophages to endothelial cells was shown to be not entirely due to increased adhesion molecules. In one study, Cpn infection induced depletion of macrophage membrane cholesterol, increased phospholipids and membrane fluidity and caused a more profound adherence to endothelial cells despite the use of adhesion molecule inhibitors (Azenabor et al. 2005). Tocotrienol, especially delta-tocotrienol, reduced monocyte-endothelial cell interaction by inhibiting surface expression of adhesion molecules. Delta-tocotrienol was shown to be a potent and effective agent for the reduction of vascular cell adhesion molecule 1 (VCAM-1) and E-selectin expression (Theriault et al. 2002; Naito et al. 2005). Thus, tocotrienol may also reduce endothelial cell adhesion of macrophages infected with *Chlamydia*.

Cpn could also have a negative effect on blood pressure. In apo E deficient mice, Cpn infection impaired arterial relaxation due to a reduction in availability of nitric oxide, an essential requirement for arterial integrity (Liuba et al. 2000). Tocotrienol has the opposite effect on arterial integrity, improving nitric oxide synthase activity (Newaz and Nawal, 1999; Newaz et al. 2003) and reducing aortic systolic blood pressure in humans (Rasool et al. 2006).

TABLE 25.2
Impact of *Chlamydia* and Tocotrienol on Atherosclerosis Markers

Condition/Marker	Effect by *Chlamydia*	Effect by Tocotrienol
Cholesterol	Accumulated by Cpn-infected macrophages	Degraded pathway to/downregulated cholesterol synthesis
Inflammatory response/cytokines	Induced by infection	Abolished tumor necrosis factor alpha (TNF)-induced NF-kappaB activation
LDL	Increased uptake by Cpn-infected cells, foam cell formation	Reduced LDL
Lesion size/plaque formation	Increased/accelerated by Cpn infection	Decreased 57–98%
Adhesion molecules	Upregulated expression in infected cells	Reduced monocyte-endothelial cell adhesion, inhibited surface expression effectively
Blood pressure	Impaired arterial relaxation	Improved nitric oxide synthase activity, reduced aortic systolic blood pressure

Another perspective for viewing the *Chlamydia*–atherosclerosis connection could be that *Chlamydia* not only aggravates atherosclerosis, but also makes the condition more intractable in terms of improvement once it becomes established. In a recent clinical study, researchers investigated the association between Cpn infection and atherosclerosis by comparing the effects of lipid-lowering drugs on intima-media thickness (IMT) in carotid atherosclerosis patients positive or negative for *Chlamydia*. After a 2-year period, IMT in Cpn-negative patients improved significantly, while there was no significant change of IMT in Cpn-positive patients (Sawayama et al. 2007). Here, Cpn was found to be the most important independent factor associated with the rate of IMT progression and Cpn is thought to reduce the effect of lipid-lowering drugs on hyperlipidemia (Sawayama et al. 2003). This correlation was previously shown in rabbits, where repeated Cpn infection of the animals increased intimal thickening (Coombes et al. 2002). The effects of tocotrienol were also tested on carotid atherosclerosis in a 4-year clinical study. In this study, carotid artery stenosis regressed or stabilized in 88% of patients with tocotrienol supplementation, whereas in the control group, 60% deteriorated (Kooyenga et al. 2001).

Clearly, there is a strong case for the acceleration and aggravation of atherosclerosis by *Chlamydia*. Tocotrienol, which in preliminary studies was shown to inhibit chlamydial infection, thus may have multiple roles in atherosclerosis reduction. These may include reduction of cholesterol levels, hypertension and carotid atherosclerosis (including initiation of regression), as well as the most recent findings suggesting an effect on *Chlamydia* infection itself. A comparison of the impact of *Chlamydia* and tocotrienol on atherosclerosis is presented in Table 25.2.

25.7 CONCLUSION

Tocotrienol, with its hypocholesterolemic activity, may have an impact on infection by *Chlamydia*, an obligate intracellular pathogen with a requirement for host cell cholesterol that it uses for entry as well as growth and replication. Preliminary research shows that tocotrienol may reduce infection by *Chlamydia* up to 50%, with delta-tocotrienol being the most potent inhibitor. It may be that tocotrienol initiates a rearranging of lipid raft regions used by *Chlamydia* for entry, or deprives the pathogen of cholesterol necessary for growth, replication and survival. Interestingly, patients with high cholesterol were found to have a higher incidence of blood cell-borne *Chlamydia*, supporting a conclusion that *in vivo* the pathogen can flourish in this environment. Other cholesterol-reducing agents (e.g., EGCG, statins) also may have an impact on infection by *Chlamydia*. Infection by other cholesterol-requiring bacteria, parasites and viruses (e.g., Coxiella, Leishmania, alphavirus) may also be mitigated by cholesterol-reducing agents and this provides rich grounds for future research.

These findings appear relevant to a potential treatment for *Chlamydia* infections, as well as atherosclerosis risk factor reductions. Tocotrienol, in addition to reducing commonly known chronic inflammatory risk factors of atherosclerosis, may also have an impact on the less frequently mentioned pathogenic infection risk factor of atherosclerosis. Chronic infections by *Chlamydia* have been shown to contribute to atherosclerosis acceleration and may also attenuate treatment or improvement of this condition. Thus, tocotrienol has many therapeutic roles and may be an important agent in reducing the incidence and duration of atherosclerosis.

REFERENCES

Ahn, K. S., G. Sethi, et al. 2007. Gamma-tocotrienol inhibits nuclear factor-kappaB signaling pathway through inhibition of receptor-interacting protein and TAK1 leading to suppression of antiapoptotic gene products and potentiation of apoptosis. *J Biol Chem* 2821: 809–20.

Arias, C. F., P. Isa et al. 2002. Molecular biology of rotavirus cell entry. *Arch Med Res* 334: 356–61.

Azenabor, A. A., G. Job et al. 2005. *Chlamydia pneumoniae* infected macrophages exhibit enhanced plasma membrane fluidity and show increased adherence to endothelial cells. *Mol Cell Biochem* 2691–2: 69–84.

Balin, B. J., H. C. Gerard et al. 1998. Identification and localization of *Chlamydia pneumoniae* in the Alzheimer's brain. *Med Microbiol Immunol Berl* 1871: 23–42.

Bano, N., J. D. Romano et al. 2007. Cellular interactions of plasmodium liver stage with its host mammalian cell. *Int J Parasitol* 3712: 1329–41.

Bansal, D., H. S. Bhatti et al. 2005. Role of cholesterol in parasitic infections. *Lipids Health Dis* 41: 10.

Beckman, M. 2005. Living off the fat of the cell. *Science NOW Daily News*, Dec. 12, American Association for the Advancement of Science (AAAS).

Black, T. M., P. Wang et al. 2000. Palm tocotrienols protect ApoE +/– mice from diet-induced atheroma formation. *J Nutr* 13010: 2420–6.

Blessing, E., C. C. Kuo et al. 2002. Foam cell formation inhibits growth of *Chlamydia pneumoniae* but does not attenuate *Chlamydia pneumoniae*-induced secretion of proinflammatory cytokines. *Circulation* 10516: 1976–82.

Blessing, E., T. M. Lin et al. 2000. *Chlamydia pneumoniae* induces inflammatory changes in the heart and aorta of normocholesterolemic C57BL/6J mice. *Infect Immun* 688: 4765–8.

Byrne, G. I. and M. V. Kalayoglu. 1999. *Chlamydia pneumoniae* and atherosclerosis: Links to the disease process. *Am Heart J* 1385 Pt 2: S488–90.

Campbell, L. A. and C. C. Kuo. 2004. *Chlamydia pneumoniae*––an infectious risk factor for atherosclerosis? *Nat Rev Microbiol* 21: 23–32.

Cantin, C., J. Holguera et al. 2007. Newcastle disease virus may enter cells by caveolae-mediated endocytosis. *J Gen Virol* 88 Pt 2: 559–69.

Carabeo, R. A., D. J. Mead et al. 2003. Golgi-dependent transport of cholesterol to the *Chlamydia trachomatis* inclusion. *PNAS* 10011: 6771–6776.

Chung, H. C., J. T. Wang et al. 2007. Clinical experience of 17 cases of imported malaria at a Taiwan university hospital, 1999–2005. *J Microbiol Immunol Infect* 403: 209–15.

Cirino, F., W. C. Webley et al. 2006. Detection of *Chlamydia* in the peripheral blood cells of normal donors using in vitro culture, immunofluorescence microscopy and flow cytometry techniques. *BMC Infect Dis* 6: 23.

Coombes, B. K., B. Chiu et al. 2002. *Chlamydia pneumoniae* infection of endothelial cells induces transcriptional activation of platelet-derived growth factor-B: A potential link to intimal thickening in a rabbit model of atherosclerosis. *J Infect Dis* 18511: 1621–30.

Coppens, I. and K. A. Joiner. 2003. Host but not parasite cholesterol controls Toxoplasma cell entry by modulating organelle discharge. *Mol Biol Cell* 149: 3804–20.

Erkkila, L., M. Jauhiainen et al. 2005. Effect of simvastatin, an established lipid-lowering drug, on pulmonary *Chlamydia pneumoniae* infection in mice. *Antimicrob Agents Chemother* 499: 3959–62.

Escalante-Ochoa, C., R. Ducatelle et al. 2000. Optimal development of *Chlamydophila psittaci* in L929 fibroblast and BGM epithelial cells requires the participation of microfilaments and microtubule–motor proteins. *Microb Pathog* 286: 321–33.

Ezzahiri, R., F. R. Stassen et al. 2006. Chlamydia pneumoniae infections augment atherosclerotic lesion formation: A role for serum amyloid P. *Apmis* 1142: 117–26.

Fukuda, E. Y., S. P. Lad et al. 2005. Activation of lipid metabolism contributes to interleukin–8 production during Chlamydia trachomatis infection of cervical epithelial cells. *Infect Immun* 737: 4017–24.

Hackstadt, T., D. D. Rockey et al. 1996. Chlamydia trachomatis interrupts an exocytic pathway to acquire endogenously synthesized sphingomyelin in transit from the Golgi apparatus to the plasma membrane. *Embo J* 155: 964–77.

Hahn, D. L. 2004. Chlamydia pneumoniae and asthma: More than just exacerbations. *J Allergy Clin Immunol* 1133: 568.

Hawkes, D. J. and J. Mak 2006. Lipid membrane; a novel target for viral and bacterial pathogens. *Curr Drug Targets* 712: 1615–21.

Hodinka, R. L., C. H. Davis et al. 1988. Ultrastructural study of endocytosis of Chlamydia trachomatis by McCoy cells. *Infect Immun* 566: 1456–63.

Holub, B. 1989. Inhibition of platelet aggregation by tocotrienols. University of Guelph, Ontario. PORIM presentation, Kuala Lumpur, Malaysia.

Howe, D. and R. A. Heinzen 2005. Replication of Coxiella burnetii is inhibited in CHO K–1 cells treated with inhibitors of cholesterol metabolism. *Ann NY Acad Sci* 1063: 123–9.

Howe, D. and R. A. Heinzen 2006. Coxiella burnetii inhabits a cholesterol-rich vacuole and influences cellular cholesterol metabolism. *Cell Microbiol* 83: 496–507.

Kalayoglu, M. V. and G. I. Byrne 1998. Induction of macrophage foam cell formation by Chlamydia pneumoniae. *J Infect Dis* 1773: 725–9.

Kalayoglu, M. V., G. S. Miranpuri et al. 1999. Characterization of low-density lipoprotein uptake by murine macrophages exposed to Chlamydia pneumoniae. *Microbes Infect* 16: 409–18.

Kalayoglu, M. V., B. N. Perkins et al. 2001. Chlamydia pneumoniae-infected monocytes exhibit increased adherence to human aortic endothelial cells. *Microbes Infect* 312: 963–9.

Kaukoranta-Tolvanen, S. S., T. Ronni et al. 1996. Expression of adhesion molecules on endothelial cells stimulated by Chlamydia pneumoniae. *Microb Pathog* 215: 407–11.

Kooyenga, D. K., T. R. Watson et al. 2001. Antioxidants modulate the course of carotid atherosclerosis: A four-year report. Micronut Hlth. K. Nesaretnam and L. Packer (Eds.). Illinois, AOCS Press: 366–375.

Kumar, Y., J. Cocchiaro et al. 2006. The obligate intracellular pathogen Chlamydia trachomatis targets host lipid droplets. *Curr Biol* 1616: 1646–51.

Kuo, C. and L. A. Campbell. 2000. Detection of Chlamydia pneumoniae in arterial tissues. *J Infect Dis* 181 Suppl 3: S432–6.

Kuo, C. C., A. M. Gown et al. 1993. Detection of Chlamydia pneumoniae in aortic lesions of atherosclerosis by immunocytochemical stain. *Arterioscler Thromb* 1310: 1501–4.

Kuroda, Y. and Y. Hara 1999. Antimutagenic and anticarcinogenic activity of tea polyphenols. *Mutat Res* 4361: 69–97.

Lin, M. and Y. Rikihisa. 2003. Ehrlichia chaffeensis and Anaplasma phagocytophilum lack genes for lipid A biosynthesis and incorporate cholesterol for their survival. *Infect Immun* 719: 5324–31.

Lin, M. and Y. Rikihisa. 2003. Obligatory intracellular parasitism by Ehrlichia chaffeensis and Anaplasma phagocytophilum involves caveolae and glycosylphosphatidylinositol–anchored proteins. *Cell Microbiol* 511: 809–20.

Liuba, P., P. Karnani et al. 2000. Endothelial dysfunction after repeated Chlamydia pneumoniae infection in apolipoprotein E–knockout mice. *Circulation* 1029: 1039–44.

Lu, Y. E. and M. Kielian. 2000. Semliki forest virus budding: Assay, mechanisms and cholesterol requirement. *J Virol* 7417: 7708–19.

Lund, E. D., F. L. Chu et al. 2007. Perkinsus marinus, a protozoan parasite of the eastern oyster, has a requirement for dietary sterols. *Comp Biochem Physiol A Mol Integr Physiol* 1461: 141–7.

Malinverni, R., C. C. Kuo et al. 1995a. Reactivation of Chlamydia pneumoniae lung infection in mice by cortisone. *J Infect Dis* 1722: 593–4.

Malinverni, R., C. C. Kuo et al. 1995b. Effects of two antibiotic regimens on course and persistence of experimental Chlamydia pneumoniae TWAR pneumonitis. *Antimicrob Agents Chemother* 391: 45–9.

McIntyre, B. S., K. P. Briski et al. 2000. Antiproliferative and apoptotic effects of tocopherols and tocotrienols on normal mouse mammary epithelial cells. *Lipids* 352: 171–80.

Moazed, T. C., L. A. Campbell et al. 1999. Chlamydia pneumoniae infection accelerates the progression of atherosclerosis in apolipoprotein E-deficient mice. *J Infect Dis* 1801: 238–41.

Mpiga, P. and M. Ravaoarinoro. 2006. Chlamydia trachomatis persistence: An update. *Microbiol Res* 1611: 9–19.

Mueller, A. M., E. S. Stuart and B. Tan 2006. Vitamin E tocotrienols inhibition of intracellularly obligate pathogen Chlamydia and methods of use. U.S. Patent Office.

Naito, Y., M. Shimozawa et al. 2005. Tocotrienols reduce 25-hydroxycholesterol-induced monocyte-endothelial cell interaction by inhibiting the surface expression of adhesion molecules. *Atherosclerosis* 1801: 19–25.

Nakashima, Y., A. S. Plump et al. 1994. ApoE-deficient mice develop lesions of all phases of atherosclerosis throughout the arterial tree. *Arterioscler Thromb* 141: 133–40.

Newaz, M. A. and N. N. Nawal. 1999. Effect of gamma-tocotrienol on blood pressure, lipid peroxidation and total antioxidant status in spontaneously hypertensive rats SHR. *Clin Exp Hypertens* 218: 1297–313.

Newaz, M. A., Z. Yousefipour et al. 2003. Nitric oxide synthase activity in blood vessels of spontaneously hypertensive rats: Antioxidant protection by gamma-tocotrienol. *J Physiol Pharmacol* 543: 319–27.

Ngeh, J., V. Anand et al. 2002. Chlamydia pneumoniae and atherosclerosis––what we know and what we don't. *Clin Microbiol Infect* 81: 2–13.

Paavonen, J. and W. Eggert-Kruse. 1999. Chlamydia trachomatis: Impact on human reproduction. *Hum Reprod Update* 55: 433–47.

Paretsky, D., C. M. Downs et al. 1964. Some biochemical changes in the guinea pig during infection with *Coxiella burnetii*. *J Bacteriol* 88: 137–42.

Pearce, B. C., R. A. Parker et al. 1992. Hypocholesterolemic activity of synthetic and natural tocotrienols. *J Med Chem* 3520: 3595–606.

Pucadyil, T. J., P. Tewary et al. 2004. Cholesterol is required for *Leishmania donovani* infection: Implications in leishmaniasis. *Mol Biochem Parasitol* 1332: 145–52.

Qureshi, A. A., N. Qureshi et al. 1991. Dietary tocotrienols reduce concentrations of plasma cholesterol, apolipoprotein B, thromboxane B2 and platelet factor 4 in pigs with inherited hyperlipidemias. *Am J Clin Nutr* 534 Suppl: 1042S–1046S.

Qureshi, A. A., W. A. Salser et al. 2001. Novel tocotrienols of rice bran inhibit atherosclerotic lesions in C57BL/6 ApoE-deficient mice. *J Nutr* 13110: 2606–18.

Ramirez, J. A. 1996. Isolation of Chlamydia pneumoniae from the coronary artery of a patient with coronary atherosclerosis. The Chlamydia pneumoniae/Atherosclerosis Study Group. *Ann Intern Med* 12512: 979–82.

Rasool, A. H., K. H. Yuen et al. 2006. Dose dependent elevation of plasma tocotrienol levels and its effect on arterial compliance, plasma total antioxidant status and lipid profile in healthy humans supplemented with tocotrienol rich vitamin E. *J Nutr Sci Vitaminol Tokyo* 526: 473–8.

Razin, S. and J. G. Tully. 1970. Cholesterol requirement of mycoplasmas. *J Bacteriol* 1022: 306–10.

Reddick, R. L., S. H. Zhang et al. 1994. Atherosclerosis in mice lacking apo E: Evaluation of lesional development and progression. *Arterioscler Thromb* 141: 141–7.

Ross, R. 1999. Atherosclerosis—an inflammatory disease. *N Engl J Med* 3402: 115–26.

Saikku, P., M. Leinonen et al. 1988. Serological evidence of an association of a novel Chlamydia, TWAR, with chronic coronary heart disease and acute myocardial infarction. *Lancet* 28618: 983–6.

Sawayama, Y., M. Tatsukawa et al. 2007. Effect on carotid atherosclerosis of probucol plus levofloxacin for Chlamydia pneumoniae infection. *J Infect Chemother* 132: 92–8.

Sawayama, Y., M. Tatsukawa et al. 2003. Association of Chlamydia pneumoniae antibody with the cholesterol-lowering effect of statins. *Atherosclerosis* 1712: 281–5.

Schachter, J. 1999. Infection and disease epidemiology. In Chlamydia: Intracellular biology, pathogenesis and immunity. R. S. Stevens (Ed.) Washington D.C., ASM Press. I: 139–169.

Sehgal, A., S. Bettiol et al. 2005. Peculiarities of host cholesterol transport to the unique intracellular vacuole containing Toxoplasma. *Traffic* 612: 1125–41.

Shor, A., C. C. Kuo et al. 1992. Detection of Chlamydia pneumoniae in coronary arterial fatty streaks and atheromatous plaques. *S Afr Med J* 823: 158–61.

Silvie, O., S. Charrin et al. 2006. Cholesterol contributes to the organization of tetraspanin-enriched microdomains and to CD81-dependent infection by malaria sporozoites. *J Cell Sci* 119Pt 10: 1992–2002.

Song, B. L. and R. A. DeBose-Boyd 2006. Insig-dependent ubiquitination and degradation of 3-hydroxy-3-methylglutaryl coenzyme a reductase stimulated by delta- and gamma-tocotrienols. *J Biol Chem* 28135: 25054–61.

Sriram, S., C. W. Stratton et al. 1999. Chlamydia pneumoniae infection of the central nervous system in multiple sclerosis. *Ann Neurol* 461: 6–14.

Stiasny, K., C. Koessl et al. 2003. Involvement of lipids in different steps of the flavivirus fusion mechanism. *J Virol* 7714: 7856–62.

Stratton, C. W. and S. Sriram. 2003. Association of Chlamydia pneumoniae with central nervous system disease. *Microbes Infect* 513: 1249–53.

Stuart, A. D., H. E. Eustace et al. 2002. A novel cell entry pathway for a DAF: Using human enterovirus is dependent on lipid rafts. *J Virol* 7618: 9307–22.

Stuart, E. S., W. C. Webley et al. 2003. Lipid rafts, caveolae, caveolin-1 and entry by Chlamydiae into host cells. *Exp Cell Res* 2871: 67–78.

Summersgill, J. T., R. E. Molestina et al. 2000. Interactions of Chlamydia pneumoniae with human endothelial cells. *J Infect Dis* 181 Suppl 3: S479–82.

Tamai, R., Y. Asai et al. 2005. Requirement for intercellular adhesion molecule 1 and caveolae in invasion of human oral epithelial cells by Porphyromonas gingivalis. *Infect Immun* 7310: 6290–8.

Theriault, A., J. T. Chao et al. 2002. Tocotrienol is the most effective vitamin E for reducing endothelial expression of adhesion molecules and adhesion to monocytes. *Atherosclerosis* 1601: 21–30.

Thorp, E. B. and T. M. Gallagher. 2004. Requirements for CEACAMs and cholesterol during murine coronavirus cell entry. *J Virol* 786: 2682–92.

Thylefors, B., A. D. Negrel et al. 1995. Global data on blindness. *Bull World Health Organ* 731: 115–21.

Triantafilou, M., F. G. Gamper et al. 2007. Lipopolysaccharides from atherosclerosis-associated bacteria antagonize TLR4, induce formation of TLR2/1/CD36 complexes in lipid rafts and trigger TLR2-induced inflammatory responses in human vascular endothelial cells. *Cell Microbiol* 98: 2030–9.

Ward, M. E. and A. Murray. 1984. Control mechanisms governing the infectivity of Chlamydia trachomatis for HeLa cells: Mechanisms of endocytosis. *J Gen Microbiol* 1307: 1765–80.

Webley, W. C., P. S. Salva et al. 2005. The bronchial lavage of pediatric patients with asthma contains infectious Chlamydia. *Am J Respir Crit Care Med* 17110: 1083–8.

Yamaguchi, H., M. Yamada et al. 2004. Prevalence of viable Chlamydia pneumoniae in peripheral blood mononuclear cells of healthy blood donors. *Transfusion* 447: 1072–8.

Yamazaki, K., T. Honda et al. 2007. Relationship of periodontal infection to serum antibody levels to periodontopathic bacteria and inflammatory markers in periodontitis patients with coronary heart disease. *Clin Exp Immunol* 1493: 445–52.

Yamazaki, T., T. Kishimoto et al. 2005. Biosynthesized tea polyphenols inactivate Chlamydia trachomatis in vitro. *Antimicrob Agents Chemother* 496: 2501–3.

Yu, S. G., A. M. Thomas et al. 2006. Dose–response impact of various tocotrienols on serum lipid parameters in 5-week-old female chickens. *Lipids* 415: 453–61.

26 Tocotrienols as Natural Neuroprotective Vitamins

Chandan K. Sen, Savita Khanna and Sashwati Roy

CONTENTS

26.1 INTRODUCTION

Vitamin E is essential for normal neurological function (Muller and Goss-Sampson 1989; Muller and Goss-Sampson 1990). The following characteristics make the brain and neural cells highly susceptible to oxidative damage:

1. Contains high amounts of polyunsaturated (20:4 and 22:6) fatty acids that are susceptible to lipid peroxidation.
2. Receives a large percentage of oxygen.
3. Is relatively deficient in certain antioxidant enzymes.
4. Specific regions of the brain have high iron concentrations.

Thus, antioxidant defenses are critically important to protect the brain and neural tissues from oxidative damage. Indeed, numerous pathophysiological conditions have been associated with increased levels of oxidative stress indices (Lehtinen and Bonni 2006). Neuroprotection by antioxidants has therefore drawn much interest. The majority of available research on the role of antioxidant nutrients in neurological function and disease has focused on vitamin E. Vitamin E is the major lipid-soluble, chain-breaking antioxidant in the body, protecting the integrity of membranes by inhibiting lipid peroxidation. Mostly based on symptoms of primary vitamin E deficiency, it has been demonstrated that vitamin E has a central role in maintaining neurological structure and function (Muller and Goss-Sampson 1990). Most vitamin E-sensitive neurological disorders are associated with elevated levels of oxidative damage markers. During the last decade, this led to the popular hypothesis that the neuroprotective effects of vitamin E are mediated by its antioxidant property (Vatassery 1998).

The natural vitamin E family includes eight chemically distinct molecules: α-, β-, γ- and δ-tocopherol; and α-, β-, γ- and δ-tocotrienol. Tocochromanols contain a polar chromanol head group with a long isoprenoid side chain. Depending on the nature of the isoprenoid chain, tocopherols (containing a phytyl chain) or tocotrienols (geranylgeranyl chain) can be distinguished from each other (Dormann 2007). A striking asymmetry in our understanding of the eight-member natural vitamin E tocol family has deprived us of the full complement of benefits offered by the natural vitamin E molecules. Only approximately 1% of the entire literature on vitamin E addresses tocotrienols. A review of the NIH CRISP database shows that funding for tocotrienol research represents less than 1% of all vitamin E research during the last 30-plus years. Within the tocopherol literature, the non-α forms remain poorly studied (Dietrich et al. 2006; Hensley et al. 2004; O'Byrne et al. 2000). This represents a major void in vitamin E research. The significance of the void is substantially enhanced by the observation that the biological functions of the different homologues of natural vitamin E are not identical. During the last 5 years, tocotrienol research has gained substantial momentum. Well over two thirds of the entire PubMed literature on tocotrienols has been published on or after 2000. This represents a major swing in the overall direction of vitamin E research. The objective of this chapter is to highlight the potential significance of the tocotrienol half of the vitamin E family as a natural neuroprotective agent.

26.2 EIGHT FORMS OF NATURAL VITAMIN E: TOCOTRIENOLS AND TOCOPHEROLS ARE NOT REDUNDANT

All eight tocols in the natural vitamin E family share close structural homology and hence possess comparable antioxidant efficacy. Yet, current studies of the biological functions of vitamin E continue to indicate that members of the vitamin E family possess unique biological functions often not shared by other family members. One of the earliest observations suggesting that α-tocopherol may have functions independent of its antioxidant property came from the observation that α-tocopherol strongly inhibited platelet adhesion. The antiadhesive effect of α-tocopherol appeared to be related to a reduction in the number and size of pseudopodia upon platelet activation, a finding that led to the hypothesis that within the human body vitamin E may exert functions beyond its antioxidant property (Steiner 1993).

That members of the tocopherol family may have functions independent of their antioxidant properties gained more prominence when vitamin E molecules with comparable antioxidant properties exhibited contrasting biological effects (Boscoboinik et al. 1991). At the posttranslational level, α-tocopherol inhibits protein kinase C, 5-lipoxygenase and phospholipase A2 and activates protein phosphatase 2A and diacylglycerol kinase. Some genes (e.g., scavenger receptors, α-tocopherol transfer protein, α-tropomyosin, matrix metalloproteinase-19 and collagenase) are specifically modulated by α-tocopherol at the transcriptional level. α-Tocopherol also inhibits cell proliferation, platelet aggregation and monocyte adhesion. These effects have been characterized to be unrelated to the antioxidant activity of vitamin E and possibly reflect specific interactions of α-tocopherol with enzymes, structural proteins, lipids and transcription factors (Zingg and Azzi 2004).

γ-Tocopherol represents the major form of vitamin E in the diet in the USA, but not in Europe. Desmethyl tocopherols, such as γ-tocopherol and specific tocopherol metabolites, most notably the carboxyethyl-hydroxychroman (CEHC) products, exhibit functions that are not shared by α-tocopherol. The activities of these other tocopherols do not map directly to their chemical antioxidant behavior but rather reflect anti-inflammatory, antineoplastic and natriuretic functions possibly mediated through specific binding interactions (Hensley et al. 2004). Metabolites of γ-tocopherol (2,7,8-trimethyl-2-(β-carboxyethyl)-6-hydroxychroman), but not that of α-tocopherol, provides natriuretic activity. Moreover, a nascent body of epidemiological data suggests that γ-tocopherol is a better negative risk factor for certain types of cancer and myocardial infarction than is α-tocopherol (Wagner et al. 2004).

Structurally, tocotrienols differ from tocopherols by the presence of three *trans* double bonds in the hydrocarbon tail. Because of these unsaturations in the isoprenoid side chain, tocotrienols are thought to assume a unique conformation. Indeed, α-tocotrienol possesses numerous functions that are not shared by α-tocopherol (Sen et al. 2006). For example, nanomolar concentrations of α-tocotrienol uniquely prevent inducible neurodegeneration by regulating specific mediators of cell death (Khanna, Roy, Parinandi et al. 2006; Khanna, Roy, Ryu et al. 2003; Sen et al. 2000). Oral supplementation of tocotrienol protects against stroke (Khanna, Roy, Slivka et al. 2005b). Micromolar amounts of tocotrienol suppress the activity of 3-hydroxy-3-methylglutaryl coenzyme A (HMG-CoA) reductase, the hepatic enzyme responsible for cholesterol synthesis (Pearce et al. 1994; Pearce et al. 1992). Tocopherols do not share the cholesterol-lowering properties of tocotrienol (Qureshi, Burger et al. 1986; Qureshi, Sami et al. 2002). Sterol-regulated ubiquitination marks HMG-CoA reductase for endoplasmic reticulum (ER)-associated degradation by 26S proteasomes. This degradation, which results from sterol-induced binding of reductase to ER membrane proteins called Insigs, contributes to the complex multivalent feedback regulation of the enzyme. Recently, it has been demonstrated that δ-tocotrienol stimulates ubiquitination and degradation of reductase and blocks processing of sterol regulatory element-binding proteins (SREBPs), another sterol-mediated action of Insigs. The γ-tocotrienol analog is more selective in enhancing reductase ubiquitination and degradation than blocking SREBP processing. Other forms of vitamin E neither accelerate reductase degradation nor block SREBP processing (Song and DeBose-Boyd 2006).

Tocotrienol, not tocopherol, administration reduces oxidative protein damage and extends the mean life span of *C. elegans* (Adachi and Ishii 2000). Tocotrienols are thought to have more potent antioxidant properties than α-tocopherol (Serbinova et al. 1991; Serbinova and Packer 1994). Reportedly, the unsaturated side chain of tocotrienol allows for more efficient penetration into tissues that have saturated fatty layers such as the brain and liver (Suzuki et al. 1993). Experimental research examining the antioxidant free radical scavenging effects of tocopherol and tocotrienols revealed that tocotrienols appear superior due to their better distribution in the fatty layers of the cell membrane (Suzuki et al. 1993). Furthermore, tocotrienol, but not tocopherol, suppresses growth of human breast cancer cells (Nesaretnam et al. 1995).

26.3 TOCOTRIENOL: THE SEED FORM OF NATURAL VITAMIN E

Tocotrienols are the primary form of vitamin E in the seed endosperm of most monocots, including agronomically important cereal grains such as wheat, rice and barley. Palm oil contains significant quantities of tocotrienol (Sundram et al. 2003). Tocotrienols are also found in the seed endosperm of a limited number of dicots, including *Apiaceae* species and certain *Solanaeceae* species, such as tobacco. These molecules are found only rarely in vegetative tissues of plants. Crude palm oil extracted from the fruits of *Elaeis guineensis* particularly contains a high amount of tocotrienols (up to 800 mg/kg), mainly consisting of γ-tocotrienol and α-tocotrienol. Compared to tocopherols, tocotrienols are considerably less widespread in the plant kingdom (Horvath et al. 2006). In 80 different plant species studied, 24 were found to contain significant amounts of tocotrienols. No taxonomic relation was apparent among the 16 dicotyledonous species that were found to contain tocotrienol. The eight monocotyledonous species belonged either to the *Poaceae* (six species) or the *Aracaceae* (two species). A more detailed analysis of tocotrienol accumulation revealed the presence of this natural vitamin E in several non-photosynthetic tissues and organs, i.e., seeds, fruits and in latex. No tocotrienols could be detected in mature photosynthetic tissues. Transient accumulation of low levels of tocotrienols is found in the young coleoptiles of plant species whose seeds contained tocotrienols. No measurable tocotrienol biosynthesis was apparent in coleoptiles, or in chloroplasts isolated from coleoptiles. Tocotrienol accumulation in coleoptiles was not associated with chloroplasts. Tocotrienols seem to be transiently present in photosynthetically active tissues; however, it remains to be proven whether they are biosynthesized in such tissues or imported from elsewhere in the plant (Horvath et al. 2006).

In contrast to tocotrienols, tocopherols occur ubiquitously in plant tissues and are the exclusive form of vitamin E in leaves of plants and seeds of most monocot plants. Transgenic expression of the barley HGGT (homogentisic acid transferase, which catalyzes the committed step of tocotrienol biosynthesis) in *Arabidopsis thaliana* leaves resulted in accumulation of tocotrienols, which were absent from leaves of non-transformed plants and a ten- to fifteenfold increase in total vitamin E antioxidants (tocotrienols plus tocopherols). Overexpression of the barley HGGT in corn seeds increased tocotrienol and tocopherol content by as much as sixfold. These results provide insight into the genetic basis for tocotrienol biosynthesis in plants and demonstrate the ability to enhance the antioxidant content of crops by introduction of an enzyme that redirects metabolic flux (Cahoon et al. 2003).

More recently, another strategy involving genetic engineering of metabolic pathways in plants has proven to be efficient in bolstering tocotrienol biosynthesis (Rippert et al. 2004). In plants, phenylalanine is the precursor of a myriad of secondary compounds termed phenylpropanoids. In contrast, much less carbon is incorporated into tyrosine that provides p-hydroxyphenylpyruvate and homogentisate, the aromatic precursors of vitamin E. The flux of these two compounds has been upregulated by deriving their synthesis directly at the level of prephenate. This was achieved by the expression of the yeast prephenate dehydrogenase gene in tobacco plants that already overexpress the *Arabidopsis* p-hydroxyphenylpyruvate dioxygenase coding sequence. Massive accumulation of tocotrienols was observed in leaves. These molecules, which were undetectable in wild-type leaves, became the major forms of vitamin E in the leaves of the transgenic lines. An increased resistance of the transgenic plants toward the herbicidal p-hydroxyphenylpyruvate dioxygenase inhibitor diketonitril was also observed. Thus, the synthesis of p-hydroxyphenylpyruvate is a limiting step for the accumulation of vitamin E in plants (Rippert et al. 2004).

Palm oil represents one of the most abundant natural sources of tocotrienols (Elson 1992). The distribution of vitamin E in palm oil is 30% tocopherols and 70% tocotrienols (Sundram et al. 2003). The oil palm (Elaeis guineensis) is native to many West African countries, where local populations have used its oil for culinary and other purposes. Large-scale plantations, established principally in tropical regions of Asia, Africa and Latin America, are mostly aimed at the production of oil (Solomons and Orozco 2003), which is extracted from the fleshy mesocarp of the palm fruit and endosperm or kernel oil. Palm oil is different from other plant and animal oils in that it contains 50% saturated fatty acids, 40% unsaturated fatty acids and 10% polyunsaturated fatty acids. Because of its high saturated fat content, palm oil has not been very popular in the United States. Hydrogenated fats contain high levels of trans-fatty acids, which are now thought to have adverse health effects. The US Food and Drug Administration's final ruling on trans-fatty acid labeling issued in 2003 has caused a rapid transformation in the fat and oil industries (Tarrago-Trani et al. 2006). Palm oil is free of trans-fatty acid and is rapidly gaining wider acceptance by the food industry in the country. Primary applications include bakery products, breakfast cereals, wafers and candies.

Rice bran oil, a by-product of the rice milling industry, is a major natural source of γ-tocotrienol but a poor source of α-tocotrienol. In addition, rice bran oil provides desmethyl tocotrienols. Two novel tocotrienols, apart from the known α-, β-, γ- and δ-tocopherols and tocotrienols, were isolated from stabilized and heated rice bran. These new tocotrienols are known as desmethyl tocotrienol [3, 4-dihydro-2-methyl-2-(4,8,12-trimethyltrideca-3'(E),7'(E), 11'-trienyl)-2H-1-benzopyran-6-ol] and didesmethy tocotrienol [3, 4-dihydro-2-(4,8,12-trimethyltrideca-3'(E),7'(E), 11'-trienyl)-2H-1-benzopyran-6-ol] (Qureshi, Mo et al. 2000). Although scientific evidence is relatively limited, rice bran oil is believed to be a healthy vegetable oil in Asian countries (Sugano et al. 1999).

Cereals such as oat, rye and barley contain small amounts of tocotrienol. α-Tocotrienol is the predominant form of tocotrienol in oat (*Avena sativa L.*) and barley (56 and 40 mg/kg of dry weight, respectively). β-Tocotrienol is the major form of tocotrienol found in hulled and dehulled wheats (from 33 to 43 mg/kg of dry weight) (Panfili et al. 2003). Steaming and flaking of dehulled oat groats results in moderate losses of tocotrienols but not of tocopherols (Bryngelsson et al. 2002). Although tocotrienols are present in edible natural products, it is questionable whether these dietary sources could provide sufficient amounts of tocotrienol to humans. For example, the processing of 1000 kg of crude palm oil is necessary to derive 1 kg of the commercial product Tocomin 50% (Carotech,

NJ). Roughly, one would have to consume 100–200g of palm/rice-bran oil or 1.5–4 kg of wheat-germ, barley or oat to achieve doses that have been published to be effective biologically. With this consideration in mind, appropriately configured dietary supplements seem to be a prudent choice.

26.4 ORAL SUPPLEMENTATION AND TISSUE DELIVERY

During the last two decades, efforts to understand how dietary vitamin E is transported to the tissues have focused on α-tocopherol transport (Blatt et al. 2001; Kaempf-Rotzoll et al. 2003; Traber and Arai 1999; Traber et al. 2004). α-Tocopherol transfer protein (TTP) has been identified to mediate α-tocopherol secretion into the plasma while other tocopherol-binding proteins seem to play a less important role (Kaempf-Rotzoll et al. 2003). Tocotrienols have been known for decades but why have they not been studied as well as α-tocopherol? Although there does not seem to be a straightforward rational answer to this question, one contributing factor is whether tocotrienol taken orally reaches vital organs of the body. This concern was primarily based on a 1997 finding that the transport system, TTP, responsible for carrying α-tocopherol to vital organs has a poorer efficiency to transport tocotrienols to tissues (Hosomi et al. 1997). The lack of relative specific affinity of TTP for tocotrienols led to the urban legend that availability of dietary tocotrienol to vital organs is negligible.

Although TTP is known to bind to α-tocotrienol with 8.5-fold lower affinity than that for α-tocopherol (Hosomi et al. 1997), it has not been clear whether, or to what extent, the delivery of orally supplemented α-tocotrienol to vital organs is dependent on TTP. Previously, it has been reported that TTP-deficient females are infertile presumably because of vitamin E deficiency (Terasawa et al. 2000). This important observation was confirmed in a lineage of TTP-deficient mice. Placentas of pregnant TTP-deficient females were severely impaired with marked reduction of labyrinthine trophoblasts, and the embryos died at mid-gestation even when fertilized eggs of TTP-containing wild-type mice were transferred into TTP-deficient recipients (Jishage et al. 2001). Even in the presence of dietary α-tocopherol, TTP knock-out mice are known to suffer from α-tocopherol deficiency (Jishage et al. 2001; Terasawa et al. 2000). Recently it has been noted that oral supplementation of female mice with α-tocotrienol restored fertility of TTP knock-out mice suggesting that tocotrienol was successfully delivered to the relevant tissues and that tocotrienol supported reproductive function under conditions of α–tocopherol deficiency (Khanna, Patel et al. 2005a). This observation was consistent with another line of evidence from rats where tocotrienol supplementation spared loss of fertility caused by long-term vitamin E deficiency in the diet (Khanna, Patel et al. 2005a).

TTP continues to be a key transport mechanism for the deliver of α-tocopherol to tissues. The significance of TTP in the transport of other forms of vitamin E remains unclear at present. It is clear, however, that natural isomers of vitamin E do get transported to vital organs even in the absence of TTP. Identification and characterization of TTP-independent vitamin E transport mechanisms *in vivo* is warranted.

Current findings support that oral tocotrienol (Carotech Inc., NJ) not only reaches the brain (Khanna, Patel et al. 2005a; Khanna, Roy et al. 2005b; Roy et al. 2002) but it does so in amounts sufficient to protect against stroke (Khanna, Roy et al. 2005b). The standard laboratory chow contains excessive amounts of α-tocopherol (Khosla et al. 2006; van der Worp et al. 1998) but negligible amounts of tocotrienol. Long-term lack of tocotrienol in the diet may repress any putative tocotrienol transport mechanism *in vivo*. Thus, long-term supplementation studies are needed. In light of the knowledge that natural analogs of vitamin E may compete for specific transporting mechanisms (Hosomi et al. 1997), it is important that tocotrienol supplementation be performed under conditions of minimized co-presence of tocopherols. Another related consideration is that although incorporation of orally supplemented vitamin E into tissues is a slow and progressive process, rapid incorporation of the supplement into tissues of newborns may occur in response to gavaging of pregnant mother rats (Roy et al. 2002). Thus, an experimental design incorporating long-term tocotrienol supplementation under conditions of minimal dietary co-presence of tocopherols and breeding of the supplemented colony would be a valuable approach to generate proof of principle testing whether dietary α–tocotrienol is capable of being transported to vital organs *in vivo*.

In a recent study, rats were maintained on a vitamin E-deficient diet and gavaged with α-tocotrienol alone, α-tocopherol alone or in combination. Five generations of rats were studied over 60 weeks (Khanna et al. 2005a). Skin, adipose, heart, lungs, skeletal muscle brain, spinal cord, liver and blood were studied. Oral tocotrienol was delivered to all vital organs. In some tissues, the level of tocotrienol exceeded that of tocopherols, indicating the presence of an efficient tocotrienol transport system *in vivo*. Baseline levels of α–tocotrienol in the skin of tocopherol-fed rats that never received any tocotrienol supplementation were negligible. Orally supplemented tocotrienol was rapidly taken up by the skin. Already in second generation rats, α-tocotrienol levels in the skin of tocotrienol supplemented rats exceeded twice the α-tocopherol levels in that organ. Of note, the α-tocotrienol level in the skin matched the α-tocotrienol level in the skin of rats fed with a comparable amount of tocopherol. When tocotrienol and tocopherol were co-supplemented, the uptake of α-tocotrienol by the skin was clearly blunted. In this group, α-tocotrienol levels were lower than α-tocotrienol levels in the skin, suggesting a direct competition between orally taken tocotrienol and tocopherol for delivery to the skin. Longer supplementation resulted in a marked increase in the α-tocotrienol levels in the skin of tocotrienol-fed rats indicating a build-up of α-tocotrienol over time. Interestingly, the levels of α-tocotrienol in the skin of these rats were folds higher than that in the skin of tocopherol-fed rats. This observation suggests the presence of an effective transport mechanism delivering α–tocotrienol to the skin and efficient retention of α-tocotrienol in the skin over time. Co-supplementation of tocotrienol and tocopherol demonstrated favorable uptake of α–tocopherol over α–tocotrienol. Adipose tissue serves as storage organ for vitamin E (Adachi et al. 1990). Analysis of adipose tissue vitamin E content of fifth-generation rats revealed substantially more accumulation of α-tocotrienol in that tissue than α-tocopherol.

In the case of tocotrienol as well as of tocopherol feeding, results from third- and fifth-generation rats indicate higher levels of vitamin E in the skin of female compared with that of male rats. This gender-specific effect suggesting better transport of tocotrienol in females than in males was noted as a general trend across all organs studied. Gender-based differences in the transport of dietary vitamins are known to exist in specific cases (Garry et al. 1987). Although the effect of several physiological factors on vitamin E transport has been studied, the gender factor remains to be specifically addressed (Lodge et al. 2004). It has been demonstrated that γ-tocopherol is more rapidly metabolized in women than in men (Leonard et al. 2005). The level of α-tocotrienol in the ovary was over fivefold higher than that in the testes from the corresponding males rats (Khanna et al. 2005a). In the ovary, tocopherol is known to accumulate via a lipoprotein receptor dependent mechanism (Aten et al. 1994). Whether tocotrienol shares that mechanism remain to be tested.

Vitamin E enters the circulation from the intestine in chylomicrons. The conversion of chylomicrons to remnant particles results in the distribution of newly absorbed vitamin E to all of the circulating lipoproteins and ultimately to tissues. This enrichment of lipoproteins with vitamin E is a key mechanism by which vitamin E is delivered to tissues (Traber et al. 2004). In the liver, newly absorbed dietary lipids are incorporated into nascent very low density lipoproteins. The liver is responsible for the control and release of α-tocopherol into blood plasma. In the absence of TTP, α-tocopherol is not secreted back into the plasma. Excess vitamin E is not accumulated in the liver, but is excreted, mostly in bile (Traber et al. 2004). It has been noted that α-tocotrienol levels in the liver of rats and of TTP-deficient mice was much lower than the levels of this vitamin E isoform in most peripheral tissues studied (Khanna, Patel et al. 2005a). Such observation argues against a central role of the liver in delivering oral α-tocotrienol to peripheral tissues.

TTP has the ability to bind to both α-tocopherol as well as α-tocotrienol. The affinity to bind α-tocopherol is several-fold higher than that for α-tocotrienol (Hosomi et al. 1997). Thus, under conditions of coexistence, α-tocopherol is expected to out-compete α-tocotrienol for binding. Although studies with the TTP-deficient mice (Khanna et al. 2005a) indicate the existence of a TTP-independent mechanisms for the tissue delivery of oral α-tocotrienol, observations in the rat (Khanna et al. 2005a) indicate that the mechanisms for transporting α-tocopherol and α-tocotrienol seem to compete such that transport of α-tocopherol is favored. Thus, co-supplementation of α-tocopherol and α-tocotrienol is likely to compromise tissue delivery of α-tocotrienol (Khanna et al. 2005a).

Few studies have specifically looked at the fate of oral tocotrienol supplementation in humans. In a study investigating the pharmacokinetics and bioavailability of α-, γ- and δ-tocotrienols under fed and fasted conditions in eight healthy volunteers, subjects were administered a single 300 mg oral dose of mixed tocotrienols under fed or fasted conditions. The peak concentration of α-tocotrienol in the blood plasma was just over 1μM (Yap et al. 2001). The fed state increased the onset as well as the extent of absorption of tocotrienols by more than twofold. In addition, the mean apparent elimination half-life of α-, γ- and δ-tocotrienols was estimated to be 4.4, 4.3 and 2.3 h, respectively, being between 4.5- to 8.7-fold shorter than that reported for α-tocopherol (Yap et al. 2001).

In another study, human subjects took tocotrienyl acetate supplements (250 mg/d) for 8 weeks while on a low-fat diet. In response to supplementation, the concentrations of tocotrienol in the mean blood plasma were as follows: α-tocotrienol, 0.98 μM; γ-tocotrienol, 0.54 μM; and δ-tocotrienol 0.09 μM (O'Byrne et al. 2000). Thus, tocotrienyl acetate supplements were observed to be hydrolyzed, absorbed and detectable in human plasma. A novel formulation for improved absorption of tocotrienols has been developed (Ho et al. 2003). Emulsions are known to increase absorption of fat-soluble drugs. This invention is based on SEDDS (self-emulsifying drug delivery systems) technology (Araya et al. 2006; Gao and Morozowich 2006; Hong et al. 2006). Soft gelatin capsules (Tocovid Suprabio™, Carotech Inc., NJ) containing tocotrienol have been produced. Once ingested, the tocotrienols form emulsion when the contents are released and mixed with human gastrointestinal fluid. In a recent study using Tocovid Suprabio™ the post-absorptive fate of tocotrienol isomers and their association with lipoprotein subfractions was examined in humans (Khosla et al. 2006). The peak α-tocotrienol concentrations in supplemented individuals averaged approximately 3 microM in blood plasma, 1.7 microM in LDL, 0.9 microM in triglyceride-rich lipoprotein and 0.5 microM in HDL. This peak plasma concentration of α-tocotrienol is 2-3 times more than the peak concentration reported in previous studies using generic supplements not based on SEDDS (O'Byrne et al. 2000; Yap et al. 2001).

26.5 DEFENDING NEURAL CELLS AND THE NERVOUS SYSTEM

On a concentration basis, the neuroprotective effects of nM tocotrienol represent the most potent biological function of all natural forms of vitamin E. Glutamate-toxicity is a major contributor to neurodegeneration. It includes excitotoxicity and an oxidative stress component also known as oxytosis (Schubert and Piasecki 2001; Tan et al. 2001). Murine HT hippocampal neuronal cells, lacking an intrinsic excitotoxicity-pathway, have been used as a standard model to characterize the oxidant-dependent component of glutamate toxicity.

In 1999, we conducted a side-by-side comparison of all eight forms of natural vitamin E in a model of glutamate-induced neurodegeneration of HT neural cells. In subsequent experiments, it was observed that the neuroprotective property of tocotrienol applies not only to neural cell lines but also to primary cortical neurons. This line of experimentation led to an observation that eventually turned out to be the most potent function of any natural form of vitamin E on a concentration basis reported. Until then, all biological functions of vitamin E studied *in vitro* were observed at micromolar concentration. Our studies led to the first evidence that α-tocotrienol was the most potent neuroprotective form of vitamin E in glutamate-induced degeneration of HT4 (Figure 26.1) hippocampal neural cells (Sen et al. 2000). What was striking in this study was the observation that nanomolar concentrations of α-tocotrienol, not α-tocopherol, provide complete neuroprotection. At such low dose, tocotrienol was not protective against direct oxidant insult, suggesting that the observed neuroprotective effect of nanomolar tocotrienol was not dependent on the widely known antioxidant property of vitamin E.

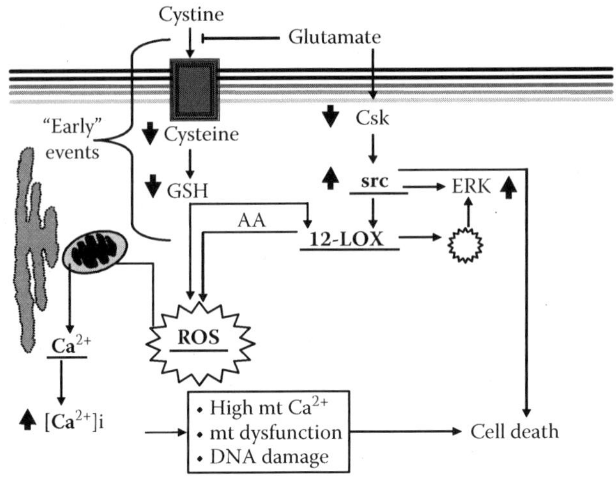

FIGURE 26.1 Sequence of events in glutamate-induced death of HT4 neural cells. ↑, activation/increase; ↓, inhibition/ decrease. Death mediators, inhibition of which has been found to rescue from death are underscored. In HT4 cells lacking the excitotoxicity pathway, high glutamate inhibits cystine entry and therefore cysteine availability within the cell. Low [cysteine]i limits GSH synthesis. Lowered [GSH]i impairs antioxidant defenses and also triggers 12-LOX (lipoxygenase) activation. Both of the above events lead to oxidant (ROS, reactive oxygen species) accumulation. Increased [ROS]i is associated with elevated $[Ca^{2+}]i$. Cytosolic Ca^{2+} enters mitochondria resulting in MPT, water entry and mitochondrial swelling. Eventually, mitochondrial outer membrane disintegrates. Rapid activation of c-Src is another key response to elevated glutamate. c-Src phosphorylates 12-Lox which migratesto the membrane.

That tocotrienol-dependent neuroprotection includes a significant antioxidant-independent mechanism has been now established (Khanna et al. 2006). The neuroprotective property of tocotrienol holds good not only in response to glutamate challenge but also in response to other insults such as homocysteic acid, glutathione deficiency and linoleic acid-induced oxidative stress (Khanna, Roy, Parinandi et al. 2006; Sen et al. 2000). It is now evident that at micromolar concentrations tocotrienol protects neural cells by virtue of its antioxidant property. At nanomolar concentrations, however, tocotrienol regulates specific neurodegenerative signaling processes.

The major tocotrienol-sensitive signaling pathways that are known to be involved in glutamate-induced neurodegeneration include c-Src and 12-lipoxygenase (Khanna, Roy, Parinandi et al. 2006; Khanna, Roy, Ryu et al. 2003; Khanna, Roy, Slivka et al. 2005b; Sen, Khanna and Roy 2004; Sen, Khanna, Roy et al. 2000). In our initial search for signaling pathways that are sensitive to tocotrienol and play a decisive role in neurodegeneration we were led to c-Src kinase (Sen, Khanna, Roy et al. 2000). c-Src and the structurally related members of the Src family are non-receptor tyrosine kinases that reside within the cell associated with cell membranes and appear to transduce signals from transmembrane receptors to the cell interior. SH2 and SH3 domains are known to play a central role in regulating the catalytic activity of src protein tyrosine kinase. High-resolution crystal structures of human Src, in their repressed state, have provided a structural explanation for how intramolecular interactions of the SH3 and SH2 domains stabilize the inactive conformation of Src (Thomas and Brugge 1997).

Our hypothesis that tocotrienol prevents neurodegeneration by regulating specific signaling processes involved in neurotoxicity led to screening for potential tocotrienol-sensitive candidate death pathways in HT4 cells. During such screening studies, inhibitors of the protein tyrosine kinase activity completely prevented glutamate-induced cell death. Herbimycin and geldanamycin potently inhibit c-Src tyrosine kinase activity (Hall et al. 1994; Yoneda et al. 1993) whereas lavendustin A is an inhibitor of extracellular growth factor receptor protein tyrosine kinase activity (Hsu et al. 1991). The observation that herbimycin and geldanamycin, but not lavendustin A prevented glutamate-induced death of HT4 neuronal cells hinted the involvement of c-Src kinase activity in the death pathway. Immunoprecipitation of tyrosine phosphorylated protein from cellular extracts confirmed that protein tyrosine phosphorylation reactions were indeed triggered by exposure of cells to elevated levels of glutamate and that such reactions were inhibited by nanomolar concentrations of α-tocotrienol (Sen, Khanna, Roy et al. 2000). These results, however, did not provide any information regarding the specific kinases involved.

The involvement of c-Src kinase activity in the death pathway was verified by experiments involving the overexpression of catalytically active or inactive Src kinase. Indeed, overexpression of catalytically active Src-kinase markedly sensitized the cells to HT4 induced death. Tocotrienol treatment completely prevented glutamate-induced death even in active c-Src kinase overexpressing cells, indicating that it either inhibited c-Src kinase activity or regulated one or more events upstream of c-Src kinase activation. Further evidence supporting this contention was provided by results obtained from the determination of c-Src kinase activity in HT4 cells. Glutamate treatment resulted in marked enhancement of c-Src kinase activity and this change was completely blocked in cells treated with nanomolar amounts of α-tocotrienol.

Further evidence establishing that signal transduction processes related to the cell death pathway are involved in glutamate-induced cytotoxicity was obtained from the study of ERK1 and ERK2 activation. Mitogen-activated/extracellular response kinase kinase (MEK) kinase (MEKK) is a serine-threonine kinase that regulates sequential protein phosphorylation pathways, leading to the activation of mitogen- activated protein kinases (MAPK), including members of the extracellular signal-regulated kinases (ERKs). MEKK selectively regulates signal transduction pathways that contribute to the apoptotic response (Johnson et al. 1996). When activated, p44 and p42 MAPK (ERK1 and ERK2) are phosphorylated at specific threonine and tyrosine residues. ERK has been implicated in mediating the signaling events that precede apoptosis. ERK2 plays an active role in mediating anti-IgM-induced apoptosis of B cells (Lee and Koretzky 1998). It has been also shown that H_2O_2 induces the activation of multiple MAPKs in oligodendrocyte progenitors and that the activation of ERK is associated with oxidant- mediated cytotoxicity (Bhat and Zhang 1999). Our studies showed that ERK1 and 2 are sensitive to elevated levels of extracellular glutamate. Rapid activation of ERK, particularly ERK2, was observed in response to glutamate treatment. Such response of ERK was completely inhibited in cells treated with α-tocotrienol suggesting that α-tocotrienol influences an early event in the glutamate-induced death pathway (Sen, Khanna, Roy et al. 2000). In some cases Src kinase activity is known to be required for the activation of ERK (Aikawa et al. 1997). Thus, it is likely tocotrienol inhibits inducible ERK activation by down-regulating Src kinase activity (Sen, Khanna, Roy et al. 2000).

c-Src is heavily expressed in the brain (Soriano et al. 1991) and in human neural tissues (Pyper and Bolen 1989). Differentiating rodent neurons are known to express high levels of c-Src. In neurons and astrocytes, c-Src is present at 15–20 times higher levels than that found in fibroblasts. The specific activity of the c-Src protein from neuronal cultures is 6–12 times higher than that from the astrocyte cultures suggesting a key function of this protein in neurons (Brugge et al. 1985). Initially, c-Src was identified as being important in growth cone-mediated neurite extension and synaptic plasticity (Maness et al. 1988) and in neuronal differentiation (Ingraham et al. 1989). Targeted disruption of c-Src, however, did not cause any abnormality in the brain (Soriano et al. 1991).

Our pursuit for the neuroprotective mechanisms of tocotrienols led to the first evidence demonstrating that rapid c-Src activation (Khanna et al. 2002; Sen, Khanna, Roy et al. 2000) plays a central role in executing neurodegeneration. Consistently, it was demonstrated in a subsequent report that Src deficiency or blockade of Src activity in mice provides cerebral protection following stroke (Paul et al. 2001). Further support of our claim that c-Src is a key player in neurodegeneration is provided by observation that the Src family kinase-inhibitor PP2 reduces focal ischemic brain injury (Lennmyr et al. 2004). Our observation that tocotrienol-dependent inhibition of c-Src is beneficial for neuroprotection has now been extended to the heart. A later study showed that c-Src mediates post-ischemic cardiac injury and dysfunction. Tocotrienol supplementation inhibited c-Src activation and protected the heart (Das et al. 2005). Many intracellular pathways can be stimulated upon Src activation and a variety of cellular consequences can result. High c-Src is tightly associated with carcinogenesis. c-Src inhibitors are being actively studied for cancer therapy (Alper and Bowden 2005; Ishizawar and Parsons 2004; Lau 2005; Shupnik 2004). Based on the inducible c-Src inhibitory properties of tocotrienol one may postulate that tocotrienol has anticancer properties. The anti-cancer properties of tocotrienol are discussed in another section.

GSH, the major cellular thiol present in mammalian cells, is critical for maintenance of redox homeostasis (Sun et al. 2006). GSH is a key survival factor in cells of the nervous system and lowered [GSH]i is one of the early markers of neurotoxicity induced by a variety of agonists (Bains and Shaw 1997; Dringen et al. 2000). We observed that α-tocotrienol clearly protects primary cortical neurons against a number of GSH-lowering neurotoxins (Khanna, Roy, Ryu et al. 2003). Of interest, the neurons survived even in the face of GSH loss. These observations led to the hypothesis that loss of [GSH]i alone is not lethal (Khanna, Roy, Ryu et al. 2003). Given that pro-GSH agents are known to be neuroprotective in a variety of scenarios (Bains and Shaw 1997; Han et al. 1997; Schulz et al. 2000) it becomes reasonable to hypothesize that glutamate-induced lowering of [GSH]i triggers downstream responses that execute cell death.

Our works led to the identification of 12-lipoxygenase (12-Lox) as a key tocotrienol-sensitive mediator of neurodegeneration (Khanna, Roy, Ryu et al. 2003). Specific inhibition of 12-Lox by BL15 protected neurons from glutamate-induced degeneration although [GSH]i is compromised by 80%. Similar protective effects of BL15 were noted when BSO, a specific inhibitor of GSH synthesis, was used as the agonist. Importantly, neurons isolated from mice lacking the 12-lipoxygenase gene were observed to be resistant to glutamate-induced loss of viability (Khanna et al. 2003). This key piece of evidence established that indeed 12-Lox represents a critical checkpoint in glutamate-induced neurodegeneration.

Understanding of the intracellular regulation of 12-lipoxygenase requires knowledge of the distribution of both enzyme protein and its activity. For example, in human erythroleukemia cells, the membrane fraction contains about 90% of the total cellular 12-Lox activity, whereas only 10% of 12-Lox activity resides in the cytosol. However, the majority of cellular 12-Lox protein is found in the cytosol (Hagmann et al. 1993). Upon activation, 12-Lox may translocate to the membrane (Hagmann et al. 1993). Consistently, we have observed the decreased presence of 12-Lox in the cytosol and increased presence in the membrane of glutamate-treated cells. For 5-lipoxygenase, both catalytic function and translocation of the enzyme from the cytosol to the membrane are known to be regulated by tyrosine kinases (Lepley et al. 1996). We have noted that 12-Lox is subject to rapid tyrosine phosphorylation in neuronal cells challenged with glutamate or GSH-lowering agents. Such rapid phosphorylation coincides with the timeline of c-Src activation (Khanna, Roy, Slivka et al. 2005b). Inhibitors of c-Src abrogated inducible 12-Lox tyrosine phosphorylation supporting the notion that c-Src may directly phosphorylate 12-Lox in challenged neurons. To test this hypothesis we utilized genetic approaches of overexpressing kinase-active, kinase-dead or dominant negative c-Src in neuronal cells. Findings from cell biology studies as well as from the study of c-Src and 12-Lox in cell-free systems indicate that in response to challenge by glutamate or GSH-lowering agents, c-Src is rapidly activated and phosphorylates 12-Lox.(Khanna, Roy, Slivka et al. 2005b).

Neurons and the brain are rich in arachidonic acid (AA; 20:4ω-6). Massive amounts of AA are released from the membranes in response to brain ischemia or trauma (Bazan 1976, 1970, 1971a, 1971b; Bazan and Rakowski 1970). Subsequent work has established that AA and its metabolites may be neurotoxic. There are three major pathways of AA metabolism: lipoxygenases, cycloxygenases and cytochrome P450. The cycloxygenase pathway has been preliminarily ruled out from being a contributor to neurodegeneration (Kwon et al. 2005). In the lipoxygenase pathway, metabolites of 12-Lox seem to be the major metabolite of arachidonic acid in the brain (Adesuyi et al. 1985; Carlen et al. 1994) as well as in cultured cortical neurons (Ishizaki and Murota 1991; Miyamoto et al. 1987a, 1987b). Lipoxygenases, mainly 5-, 12- and 15-Lox, are named for their ability to insert molecular oxygen at the 5, 12, or 15-carbon atom of arachidonic acid forming a distinct hydroperoxy-eicosatetraenoic (HPETE) acid (Yamamoto 1992). 12-Lox produces 12(S)-HPETE which is further metabolized into four distinct products: an alcohol [12(S)-HETE], a ketone (12-keto-eicosatetraenoic acid), or two epoxy alcohols (hepoxilin A3 and B3).

Immunohistochemical studies revealed the occurrence of 12-Lox in neurons; particularly in hippocampus, striatum, olivary nucleus, as well as in glial and in cerebral endothelial cells (Nishiyama, Okamoto et al. 1992; Nishiyama, Watanabe et al. 1993). Using immature cortical neurons and HT cells, it has been shown that a decrease in [GSH]i triggers the activation of neuronal 12-Lox, which leads to the production of peroxides, the influx of Ca^{2+} and ultimately to cell death (Li et al. 1997; Tan et al. 2001). The 12-Lox metabolite 12-HPETE proved to be capable of causing cell death (Gu et al. 2001). Inhibition of 12-Lox protected cortical neurons from β-amyloid induced toxicity (Lebeau et al. 2001). Intracellular calcium chelation delayed cell death by lipoxygenase-mediated free radicals in mouse cortical cultures (Wie et al. 2001). In sum, 12-Lox poses clear threat to neuronal survival especially under GSH-deficient conditions.

Lipoxygenase activity is sensitive to vitamin E. α-tocopherol strongly inhibits purified 5-Lox with a IC_{50} of 5 μM. The inhibition is independent of the antioxidant property of tocopherol. Tryptic digestion and peptide mapping of the 5-Lox-tocopherol complex indicated that tocopherol binds strongly to a single peptide (Reddanna et al. 1985). Another study reported inhibition of 15-Lox by tocopherol *via* specific interaction with the enzyme protein (Grossman and Waksman 1984). Of interest, inhibitors specific for cycloxygenase or 5-Lox are not effective in protecting neuronal cells against glutamate-induced death suggesting a specific role of 12-Lox in glutamate-induced death (Khanna, Roy, Ryu et al. 2003; Khanna, Roy, Slivka et al. 2005b).

Our studies addressing the effect of α-tocotrienol on pure 12-Lox indicate that α-tocotrienol directly interacts with the enzyme to suppress arachidonic acid metabolism. *In silico* studies examining possible docking sites of α-tocotrienol to 12-Lox support the presence of a α-tocotrienol binding solvent cavity close to the active site. Previously it has been demonstrated in 15-Lox that COOH terminal of arachidonic acid enters this solvent cavity while accessing the catalytic site (Borngraber et al. 1999). It is therefore plausible that the binding position of α-tocotrienol prevents access of the natural substrate arachidonic acid to the active site of 12-Lox (Khanna et al. 2003). Does 12-Lox have a tangible impact on neurodegenerative processes *in vivo*? In 1992, it was reported that a mixed lipoxygenase/cyclooxygenase inhibitor SK&F 105809 reduced cerebral edema after closed head injury in rat (Shohami et al. 1992). We noted that 12-Lox, but not 5-Lox (Kitagawa et al. 2004), deficient mice were significantly protected against stroke-related injury of the brain (Khanna, Roy, Slivka et al. 2005b). The case for 12-Lox as an important mediator of neurodegeneration in vivo is gaining additional support from independent studies (Musiek et al. 2006). 12-Lox has been also implicated in the pathogenesis of Alzheimer's (Yao et al. 2005). α-Tocotrienol is capable of resisting neurodegeneration *in vivo* by opposing the c-Src and 12-Lox pathways.

Other than stroke, another area where tocotrienol-based therapeutics shows promise is in the treatment of familial dysautonomia (FD), a neurodegenerative genetic disorder primarily affecting individuals of Ashkenazi Jewish descent. FD is a neurodevelopmental genetic disorder within the larger classification of hereditary sensory and autonomic neuropathies, each caused by a different genetic error. Clinical features reflect widespread involvement of sensory and autonomic neurons. The FD gene has been identified as IKBKAP, a gene that encodes the IkappaB kinase complex-associated protein (IKAP). Mutations result in tissue-specific expression of mutant IkappaB kinase-associated protein (IKAP). The genetic error probably affects development, as well as maintenance, of neurons because there is neuropathological and clinical progression. Pathological alterations consist of decreased unmyelinated and small-fiber neurons.

In 2003, it was first reported that tocotrienols may induce the transcription of IKAP mRNA in FD-derived cells such that expression of correctly spliced transcript and normal protein is increased (Anderson, 2003 #453). These findings suggested that *in vivo* supplementation with tocotrienols may elevate IKBKAP gene expression and in turn increase the amount of functional IKAP protein produced in FD patients. FD is associated with elevated plasma levels of norepinephrine (NE) and dopamine. These changes are observed during autonomic crises. Fetal tissue homozygous for the common FD-causing mutation and peripheral blood cells of individuals with FD have reduced monoamine oxidase (MAO) A mRNA levels. FD-derived cells, stimulated with tocotrienols produced increased levels of functional IKAP, and expressed increased amounts of MAO A mRNA transcript and protein. Administration of tocotrienol to individuals with FD resulted in increased expression of both functional IKAP and MAO A transcripts in their peripheral blood cells. Thus, tocotrienols may be useful for patients suffering from FD. Randomized placebo controlled clinical studies are warranted.

26.6 SUMMARY

Members of the natural vitamin E family possess overlapping as well as unique functional properties. Our knowledge about the biology and significance is limited but rapidly expanding. Among the natural vitamin E molecules, d-α-Tocopherol (RRR-α-tocopherol) has the highest bioavailability and is the standard against which all the others are compared. However, it is only one out of eight natural forms of vitamin E. Interestingly, symptoms caused by α-tocopherol deficiency can be alleviated by tocotrienols. Thus, tocotrienols can be viewed as being members of the natural vitamin E family not only structurally but also functionally. Disappointments with outcomes-based studies investigating α-tocopherol (Friedrich 2004; Greenberg 2005) need to be cautiously handled, recognizing the untapped opportunities offered by the other forms of natural vitamin E. It has been suggested that the safe dose of various tocotrienols for human consumption is 200–1000 mg/d (Yu et al. 2006). Vitamin E represents one of the most fascinating natural resources that have the potential to influence a broad range of mechanisms underlying human health and disease. The current state of knowledge warrants strategic investment into the lesser-known forms of vitamin E, with emphasis on uncovering the specific conditions that govern the function of vitamin E molecules *in vivo*. Outcome studies designed in light of such information have the clear potential of returning dividends that are more lucrative than findings of the current clinical outcome studies.

ACKNOWLEDGMENT

Tocotrienol research in the laboratory is supported by NIH RO1NS42617.

REFERENCES

Adachi H, Ishii N. 2000. Effects of tocotrienols on life span and protein carbonylation in *Caenorhabditis elegans*. *J Gerontol. Series A: Biological Sciences and Medical Sciences,* Vol. 55A, No. 6. Washington, DC: The Gerontological Society of America. B280–5.

Adachi K, Miki M, Tamai H, Tokuda M, Mino M. 1990. Adipose tissues and vitamin E. *J Nutr Sci Vitaminol* Tokyo 36(4):327–37.

Adesuyi SA, Cockrell CS, Gamache DA, Ellis EF. 1985. Lipoxygenase metabolism of arachidonic acid in brain. *J Neurochem* 45(3):770–6.

Aikawa R, Komuro I, Yamazaki T, Zou Y, Kudoh S, Tanaka M, Shiojima I, Hiroi Y, Yazaki Y. 1997. Oxidative stress activates extracellular signal-regulated kinases through Src and Ras in cultured cardiac myocytes of neonatal rats. *J Clin Invest* 100(7):1813–21.

Alper O, Bowden ET. 2005. Novel insights into c–Src. *Curr Pharm Des* 11(9):1119–30.

Anderson SL, Qiu J, Rubin BY. 2003. Tocotrienols induce IKBKAP expression: A possible therapy for familial dysautonomia. *Biochem Biophys Res Commun* 306(1):303–309.

Araya H, Tomita M, Hayashi M. 2006. The novel formulation design of self-emulsifying drug delivery systems SEDDS type O/W microemulsion III: The permeation mechanism of a poorly water soluble drug entrapped O/W microemulsion in rat isolated intestinal membrane by the Ussing chamber method. *Drug Metab Pharmacokinet* 21(1):45–53.

Aten RF, Kolodecik TR, Behrman HR. 1994. Ovarian vitamin E accumulation: Evidence for a role of lipoproteins. *Endocrinology* 135(2):533–9.

Bains JS, Shaw CA. 1997. Neurodegenerative disorders in humans: the role of glutathione in oxidative stress-mediated neuronal death. *Brain Res Rev* 25(3):335–58.

Bazan NG. 1976. Free arachidonic acid and other lipids in the nervous system during early ischemia and after electroshock. *Adv Exp Med Biol* 7(2):317–35.

Bazan NG, Jr. 1970. Effects of ischemia and electroconvulsive shock on free fatty acid pool in the brain. *Biochim Biophys Acta* 218(1):1–10.

Bazan NG, Jr. 1971a. Changes in free fatty acids of brain by drug–induced convulsions, electroshock and anaesthesia. *J Neurochem* 18(8):1379–85.

Bazan NG, Jr. 1971b. Phospholipases A 1 and A 2 in brain subcellular fractions. *Acta Physiol Lat Am* 21(2):101–6.

Bazan NG, Jr., Rakowski H. 1970. Increased levels of brain free fatty acids after electroconvulsive shock. *Life Sci* 9(9):501–7.

Bhat NR, Zhang P. 1999. Hydrogen peroxide activation of multiple mitogen-activated protein kinases in an oligodendrocyte cell line: Role of extracellular signal-regulated kinase in hydrogen peroxide-induced cell death. *J Neurochem* 72(1):112–9.

Blatt DH, Leonard SW, Traber MG. 2001. Vitamin E kinetics and the function of tocopherol regulatory proteins. *Nutrition* 17(10):799–805.

Borngraber S, Browner M, Gillmor S, Gerth C, Anton M, Fletterick R, Kuhn H. 1999. Shape and specificity in mammalian 15-lipoxygenase active site. The functional interplay of sequence determinants for the reaction specificity. *J Biol Chem* 274(52):37345–50.

Boscoboinik D, Szewczyk A, Hensey C, Azzi A. 1991. Inhibition of cell proliferation by alpha-tocopherol. Role of protein kinase C. *J Biol Chem* 266(10):6188–94.

Brugge JS, Cotton PC, Queral AE, Barrett JN, Nonner D, Keane RW. 1985. Neurones express high levels of a structurally modified, activated form of pp60c-Src. *Nature* 316(6028):554–7.

Bryngelsson S, Dimberg LH, Kamal-Eldin A. 2002. Effects of commercial processing on levels of antioxidants in oats Avena sativa L. *J Agric Food Chem* 50(7):1890–6.

Cahoon EB, Hall SE, Ripp KG, Ganzke TS, Hitz WD, Coughlan SJ. 2003. Metabolic redesign of vitamin E biosynthesis in plants for tocotrienol production and increased antioxidant content. *Nat Biotechnol* 21(9):1082–7.

Carlen PL, Gurevich N, Zhang L, Wu PH, Reynaud D, Pace-Asciak CR. 1994. Formation and electrophysiological actions of the arachidonic acid metabolites, hepoxilins, at nanomolar concentrations in rat hippocampal slices. *Neuroscience* 58(3):493–502.

Das S, Powell SR, Wang P, Divald A, Nesaretnam K, Tosaki A, Cordis GA, Maulik N, Das DK. 2005. Cardioprotection with palm tocotrienol: Antioxidant activity of tocotrienol is linked with its ability to stabilize proteasomes. *Am J Physiol Heart Circ Physiol* 289(1):H361–7.

Dietrich M, Traber MG, Jacques PF, Cross CE, Hu Y, Block G. 2006. Does {gamma}–tocopherol play a role in the primary prevention of heart disease and cancer? A review. *J Am Coll Nutr* 25(4):292–9.

Dormann P. 2007. Functional diversity of tocochromanols in plants. *Planta* 225(2):269–76.

Dringen R, Gutterer JM, Hirrlinger J. 2000. Glutathione metabolism in brain metabolic interaction between astrocytes and neurons in the defense against reactive oxygen species. *Eur J Biochem* 267(16):4912–6.

Elson CE. 1992. Tropical oils: Nutritional and scientific issues. *Crit Rev Food Sci Nutr* 31(1–2):79–102.

Friedrich MJ. 2004. To "E" or not to "E," vitamin E's role in health and disease is the question. *JAMA* 292(6):671–3.

Gao P, Morozowich W. 2006. Development of supersaturatable self-emulsifying drug delivery system formulations for improving the oral absorption of poorly soluble drugs. *Expert Opin Drug Deliv* 3(1):97–110.

Garry PJ, Hunt WC, Bandrofchak JL, VanderJagt D, Goodwin JS. 1987. Vitamin A intake and plasma retinol levels in healthy elderly men and women. *Am J Clin Nutr* 46(6):989–94.

Greenberg ER. 2005. Vitamin E supplements: Good in theory, but is the theory good? *Ann Intern Med* 142(1):75–6.

Grossman S, Waksman EG. 1984. New aspects of the inhibition of soybean lipoxygenase by alpha-tocopherol. Evidence for the existence of a specific complex. *Int J Biochem* 16(3):281–9.

Gu J, Liu Y, Wen Y, Natarajan R, Lanting L, Nadler JL. 2001. Evidence that increased 12-lipoxygenase activity induces apoptosis in fibroblasts. *J Cell Physiol* 186(3):357–65.

Hagmann W, Kagawa D, Renaud C, Honn KV. 1993. Activity and protein distribution of 12–lipoxygenase in HEL cells: Induction of membrane–association by phorbol ester TPA, modulation of activity by glutathione and 13-HPODE and Ca^{2+}-dependent translocation to membranes. *Prostaglandins* 46(6):471–7.

Hall TJ, Schaeublin M, Missbach M. 1994. Evidence that c-Src is involved in the process of osteoclastic bone resorption. *Biochem Biophys Res Commun* 199(3):1237–44.

Han D, Sen CK, Roy S, Kobayashi MS, Tritschler HJ, Packer L. 1997. Protection against glutamate-induced cytotoxicity in C6 glial cells by thiol antioxidants. *Am J Physiol* 273(5 Pt 2):R1771–8.

Hensley K, Benaksas EJ, Bolli R, Comp P, Grammas P, Hamdheydari L, Mou S, Pye QN, Stoddard MF, Wallis G and others. 2004. New perspectives on vitamin E: Gamma-tocopherol and carboxyelthylhydroxychroman metabolites in biology and medicine. *Free Radic Biol Med* 36(1):1–15.

Ho D, Yuen KH, Yap SP; 2003. Drug delivery system: Formulation for fat-soluble drugs. US patent 6,596,306.

Hong JY, Kim JK, Song YK, Park JS, Kim CK. 2006. A new self-emulsifying formulation of itraconazole with improved dissolution and oral absorption. *J Control Release* 110(2):332–8.

Horvath G, Wessjohann L, Bigirimana J, Jansen M, Guisez Y, Caubergs R, Horemans N. 2006. Differential distribution of tocopherols and tocotrienols in photosynthetic and non-photosynthetic tissues. *Phytochemistry* 67(12):1185–95.

Hosomi A, Arita M, Sato Y, Kiyose C, Ueda T, Igarashi O, Arai H, Inoue K. 1997. Affinity for alpha-tocopherol transfer protein as a determinant of the biological activities of vitamin E analogs. *FEBS Lett* 409(1):105–8.

Hsu CY, Persons PE, Spada AP, Bednar RA, Levitzki A, Zilberstein A. 1991. Kinetic analysis of the inhibition of the epidermal growth factor receptor tyrosine kinase by Lavendustin-A and its analogue. *J Biol Chem* 266(31):21105–12.

Ingraham CA, Cox ME, Ward DC, Fults DW, Maness PF. 1989. c-src and other proto-oncogenes implicated in neuronal differentiation. *Mol Chem Neuropathol* 10(1):1–14.

Ishizaki Y, Murota S. 1991. Arachidonic acid metabolism in cultured astrocytes: Presence of 12-lipoxygenase activity in the intact cells. *Neurosci Lett* 131(2):149–52.

Ishizawar R, Parsons SJ. 2004. c-Src and cooperating partners in human cancer. *Cancer Cell* 6(3):209–14.

Jishage K, Arita M, Igarashi K, Iwata T, Watanabe M, Ogawa M, Ueda O, Kamada N, Inoue K, Arai H and others. 2001. Alpha-tocopherol transfer protein is important for the normal development of placental labyrinthine trophoblasts in mice. *J Biol Chem* 276(3):1669–72.

Johnson NL, Gardner AM, Diener KM, Lange-Carter CA, Gleavy J, Jarpe MB, Minden A, Karin M, Zon LI, Johnson GL. 1996. Signal transduction pathways regulated by mitogen-activated/extracellular response kinase kinase kinase induce cell death. *J Biol Chem* 271(6):3229–37.

Kaempf-Rotzoll DE, Traber MG, Arai H. 2003. Vitamin E and transfer proteins. *Curr Opin Lipid* 14(3):249–54.

Khanna S, Patel V, Rink C, Roy S, Sen CK. 2005a. Delivery of orally supplemented alpha-tocotrienol to vital organs of rats and tocopherol-transport protein deficient mice. *Free Radic Biol Med* 39(10):1310–9.

Khanna S, Roy S, Parinandi NL, Maurer M, Sen CK. 2006. Characterization of the potent neuroprotective properties of the natural vitamin E alpha-tocotrienol. *J Neurochem* 98(5):1474–1486.

Khanna S, Roy S, Ryu H, Bahadduri P, Swaan PW, Ratan RR, Sen CK. 2003. Molecular basis of vitamin E action: Tocotrienol modulates 12-lipoxygenase, a key mediator of glutamate-induced neurodegeneration. *J Biol Chem* 278(44):43508–15.

Khanna S, Roy S, Slivka A, Craft TK, Chaki S, Rink C, Notestine MA, DeVries AC, Parinandi NL, Sen CK. 2005b. Neuroprotective properties of the natural vitamin E alpha-tocotrienol. *Stroke* 36(10):2258–64.

Khanna S, Venojarvi M, Roy S, Sen CK. 2002. Glutamate-induced c-Src activation in neuronal cells. *Meth Enzymol* 35(2):191–8.

Khosla P, Patel V, Whinter JM, Khanna S, Rakhkovskaya M, Roy S, Sen CK. 2006. Postprandial levels of the natural vitamin E tocotrienol in human circulation. *Antioxid Redox Signal* 8(5–6):1059–68.

Kitagawa K, Matsumoto M, Hori M. 2004. Cerebral ischemia in 5-lipoxygenase knockout mice. *Brain Res* 1004(1–2):198–202.

Kwon KJ, Jung YS, Lee SH, Moon CH, Baik EJ. 2005. Arachidonic acid induces neuronal death through lipoxygenase and cytochrome P450 rather than cyclooxygenase. *J Neurosci Res* 81(1):73–84.

Lau AF. 2005. c-Src: Bridging the gap between phosphorylation- and acidification-induced gap junction channel closure. *Sci STKE* 2005(291):pe33.

Lebeau A, Esclaire F, Rostene W, Pelaprat D. 2001. Baicalein protects cortical neurons from beta-amyloid 25-35 induced toxicity. *Neuroreport* 12(10):2199–202.

Lee JR, Koretzky GA. 1998. Extracellular signal-regulated kinase-2, but not c-Jun NH2–terminal kinase, activation correlates with surface IgM-mediated apoptosis in the WEHI 231 B cell line. *J Immunol* 161(4):1637–44.

Lehtinen MK, Bonni A. 2006. Modeling oxidative stress in the central nervous system. *Curr Mol Med* 6(8):871–81.

Lennmyr F, Ericsson A, Gerwins P, Akterin S, Ahlstrom H, Terent A. 2004. Src family kinase-inhibitor PP2 reduces focal ischemic brain injury. *Acta Neurol Scand* 110(3):175–9.

Leonard SW, Paterson E, Atkinson JK, Ramakrishnan R, Cross CE, Traber MG. 2005. Studies in humans using deuterium-labeled alpha- and gamma-tocopherols demonstrate faster plasma gamma-tocopherol disappearance and greater gamma-metabolite production. *Free Radic Biol Med* 38(7):857–66.

Lepley RA, Muskardin DT, Fitzpatrick FA. 1996. Tyrosine kinase activity modulates catalysis and translocation of cellular 5-lipoxygenase. *J Biol Chem* 271(11):6179–84.

Li Y, Maher P, Schubert D. 1997. A role for 12-lipoxygenase in nerve cell death caused by glutathione depletion. *Neuron* 19(2):453–63.

Lodge JK, Hall WL, Jeanes YM, Proteggente AR. 2004. Physiological factors influencing vitamin E biokinetics. *Ann N Y Acad Sci* 1031:60–73.

Maness PF, Aubry M, Shores CG, Frame L, Pfenninger KH. 1988. c-Src gene product in developing rat brain is enriched in nerve growth cone membranes. *Proc Natl Acad Sci USA* 85(14):5001–5.

Miyamoto T, Lindgren JA, Hokfelt T, Samuelsson B. 1987a. Formation of lipoxygenase products in the rat brain. *Adv Prostaglandin Thromboxane Leukot Res* 17B:929–33.

Miyamoto T, Lindgren JA, Hokfelt T, Samuelsson B. 1987b. Regional distribution of leukotriene and monohydroxyeicosatetraenoic acid production in the rat brain. Highest leukotriene C4 formation in the hypothalamus. *FEBS Lett* 216(1):123–7.

Muller DP, Goss-Sampson MA. 1989. Role of vitamin E in neural tissue. *Ann NY Acad Sci* 570:146–55.

Muller DP, Goss-Sampson MA. 1990. Neurochemical, neurophysiological and neuropathological studies in vitamin E deficiency. *Crit Rev Neurobiol* 5(3):239–63.

Musiek ES, Breeding RS, Milne GL, Zanoni G, Morrow JD, McLaughlin B. 2006. Cyclopentenone isoprostanes are novel bioactive products of lipid oxidation which enhance neurodegeneration. *J Neurochem* 97(5):1301–13.

Nesaretnam K, Guthrie N, Chambers AF, Carroll KK. 1995. Effect of tocotrienols on the growth of a human breast cancer cell line in culture. *Lipids* 30(12):1139–43.

Nishiyama M, Okamoto H, Watanabe T, Hori T, Hada T, Ueda N, Yamamoto S, Tsukamoto H, Watanabe K, Kirino T. 1992. Localization of arachidonate 12-lipoxygenase in canine brain tissues. *J Neurochem* 58(4):1395–400.

Nishiyama M, Watanabe T, Ueda N, Tsukamoto H, Watanabe K. 1993. Arachidonate 12-lipoxygenase is localized in neurons, glial cells and endothelial cells of the canine brain. *J Histochem Cytochem* 41(1):111–7.

O'Byrne D, Grundy S, Packer L, Devaraj S, Baldenius K, Hoppe PP, Kraemer K, Jialal I, Traber MG. 2000. Studies of LDL oxidation following alpha-, gamma-, or delta-tocotrienyl acetate supplementation of hypercholesterolemic humans. *Free Rad Biol Med* 29(9):834–845.

Panfili G, Fratianni A, Irano M. 2003. Normal phase high-performance liquid chromatography method for the determination of tocopherols and tocotrienols in cereals. *J Agric Food Chem* 51(14):3940–4.

Paul R, Zhang ZG, Eliceiri BP, Jiang Q, Boccia AD, Zhang RL, Chopp M, Cheresh DA. 2001. Src deficiency or blockade of Src activity in mice provides cerebral protection following stroke. *Nat Med* 7(2):222–7.

Pearce BC, Parker RA, Deason ME, Dischino DD, Gillespie E, Qureshi AA, Volk K, Wright JJ. 1994. Inhibitors of cholesterol biosynthesis. 2. Hypocholesterolemic and antioxidant activities of benzopyran and tetrahydronaphthalene analogues of the tocotrienols. *J Med Chem* 37(4):526–41.

Pearce BC, Parker RA, Deason ME, Qureshi AA, Wright JJ. 1992. Hypocholesterolemic activity of synthetic and natural tocotrienols. *J Med Chem* 35(20):3595–606.

Pyper JM, Bolen JB. 1989. Neuron-specific splicing of c-Src RNA in human brain. *J Neurosci Res* 24(1):89–96.

Qureshi AA, Burger WC, Peterson DM, Elson CE. 1986. The structure of an inhibitor of cholesterol biosynthesis isolated from barley. *J Biol Chem* 261(23):10544–50.

Qureshi AA, Mo H, Packer L, Peterson DM. 2000. Isolation and identification of novel tocotrienols from rice bran with hypocholesterolemic, antioxidant and antitumor properties. *J Agric Food Chem* 48(8):3130–40.

Qureshi AA, Sami SA, Salser WA, Khan FA. 2002. Dose-dependent suppression of serum cholesterol by tocotrienol-rich fraction TRF25 of rice bran in hypercholesterolemic humans. *Atherosclerosis* 161(1):199–207.

Reddanna P, Rao MK, Reddy CC. 1985. Inhibition of 5-lipoxygenase by vitamin E. *FEBS Lett* 193(1):39–43.

Rippert P, Scimemi C, Dubald M, Matringe M. 2004. Engineering plant shikimate pathway for production of tocotrienol and improving herbicide resistance. *Plant Physiol* 134(1):92–100.

Roy S, Lado BH, Khanna S, Sen CK. 2002. Vitamin E sensitive genes in the developing rat fetal brain: A high-density oligonucleotide microarray analysis. *FEBS Lett* 530(1)–3:17–23.

Schubert D, Piasecki D. 2001. Oxidative glutamate toxicity can be a component of the excitotoxicity cascade. *J Neurosci* 21(19):7455–62.

Schulz JB, Lindenau J, Seyfried J, Dichgans J. 2000. Glutathione, oxidative stress and neurodegeneration. *Eur J Biochem* 267(16):4904–11.

Sen CK, Khanna S, Roy S. 2004. Tocotrienol: The natural vitamin E to defend the nervous system? *Ann N Y Acad Sci* 1031:127–42.

Sen CK, Khanna S, Roy S. 2006. Tocotrienols: Vitamin E beyond tocopherols. *Life Sci* 78(18):2088–98.

Sen CK, Khanna S, Roy S, Packer L. 2000. Molecular basis of vitamin E action. Tocotrienol potently inhibits glutamate-induced pp60c-Src kinase activation and death of HT4 neuronal cells. *J Biol Chem* 275(17):13049–55.

Serbinova E, Kagan V, Han D, Packer L. 1991. Free radical recycling and intramembrane mobility in the antioxidant properties of alpha-tocopherol and alpha-tocotrienol. *Free Rad Biol Med* 10(5):263–75.

Serbinova EA, Packer L. 1994. Antioxidant properties of alpha-tocopherol and alpha-tocotrienol. *Meth Enzymol* 234:354–66.

Shohami E, Glantz L, Nates J, Feuerstein G. 1992. The mixed lipoxygenase/cyclooxygenase inhibitor SK&F 105809 reduces cerebral edema after closed head injury in rat. *J Basic Clin Physiol Pharmacol* 3(2):99–107.

Shupnik MA. 2004. Crosstalk between steroid receptors and the c-Src-receptor tyrosine kinase pathways: Implications for cell proliferation. *Oncogene* 23(48):7979–89.

Solomons NW, Orozco M. 2003. Alleviation of vitamin A deficiency with palm fruit and its products. *Asia Pac J Clin Nutr* 12(3):373–84.

Song BL, DeBose-Boyd RA. 2006. Insig-dependent ubiquitination and degradation of 3-hydroxy-3-methylglutaryl coenzyme A reductase stimulated by delta- and gamma-tocotrienols. *J Biol Chem* 281, 25054–25061.

Soriano P, Montgomery C, Geske R, Bradley A. 1991. Targeted disruption of the c-Src proto-oncogene leads to osteopetrosis in mice. *Cell* 64(4):693–702.

Steiner M. 1993. Vitamin E: More than an antioxidant. *Clin Cardiol* 16(4 Suppl 1):I16–8.

Sugano M, Koba K, Tsuji E. 1999. Health benefits of rice bran oil. *Anticancer Res* 19(5A):3651–7.

Sun X, Shih AY, Johannssen HC, Erb H, Li P, Murphy TH. 2006. Two-photon imaging of glutathione levels in intact brain indicates enhanced redox buffering in developing neurons and cells at the cerebrospinal fluid and blood–brain interface. *J Biol Chem* 281(25):17420–31.

Sundram K, Sambanthamurthi R, Tan YA. 2003. Palm fruit chemistry and nutrition. *Asia Pac J Clin Nutr* 12(3):355–62.

Suzuki YJ, Tsuchiya M, Wassall SR, Choo YM, Govil G, Kagan VE, Packer L. 1993. Structural and dynamic membrane properties of alpha-tocopherol and alpha-tocotrienol: Implication to the molecular mechanism of their antioxidant potency. *Biochemistry* 32(40):10692–9.

Tan S, Schubert D, Maher P. 2001. Oxytosis: A novel form of programmed cell death. *Curr Top Med Chem* 1(6):497–506.

Tarrago-Trani MT, Phillips KM, Lemar LE, Holden JM. 2006. New and existing oils and fats used in products with reduced trans-fatty acid content. *J Am Diet Assoc* 106(6):867–80.

Terasawa Y, Ladha Z, Leonard SW, Morrow JD, Newland D, Sanan D, Packer L, Traber MG, Farese RV, Jr. 2000. Increased atherosclerosis in hyperlipidemic mice deficient in alpha-tocopherol transfer protein and vitamin E. *Proc Nat Acad Sci USA* 97(25):13830–4.

Thomas SM, Brugge, JS. 1997. Cellular functions regulated by Src family kinases. *Ann Rev Cell Devel Biol* 13:513–609.

Traber MG, Arai H. 1999. Molecular mechanisms of vitamin E transport. *Ann Rev Nutr* 19:343–55.

Traber MG, Burton GW, Hamilton RL. 2004. Vitamin E trafficking. *Ann NY Acad Sci* 1031:1–12.

van der Worp HB, Bar PR, Kappelle LJ, de Wildt DJ. 1998. Dietary vitamin E levels affect outcome of permanent focal cerebral ischemia in rats. *Stroke* 29(5):1002–5; discussion 1005–6.

Vatassery GT. 1998. Vitamin E and other endogenous antioxidants in the central nervous system. *Geriatrics* 5(3 Suppl 1):S25–7.

Wagner KH, Kamal–Eldin A, Elmadfa I. 2004. Gamma-tocopherol––an underestimated vitamin? *Ann Nutr Metab* 48(3):169–88.

Wie MB, Koh JY, Won MH, Lee JC, Shin TK, Moon CJ, Ha HJ, Park SM, Kim HC. 2001. BAPTA/AM, an intracellular calcium chelator, induces delayed necrosis by lipoxygenase-mediated free radicals in mouse cortical cultures. *Prog Neuropsychopharmacol Biol Psych* 25(8):1641–59.

Yamamoto S. 1992. Mammalian lipoxygenases: Molecular structures and functions. *Biochim Biophys Acta* 1128(2–3):117–31.

Yao Y, Clark CM, Trojanowski JQ, Lee VM, Pratico D. 2005. Elevation of 12/15 lipoxygenase products in AD and mild cognitive impairment. *Ann Neurol* 58(4):623–6.

Yap SP, Yuen KH, Wong JW. 2001. Pharmacokinetics and bioavailability of alpha-, gamma- and delta-tocotrienols under different food status. *J Pharm Pharmacol* 53(1):67–71.

Yoneda T, Lowe C, Lee CH, Gutierrez G, Niewolna M, Williams PJ, Izbicka E, Uehara Y, Mundy GR. 1993. Herbimycin A, a pp60c-Src tyrosine kinase inhibitor, inhibits osteoclastic bone resorption in vitro and hypercalcemia in vivo. *J Clin Invest* 91(6):2791–5.

Yu SG, Thomas AM, Gapor A, Tan B, Qureshi N, Qureshi AA. 2006. Dose–response impact of various tocotrienols on serum lipid parameters in 5-week-old female chickens. *Lipids* 41(5):453–61.

Zingg JM, Azzi A. 2004. Non-antioxidant activities of vitamin E. *Curr Med Chem* 11(9):1113–33.

27 Gamma-Tocotrienol: Potential as a Countermeasure against Radiological Threat

K. Sree Kumar, Sanchita P. Ghosh and Martin Hauer-Jensen

CONTENTS

27.1 INTRODUCTION

Tocotrienols exist in nature as four tocol isoforms of the vitamin E family — α, β, γ and δ tocotrienols. Among them, gamma (γ)-tocotrienol (GT3), a better antioxidant than alpha-tocopherol (AT, also commonly known as vitamin E), has gained importance due to its potent inhibition of hydroxymethyl glutaryl coenzyme A (HMG-CoA) reductase enzyme. GT3 has almost 30-fold greater inhibitory activity than alpha-tocotrienol. HMG-CoA reductase is the pivotal enzyme in the synthesis of mevalonic acid, a key metabolic intermediate in the biosynthetic pathway of cholesterol. Regulation of this enzyme has been the basis for developing cholesterol-lowering drugs—statins—for nearly two decades (Pearce et al., 1992).

TABLE 27.1
Dose-Dependent Hazards of Exposure to Radiation

Dose-rem	Effects
5–20	Possible late effects; possible chromosomal damage
20–100	Temporary reduction in white blood cells
100–200	Mild radiation sickness within a few hours: vomiting, diarrhea, fatigue; reduction in resistance to infection
200–300	Serious radiation sickness effects (as in 100–200 rem) and hemorrhage; exposure is a lethal dose to 10–35% of the population after 30 days (LD 10–35/30)
300–400	Serious radiation sickness; also marrow and intestine destruction; LD 50–70/30
400–1000	Acute illness, early death; LD 60–95/30
1000–5000	Acute illness, death in days; LD 100/10

Source: ©Copyright 2007, atomicarchive.com; reproduced with permission

Another important property of GT3 is its potent radioprotective activity. Tocol antioxidants, particularly alpha-tocopherol and its hemisuccinate ester, show varying levels of radioprotection in rodents (Kumar, Srinivasan et al., 2002; Kumar et al., 2007; Singh et al., 2005). This chapter provides an overview of protection provided by one of the tocotrienols, GT3, against radiation-induced lethality, as well as its possible mechanisms of protection. These may involve radiation-induced reactive oxygen and nitrogen species, among other things. The chapter will first address the need for radioprotection, types of radiation injuries, available radiation countermeasures and the role of GT3 as a radiation countermeasure, possibly against more than one type of radiation injury. For the sake of convenience, throughout this chapter "radioprotectant" or "radioprotector" may be used instead of "radiation countermeasure."

27.2 NEED FOR RADIATION COUNTERMEASURES

27.2.1 Nuclear-Radiological Threat

An insidious yet enduring terrorist threat is use of a nuclear/radiological device. Nuclear threat generally refers to a nuclear warfare device involving many casualties. For survivors of a nuclear blast, the radiation hazard may last 1–5 years or even longer, depending on a victim's distance from the radiation source, which determines the dose and dose rate. Radiological threats can vary from exposures caused by detonation of radiological dispersion devices (RDDs or "dirty bombs") to attacks on facilities such as nuclear power plants. Detonation of a nuclear/biological device can cause levels of radiation hazards varying from minimal or no immediate effect to mortality within a few days (Table 27.1). The apparent lack of effect with low doses of radiation should not be misconstrued as harmless because exposure can cause effects such as carcinogenesis later in life.

Although, to date, few attacks on nuclear facilities have been attempted and no actual use of RDDs, global governments and their citizens have become increasingly anxious about the threat of such attacks. Terrorists' global activities since 9/11 have shown that they are capable of causing mass casualties and are prepared to do so. Radiological terrorism is a more attractive option than nuclear terrorism because of the relative ease with which a radiological device can be made and used; whereas nuclear terrorism requires obtaining or constructing a nuclear weapon to produce a nuclear explosion.

27.2.2 Types of Radiation Damage

Because radioprotection studies discussed herein are based on a mouse model, the radiation doses described correspond to those responsive in mice. Depending on the strain of mice, human doses will be 0.4 to 0.5 times less than doses used for mice.

27.2.2.1 Hematopoietic Effects (Syndrome)

The hematopoietic system is highly sensitive to ionizing radiation (IR) in the range of 3 to 8 Gy. These effects are characterized as hematopoietic syndrome. Bone marrow injury is the primary determinant of survival because of its rapidly proliferating stem/progenitor cell compartments, which are readily susceptible to radiation damage. Radiation sterilizes bone marrow's mitotically active progenitor cells. It diminishes the marrow's supply of mature red blood cells, white blood cells and platelets, making victims susceptible to secondary infections. Peripheral blood neutropenia (absolute neutrophils less than 500 per microliter) and thrombocytopenia (platelets less than 20,000 per microliter) resulting from radiation exposure cause infectious and hemorrhagic complications. If these complications are not prevented, they can lead to lethality in the short term or to adverse long-term health effects. Thus, protection or reconstitution of the hematopoietic and immune systems is a major concern in the development of radiation countermeasures and therapeutic agents.

Significant progress has been made in the post-exposure management of radiation-induced bone marrow injury, using hematopoietic cytokines, blood transfusions, antimicrobial therapy and stem cell reconstitution. The use of cytokines and growth factors in radiation injury results from a focus on enhancing recovery from neutropenia and thrombocytopenia. A number of cytokines and growth factors have shown significant *in vivo* and *in vitro* preclinical efficacy against radiation-induced depletion of blood cells. The Food and Drug Administration (FDA) has approved some of them for treating profound neutropenia and thrombocytopenia resulting from cancer chemotherapy and some are in different stages of clinical trials for radiation injury (MacVittie and Farese, 2002; Pellmar and Rockwell, 2005; Singh and Seed, 2003)

27.2.2.2 Gastrointestinal (GI) Effects (Syndrome)

Classical acute GI radiation syndrome occurs after whole body radiation of more than 10 Gy of gamma-rays. It causes loss of intestinal mucosa, secretory diarrhea and massive loss of fluids and electrolytes. However, GI radiation injury also results from lower doses of radiation. Mucosal inflammation and dysfunction of the epithelial barrier occur after many lower radiation doses, resulting in output of inflammatory mediators from the mucosa and translocation of bacteria from the gut lumen into the systemic circulation. Depending on radiation dose, GI syndrome is characterized by loss of appetite, diarrhea, luminal hemorrhage, loss of ionic and electrolyte balance, dehydration, infection and death. Symptoms of full-blown GI radiation syndrome and death that may follow are attributable to the depopulation of the epithelial lining of the gastrointestinal tract caused by radiation.

Dividing cells are confined to the GI tract's crypts, which provide a continuous supply of new cells; these cells move up the villi, differentiate and become the functioning cells. Cells at the top of the villi folds are sloughed off slowly but continuously in the normal course of events and the villus epithelium are continuously replaced by cells that originate from mitoses in the crypts. A 10-Gy to 15-Gy dose of radiation sterilizes a large proportion of the dividing cells in the crypts. As the surface of the villi is sloughed off and rubbed away by normal use, no replacement cells are produced in the crypts. Consequently, after a few days, the villi begin to shorten and shrink and eventually the surface lining of the intestine is completely denuded of villi. At the time of GI death, the villi are flat and almost completely devoid of cells.

In humans, the GI radiation syndrome occurs after whole-body radiation exposures to doses in excess of 6 Gy. Survival is very unlikely. Destructive changes of the intestinal epithelial lining cause breakdown of the mucosal barrier that normally separates the contents of the intestinal lumen from the gastrointestinal tissue, resulting in severe secretory diarrhea, dehydration and electrolyte imbalance. Even after lower doses of radiation, the GI tract plays a major role in the pathophysiology of toxicity and clinical outcome. Hence, sepsis from enteric bacteria is an important cause of lethality after radiation exposure. This is because, as a result of hematopoietic failure, bacterial translocation (i.e., passage of bacteria from the intestinal lumen through the defective mucosal barrier and into the blood stream) occurs during a period of severe, radiation-induced immune system compromise.

The risk of intestinal complications and the severity of injury after radiation exposure may be further accentuated by concomitant injuries that result in the so-called combined injury syndrome. While the biological mechanisms underlying interactions between radiation and other types of injury are largely unknown, there is a synergistic response to lethality in a combined injury situation. A non-lethal radiation exposure often can become potentially super-lethal by concomitant exposure with other types of injury. Thus, elucidating the mechanisms of synergy between radiation and other traumatic injuries and developing effective countermeasures for use in the combined injury situation are vital priorities. Moreover, because the GI tract is involved in the pathophysiological response to burns, trauma, sepsis and multiple organ dysfunction syndromes (MODS) as well as in isolated radiation syndromes, it likely plays a key role in combined injury and represents a particularly promising target for countermeasure development. The synergistic response to combined injury occasionally can be alleviated to a non-lethal event if a countermeasure can be developed for radiation injury alone.

27.2.2.3 Central Nervous System (CNS) Effects (Syndrome)

High dose gamma-radiation (>20 Gy) to the whole body produces central nervous system damage resulting in death within days. At very high doses (i.e., in excess of about 100 Gy), death occurs 24 to 48 hr after exposure and appears to result from neurologic and cardiovascular breakdown in addition to the severe hematopoietic and GI symptoms manifest at this dose level. The exact cause of death from the CNS syndrome is not clear. In the cases of the other two modes of death—the gastrointestinal and the hematopoietic syndromes—the principal mechanisms that lead to organism death are more or less defined. Death is caused by the depletion of the stem cells of a critical self-renewal tissue: the bone marrow or epithelium of the gut.

27.3 RADIATION COUNTERMEASURES

In the event of a radiological/nuclear terrorist attack, three groups will require a radiation countermeasure to mitigate the effects of harmful IR exposure: first responders, remediation workers and, if there is advance warning, the resident population. Thus, developing radiation countermeasures, applicable prior to or during exposure to prevent or limit injury, is a high-priority research area (Pellmar and Rockwell, 2005). Therapeutic agents for treating IR victims also are important. The ideal radiation countermeasure (i.e., radioprotectant or therapeutic agent) must be safe for all populations at risk of radiation exposure, even with repeated doses (as needed), easily administered, rapidly effective, and chemically stable. It also must be simple and inexpensive to manufacture and easily stored.

27.3.1 Historical Development of Radiation Countermeasures

The search for radioprotectors has been dominated by the study of sulphydryl compounds (Davidson et al., 1980). Most prominent among them is amifostine, shown in animal studies to be an effective radioprotectant. Although approved by the FDA for specific consequences of radiation therapy under supervised clinical scenarios (Capizzi and Oster, 1995), amifostine has significant side effects due to toxicity and a limited window of effectiveness. As a result, amifostine has not been accepted and approved as a radioprotector for military personnel. Moreover, it may not be useful for first responders against terrorist attacks because of its aforementioned performance-degrading toxicity (Landauer et al., 1992) and hypocalcaemia (Glover et al., 1983). In unsupervised situations such as in a potential terrorist scenario, amifostine virtually has no use for healthy individuals as a radiation countermeasure.

In an effort to identify other suitable radiation countermeasures (i.e., prophylactic agents to prevent radiation-induced tissue injuries), a number of compounds of diverse chemical structures have been considered as radioprotectors. These compounds include, in addition to thiols, cytokines (Waddick et al., 1991), steroids (Whitnall et al., 2001), prostaglandin analogs (Hanson et al., 1988), antioxidants (Kumar, Vaishnav and Weiss 1988; Weiss and Kumar, 1988), nutraceuticals (Davis et al., 2007; Kumar, Srinivasan, Toles, Miner et al., 2002; Landauer et al., 2003; Srinivasan and Weiss, 1992; Weiss et al., 1992; Weiss and Landauer, 2003) and other phytoceuticals (Devi et al., 1998; Goel et al., 2007; Maurya, Devasagayam and Nair 2006; Maurya, Adhikari et al., 2007).

Nutraceuticals include soy isoflavone, genistein and various tocol (tocopherols and tocotrienols) isoforms. Some have been shown to provide moderate protection against hematological deficits and lethality in rodents (Kumar, Srinivasan, Toles, Jobe et al., 2002; Kumar, Srinivasan, Toles, Miner et al., 2003; Kumar et al., 2007). This chapter will review the potential use of GT3 as a nutraceutical radiation countermeasure.

27.3.2 Biochemistry of Radiation Damage—Reactive Oxygen Species (ROS) and Reactive Nitrogen Species (RNS)

The transfer of energy from radiation exposure to biomolecules is followed, in less than 10^{-12} seconds, by a variety of physicochemical reactions (Weiss and Kumar, 1988). These changes can cause excitation and ionization by the *direct action* of radiation with critical biomolecules (e.g., DNA, enzymes, plasma and nuclear membrane constituents):

$$\text{Radiation} + \text{TH (target biomolecule)} \rightarrow \text{T}^{\cdot}\text{(target free radical)} + \text{H}^+ + e^-$$

Ionization also can occur by *indirect reaction* as a result of radiolysis of water and the subsequent reaction of free radicals formed within the cellular milieu:

$$\text{Radiation} + H_2O \rightarrow H_2O^+ + e^-$$

$$H_2O + e^- \rightarrow H^{\cdot} + OH^{\cdot}\text{(hydroxyl radical)}$$

Also

$$H_2O + e^- \rightarrow e_{aq}^-\ \text{(hydrated electron)}$$

$$e_{aq}^- + O_2 \rightarrow O_2^{-\cdot}\text{(superoxide)}$$

In the order of toxicities, the hydroxyl radical is believed to be the most toxic followed by the superoxide and hydrogen peroxide.

Radiation also induces production of RNS such as nitric oxide, possibly by stimulating nitric oxide synthase (NOS) enzyme (Deliconstantinos et al., 1996a; Leach et al., 2001) using arginine in the cell as the substrate. Nitric oxide (NO) and superoxide formed by radiation can react together to form more toxic peroxynitrite (–OONO) (Deliconstantinos et al., 1996b). Thus, radiation's ultimate damaging effect may result from a combination of events set in motion by permutations and combinations of interactions among the hydroxyl radical, superoxide, NO and peroxynitrite (Figure 27.1).

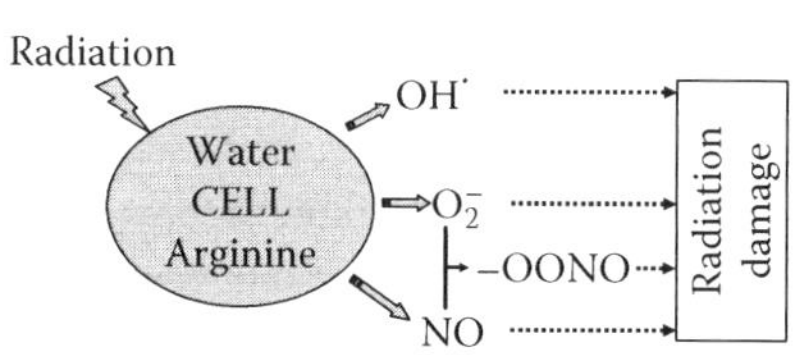

FIGURE 27.1 Proposed roles of ROS and RNS in radiation damage.

It is imperative from the proposed scheme that scavengers of ROS and RNS can function as potential radioprotective agents.

27.3.3 Tocol Nutraceutical Antioxidants as Radiation Countermeasures

Studies on radioprotection provided by tocols have focused mainly on alpha-tocopherol and its acetate and hemisuccinate esters. Probably one of the earliest indications of AT-provided radioprotection was report by Prince and Little (1973), who showed that AT protects erythrocytes from radiation-induced hemolysis. Their findings were confirmed by Brown (1983), who reported that elevated levels of AT in human erythrocytes render them more resistant to radiation.

Subsequently, Srinivasan et al. (1983) demonstrated that AT prevents radiation-induced, delayed-type hypersensitivity. We reported that among mice given 400 IU/kg of AT subcutaneously 24 hr before cobalt-60 irradiation (10.5 Gy), their 30-day postirradiation survival was 70-80%, whereas none survived among control animals (Kumar et al., 2002). When AT was given 12 hr before irradiation, protection was only 45%. We later showed that AT ameliorates radiation-induced peripheral blood cytopenia induced by sublethal irradiation of mice (Kumar et al., 2007). In addition to cellular and whole-animal protection, Felemovicius et al. (1995) reported organ-specific partial protection of exteriorized intestine by AT from radiation-induced enteritis.

Protective effects were also provided by the acetate, phosphate and hemisuccinate esters, as well as with other derivative forms of AT. Tocopherol acetate protected against ultraviolet B(UVB)-radiation-induced *in vitro* inactivation of rat lens enzymes (Reddy and Bhat, 1999). Phosphorylated tocopherol significantly repressed age-related shortening of the chromosome telomere and enlarged cell diameters in neonatal human brain microvascular endotheliocytes (Tanaka et al., 2007). Preliminary studies indicate that tocopherol succinate (ATS) is a better radiation countermeasure than its parent compound, alpha-tocopherol (Singh et al., 2005). The most studied aspect of tocopherol succinate is its effect on cancer cells. In experimental models, there is convincing evidence that ATS reduces human prostate growth significantly more than AT or its acetate ester (Basu et al., 2006). The mechanism of ATS' antitumor effect is believed to result from the induction of apoptosis in tumor cells by inhibiting the BCL-XL-BCL2 function (Shiau et al., 2006).

27.4 TOCOTRIENOL AS A RADIATION COUNTERMEASURE

Compared to the vast number of studies done with AT, radioprotective studies done with tocotrienols are few and results are preliminary. Recent research at the Armed Forces Radiobiology Research Institute (AFRRI) has focused on one of the tocotrienols, gamma-tocotrienol (GT3). We compared the efficacies of AT and GT3 using an 11-Gy radiation dose in mice (LD50/30; the radiation dose at which 50% of animals will die in 30 days for this strain of mice is 8.7 Gy). At this dose (11 Gy), death results primarily from gastrointestinal syndrome. Dose of AT and GT3 was 400 mg/kg body weight given subcutaneously 24 hr before irradiation with Cobalt-60. None of the mice given the vehicle or AT survived. Forty percent of mice receiving GT3 survived, indicating that it is a better radioprotectant than AT (Figure 27.2). Protection observed at this high radiation dose may result from the ability of intestinal epithelial cells to absorb GT3 faster than AT (Tsuzuki et al., 2007). They reported that there is a more rapid transepithelial transport of GT3 than AT in intestinal epithelial CaCO2 cells. They also observed GT3 was absorbed at a faster rate than AT.

AFRRI researchers are studying the possible mechanisms of the superior protection provided by GT3. Some are described below:

1. Measured in terms of International Units or tocopherol equivalent, GT3 has no biological equivalent value as do tocopherols or its esters. But the antioxidant activities of tocotri-

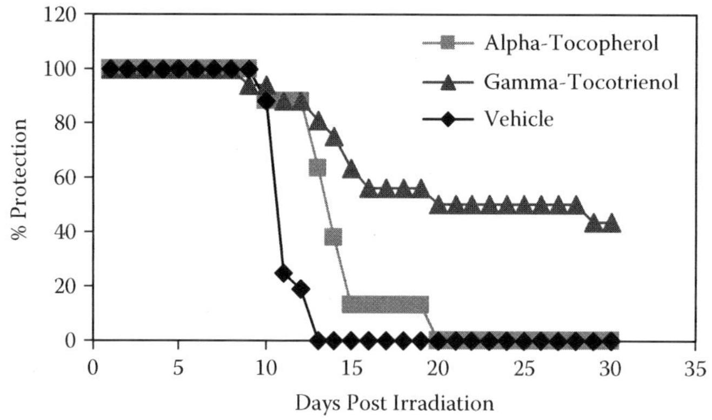

FIGURE 27.2 Comparison of the radioprotective effects of AT and GT3 at 11 Gy.

enols, particularly those of the gamma and delta tocotrienols, are greater than tocopherols (Watkins et al., 1999). GT3's higher levels of antioxidant activity will enhance the efficiency of scavenging free radicals in terms of the variety of ROS scavenged (see Figure 27.1) and, hence, the possibility of increased radioprotection.

2. GT3 more efficiently scavenges RNS induced by radiation exposure. In addition to ROS, radiation also induces RNS (Figure 27.1). Nitric oxide, peroxynitrite and nitroso compounds are formed in human endothelial cells on exposure to ultraviolet radiation and also in human squamous-cell carcinoma (Deliconstantinos et al., 1996b; Villiotou and Deliconstantinos, 1995). Radiation activates xanthine oxidase and nitric oxide synthase in endothelial cells. Superoxide formed from xanthine oxidase and nitric oxide formed by the action of nitric oxide synthase react together to produce peroxynitrite (Figure 27.1), which is more toxic than superoxide or nitric oxide. The specificity of the involvement of nitric oxide synthase is confirmed by use of N-monomethyl-L-arginine (L-NMMA), a compound that inhibits NO synthase activity, which decreases nitric oxide production (Villiotou and Deliconstantinos, 1995). While any agent that decreases the steady-state levels of superoxide or nitric oxide can decrease the generation of peroxynitrite, superior radioprotection by GT3 can be surmised on the assumption that GT3 by itself also is a scavenger of peroxynitrite. This is an area that needs further examination. GT3 also reduced hypertension in SHRs (spontaneously hypertensive rats) by stimulating nitric oxide synthase and increasing the production of nitric oxide, which ultimately reduced hypertension (Newaz et al., 2003).
3. GT3-rich natural sources as well as pure GT3 have anticancer activities. One of the serious long-term effect of radiation is carcinogenesis. Any radioprotectant that can prevent carcinogenesis in addition to short-term lethality will be more desirable than those with only short-term protection. There are extensive reviews about the anticancer effects of tocotrienol (Sen et al., 2007) and three chapters in this book are devoted to tocotrienols and cancer. The tumor-suppressive effects of tocotrienol were demonstrated both *in vitro* and *in vivo*. Wada et al., (2005) showed the *in vitro* antiproliferative effect of GT3 in HepG2 human hepatocellular carcinoma cells and *in vivo* tocotrienols significantly suppressed liver and lung carcinogenesis in mice. Tocotrienol-rich fraction from palm oil is equally effective at suppressing breast cancer (Nesaretnam et al., 2004) as well as promoting the antiproliferative effect in breast cancer cells (Nesaretnam et al., 1995). GT3's antiproliferative activity had been attributed to the inhibition of Akt and NFkB activity in mammary epithelial cells (Sylvester et al., 2005). GT3 also suppressed epidermal growth factor-dependent phosphatidyl inositol-3 kinase mitogenic signaling pathway in neoplastic mammary epithelial cells (Samant and Sylvester, 2006).

In addition to GT3's antiproliferative effect, the anticarcinogenic property of tocotrienols is due to the induction of apoptosis. While lower tocotrienol doses inhibited signaling pathways necessary for the proliferation of tumor cells, higher concentrations of GT3 activated initiator caspase-8 and effecter caspase-3, which are involved in apoptotic processes (Sylvester et al., 2005). Tocotrienol-rich fraction of palm oil responded differentially to normal prostate cells and prostate cancer cells. Normal cells had only marginal growth inhibitory effects with tocotrienol-rich fraction with no G0/G1 arrest and no sub-G1 accumulation of cells, whereas there was G0/G1 arrest and sub-G1 accumulation of prostate cancer cells with tocotrienol-rich fraction of palm oil (Srivastava and Gupta, 2006).

Nesaretnam et al. (2004) provided the most convincing evidence of the effect of tocotrienols on tumor regression from studies using nude mice. They injected MCF-7 breast cancer cells into animals fed orally for 20 weeks with 1 mg/d of tocotrienol-rich fraction (TRF). Compared with control animals, there was significant delay in the onset and incidence of tumors as well as tumor size in mice supplemented with TRF. When the tumor tissue was analyzed for gene expression profiles, 30 out of 1176 genes were affected significantly. Of these 30 genes, 10 were downregulated and 20 upregulated with respect to control. Because immune function is related closely to tumorigenesis, these authors sought to identify genes involved in regulating immune system functions. Among the genes involved in immune function, they found that the expression of the interferon-inducible transmembrane protein-1 and CD59 gene were significantly upregulated in tumors from TRF-fed animals compared to control animals. The c-myc gene was downregulated significantly in tumors from treated mice. These studies establish the significant role of tocotrienols on the host immune system, thereby reducing or aborting tumor growth. They also emphasize reactions of tocotrienol that are independent of antioxidant functions.

We obtained similar results when prostate cancer cells were injected subcutaneously into nude mice (Kumar, Raghavan et al., 2006). In a pilot study using a limited number of animals, eight mice were selected from a group injected with prostate cancer bone-metastasizing (PC3) cells in which the tumor had grown to at least 5 mm in diameter. These were divided into four groups of two animals each. The first group received no treatment, the second and fourth groups were given 400 mg/kg of GT3 subcutaneously. Twenty-four hours later, the third and fourth groups were irradiated with 12 Gy of gamma-irradiation at the site of the tumor.

Tumor growth was monitored for 24 days and, in spite of the small number of mice in each group, the results were convincing. The tumors grew continually for 12 days in unirradiated mice not treated with GT3 but did not grow further for the remaining 12 days. In the group given tocotrienol, tumor size did not increase at all over the 24-day period. In the irradiated group not given tocotrienol, the size of the tumor did not increase for 12 days but then did increase after 12 days, almost the same as the untreated, unirradiated group. When mice were treated with tocotrienol and irradiated, the size of the tumor decreased until the study's final day. With the combined modality of tocotrienol treatment and irradiation, the tumor decreased in size by almost 40% (Figure 27.3).

We also determined the lipid peroxidation in the liver, kidney, rectum and tumor from these mice. The liver was selected as a tissue distal from the prostate tumor irradiation and the kidney and rectum were selected due to their proximity to prostate tumor irradiation. Using ferrous ammonium sulfate (Fe-stimulated), lipid peroxidation was studied in two modes: unstimulated and stimulated. Peroxide was generated *in situ* in homogenates of these tissues by co-incubating with xanthine oxidase and hypoxanthine. Lipid peroxidation was monitored spectrophotometrically by the formation of thiobarbituric acid reactive substances (TBRS) and monitored for 4 (short-term) and 24 (long-term) days after irradiation (Table 27.2).

In the unstimulated groups, 4 days after irradiation, tumor tissue from irradiated mice had the highest amounts of TBRS and liver tissue had the lowest. Mice treated with tocotrienol before irradiation showed a 135% increase in TBRS in tumors, whereas there was no effect in kidney and rectum tissue. Lipid peroxidation was inhibited in liver tissue by 76%. In the long term, the tumor had a higher level of lipid peroxidation even 24 days after irradiation. Tocotrienol caused

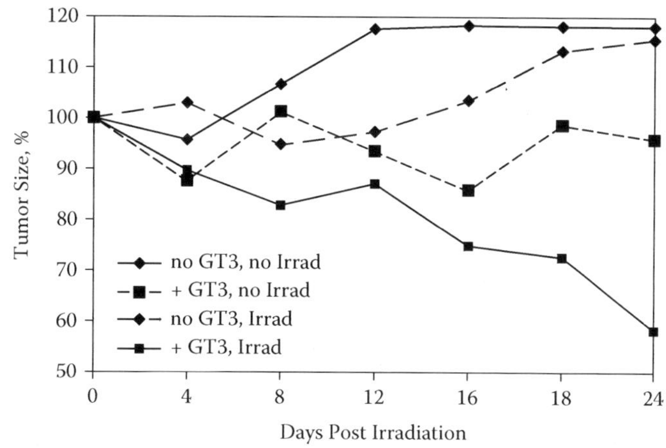

FIGURE 27.3 GT3/irradiation induced regression of prostrate tumor induced by PC3 cells.

TABLE 27.2
Lipid Peroxidation of Tumor and Tissues from Nude Mice with PC3 Cells-Induced Tumor: The Effect of GT3 on Local Radiation (12 Gy)

		Lipid peroxidation (nmoles TBRS/mg protein)			
		Unstimulated		Fe-stimulated	
Tissue	Treatment	Day 4	Day 24	Day 4	Day 24
Liver	Irradiated	212.2 ± 17.7	127.3 ± 1.7	572.9 ± 51.8	185.1 ± 11.4
	γ-T + Irrad.	50.6 ± 4.4	137.0 ± 2.3	150.5 ± 5.1	193.1 ± 4.0
Kidney	Irradiated	254.4 ± 5.1	388.9 ± 20	1034.9 ± 37.2	1066.2 ± 36.7
	γ-T + Irrad.	276 ± 9.6	556.2 ± 33.7	914 ± 56.7	1728 ± 35.7
Rectum	Irradiated	171.8 ± 10.7	553.0 ± 28.9	213.7 ± 21.6	1722.6 ± 414
	γ-T + Irrad.	165.6 ± 14.2	497.8 ± 4.1	276.5 ± 9.4	815.5 ± 124.1
Tumor	Irradiated	560.2 ± 24.5	1181.5 ± 75.7	2178.1 ± 222	3088.5 ± 163.3
	γ-T + Irrad.	1317.7 ± 260.5	1573.5 ± 370.5	5458.9 ± 205.7	5113.0 ± 1621

an increase of lipid peroxidation in tumor tissue (33%) as well as in kidney tissue (43%). Tocotrienol had no effect on lipid peroxidation in the liver and rectum. In the Fe-stimulated groups, TBRS values were very high in tumor tissue in both the short term (4 days) and long term (24 days) after irradiation in comparison with other tissue. Short-term (4 days after irradiation) treatment with tocotrienol resulted in a 150% increase in lipid peroxidation in tumor tissue. There was no significant effect on the kidney or rectum, and lipid peroxidation in the liver was inhibited by 74%. Even 24 days after irradiation, treatment with tocotrienol increased the lipid peroxidation in the kidney and the tumor by 62% and 66%, respectively. There was no effect in the liver but in the rectum there was a 53% inhibition.

Because this was a pilot experiment using a limited number of mice, these data should be interpreted cautiously. However, results indicate a new paradigm of increased lipid peroxidation in tumor tissue of mice injected with GT3, an antioxidant, and irradiated. In addition to suppressing signaling pathways necessary for cell proliferation and stimulating initiator caspase-8 and effecter caspase-3 by GT3 that leads to apoptosis (Sylvester et al., 2005), these findings indicate GT3's pro-oxidant mechanism in tumors and its antioxidant mechanism in normal cells. Thus, it appears that

GT3 responds differently to normal and malignant tissues. A possible explanation may be the differential ability of the normal and cancer cells in handling GT3's metabolic product.

Tocotrienols and tocopherols are oxidized, as a result of free-radical scavenging, to corresponding quinones, which are pro-oxidants (Yoshida et al., 2003). Cancer tissues may not be able to detoxify the pro-oxidant quinones. If they accumulate in the tumor, pro-oxidant quinones can initiate new peroxidation locales and increase the lipid peroxidation of tumor tissue. So, the preferential sensitization of tumor tissues to lipid peroxidation appears to be due to the unmetabolized pro-oxidant products of tocotrienol. In addition to increased lipid peroxidation, other non-oxidant mechanisms related to signal transduction mechanisms may also play a role in reducing tumor size. These include apoptosis by different mechanisms (Shah et al., 2003; Takashi, 2004), inhibition of cell proliferation (Sakai et al., 2004) and modulation of p53, Bax/Bcl2 (Agarwal et al., 2004). However, it seems that alpha-tocopherol does not provide any protection against breast cancer. Moreover, alpha-tocopherol supplementation in the diet alone has little effect on mammary tumors. All tocotrienol isoforms except beta-tocotrienol and to a certain degree delta-tocopherol have potent antiproliferative and proapoptotic effects in breast cancer cells that can reduce risk.

The reported antiproliferative effects of GT3 on cancer cells *in vitro* along with our report on the reduction of tumor size indicate that GT3 may have both prophylactic and therapeutic effects in treating cancer.

27.4.1 Gamma-Tocotrienol and Microvascular Endothelium-Oriented Countermeasures

Radiation affects endothelial function by shifting the thrombohemorrhagic balance from the normal anti-coagulant state to a pro-coagulant state. According to Wang et al., (2002), this results from an increase of the tissue factor (Verheij et al., 1995) and the von Willebrand factor (Jahroudi et al., 1996), as well as from a decrease of prostacyclin (Dunn et al., 1986) and thrombomodulin (TM). Our studies indicate that TM deficiency is an important aspect of radiation-induced endothelial dysfunction. Also that the TM-protein C system is involved in the pathogenesis of both acute and chronic intestinal radiation toxicity (Hauer-Jensen et al., 2004; Richter et al., 1997; Richter et al., 1998; Wang et al., 2002; Wang et al., 2003).

When bound to TM, thrombin loses its pro-coagulant activities and its ability to activate cellular thrombin-receptors (e.g., proteinase-activated receptors, PARs). Instead, thrombin acquires the ability to activate protein C. Activated protein C (APC) limits further thrombin generation and counteracts thrombin's many coagulant, inflammatory and fibroproliferative effects (Esmon et al., 1991). It also has potent intrinsic anti-inflammatory and cytoprotective properties (Mosnier et al., 2004). Moreover, TM exerts protein C-independent anti-inflammatory effects via its ability to bind high mobility group box 1 (HMGB1) protein (Abeyama et al., 2005).

Thrombin exerts its cellular effects by activating proteinase-activated receptors (PARs) on the cell surface. PARs, a four-member subgroup of the G-protein-coupled receptor family, are activated by proteolytic cleavage of the extracellular aminoterminal end. After being cleaved by specific proteinases, the new amino-terminal end activates the ligand binding site on the receptor by a so-called tethered ligand mechanism. Thrombin activates PAR1, PAR3 and PAR4 although PAR1 is the most relevant receptor in inflammation and fibrosis. PAR1 activation promotes endothelial permeability (DeMichele and Minnear, 1992); chemotaxis of neutrophils (Bizios et al., 1986) and monocytes; production of transforming growth factor beta-1 (TGFβ1); and proliferation, migration and collagen production by fibroblasts and smooth muscle cells (Dabbagh et al., 1998; Noda-Heiny and Sobel, 1995; Ragosta et al., 1996). Studies in our laboratory show that intestinal radiation injury is associated with a striking upregulation of PAR1 in endothelium, smooth muscle cells and myofibroblasts, particularly in areas of fibrosis (Wang et al., 2002). Moreover, experiments using PAR1 knockout mice with a small molecule inhibitor of PAR1 activation have confirmed a role for PAR1 in certain aspects of intestinal radiation injury (unpublished data).

Some of these changes in the microvascular endothelium are transient but may be involved mechanistically in developing various aspects of acute radiation injury and lethality. Other changes are more sustained and may play direct roles in radiation fibrosis and in the mechanisms of chronic injury. Particularly promising targets for modulation are the post-radiation shift in thrombohemorrhagic balance toward procoagulation and the accompanying cellular effects of thrombin.

Administration of "traditional" antithrombotics, such as heparin, warfarin, or acetylsalicylic acid, confer some, albeit inconsistent, protection against radiation injury in some organs, including the intestine. Recent studies also have shown that inhibition of ADP-induced platelet aggregation with clopidogrel, as well as direct thrombin inhibition with hirudin, markedly reduce acute and chronic intestinal radiation injury in a rat model (Wang et al., 2002; Wang et al., 2004b). However, when these agents are administered in effective doses, their use also is associated with a significant risk of bleeding complications. Thus, the potential for clinical use is likely limited, particularly in a combined injury situation where optimal hemostasis may be critical (Boegelein et al., 1980). These agents may have potential application as adjuvants in excipients for other radioprotection drugs and may result in synergy for survival-protection from lethality. On the other hand, restoring the TM-protein C pathway or blocking PAR1 present more attractive and presumably safer alternatives for preventing or reducing radiation-induced endothelial dysfunction and its downstream detrimental effects.

Recently, cholesterol-lowering drugs, statins, have emerged as a promising intervention for counteracting radiation-induced endothelial dysfunction. Statins, among the most commonly prescribed drugs in the Western world, are extremely safe. Statins lower cholesterol by inhibiting the conversion of HMG-CoA to mevalonic acid, the rate-limiting step in cholesterol biosynthesis. Also, by decreasing the generation of various mevalonate pathway intermediates, statins reduce the isoprenylation of small GTP-binding proteins (e.g., Rho, Ras, Rac) and other proteins, resulting in effects that are unrelated to lipid-lowering. Through these pleiotropic effects, statins influence a vast array of metabolic and physiological processes, including cell proliferation, apoptosis, immune function, inflammation, coagulation and fibrinolysis.

The vascular endothelium is a major effector cell compartment for the pleiotropic effects of statins. The mechanism underlying most of these effects is related to increased expression and enhanced activity of endothelial nitric oxide synthase (eNOS). Statins prominently upregulate endothelial TM *in vitro*, in an eNOS-dependent manner (Masamura et al., 2003; Shi et al., 2003). This occurs via a mechanism involving S-nitrosylation, dissociation of heat shock protein 90 (HSP90) from heat shock factor 1 (HSF1) and binding of HSF1 to specific heat shock elements in the TM promoter (Fu et al., 2006). Statins ameliorate gut toxicity *in vivo* after localized irradiation of the exteriorized small intestine in mice; after localized, fractionated small bowel irradiation in rats (Wang, Qui et al., 2004a; Wang, Boerma et al., 2007); and lung injury in mice after irradiation of the chest (Williams et al., 2004).

Researchers are currently investigating the use of statins as radiation response modifiers after total body irradiation. Interestingly, modulation of nitric oxide ameliorates the hematopoietic radiation syndrome in mice (Liebmann et al., 1994) and eNOS is absolutely required for appropriate hematopoietic progenitor cell mobilization and recovery after myelosuppressive insults (Aicher et al., 2003). Hence, the fact that most of the pleiotropic statin effects, including the regulation of TM, are eNOS-dependent, provide a strong rationale for testing statins in hematopoietic injury as well.

Tocols (tocopherols and tocotrienols) protect progenitor cells in the GI tract and the hematopoietic system from the effects of ionizing radiation by virtue of their antioxidant properties and by preventing endothelial dysfunction (Schulz et al., 2004). Although comparative studies of antioxidant activity of tocols suggest that their antioxidant properties are similar (Suarna et al., 1993; Yoshida et al., 2003), there are substantial differences among tocols in terms of their radioprotective efficacies. We have evidence to suggest that GT3 is significantly more potent as a radiation prophylactic agent than other alpha-tocopherol (Figure 27.2).

An important feature distinguishing GT3 from other tocols relates to its ability to inhibit HMG-CoA reductase (Qureshi et al., 1986). Hence, compared to tocopherols, tocotrienols accumulate in endothelial cells to levels that are 25- to 95-fold greater (Naito et al., 2005) and are 10-fold

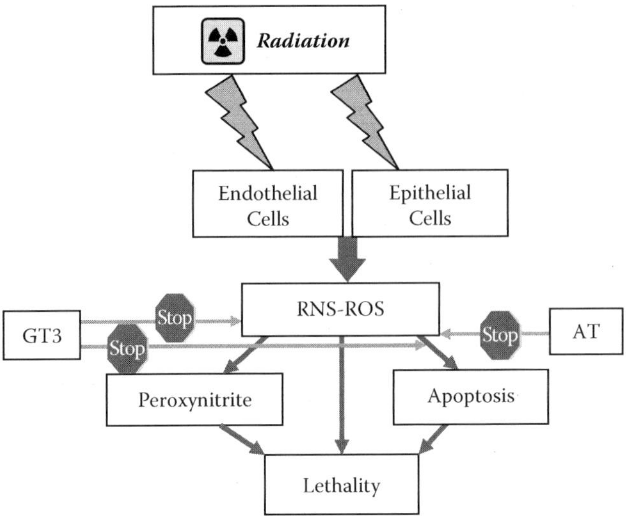

FIGURE 27.4 Schematic diagram showing interactions between epithelial and endothelial radiation injury and the possible superior role of GT3 to AT in radiation protection.

more effective in reducing adhesion molecule expression (Theriault et al., 1999). GT3's HMG-CoA reductase inhibitory activity is 30-fold greater than that of alpha-tocotrienol (Pearce et al., 1992). This feature places GT3 in a unique position among the tocols.

Ongoing studies support the notion that some of GT3's radioprotective effects are attributable to HMG-CoA reductase inhibition (unpublished data). A recent study showed that GT3 reduces the activity of HMG-CoA reductase by triggering ubiquitination of the enzyme, resulting in endoplasmic reticulum-associated degradation by 26 S proteasomes (Song and DeBose-Boyd, 2006). Hence, there are interesting possibilities for combining GT3 with statins to take advantage of the potential synergy from simultaneously increasing enzyme degradation and inhibiting enzyme activity. Although it was suggested recently that AT functions only as an antioxidant, GT3 activities reveal properties other than antioxidant functions. Figure 27.4 shows these reactions schematically.

27.4.2 Gamma-Tocotrienol and Pentoxifylline

The phosphodiesterase inhibitor pentoxifylline, in addition to exhibiting antioxidant properties, has a variety of other biochemical, immunomodulatory, anti-cytokine, vascular and rheologic effects. While the initial impetus for investigating this compound in the context of radiation injury was its presumed rheological properties (Dion et al., 1989; Dion et al., 1990), other effects more likely are responsible for its efficacy, particularly its endothelial effects. Hence, pentoxifylline is one of relatively few drugs shown to strongly upregulate endothelial TM (Ohdama et al., 1991; Seigneur et al., 1995) and downregulate tissue factor expression (Leclerc et al., 1995).

In the context of radiation toxicity, pentoxifylline has been used, mostly with vitamin E, to treat established radiation-induced fibrosis and found to be effective in some studies (Delanian et al., 2003; Okunieff et al., 2004). The effectiveness of pentoxifylline to prevent early radiation toxicity in general and specifically in the gut is unclear. However, because pentoxifylline also appears to have benefits in trauma, shock and critical care (Akgur et al., 1999; Boldt et al., 1996; Coe et al., 1997), it may be of particular benefit in combined injury situations.

27.4.3 GT3 and Shock-Induced Neuronal and Pulmonary Damage

For several reasons, the nervous system is vulnerable to the damaging effects of highly reactive free radicals. The brain contains large amounts of polyunsaturated fatty acids that are susceptible to lipid peroxidation, receives a large percentage of oxygen and is relatively deficient in certain antioxidant enzymes. In addition, specific regions of the brain have high iron concentrations. So, antioxidant defenses are critically important to protect the brain and neural tissues from oxidative damage (Floyd, 1999).

Most available research on the role of antioxidant nutrients in neurological function has focused on vitamin E because it is the major lipid-soluble, chain-breaking antioxidant in the body, protecting the membrane integrity by inhibiting lipid peroxidation. Orally supplemented vitamin E reaches the cerebrospinal fluid and brain (Vatassery, 1998). Most vitamin E-sensitive neurological disorders are associated with elevated levels of oxidative damage markers, indicating that vitamin E's neuroprotective effects are wholly mediated by its antioxidant property.

However, alpha-tocotrienol has been shown to protect neuronal cells from glutamate-, homocysteine- and L-buthionine sulfoximine-induced toxicity (Khanna, Roy, Ryu et al., 2003). The buthionine sulfoximine-induced toxicity indicates that toxicity results from depletion of glutathione, which also has been observed in radiation exposure scenarios. Long-term time-lapse imaging studies reveal that neurons and their axo-dendritic network are fairly motile under standard culture conditions. Such motility was arrested in response to glutamate challenge. Tocotrienol-treated primary neurons maintained healthy growth and motility even in the presence of excess glutamate.

Pulmonary injury and neurotrauma are associated with shock and trauma and it is reported that in blast-injured rats, there was a significant elevation of total nitrite/nitrate levels 3 and 24 hours after injury (Cernak et al., 1996; Cernak et al., 2001). Elevated NO levels were accompanied by changes in the expression of inducible nitric oxide synthase mRNA. The effect of AT and GT3 in minimizing oxidative damage by hydrogen peroxide was compared in astrocytes, which support the survival of central nervous system (CNS) neurons (Mazlan et al., 2006). Although gamma-tocotrienol was toxic at concentrations >200 microM, it protected cells against hydrogen peroxide-induced cell loss and apoptosis in a dose-dependent manner up to 100 microM. AT was not cytotoxic up to 750 microM and, like GT3, reduced apoptosis but was less effective than GT3 in maintaining viable cell numbers.

These studies show the possibility of using GT3 to protect the brain from neuronal damage induced by a combined injury radiation-trauma model. GT3's improved protection of astrocytes from oxidative damage may be due to the unsaturated side chain of tocotrienol that allows for more efficient penetration into tissues, such as brain having saturated fatty layers (Suzuki et al., 1993).

2.74.4 GT3 and Other Agents—Potential for Synergism

Decreased expression of prostacyclin is one of the factors that causes a pronounced shift in the thrombohemorrhagic balance from the normal anti-coagulant state to a pro-coagulant state on irradiation (Rubin et al., 1985). We reported that combining iloprost (a prostacyclin) with misoprostol results in a synergistic increase in radioprotection (Kumar et al., 1997). When doses of iloprost and misoprostol were administered subcutaneously to mice before irradiation, neither provided significant protection. But when the two compounds were combined, the synergistic protection was almost 100%. This indicates that prostacyclin synergistically can increase protection with a radioprotectant that functions with a different mechanism, such as GT3. Srinivasan and Weiss (1992) reported that AT enhances protection when combined with a methylated derivative of amifostine (WR-3689). Mice treated with AT 1 hr before irradiation were also given WR-3689 intraperitoneally 30 min before irradiation. Survival increased in mice given AT and WR-3689 compared with mice given WR-3689 alone: the DRF for WR-3689 (150 mg) was 1.35 [1.32, 1.38]; for WR-3689 combined with vitamin E (100 IU), the DRF was 1.49 [1.45, 1.53]. Because GT3 is a more effective radioprotectant than AT, such combinations could elicit greater protection.

27.4.5 Better Excipient Formulations to Increase Radioprotective Efficacy

Drug formulation is an important and integral concern, especially for lipophilic drugs such as GT3. Improved formulation of AT increased its radioprotective efficacy, probably resulting from better solubilization that enabled AT to be absorbed easily from the site of injection to attain a steady level in blood affording better protection (Kumar et al., 2002). Formulation will be a crucial factor in oral preparations, particularly in patients with symptoms of malabsorption due to cystic fibrosis (Papas et al., 2007). These authors reported a 2.5-fold increase in absorption of tocols given a water-soluble preparation as compared to oil-based soft gels. The absorption of one tocol, gamma-tocopherol, was 4.5-fold greater with the water-based formulations than with oil-based soft gels.

Increasing a drug's hydrophilicity-lipohilicity balance (HLB) has become an important challenge to pharmaceutical product manufacturers. Several excipients have been developed to increase the HLB numbers, i.e., to achieve improved solubilization. Solubilizing excipients that may be relevant to GT3 are (1) water-soluble organic solvents (polyethylene glycols, PEG-300, PEG-400; dimethylacetamide, DMA), (2) non-ionic surfactants (Cremaphors, Tween 80, Tween 20, Labrasol, etc.) and (3) cyclodextrins (alpha- and beta-cyclodextrin; sulfobutylether-beta-cyclodextrin, also called SBE-gamma-CD or Captisol) (Strickley, 2004).

Our studies with another radioprotectant indicate that use of Tween-80 as an excipient enables 100% protection at lethal radiation dose, compared to inconsistent values obtained without Tween-80. Although we used subcutaneous administration, Tween-80 can be used orally, intramuscularly and intravenously (Cercueil et al., 2004; Strickley, 2004) and at concentrations from 0.4% (intravenous) to 12% (intramuscular). Formulation with Captisol also can be used for both oral and parenteral formulations (Ma et al., 1999). If necessary, its penetrating power can be increased by 4% limonene in 2% Captisol (Krishnaiah et al., 2004).

Preparation of water soluble prodrugs is a strategy used to increase the bioavailability of fat-soluble tocols like GT3. Akaho et al., synthesized three kinds of ester derivatives of GT3 and evaluated their use as hydrophilic GT3 prodrugs *in vitro* and *in vivo* (Akaho et al., 2007). One derivative, N,N-dimethylaminoacetate hydrochloride, was a solid compound with high solubility and stability in water. It was converted to GT3 by esterases in rat and human liver. Intravenous administration of this derivative to rats led to a rapid increase of GT3 in the plasma, liver, heart and kidney. Although there was no significant difference in the bioavailability (plasma level) of the derivative as compared to GT3 in surfactant, the availability in liver was twofold greater than with GT3 in a surfactant. The plasma level of the metabolic product of GT3, 2,7,8-trimethyl-2S-(beta-carboxyethyl)-6-hydroxychroman (S-gamma-CEHC), was almost twofold higher with the derivative than with GT3 in surfactant. Similar results were obtained using a water-soluble derivative of AT, alpha-tocopherol monoglucoside (TMG; Nadezda et al., 2005). TMG was effective even when given after radiation. TMG ameliorated peripheral blood cytopenia observed after irradiation.

27.5 CONCLUSIONS

Preliminary studies indicate that GT3 is an effective radiation countermeasure. It could be further developed for use by first responders and remedial workers in a nuclear/radiological fallout field and for astronauts engaged in extravehicular activity in space. Increasing studies also indicate that GT3 is an antiproliferative and pro-apoptotic drug for cancer cells but not for normal cells. A pilot study using a limited number of animals supports this concept.

These studies indicate that GT3 not only is an effective countermeasure against radiation-induced short-term lethality but also could prevent long-term effects like cancer. Another interesting aspect of GT3 is its profound inhibition of the HMG-CoA reductase enzyme, which is linked to protection against radiation-induced injury of the endothelium. GT3 also inhibits shock-induced peroxidative changes in neurons.

Based on available data, it appears that GT3's radiation protection may result from its ability not only to detoxify/terminate radiation-induced ROS but also to scavenge or degrade RNS and the products of their interactions. These studies indicate that GT3 can be useful as a radiation countermeasure for radiation-induced hematopoietic and gastrointestinal syndromes and ameliorate some of the adverse effects of radiation injury combined with shock and trauma. Finally, combining GT3 with other countermeasures (e.g., pentoxifylline) holds particular promise.

27.6 FUTURE DIRECTIONS

Clearly, findings reported here should be reinforced with additional experiments. The current focus is on developing GT3 as a prophylactic countermeasure for ionizing radiation (IR) exposure scenarios. But in a civilian mass-casualty scenario, there would be an urgent need for therapeutic measures available for victims of IR exposure. Therefore, extensive studies are needed to test its efficacy as a radiation therapeutic agent.

Treating combined injuries resulting from a nuclear/radiological scenario is complicated, unpredictable and multifaceted. Thus, there is a clear need for an improved understanding of the pathophysiology underlying interactions between radiation and other types of tissue injury and their mechanisms. Research is needed to test the efficacy of GT3, if any, under these circumstances.

A serious concern with lipophilic agents such as GT3 is the extent to which they are absorbed from the intestine to provide sufficient levels in blood to be effective. Pharmacokinetic and pharmacodynamic studies with formulations using novel excipients will be able to address this question and recommend effective formulations for testing GT3's efficacy as a radiation therapeutic agent.

ACKNOWLEDGMENTS

The authors acknowledge editorial help by Frank Duffy and help with reference management by Nancy Morell. Financial support: Defense Threat Reduction Agency grants number H.10027_07_AR_R to KSK and HDTRA1-07-C-0028 to MH-J and a University Technology Development Award to KSK by the Maryland Technology Development Corporation (TEDCO). All grants were awarded through The Henry M. Jackson Foundation for the Advancement of Military Medicine Inc., Rockville, MD. KSK was also supported by Armed Forces Radiobiology Research Institute grant RAB2AA. MH-J was also supported by the National Institutes of Health grant CA83719.

REFERENCES

Abeyama, K., D.M. Stern, Y. Ito, K. Kawahara, Y. Yoshimoto, M. Tanaka, T. Uchimura, N. Ida, Y. Yamazaki, S. Yamada, Y. Yamamoto, H. Yamamoto, S. Iino, N. Taniguchi, I. Maruyama. 2005. The N-terminal domain of thrombomodulin sequesters high-mobility group-B1 protein, a novel antiinflammatory mechanism. *J Clin Invest*, 115, 1267–74.

Agarwal, M.K., M.L. Agarwal, M. Athar, S. Gupta. 2004. Tocotrienol-rich fraction of palm oil activates p53, modulates Bax/Bcl2 ratio and induces apoptosis independent of cell cycle association. *Cell Cycle*, 3, 205–11.

Aicher, A., C. Heeschen, C. Mildner–Rihm, C. Urbich, C. Ihling, K. Technau–Ihling, A.M. Zeiher, S. Dimmeler. 2003. Essential role of endothelial nitric oxide synthase for mobilization of stem and progenitor cells. *Nat Med*, 9, 1370–6.

Akaho, N., J. Takata, T. Fukushima, K. Matsunaga, A. Hattori, R. Hidaka, K. Fukui, M. Yoshida, T. Fujioka, Y. Karube, K. Imai. 2007. Preparation and in vivo evaluation of a water–soluble prodrug for 2R–{gamma}tocotrienol and as a two–step prodrug for S–{gamma}–CEHC in rat. *Drug Metab Dispos*.

Akgur, F.M., G.B. Zibari, J.C. McDonald, D.N. Granger, M.F. Brown. 1999. Effects of dextran and pentoxifylline on hemorrhagic shock-induced P-selectin expression. *J Surg Res*, 87, 232–8.

Basu, A., B. Grossie, M. Bennett, N. Mills, V. Imrhan. 2006. Alpha-tocopheryl succinate (alpha-TOS) modulates human prostate LNCaP xenograft growth and gene expression in BALB/c nude mice fed two levels of dietary soybean oil. *Eur J Nutr*.

Bizios, R., L. Lai, J.W. Fenton, 2nd, A.B. Malik. 1986. Thrombin-induced chemotaxis and aggregation of neutrophils. *J Cell Physiol*, 128, 485–90.

Boegelein, K., K.E. Reichenbach–Klinke, O. Messerschmidt. 1980. [Investigations of combined injuries, 28th communication: Troubles of hemostatic equilibrium arising from radiation and combined injuries (author's trans)]. *Strahlentherapie*, 156, 430–6.

Boldt, J., M. Muller, S. Heyn, I. Welters, G. Hempelmann. 1996. Influence of long–term continuous intravenous administration of pentoxifylline on endothelial–related coagulation in critically ill patients. *Crit Care Med*, 24, 940–6.

Brown, M.A. 1983. Resistance of human erythrocytes containing elevated levels of vitamin E to radiation-induced hemolysis. *Radiat Res*, 95, 303–16.

Capizzi, R.L., W. Oster. 1995. Protection of normal tissue from the cytotoxic effects of chemotherapy and radiation by amifostine: Clinical experiences. *Eur J Cancer*, 31A Suppl 1, S8–13.

Cercueil, J.P., E. Ferrant, N. Isambert, J.L. Jouve, M. Flesch, D. Krause, L. Bedenne, B. Chauffert. 2004. Sustained clinical response of large hepatocellular carcinoma after chemoembolization with pirarubicin, amiodarone and Lipiodol. *Gastroenterol Clin Biol,* 28, 1281–3.

Cernak, I., J. Savic, Z. Malicevic, G. Zunic, P. Radosevic, I. Ivanovic, L. Davidovic. 1996. Involvement of the central nervous system in the general response to pulmonary blast injury. *J Trauma,* 40, S100–4.

Cernak, I., Z. Wang, J. Jiang, X. Bian, J. Savic. 2001. Cognitive deficits following blast injury-induced neurotrauma: possible involvement of nitric oxide. *Brain Inj,* 15, 593–612.

Coe, D.A., J.A. Freischlag, D. Johnson, J.H. Mudaliar, S.A. Kosciesza, D.K. Traul, P.C. Chiang, R.A. Cambria, G.R. Seabrook, J.B. Towne. 1997. Pentoxifylline prevents endothelial damage due to ischemia and reperfusion injury. *J Surg Res,* 67, 21–5.

Dabbagh, K., G.J. Laurent, R.J. McAnulty, R.C. Chambers. 1998. Thrombin stimulates smooth muscle cell procollagen synthesis and mRNA levels via a PAR–1 mediated mechanism. *Thromb Haemost,* 79, 405–9.

Davidson, D.E., M.M. Greenan, T.R. Sweeney. 1980. Biological characteristics of some improved radioprotectors. In *Radiation sensitizers, their use in the clinical management of cancer,* Brady, L.W. (Ed.) Masson: New York, 309–320.

Davis, T.A., T.K. Clarke, S.R. Mog, M.R. Landauer. 2007. Subcutaneous administration of genistein prior to lethal irradiation supports multilineage, hematopoietic progenitor cell recovery and survival. *Int J Radiat Biol,* 83, 141–51.

Delanian, S., R. Porcher, S. Balla-Mekias, J.L. Lefaix. 2003. Randomized, placebo-controlled trial of combined pentoxifylline and tocopherol for regression of superficial radiation-induced fibrosis. *J Clin Oncol,* 21, 2545–50.

Deliconstantinos, G., V. Villiotou, J.C. Stavrides. 1996a. Alterations of nitric oxide synthase and xanthine oxidase activities of human keratinocytes by ultraviolet B radiation. Potential role for peroxynitrite in skin inflammation. *Biochem Pharmacol,* 51, 1727–38.

Deliconstantinos, G., V. Villiotou, J. C. Stavrides. 1996b. Nitric oxide and peroxynitrite released by ultraviolet B–irradiated human endothelial cells are possibly involved in skin erythema and inflammation. *Exp Physiol,* 81, 1021–33.

DeMichele, M.A., F.L. Minnear. 1992. Modulation of vascular endothelial permeability by thrombin. *Semin Thromb Hemost,* 18, 287–95.

Devi, P.U., K.S. Bisht, M. Vinitha. 1998. A comparative study of radioprotection by Ocimum flavonoids and synthetic aminothiol protectors in the mouse. *Br J Radiol,* 71, 782–4.

Dion, M.W., D.H. Hussey, J.W. Osborne. 1989. The effect of pentoxifylline on early and late radiation injury following fractionated irradiation in C3H mice. *Int J Radiat Oncol Biol Phys,* 17, 101–7.

Dion, M.W., D.H. Hussey, J.F. Doornbos, A.P. Vigliotti, B.C. Wen, B. Anderson. 1990. Preliminary results of a pilot study of pentoxifylline in the treatment of late radiation soft tissue necrosis. *Int J Radiat Oncol Biol Phys,* 19, 401–7.

Dunn, M.M., E.A. Drab, D.B. Rubin. 1986. Effects of irradiation on endothelial cell–polymorphonuclear leukocyte interactions. *J Appl Physiol,* 60, 1932–7.

Esmon, C.T., F.B. Taylor, Jr., T.R. Snow. 1991. Inflammation and coagulation: Linked processes potentially regulated through a common pathway mediated by protein C. *Thromb Haemost,* 66, 160–5.

Felemovicius, I., M.E. Bonsack, M.L. Baptista, J.P. Delaney. 1995. Intestinal radioprotection by vitamin E (alpha-tocopherol). *Ann Surg,* 222, 504–8, discussion 508–10.

Floyd, R. 1999. Antioxidants, oxidative stress and degenerative neurological disorders. *Proc. Soc. Exp. Biol. Med.,* 222, 236–245.

Fu, Q., J. Wang, X. Qiu, L.M. Fink, M. Hauer-Jensen. 2006. Mechanisms of transcriptional regulation of endothelial cell thrombomodulin by statins (Abstr.). *Radiat Res Soc,* 53, 106.

Glover, D., L.J.J. Riley, K. Carmichael, B. Spar, J.H. Glick, E. Slatopolsky, M. Attie, S. Goldfarb. 1983. Hypocalcemia and inhibition of parathyroid hormone secretion following administration of WR–2721: A radio- and chemo protective agent. *N. Engl. J. Med,* 309, 1137–1141.

Goel, H.C., H. Prakash, A. Ali, M. Bala. 2007. Podophyllum hexandrum modulates gamma radiation-induced immunosuppression in Balb/c mice: implications in radioprotection. *Mol Cell Biochem,* 295, 93–103.

Hanson, W.R., K.A. Houseman, P.W. Collins. 1988. Radiation protection in vivo by prostaglandins and related compounds of the arachidonic acid cascade. *Pharmacol Ther,* 39, 347–56.

Hauer-Jensen, M., L.M. Fink, J. Wang. 2004. Radiation injury and the protein C pathway. *Crit Care Med,* 32, S325–30.

Jahroudi, N., A.M. Ardekani, J.S. Greenberger. 1996. Ionizing irradiation increases transcription of the von Willebrand factor gene in endothelial cells. *Blood,* 88, 3801–14.

Khanna, S., S. Roy, H. Ryu, P. Bahadduri, P.W. Swaan, R.R. Ratan, C.K. Sen. 2003. Molecular basis of vitamin E action: tocotrienol modulates 12-lipoxygenase, a key mediator of glutamate-induced neurodegeneration. *J Biol Chem,* 278, 43508–15.

Krishnaiah, Y.S., P. Bhaskar, V. Satyanarayana. 2004. Formulation and evaluation of limonene-based membrane-moderated transdermal therapeutic system of nimodipine. *Drug Deliv,* 11, 1–9.

Kumar, K.S., Y.N. Vaishnav, J.F. Weiss. 1988. Radioprotection by antioxidant enzymes and enzyme mimetics. *Pharmacol Ther,* 39, 301–9.

Kumar, K.S., V. Srinivasan, D. Palazzolo, J. M. Kendrick, E. P. Clark. 1997. Synergistic protection of irradiated mice by a combination of iloprost and misoprostol. *Adv Exp Med Biol,* 400B, 831–9.

Kumar, K.S., V. Srinivasan, R. Toles, L. Jobe, T. Seed. 2002. Nutritional approaches to radioprotection: Vitamin E. *Mil Med,* 167, 57–59.

Kumar, K.S., V. Srinivasan, R. Toles, V. Miner, T. Seed. 2003. Recovery of reticulocytes and prevention of radiation-induced weight loss in mice by gamma-tocotrienol: Possible application to cancer therapy. In *Book of Abstracts. 12th International Congress of Radiation Research,* p153., Brisbane, Australia.

Kumar, K.S., M. Raghavan, K. Hieber, C. Ege, S. Mog, N. Parra, A. Hildabrand, V. Singh, V. Srinivasan, R. Toles, P. Karikari, G. Petrovics, T. Seed, S. Srivastava, A. Papas. 2006. Preferential radiation sensitization of prostate cancer in nude mice by nutraceutical antioxidant gamma-tocotrienol. *Life Sci,* 78, 2099–2104.

Kumar, K.S., T.Z. Kao, S. Ghosh. 2007. Radiation protection by nutraceuticals: Alpha-tocopherol. Current Problems of Radiation Research—*Proc 35th Ann Meet Eur Radiat Res Soc,* Kyiv, Ukraine, August 22–25, 2006., Grodzinsky, D., A. Dmitriev (Eds.) National Academy of Sciences of Ukraine: Kyiv, pp 199–210.

Landauer, M.R., H.D. Davis, K.S. Kumar, J.F. Weiss. 1992. Behavioral toxicity of selected radioprotectors. *Adv Space Res,* 12, 273–83.

Landauer, M.R., V. Srinivasan, T.M. Seed. 2003. Genistein treatment protects mice from ionizing radiation injury. *J Appl Toxicol,* 23, 379–85.

Leach, J.K., G. Van Tuyle, P.S. Lin, R. Schmidt-Ullrich, R.B. Mikkelsen. 2001. Ionizing radiation-induced, mitochondria-dependent generation of reactive oxygen/nitrogen. *Cancer Res,* 61, 3894–901.

Leclerc, N.E., G. HaaN-Archipoff, M. Lenoble, A. Beretz. 1995. Inhibitors of phosphodiesterase (pentoxifylline, trequinsin) inhibit apical and subcellular matrix expression of tissue factor in cultured human endothelial cells. *J Cardiovasc Pharmacol,* 25 Suppl 2, S88–91.

Liebmann, J., A.M. DeLuca, D. Coffin, L.K. Keefer, D. Venzon, D.A. Wink, J.B. Mitchell. 1994. In vivo radiation protection by nitric oxide modulation. *Cancer Res,* 54, 3365–8.

Ma, D.Q., R.A. Rajewski, V.J. Stella. 1999. New injectable melphalan formulations utilizing (SBE)(7m)-beta-CD or HP-beta-CD. *Int J Pharm,* 189, 227–34.

MacVittie, T.J., A.M. Farese. 2002. Cytokine based treatment of radiation injury: Potential benefits after low-level radiation exposure. *Mil Med,* 167, 68–70.

Masamura, K., K. Oida, H. Kanehara, J. Suzuki, S. Horie, H. Ishii, I. Miyamori. 2003. Pitavastatin-induced thrombomodulin expression by endothelial cells acts via inhibition of small G proteins of the Rho family. *Arterioscler Thromb Vasc Biol,* 23, 512–7.

Maurya, D.K., T.P. Devasagayam, C.K. Nair. 2006. Some novel approaches for radioprotection and the beneficial effect of natural products. *Indian J Exp Biol,* 44, 93–114.

Maurya, D.K., S. Adhikari, C.K. Nair, T.P. Devasagayam. 2007. DNA protective properties of vanillin against gamma-radiation under different conditions: Possible mechanisms. *Mutat Res.*

Mazlan, M., T. Sue Mian, G. Mat Top, W. Zurinah Wan Ngah. 2006. Comparative effects of alpha-tocopherol and gamma-tocotrienol against hydrogen peroxide induced apoptosis on primary-cultured astrocytes. *J Neurol Sci,* 243, 5–12.

Mosnier, L.O., A.J. Gale, S. Yegneswaran, J.H. Griffin. 2004. Activated protein C variants with normal cytoprotective but reduced anticoagulant activity. *Blood*, 104, 1740–4.

Nadezda, C., A. Shishkina, I. Butorin, H. Murase, P. Gervas, T.V. Kagiya. 2005. Effect of tocopherol-monoglucoside (TMG), a water-soluble glycosylated derivate of vitamin E, on hematopoietic recovery in irradiated mice. *J Radiat Res* (Tokyo), 46, 37–41.

Naito, Y., M. Shimozawa, M. Kuroda, N. Nakabe, H. Manabe, K. Katada, S. Kokura, H. Ichikawa, N. Yoshida, N. Noguchi, T. Yoshikawa. 2005. Tocotrienols reduce 25-hydroxycholesterol-induced monocyte-endothelial cell interaction by inhibiting the surface expression of adhesion molecules. *Atherosclerosis*, 180, 19–25.

Nesaretnam, K., N. Guthrie, A.F. Chambers, K.K. Carroll. 1995. Effect of tocotrienols on the growth of a human breast cancer cell line in culture. *Lipids*, 30, 1139–43.

Nesaretnam, K., R. Ambra, K.R. Selvaduray, A. Radhakrishnan, K. Reimann, G. Razak, F. Virgili. 2004. Tocotrienol–rich fraction from palm oil affects gene expression in tumors resulting from MCF–7 cell inoculation in athymic mice. *Lipids*, 39, 459–67.

Newaz, M.A., Z. Yousefipour, N. Nawal, N. Adeeb. 2003. Nitric oxide synthase activity in blood vessels of spontaneously hypertensive rats: Antioxidant protection by gamma-tocotrienol. *J Physiol Pharmacol,* 54, 319–27.

Noda–Heiny, H., B.E. Sobel. 1995. Vascular smooth muscle cell migration mediated by thrombin and urokinase receptor. *Am J Physiol,* 268, C1195–201.

Ohdama, S., S. Takano, K. Ohashi, S. Miyake, N. Aoki. 1991. Pentoxifylline prevents tumor necrosis factor-induced suppression of endothelial cell surface thrombomodulin. *Thromb Res,* 62, 745–55.

Okunieff, P., E. Augustine, J.E. Hicks, T.L. Cornelison, R.M. Altemus, B.G. Naydich, I. Ding, A.K. Huser, E.H. Abraham, J.J. Smith, N. Coleman, L.H. Gerber. 2004. Pentoxifylline in the treatment of radiation-induced fibrosis. *J Clin Oncol,* 22, 2207–13.

Papas, K., J. Kalbfleisch, R. Mohon. 2007. Bioavailability of a novel, water-soluble vitamin E formulation in malabsorbing patients. *Dig Dis Sci,* 52, 347–52.

Pearce, B.C., R.A. Parker, M.E. Deason, A.A. Qureshi, J.J. Wright. 1992. Hypocholesterolemic activity of synthetic and natural tocotrienols. *J Med Chem,* 35, 3595–606.

Pellmar, T.C., S. Rockwell. 2005. R.N.T.C.W. Group. Meeting report: Priority list of research areas for radiological nuclear threat countermeasures. *Radiat. Res.,* 163, 115–123.

Prince, E.W., J.B. Little. 1973. The effect of dietary fatty acids and tocopherol on the radiosensitivity of mammalian erythrocytes. *Radiat Res,* 53, 49–64.

Qureshi, A.A., W.C. Burger, D.M. Peterson, C.E. Elson. 1986. The structure of an inhibitor of cholesterol biosynthesis isolated from barley. *J Biol Chem,* 261, 10544–50.

Ragosta, M., W.L. Barry, L.W. Gimple, S.D. Gertz, K.W. McCoy, G.A. Stouffer, C.A. McNamara, E.R. Powers, G.K. Owens, I.J. Sarembock. 1996. Effect of thrombin inhibition with desulfatohirudin on early kinetics of cellular proliferation after balloon angioplasty in atherosclerotic rabbits. *Circulation*, 93, 1194–200.

Reddy, G.B., K.S. Bhat. 1999. Protection against UVB inactivation (in vitro) of rat lens enzymes by natural antioxidants. *Mol Cell Biochem,* 194, 41–5.

Richter, K.K., L.M. Fink, B.M. Hughes, C.C. Sung, M. Hauer-Jensen. 1997. Is the loss of endothelial thrombomodulin involved in the mechanism of chronicity in late radiation enteropathy? *Radiother Oncol,* 44, 65–71.

Richter, K.K., L.M. Fink, B.M. Hughes, H.M. Shmaysani, C.C. Sung, M. Hauer-Jensen. 1998. Differential effect of radiation on endothelial cell function in rectal cancer and normal rectum. *Am J Surg,* 176, 642–7.

Rubin, D.B., E.A. Drab, C.H. Ts'ao, D. Gardner, W.F. Ward. 1985. Prostacyclin synthesis in irradiated endothelial cells cultured from bovine aorta. *J Appl Physiol,* 58, 592–7.

Sakai, M., M. Okabe, M. Yamasaki, H. Tachibana, K. Yamada. 2004. Induction of apoptosis by tocotrienol in rat hepatoma dRLh–84 cells. *Anticancer Res,* 24, 1683–8.

Samant, G.V., P.W. Sylvester. 2006. Gamma-tocotrienol inhibits ErbB3–dependent PI3K/Akt mitogenic signalling in neoplastic mammary epithelial cells. *Cell Prolif,* 39, 563–74.

Schulz, E., E. Anter, J.F. Keaney, Jr. 2004. Oxidative stress, antioxidants and endothelial function. *Curr Med Chem,* 11, 1093–104.

Seigneur, M., P. Dufourcq, F. Belloc, M. Lenoble, M. Renard, M.R. Boisseau. 1995. Influence of pentoxifylline on membrane thrombomodulin levels in endothelial cells submitted to hypoxic conditions. *J Cardiovasc Pharmacol,* 25 Suppl 2, S85–7.

Sen, C.K., S. Khanna, S. Roy. 2007. Tocotrienols in health and disease: The other half of the natural vitamin E family. *Molec. Aspects Med.,* 28(5-6), 692–728.

Shah, S., A. Gapor, P.W. Sylvester. 2003. Role of caspase-8 activation in mediating vitamin E-induced apoptosis in murine mammary cancer cells. *Nutr Cancer,* 45, 236–46.

Shi, J., J. Wang, H. Zheng, W. Ling, J. Joseph, D. Li, J.L. Mehta, U. Ponnappan, P. Lin, L.M. Fink, M. Hauer-Jensen. 2003. Statins increase thrombomodulin expression and function in human endothelial cells by a nitric oxide-dependent mechanism and counteract tumor necrosis factor alpha-induced thrombomodulin downregulation. *Blood Coagul Fibrinolysis,* 14, 575–85.

Shiau, C.W., J.W. Huang, D.S. Wang, J.R. Weng, C.C. Yang, C.H. Lin, C. Li, C.S. Chen. 2006. Alpha-tocopheryl succinate induces apoptosis in prostate cancer cells in part through inhibition of Bcl-xL/Bcl-2 function. *J Biol Chem,* 281, 11819–25.

Singh, V.J., T.M. Seed. In *Radiation effects. Physicians' guide to terrorist attack radiation effects,* Roy, M.J. (Ed.) Humana Press: Totowa, NJ, 2003, pp 339–362.

Singh, V.K., V. Srinivasan, R. Toles, P. Karikari, T. Seed, A. Papas, J.A. Hyatt, K.S. Kumar. 2005. Radiation protection by the antioxidant alpha-tocopherol succinate. NATO–RTG–099–Conference presentation, AFRRI-CD-05-2.

Song, B.L., R.A. DeBose-Boyd. 2006. Insig-dependent ubiquitination and degradation of 3-hydroxy-3-methylglutaryl coenzyme A reductase stimulated by delta- and gamma-tocotrienols. *J Biol Chem,* 281, 25054–25061.

Srinivasan, V., A.J. Jacobs, S.A. Simpson, J.F. Weiss. 1983. Radioprotection by vitamin E: effects on hepatic enzymes, delayed type hypersensitivity and postirradiation survival in mice.*Modulation and mediation of cancer by vitamin E,* Meyskens, F.L., K.N. Prasad (Eds.). S. Karger: Basel., pp 119–131.

Srinivasan, V., J.F. Weiss. 1992. Radioprotection by vitamin E: Injectable vitamin E administered alone or with WR–3689 enhances survival of irradiated mice. *Int J Radiat Oncol Biol Phys,* 23, 841–5.

Srivastava, J.K., S. Gupta. 2006. Tocotrienol-rich fraction of palm oil induces cell cycle arrest and apoptosis selectively in human prostate cancer cells. *Biochem Biophys Res Commun,* 346, 447–53.

Strickley, R.G. 2004. Solubilizing excipients in oral and injectable formulations. *Pharm Res,* 21, 201–30.

Suzuki, Y.J., M. Tsuchiya, S.R. Wassall, Y.M. Choo, G. Govil, V.E. Kagan, L. Packer. 1993. Structural and dynamic membrane properties of alpha-tocopherol and alpha-tocotrienol: Implication to the molecular mechanism of their antioxidant potency. *Biochemistry,* 32, 10692–9.

Sylvester, P.W., S.J. Shah, G.V. Samant. 2005. Intracellular signaling mechanisms mediating the antiproliferative and apoptotic effects of gamma-tocotrienol in neoplastic mammary epithelial cells. *J Plant Physiol,* 162, 803–10.

Takashi, K., Loo, G. 2004. Disruption of mitochondria during tocotrienol-induced apoptosis in MDA-MB-231 human breast cancer cells. *Biochem. Pharmacol.,* 67, 315–324.

Tanaka, Y., Y. Moritoh, N. Miwa. 2007. Age-dependent telomere-shortening is repressed by phosphorylated alpha-tocopherol together with cellular longevity and intracellular oxidative-stress reduction in human brain microvascular endotheliocytes. *J Cell Biochem.*

Theriault, A., J.T. Chao, Q. Wang, A. Gapor, K. Adeli. 1999. Tocotrienol: A review of its therapeutic potential. *Clin Biochem,* 32, 309–19.

Tsuzuki, W., R. Yunoki, H. Yoshimura. 2007. Intestinal Epithelial Cells Absorb gamma-tocotrienol Faster than alpha-tocopherol. *Lipids,* 42, 163–70.

Vatassery, G.T., S. Fahn, M.A. Kuskowski. 1998. Alpha-tocopherol in CSF of subjects taking high dose of vitamin E in the DATATOP study. *Neurology: Parkinson Study Group,* 50, 1900–1902.

Verheij, M., L.G. Dewit, J.A. van Mourik. 1995. The effect of ionizing radiation on endothelial tissue factor activity and its cellular localization. *Thromb Haemost,* 73, 894–5.

Villiotou, V., G. Deliconstantinos. 1995. Nitric oxide, peroxynitrite and nitroso-compounds formation by ultraviolet A (UVA) irradiated human squamous cell carcinoma: Potential role of nitric oxide in cancer prognosis. *Anticancer Res,* 15, 931–42.

Wada, S., Y. Satomi, M. Murakoshi, N. Noguchi, T. Yoshikawa, H. Nishino. 2005. Tumor suppressive effects of tocotrienol in vivo and in vitro. *Cancer Lett,* 229, 181–91.

Waddick, K.G., C.W. Song, L. Souza, F.M. Uckun. 1991. Comparative analysis of the in vivo radioprotective effects of recombinant granulocyte colony-stimulating factor (G-CSF), recombinant granulocyte-macrophage CSF and their combination. Blood, 77, 2364–71.

Wang, J., H. Zheng, X. Ou, L. M. Fink, M. Hauer-Jensen. 2002. Deficiency of microvascular thrombomodulin and up-regulation of protease-activated receptor-1 in irradiated rat intestine: Possible link between endothelial dysfunction and chronic radiation fibrosis. *Am J Pathol,* 160, 2063–72.

Wang, J., H. Zheng, M.D. Hollenberg, S.J. Wijesuriya, X. Ou, M. Hauer-Jensen. 2003. Up-regulation and activation of proteinase-activated receptor 2 in early and delayed radiation injury in the rat intestine: Influence of biological activators of proteinase-activated receptor 2. *Radiat Res,* 160, 524–35.

Wang, J., X. Qiu, H. Zheng, J. Joseph, U. Ponnappan, J.L. Mehta, L.M. Fink, M. Hauer-Jensen. 2004. Effect of statins on endothelial thrombomodulin in vitro and the intestinal radiation exposure in vivo (Abst). *Radiat. Res. Society Abst Book,* 51, 37.

Wang, J., H. Zheng, X. Ou, C.M. Albertson, L.M. Fink, J.M. Herbert, M. Hauer–Jensen. 2004. Hirudin ameliorates intestinal radiation toxicity in the rat: support for thrombin inhibition as strategy to minimize side–effects after radiation therapy and as countermeasure against radiation exposure. *J Thromb Haemost,* 2, 2027–35.

Wang, J., M. Boerma, Q. Fu, A. Kulkarni, L.M. Fink, M. Hauer-Jensen. 2007. Simvastatin ameliorates radiation enteropathy development after localized, fractionated irradiation by a protein C-independent mechanism. *Int J Radiat Oncol Biol Phys,* in press.

Watkins, T.R., M.L. Bierenbaum, A. Giampaolo, Tocotrienols: Biological and health effects. In *Antioxidant Status, Diet, Nutrition and Health*, Papas, A.M. (Ed.). CRC Press: Boca Raton, 1999, 479–496.

Weiss, J.F., K.S. Kumar. Antioxidant Mechanisms in radiation injury and radioprotection. In *Cellular Antioxidant Defense Mechanisms,* Chow, C.K. (Ed.). CRC Press: Boca Raton, 1988, Vol. II, 163–189.

Weiss, J.F., V. Srinivasan, K.S. Kumar, M.R. Landauer. 1992. Radioprotection by metals: Selenium. *Adv Space Res,* 12, 223–31.

Weiss, J.F., M.R. Landauer. 2003. Protection against ionizing radiation by antioxidant nutrients and phytochemicals. *Toxicology*, 189, 1–20.

Whitnall, M.H., T.B. Elliott, M.R. Landauer, W.E. Jackson, 3rd, C.L. Wilhelmsen, L. McKinney, K.S. Kumar, V. Srinivasan, G.D. Ledney, T.M. Seed. 2001. In vivo protection against gamma-irradiation with 5-androstenediol. *Exp Biol Med* (Maywood), 226, 625–7.

Williams, J.P., E. Hernady, C.J. Johnston, C.M. Reed, B. Fenton, P. Okunieff, J.N. Finkelstein. 2004. Effect of administration of lovastatin on the development of late pulmonary effects after whole-lung radiation in a murine model. *Radiat. Res.,* 161, 560–7.

Yoshida, Y., E. Niki, N. Noguchi. 2003. Comparative study on the action of tocopherols and tocotrienols as antioxidant: Chemical and physical effects. *Chem Phys Lipids,* 123, 63–75.

Index